MOSBY'S
FUNDAMENTALS OF THERAPEUTIC MASSAGE

MOSBY'S FUNDAMENTALS OF THERAPEUTIC MASSAGE

SANDY FRITZ, BS

Founder, Owner, Director, and Head Instructor
Health Enrichment Center
School of Therapeutic Massage and Bodywork
Lapeer, Michigan

SECOND EDITION

with 515 illustrations

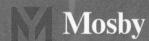

Mosby

An Affiliate of Elsevier Science

St. Louis   London   Philadelphia   Sydney   Toronto

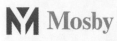
Mosby

An Affiliate of Elsevier Science

Publisher: John Schrefer
Executive Editor: Martha Sasser
Senior Developmental Editor: Amy Christopher
Associate Developmental Editor: Leslie Mosby
Project Manager: Linda McKinley
Production Editor: Jennifer Furey
Designer: Renée Duenow
Photography: Camille Gerace, Cam-Works
Line Art: Beverley Ransom
Additional Art: Alice Chin and Graphic World Illustration Services
Cover and chapter opener photos courtesy PhotoDisc, Inc.

Mosby, Inc.
An Affiliate of Elsevier Science
11830 Westline Industrial Drive
St. Louis, Missouri 63146

Printed in United States

Library of Congress Cataloging-in-Publication Data
Fritz, Sandy.
Mosby's fundamentals of therapeutic massage / Sandy Fritz. — 2nd ed.
  p.   cm.
Includes bibliographical references and index.
ISBN 0-323-00677-9
1. Massage therapy.   I. Title.   II. Title: Fundamentals of
therapeutic massage.
RM721.F75   2000
615.8'22—dc21   99-14180

02   03   /   9   8   7   6   5

Second edition dedication

To both of my Dr. G's,

who were and are my teachers and my support.

First edition dedication

To my kids—Greg, Laura, and Luke—for doing without me for so long.

To my mother, who kept the house together and worried about me.

To all my dogs, who spend countless hours by my side and in my lap, and especially

to my old bulldog, Ethan, who died quietly at my feet while I worked on rewrites.

To Eric and Christine, for "making it happen."

To my special staff, who are my friends and family, for giving me the space to write.

To all the wonderful people who teach with me.

To every client and student I have had the opportunity to touch; thank you for teaching me.

To all my teachers. To those who listened. To those who love me anyway.

FOREWORD

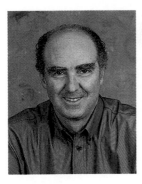

THIS revised, expanded, and improved edition of *Mosby's Fundamentals of Therapeutic Massage* takes the first version to a new degree of merit. As the text was reviewed, it became clear that just as the original version had been carefully thought out and crafted, so had the revision. This is no hasty enterprise but one that has diligently examined ways of expanding on and improving what has gone before—a truly praiseworthy piece of work. It is no longer just a fine entry-level book for prospective massage therapists, but one that addresses the needs of these times in which integration of health care approaches is advancing rapidly. As massage therapy grows into a major health care profession, society (as well as official agencies) insists that the level of training and the excellence of delivery, as well as the ethical standards of its graduates and practitioners, continue to improve.

The demands of the present are that what is offered in health care be evidence based. This is as it ought to be, since without a solid training in the ethical, theoretical, and practical components of massage and bodywork, based on what is known and not just on what is believed, confidence would erode.

The public and other health care professions, as well as government agencies and insurance companies, expect and demand no less from the massage therapy profession than any other in order to feel safe on all levels in the hands of its professionals.

If this confidence is to continue to grow, as it deservedly should, the broad spectrum of knowledge, so eloquently incorporated into this book, should be seen as a foundation on which to build. Its title is therefore a precise description of what it offers—the principal elements, the primary knowledge, the fundamentals.

This revised version of the book examines touch as a form of communication and with great insight has expanded on the importance of those offering these forms of care being able to recognize the ways in which touch therapies can be interpreted. It is vital for massage therapists to understand touch in the context of the client's life and beliefs, culture, age, gender, religion, and health status in order that delivery may be sensitively offered and accepted.

Ethics receives a justifiably expanded degree of attention in the text, accurately reflecting both the profession's own increased focus on this important topic and society's demand for excellence in the ethical arena. And rather than presenting fixed formulae in relation to either therapeutic intervention in given settings or the solution of ethical dilemmas, the author has adopted an innovative approach in which the student of therapeutic massage is encouraged (and shown how) to make effective decisions in these critical areas, building on the foundation of knowledge that their studies—and the book—encompasses.

Anatomy and physiology follow this educational pattern in which facts are identified and from these facts therapeutic choices are generated.

Analysis of the probable efficacy of such choices is then encouraged in relation to the way in which they might affect given situations, problems, and people. In this way menus and recipes are avoided and reflection and planning are encouraged.

The text contains many practical and informative case studies that highlight these approaches—showing how appropriate decisions can be arrived at after analysis of the information available.

Issues involving special population groups and associated and complementary bodywork modalities, as well as energy-based systems, have all received increased attention in this revision, as have sections that feature topics such as therapeutic change, condition management, and palliative care. Over and above new material, the text has usually been streamlined with rearrangement of the sequence and flow of the material, enhanced color in its illustrations, and a more accessible and user-friendly work-text format.

If the entry-level standards of the massage profession can universally match those incorporated into this book, then the profession as a whole will deservedly move on to a higher level of excellence.

Leon Chaitow, ND, DO
Senior Lecturer, University of Westminster, London

PREFACE

THE second edition of *Mosby's Fundamentals of Therapeutic Massage* is intended to be used by skilled therapeutic massage educators in the classroom setting. It will also be used as a continuing education resource by practitioners and as a reference text for health professionals and massage and bodywork practitioners.

More than 20 years ago, when I was exploring a career in therapeutic massage, there were few schools. Because none of them was readily accessible to me, I taught myself. I took a course of less than 100 hours, which at least provided basic skills. The rest of my massage therapy training has come from reading a multitude of books, attending hundreds of hours of workshops, apprenticeship training, taking college courses in related subjects, teaching over 3000 beginning students, and providing over 23,000 massage sessions. Since the publication of the first edition, I have completed a degree at Central Michigan University. Becoming a student again in the university environment had a great influence on my perspective about education, as well as on my professional development. I am still learning the importance of the fundamental concepts upon which all bodywork methods are based. I learn more about the elegant simplicity of massage each time I teach, and I have learned a great deal through researching and writing this textbook as well. More than ever, I am convinced that **a strong understanding of the fundamental concepts of therapeutic massage and the ability to effectively reason through a decision-making process are essential for proficient professional practice.**

There have been many exciting developments since the first edition of this text published. The changes and additions to the second edition reflect how much therapeutic massage has evolved as a profession over the past few years. One of the most exciting developments is the publication of *Mosby's Basic Science for Soft Tissue and Movement Therapies* (Fritz, 1999). This comprehensive anatomy, physiology, pathology, and clinical application text was written to complement and support the body of knowledge of *Mosby's Fundamentals of Therapeutic Massage*, second edition. What a thrill it is for me to have participated in the development of "real" textbooks written specifically for the students I serve.

Today, the profession of therapeutic massage is in the process of standardizing and organizing. Major advances in the acceptance of therapeutic massage have occurred since the first edition of this text published. This is primarily due to valid research that is now available to support the value of the simple work we do. There are many highly respected schools teaching students therapeutic applications of nurturing, safe touch that stimulates the body's various physiologic processes.

A well-rounded education includes learning all of the following: how to perform massage manipulations and bodywork techniques, the anatomy and physiology of why the methods work, and the importance of structure, intent, and purpose of touch. It is as important to touch the whole person as it is to skillfully apply techniques. The massage professional must do both. In addition, the student needs to understand the importance of sanitation, hygiene, body mechanics, business practices, and ethics and apply this knowledge through effective decision making to build a well-balanced, professional massage career.

The fundamentals of massage methods are relatively simple. A well-planned school curriculum, as developed in this textbook and instructor's manual, combined with a comprehensive science curriculum as presented in *Mosby's Basic Science for Soft Tissue and Movement Therapies,* will teach the basics in a program of 500 to 1500 class hours.

The days of self-teaching massage that I and many others experienced are over. Validation of a profession requires standardized, formal education. Although I believe that apprenticeship training is a valid and desirable way to learn, I also realize that verifiable credentials are necessary if the profession of therapeutic massage and bodywork wishes to obtain formal recognition. It is easier to standardize curriculum requirements through the formal school environment and an accepted set of teaching materials. Written and practical tests can be developed from the textbook base. These tests determine the minimal standard of practice. There is probably a better way to maintain a professional standard of expertise, but this system works. It is cost effective, simple to set in place, and easy to inspect. Massage therapy educators have found that agreement about the core body of knowledge and standardizing of the educational process will free them to teach the crucial, hands-on material that a book cannot effectively teach. I am pleased that the first edition of this text served educators and students well and hope that this expanded and revised second edition will be even more effective and useful.

Once students learn the fundamental core body of knowledge for all therapeutic massage and bodywork methods, the essential learning begins. The uniqueness of our profession is not dependent upon the methods or the technical application of massage techniques. The massage therapy profession offers skilled, structured, and safe touch in a nurturing environment. This relationship joins people in a healing partnership. A book cannot touch the student; only a teacher can.

If the general public and health care providers understand the physiologic effects of therapeutic massage, they will be better able to make decisions about when massage will be beneficial. There are many claims about the effects of massage and bodywork techniques that cannot be substantiated. Current research into alternative treatment methods will reveal the physiologic process of many of these methods. Unfortunately, the conclusive results of this research may take years to become concrete. Fortunately, there is enough existing research to support the benefits of massage. The health care community is beginning to accept the effectiveness of massage as a complement to the care they currently provide. The simple physiologic effects of massage and bodywork speak for themselves.

Therapeutic massage is a labor-intensive therapy that requires time to perform. Our knowledge base is unique. Other licensed health care professionals are often too busy to do this work. Our work can be effectively done at a paraprofessional level that is more cost effective for the public. This is the special gift our profession has to give.

Licensed medical professionals need a standardized basis of training proficiency before they can routinely incorporate therapeutic massage into their team healing approaches. Currently, the medical community cannot trust the expertise level of the massage profession because of the divergence in educational standards. While a program length of 500 to 1000 hours will prepare the graduate to work effectively in general applications of therapeutic massage to the general public outside the health care environment, this level of classroom instruction may not include enough pathology, medical terminology, evaluation skills, or specific application of methods to effectively support a medical healing team approach. Ontario and British Columbia, Canada, have developed therapeutic massage as part of the health care system. Their standards of education exceed 2200 class hours, equivalent to a typical associate's degree. Many medical technicians are trained at this level and it is a paradigm that is accepted.

I believe that massage has the most to offer in the realm of general service for the public at large and paraprofessional support in the health care environment. I do not see the formal educational requirements increasing beyond this level unless one wishes to teach in some capacity. I believe that proprietary private education and the few unique, highly focused community college programs best serve the needs of therapeutic massage education. I also believe that an increasing number of health care professionals will learn more about therapeutic massage so that they can better work with the massage professional and provide knowledgeable supervision in the health care setting.

The level of knowledge in the second edition of this text has been increased to reflect the skills necessary to be able to work effectively in the health care world with supervision. While my personal love for this profession lies in humble service to the general public in the support of their wellness and compassion and help for the daily aches and pains of life, I recognize the importance of being able to also work within the health care system. My work over the past several years with a clinical physiologist supports this observation. Because of the development of comprehensive textbooks, more schools will be better able to expand their curriculum for those who wish to pursue the more complex approach to therapeutic massage applications.

Schools that offer training programs of 500 to 1000 hours adequately prepare students for the general wellness personal service approach of therapeutic massage. Everyone can benefit from massage, not just those who are under medical care. This level of education is an entry-level point for those who wish to serve the general public and provide wellness and health-enhancing massage and bodywork. In my opinion, fewer than 500 class hours is insufficient time to cover the necessary body of knowledge to meet the emerging educational standards as set by the introduction of the National Certification Examination for Therapeutic Massage and Bodywork. I also believe that 500 class hours is barely sufficient to present the necessary information and allow adequate time for integration of the information. Programs of 1000 to 1500 hours as a standard would more effectively serve the student and the profession as a whole.

Therapeutic application of massage (structured touch) is not a new phenomenon. Very little of the information presented in this text is my original creation. The foundation for therapeutic massage was laid centuries ago and will not change provided the physiology of the human being remains constant. It is virtually impossible to acknowledge everyone who has contributed to the knowledge base. Our observations of the natural world are a good starting point for this basic knowledge. For example, animals know the value of rhythmic touch. Just watch a litter of puppies and observe the structured application of touch. The base of information goes beyond us to an innate need to rub an area that is hurt and to touch others to provide comfort, pleasure, and bonding.

ABOUT THIS BOOK

The second edition of this book has been extensively expanded and revised, using recommendations from many of my teaching colleagues, into a highly effective work-text format. Changes include but are not limited to the following: The new full-color presentation greatly enhances clarity of both the text and illustrations. A comprehensive section about the importance of touch has been added. Chapters on special populations and complementary bodywork modalities have been expanded. The historical information has been reorganized and expanded, and a helpful timeline has been added. The sections on ethics and professionalism have been completely revised and expanded. The medical terminology chapter has been reworked to support effective intake, treatment plan development, and charting procedures. More information on energy-based systems has been included. A section on the appropriateness of therapeutic change, condition management, and palliative care has been added to help in the development of treatment plans. The chapter order has been changed to support a more logical presentation for the student. A clinical reasoning model is presented as a unifying thread throughout the text. In addition, many case studies have been added.

Chapters 1 through 5 build the theory base and decision-making skills for the reader. Chapter 1 begins with an exploration of touch and builds to the historical foundations of massage. Chapter 2 introduces the clinical-reasoning problem-solving model for ethical decision making. It also covers professionalism and legal issues. Chapter 3 builds on Chapter 2 to teach readers how to develop effective record-keeping skills. Appropriate medical terminology is presented to support this process. Chapter 4 explains the scientific basis for therapeutic massage, and Chapter 5 begins the process of decision making in terms of indications and contraindications to massage. Chapters 6 through 8 present information concerning sanitation, hygiene, safety, body mechanics, massage equipment and supplies, positioning and draping procedures, various massage environments, and other information ancillary to a successful massage practice. Chapters 9 through 11 are the technical skills chapters. Each chapter builds on the previous one, beginning with the basics and expanding to therapeutic applications, as well as providing an introduction to complementary bodywork systems. As the methods and techniques of therapeutic massage and bodywork are presented, the reader will learn how and why

they work and when to use them to obtain a particular physiologic response. Chapter 12 focuses on providing massage to particular populations, whereas Chapter 13 explores the issue of wellness. Chapter 14, the final chapter, discusses business considerations for a career in massage. The text can be taught in a sequential manner, or the more technical chapters (6 through 11) can be presented simultaneously with Chapters 1 through 5 so that the student learns "hands-on skills" in conjunction with "head or thinking skills." Chapters 12 through 14 can then act as integration chapters to be presented after other chapters are covered. Many of the exercises provided throughout the text support introspection and understanding of the self to encourage "heart" learning as well.

The new work-text format of this book is highly interactive and enables the reader to learn and understand the information presented more easily. Proficiency Exercises and Think it Over exercises are provided to enhance the reader's learning experience. For many of these the reader is encouraged to answer directly in the book. Examples are often provided to help guide the student in processing the exercises. In addition, there are Workbook Sections at the end of most chapters where readers can test their knowledge through short answer questions, labeling exercises, and various other activities. Answers are provided for those questions that have correct answers. In other cases the student is asked to use the clinical-reasoning model to develop an answer to a question. In these situations, no *single* correct answer exists. Competencies can be determined by the effective justification of the answer that the student develops in response to the exercise.

While all the exercises and activities throughout the chapters and workbook sections are valuable, not all of them need to be completed by every student. In support of various learning styles, offering the students a choice among the various exercises is appropriate.

At the beginning of each chapter are chapter outlines, chapter objectives, and key terms. While complex terminology is defined within the body of the text, a specific massage glossary is included at the end of the book. Each discipline has its own language, and therapeutic massage is no exception. This common language facilitates effective communication within the field of therapeutic massage, as well as between massage practitioners and other disciplines.

There are several helpful appendices located at the end of the book. These include Appendix A: Indications and Contraindications to Massage; Appendix B: Skin Pathology; Appendix C: Common Medications and Possible Implications for Massage; Appendix D: Resource List; and Appendix E: Self-Massage. Two of these appendices are completely new to this edition.

Because the profession has not yet reached consensus on any one term used to describe the massage and bodywork professional, the following terms are all currently used: *massage therapist, massage practitioner, massage technician, bodyworker, touch therapist, bodywork practitioner, bodywork therapist, myomassologist, neuromuscular therapist,* and *massagist.* All of these terms describe a person who uses structured touch of some type to create physiologic response in the client. The use of the terms *masseuse* and *masseur* are discouraged in the United States, although these terms are still used in other countries. As an educator of therapeutic massage, I prefer the terms *massage practitioner, massage therapist, massage professional,* and *massage technician.* These terms are used interchangeably throughout this text. Early chapters tend to use the words *massage technician* and *massage professional,* middle chapters tend to use the words *massage professional* and *massage practi-* *tioner,* and end chapters tend to use the words *massage therapist.* This shows how the progression of knowledge corresponds with professional development.

As the author, my intent is to make reading this textbook an enjoyable learning experience; I hope my purpose is reflected in the personal, conversational tone in which I have written the text. My personal conviction is that *Mosby's Fundamentals of Therapeutic Massage, second edition,* effectively presents the information and reflects both the heart and the art of therapeutic massage. After all, no one cares how much you know until they know how much you care.

Sandy Fritz, BS

ACKNOWLEDGMENTS

A special thank you to:

M. James Grosenbach, EdD, Clinical psychologist and administrative director for Health Enrichment Center School of Therapeutic Massage and Bodywork, Lapeer, MI, for his extensive influence on the manuscript development of the second edition, for his contribution to the development of this text as a process model for clinical reasoning, for being a major contributor to the *Instructor's Manual,* and for his sensitivity to the learning needs of individuals.

Karen Craig and the entire educational staff at The Massage Institute of Memphis for their extensive review work.

The many additional reviewers who took the time and effort to provide feedback for this second edition.

A special thank you is extended to those contributors who generously dedicated their time and talents in working on the first edition of this text, which laid the foundation for the second edition.

Dr. Leon K. Chaitow, for his support and for writing the foreword for the text.

Emily Edith Safrona Cowall, for her contributions to the text and her extensive attention to detail in the review process.

Kathleen Maison Paholsky, for her committed work on the *Instructor's Manual* and extensive work in helping me to revise the manuscript.

Richard van Why, for his contributions to the historical information in the text.

My thanks to the following reviewers who have influenced the content and clarity of this text to ensure the accurate presentation of information:

Patricia J. Benjamin, PhD
Director of Education,
Connecticut Center for Massage Therapy,
Newington, CT

Leon K. Chaitow, ND, DO
Member of the Register of Osteopaths,
Senior Lecturer,
Center for Community Care & Primary Health,
University of Westminster;
Consultant Osteopath,
The Hale Clinic,
London, England

Emily Edith Safrona Cowall, Reg MT
Vice-Chairman (present),
National Certification Board for Therapeutic Massage
    and Bodywork,
Arlington, Virginia;
Formerly Chairman,
The College of Massage Therapists (formerly Board of
    Directors of Masseurs),
Province of Ontario, Canada

Peter A. Goldberg, DIPL AC (NCCA), LMT
National Commission on Certification of
    Acupuncturists,
Great Barrington, MA

Lucy Liben, MS, LMT
Director of Education,
Swedish Institute of Massage Therapy,
New York, NY

Jean E. Loving, BA, LMT
Director of Education,
Co-owner, Seminar Network International, Inc,
Lake Worth, FL

Karen B. Napolitano, MS
Formerly Director of Education,
Potomac Massage Training Institute,
Washington, DC

Kathleen Maison Paholsky, MS, PhD
Director of Education,
Health Enrichment Center;
Director,
Clinical Approaches Program,
Lapeer, MI

Cherie Marilyn Sohnen-Moe, BA
Instructor,
Desert Institute of the Healing Arts,
Tucson, AZ

Mary Margaret Tuchscherer, DC, PhD
Doctor of Chiropractic and Associate Professor of Basic
    Science,
Departments of Clinical and Basic Science,
Northwestern College of Chiropractic,
Bloomington, MN;
Faculty and Chairperson of Basic Science,
Northern Lights School of Massage Therapy,
Minneapolis, MN

Sherri Williamson, LMT
Founder,
Associated Bodywork & Massage Professionals (ABMP),
Evergreen, CO

Ed Wilson, PhD, LMT
Dean of Student Development,
Educator and Massage Therapist,
Educating Hands School of Massage,
Miami, FL

*In addition to the contributors and reviewers, there are several
people who also deserve special recognition for their efforts in
the publication and promotion of the first and second editions:*

Beverley Ransom, for her terrific artwork.

Martha Sasser at Mosby, for her steadfastness during transition and revision.

Amy Christopher at Mosby, for her gentle but persistent support and attention to detail.

Jennifer Furey at Mosby, for her diligence in the production of the text.

Camille Gerace, for the incredible photos and for her energy and enthusiasm during the photo shoots.

It truly has been a team effort.

CONTENTS

DETAILED CONTENTS

MOSBY'S
FUNDAMENTALS OF THERAPEUTIC MASSAGE

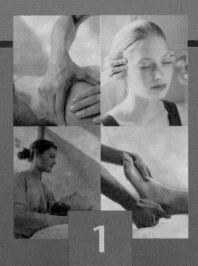

1

FOUNDATIONS OF THERAPEUTIC APPLICATIONS OF TOUCH

o b j e c t i v e s

After completing this chapter, the student will be able to perform the following:

■ Describe professional touch

■ Identify personal interpretations of touch and their influence on professional interactions

■ Explain the rich heritage and history of therapeutic massage

■ Explain the influence of historical events on the current development of therapeutic massage

EDUCATION is just as much about asking questions as it is about seeking answers. Consider the possibility that information dispensed during an educational process, coupled with the ability to formulate insightful and productive questions, allows students an opportunity to make thoughtful decisions. Are decisions answers? Do answers come from thoughtful situational decisions? Are answers the truth? Some questions seem to have easy answers. For example, "What is the color of grass?" Quickly we jump to the answer "green," but is that an always the answer? Because many questions have several answers, the truth can be difficult to determine. In what way is the professional application of touch influenced by the practitioner's ability to make thoughtful decisions and find answers that best serve the situation at a particular moment?

In massage, which is professional, structured, therapeutic touch, education begins with questions: What is the significance of touch? What is professional touch? What motivates me to study therapeutic massage? What is therapeutic? How am I served by touching others? How do the connections with others created through touch influence the professional practice of therapeutic massage? When did touch become professional? Why did touch become professional? Do therapeutic forms of touch have to be provided by a professional? In what way is professional therapeutic touch different from casual touch, friendship touch, family touch, intimate touch, or sexual (erotic) touch? How do different individuals, social groups, or cultures view touch? In what way does the past affect the present and provide guidance for the future development of the profession of massage therapy? Questions continue to arise, and the answers are not necessarily simple.

As we seek to serve others, eventually we are faced with these questions and many others. Some of the questions mentioned previously are explored in this text, especially as they relate to the professional practice of therapeutic massage. Some are not explored directly; rather, both the questions and the answers evolve for each student as the individual's information base and experience increase and the journey through education continues. This text does not provide definitive answers to any of these questions, but it does provide information to help you find your own answers to questions you may face. What will your questions be? How will your answers influence those you touch? How will your answers touch you?

These are huge issues to consider at the beginning of any course of study. As you begin to think about these issues, you might feel interested, excited, overwhelmed, or maybe even frightened as you realize how necessary, beneficial, complex, and powerful touch can be. Remember that understanding evolves. These important questions are posed at the beginning of this study and possibly before you have sufficient information to develop effective answers. Your awareness of these questions during your course of study will help you make decisions and find an-swers as you progress in your study of therapeutic massage. You will come to understand the process of developing *your* answers to the previously mentioned questions and many others that will arise by embracing the importance of *respect*—for yourself and for all those with whom you interact, both personally and professionally (Proficiency Exercise 1-1).

PROFESSIONAL TOUCH

section objectives

Using the information presented in this section, the student will be able to perform the following:

- Distinguish between professional and nonprofessional forms of touch
- List factors that influence the communication of touch
- Identify factors that constitute appropriate and inappropriate touch in the professional setting

Dictionaries define a **profession** as an occupation requiring training and specialized study. An **occupation** can be defined as a productive or creative activity that serves as one's regular source of livelihood. A **professional** is one who engages in a profession. **Professionalism** is the adherence to professional status, methods, standards, and character. This idea of professionalism is further explored in Chapter 2 in the discussion of ethics.

For the purpose of understanding the idea of professional touch, we look at specialized training that allows a person to provide a service to another. Professionals may sell a product, but usually a profession is built around the skilled ability to provide a service such as therapeutic massage. A **service** is something done for another that results

---

1 - 1

PROFICIENCY EXERCISE

Look up the words *truth* and *respect* in the dictionary, then develop your personal definition of each. Consider the cartoon in Fig. 1-1 as you develop your definitions. Write the definitions in the spaces below.

Truth

Respect

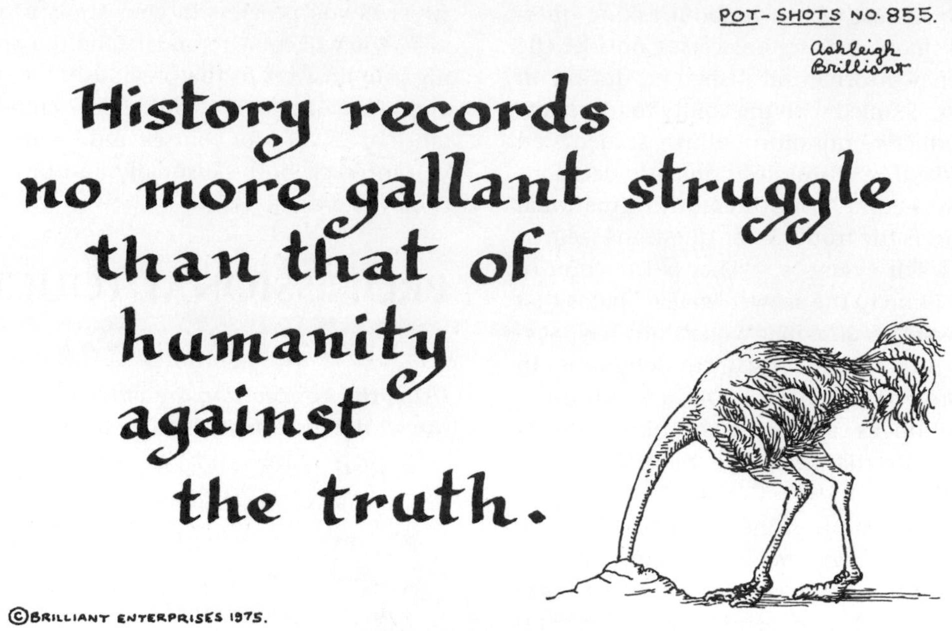

History records no more gallant struggle than that of humanity against the truth.

©BRILLIANT ENTERPRISES 1975.

fig. 1-1

Pot-Shots. (Courtesy Ashleigh Brilliant, Santa Barbara, Calif.)

in a specific outcome; for example, the car is fixed, the garden is tended, communication skills are taught, emotional problems are sorted out, changes are perceived in an unpleasant physical sensation, bodily functions are restored, and spiritual or life paths are discovered. In return, income (livelihood) is received for that service. When a professional relationship exists, certain agreed criteria apply. The person providing the service is skilled (schooled) and operates within certain standards of practice, including technical application and ethical conduct. **Professional touch,** then, is skilled touch delivered to achieve a specific outcome, and the recipient in some way reimburses the professional for services rendered.

It is the aspect of skilled or schooled touch that leads to the idea of structured touch. Professional touch is not random but purposeful. Its organization follows systems and patterns. A **system** is a group of interacting elements that functions as a complex whole. Professional touch, such as that provided by a massage practitioner, requires education in the many systems of the body, systems of massage and other forms of soft tissue methodology, and the influence of massage systems on body systems. Communication and interpersonal skills, including systems of social and cultural interaction, also are part of the education of the therapeutic massage professional.

Inherent in this understanding of skilled and structured touch is the idea of therapeutic application of touch. The term **therapeutic applications** pertains to healing or curative powers. Something that is therapeutic provides the structure for beneficial change or provides support for current healing practices. A walk in the woods or conversation with a compassionate friend can be thera-

peutic, as is the application of various bodywork modalities, medical and mental health practices, and empowering spiritual rituals. **Healing** is the restoration of well-being, and therapeutic applications promote a healing environment.

Touch

Before discussing the historical perspectives of therapeutic massage (professional, structured, therapeutic touch), we need to consider the nature of touch in order to understand the role of professional touch and the evolution of therapeutic massage throughout history. It is important to look at the idea of professionalism in the physical, emotional, social, cultural, and, in some instances, spiritual dimensions of touch. The roots of the word *massage* concern touch and the various applications of touch. It is important to explore the ideas behind the structure of touch. We must differentiate the therapeutic value of touch in the professional sense from forms of touch shared between people in life circumstances outside the professional environment. These themes are expanded on and carried throughout the text, and in some instances the information base is expanded in future chapters.

The Science of Touch

Anatomically and physiologically, touch is the collection of tactile sensations that arise from sensory stimulation, primarily of the skin but also of deeper structures of the body, such as muscles.

The skin is an amazing organ. It has many functions, but the most notable one for this discussion is its function in touch. The skin is the largest sensory organ of the body. From the outside we are always touched first on our skin, and in many ways, through the skin, we touch ourselves from the inside. Many internal somatic soft tissue structures (e.g., muscles, connective tissue) and visceral structures (e.g., the lungs, heart, digestive organs) project sensation to the skin (see Chapter 5 regarding viscerally referred pain patterns). The autonomic nervous system, which regulates the visceral and chemical homeostasis of the body, is highly responsive to skin stimulation in support of well-being. Mood (the way one is feeling) often is reflected in the skin as we touch ourselves from the inside. We blush with embarrassment, flush with excitement, or grow pale with fear.

The anatomy of the skin is described in most comprehensive anatomy texts.* The anatomic parts that make up the skin—the epidermis (top layer), dermis (inner layer), and the interlacing connective tissues of these layers—and the massive network of nerves both receive and relay information from the central nervous system. This vast network combines with the rich complex of circulatory vessels that supply the skin. Yet, even in their complexity, the anatomy and physiology of the skin cannot explain the experience of touch. In some way, the pressure, vibration, temperature, and muscle motion that move the skin enliven us with sensations and experiences of pleasure, connectedness, joy, pain, sadness, and longing.

We must be touched to survive. Touch is a hunger that must be fed, not just for well-being, but as the very essence of our survival. The importance of touch is well described in the books of Ashley Montagu, particularly *Touching: The Human Significance of the Skin,* which is recommended reading for all students of therapeutic massage. Dr. Tiffany Field is conducting scientific research on touch at the Touch Research Institute at the University of Miami Medical School. Additional research has been done or is underway at the University of South Carolina Medical School, Emory University, and Bastyr University, among others. Initially, much of this research was devoted to infant development, primarily in premature babies. Dr. Field has greatly expanded our understanding of the importance of touch by studying many different groups of people, including infants, elderly persons, people currently well but under stress, and very ill persons. Research supports the belief that touching in a structured way is a very important if not absolute need of all living beings.

Scientific technology has enabled us to describe some of the physiologic responses to touch, such as changes in the concentration of hormones, alterations in the activity of the central and peripheral nervous systems, and regulation of body rhythms. (These mechanisms are discussed more extensively in later chapters.) However, even this explosion of information falls short in helping us to understand the experience of touch. For all its scientific interpretations, the experience of touch is much more than the sum of its parts.

The Experience of Touch

Touch often is the concrete experience of more abstract sensations. For example, something that can be seen may not necessarily be real, as is the case in watching a movie, but when something can be touched, it is tangible. When the first edition of this text was written, I certainly touched all the reference books and the keyboard of the computer, but these were not the book. Even the finished manuscript that I sent away to the publisher did not feel real to me. It was not until I received the first copy of the text and held it in my hands, felt the size and weight of it, and experienced the pages turning between my fingers that the experience became real to me.

It is the same when I am touched or when I touch someone. I can listen to clients tell me their history, and I can look and observe during a physical assessment, but it is not until I touch clients and feel them that I begin to understand their bodies. In a reciprocal sense, when I lay my hands on a person's body, the understanding that I, as the practitioner, have received from the client is conveyed back to the client. Touch is a fundamental, multilayered, and powerful form of communication. It is the most personalized form of communication we know.

Touch as Communication

Touch in many ways is a more emotionally powerful form of communication than speech. Verbal communication uses specific words with specific meanings to relay a message. Touch communication is more ambiguous, relying on interpretation of its meaning through past experience and current circumstances. Delivering a clear, concise verbal message is difficult enough when both parties—the one delivering the message and the one receiving it—agree on the meaning of the words. How much more challenging it is to deliver a touch message, in which many factors are involved in the interpretation of the message. The potential for misunderstanding increases. Often, with both verbal and touch communication, the message intended is not the one received.

The communication of touch is influenced by personal, familial, and cultural contexts. Each individual defines an area around himself as personal space, and the distance encompassed by this personal space differs from person to person and culture to culture. Therapies of touch enter this personal space; therefore the professional must be sensitive to the various factors that influence people's responses when their personal space is entered. Understanding each person's culture and subculture, personal experiences in that culture, and genetically predetermined tendencies toward a large or small amount of personal

---

*Further study of the anatomy and physiology of the skin is included in comprehensive anatomy and physiology studies, as well as in the textbook *Mosby's Basic Science for Soft Tissue and Movement Therapies* (Fritz S, St Louis, 1999, Mosby).

space often becomes mind-boggling in designing individual interactions of touch.

Cultural Influences

A **culture** is defined by the arts, beliefs, customs, institutions, and all other products of human work and thought created by a specific group of people at a particular time. It is stereotypical to say that those of a certain culture act a certain way; individuals always vary. However, tendencies can be defined by culture, which may determine the way at least to begin initial touch interaction, until the person's uniqueness is better understood.

It is impossible to explore the vast diversity of cultural norms and mores in this text. Yet you, as a professional, are responsible for developing an understanding of the social, cultural, and spiritual ways of the client population you serve. This can be accomplished by doing research at the library about a particular culture or by taking a class. In your practice, observe how clients act and model from them (follow the client's lead). Ask questions, and let clients teach you about themselves and their culture.

The following personal experience demonstrates one of the ways people can teach you about their culture.

After a lecture I had given, a group of people came up to me to greet me and ask questions. By my nature and through years of conditioning in professional practice, I would reach out to take the person's hand or to touch his shoulder. A gentleman approached, and I offered my hand, but he crossed his hands over his chest and nodded slightly. I reached out to touch his arm, and he very gently became my teacher in that moment. He backed away just a bit and said, "In my country this is how we greet a woman with respect" and again crossed his arms over his chest and nodded slightly. So I asked, "How would I respond in your country?" He replied, "You would nod back and then avert your gaze so you do not look me directly in the eyes." I asked the reason for averting my eyes, and he gently explained that touching with one's eyes is a very sacred act and not for casual contact. A meeting of the eyes is a meeting of the souls. He again crossed his arms over his chest and nodded, and I nodded in return and then turned my gaze just below his eyes. It was a very poignant moment for me.

Gender Issues

The preceding story points out not only cultural but also gender issues in touch. Women and men may have different conceptions of the appropriateness of touch. The patterns of gender custom in touch are complex. Biology, survival behaviors, social learning, and cultural customs are some of the influences that affect the development of these patterns.

For example, women generally require a somewhat smaller and more permeable personal space for comfort. Until recently, child rearing was the responsibility primarily of women, and child care requires caregivers to en-

ter another's personal space or allow someone to enter theirs. Men, in general, establish territories. Personal space is entered by invitation because the territory must be protected. A man's personal space often is larger and more structured.

Although these gender trends can be viewed from biologic and survival behavior perspectives, the patterns do not necessarily hold true when cultural customs or other influences affecting gender roles or behavior patterns are factored in. It is stereotypical to state that women always act this way, and men always act that way; it simply is not true. Diversity of expression will forever exist within biologic influences and the cultural or gender rules of behavior.

Influence of Age on Touch

Age difference can be a factor in the interpretation of touch. Some may consider touching very young persons appropriate but may be more cautious about touching older people. A younger person touching an elder may be acceptable, yet when two people of the same age touch, the dynamics are different. The touch of a young practitioner may be interpreted differently from the touch of an older practitioner, even if the skill and experience levels are equivalent.

Influence of Life Events and the Interpretation of Touch

Life events can influence the response to touch experiences. People who have undergone painful and extensive medical interventions, especially at a young age, may process touch differently than might be expected. Those who have experienced touch trauma are influenced by those events. People who have experienced isolation respond uniquely to touch. Those who grew up with excessive touch stimulation outside the context of trauma (e.g., being part of a large family in small living quarters or being an only child with many adoring family members) may develop certain touch responses. Having a healthy and appropriate touch history also influences one's interpretation of touch. Any of these experiences and many more not listed affect the way in which a person understands another's experience of touch.

Spiritual Touch

Touch also can have a spiritual context. Many spiritual rituals incorporate touch, especially those that involve concepts of healing of the body (that which is organic), the mind (that which is of thought), or the spirit (that which is transcending and sacred). Each person deserves respect for his or her personal truth and individual spiritual path.

Diversity and Touch

Generalities are useless in discussing cultural orientations to touch, and it is stereotypical to imply that all those from a specific culture hold to similar customs. The same difficulties with stereotyping occur with regard to gender, age, and life or spiritual path. Gender and age probably influence the interpretation of professional touch, but in just what way varies considerably. On any given day or even at any given moment, the need, desire, interpretation, and appropriateness of touch given and received can change.

These changes occur because a person is in a constant state of flux in responding and adapting to events they encounter. The type of relationship between people and its duration influence touch. For example, a first-time client may not be receptive to the deeper pressure required in some forms of massage, especially if the goal of the session gives no indication for this type of work. However, that same client, 12 sessions later and having a tension pattern in the back, may be responsive to touch in that particular form. Although clients may be ticklish to light touch initially in the session, after they relax somewhat, they may find light stroking pleasurable.

A person's response to and need for the delivery of touch cannot be predetermined. It can be stated, however, that each individual, including you, has been influenced by many factors regarding the appropriate procedure for touch and ultimately the interpretation of the meaning of a touch. As professionals it is important to be aware, sensitive, and open to an appreciation of the magnitude of the variety of influences affecting professional touch and diligently seek a personal understanding of our own desires, motivations, and responses to touch (Proficiency Exercise 1-2). After all, it is impossible to touch clients without them in turn touching us. A touch given is at the same time a touch received.

Professional Classifications of Touch

Models have been developed for classifying touch. Touch encompasses various nuances, forms, and intentions. In the professional world, touch can be appropriate or inappropriate.

Forms of Inappropriate Touch

Hostile or aggressive touch. Hostile or aggressive touch occurs when a potential for conflict or power struggle exists. Professionals who use touch need to be aware of the underlying energy directed toward the client to prevent this intention in the touch. The obvious is easy: if you are angry with a client, it is best not to touch at that moment and vice versa; if a client is angry with you, it is best not to touch until the energy changes. A more subtle aspect is the undercurrent of conflict. Say, for example, that the client is late for the appointment, or the practitioner is hurried or angry about something at home and inadvertently is more aggressive during the massage than necessary.

The perception of holding power over another underlies hostile or aggressive touch. Careful attention must be paid to this idea of power in the therapeutic relationship between the professional and the client. In the professional relationship, a power difference between the professional and the client exists simply because of the knowledge base that defines the profession. Knowledge is power, and most of the time the professional knows more about the service rendered than the client does. In body therapies, often the client's physical position creates an environment that fosters a power differential. Clients usually lie down or are seated, and the professional is physically above the client, generating the impression of authority.

Touching is an action energy focused outside the body that has the ability to exert power. When a person is touched, energy is received and internalized; it is not overtly an act of exerting power. Although the ability to receive touch is powerful, the difference in the power base between those who give and those who receive touch must be considered. This interplays with the appropriateness or inappropriateness of touch. Careful attention must be paid during professional touch if the issue of power is to be managed appropriately.

Erotic or sexual touch. The *intention* of erotic or sexual touch is sexual arousal and expression. The issue of erotic touch cannot be sidestepped in the study of massage therapy or any other body-oriented treatment in which touch is a primary aspect of the therapy. Complex physiologic, mental, and spiritual aspects, both of the client and the practitioner, influence the ideas of erotic touch.

Inherent in many forms of massage and bodywork is the *pleasure* of being touched. Pleasure is an important therapeutic tool. In later chapters you will learn that chemicals in the body create pleasure moods and feelings of connectedness increase during massage. These chemical responses to massage are one of the main reasons for the therapeutic benefit of the methods. Constant attention must be paid to the appropriate understanding and interpretation of the feelings generated during professional touch so that pleasurable touch does not evolve into or is misinterpreted as erotic touch.

Not only in body-oriented therapies but also in psychotherapy and other health care disciplines, it is not uncommon for professionals occasionally to have sexual feelings in the context of the professional environment. Professionals are people with complex, intertwined needs, desires, and means of expressing themselves. However, it is inappropriate for professionals to foster any type of erotic feelings with a client, either within the therapeutic environment or outside that environment. *Erotic feelings should never be acted on with clients.*

Body areas of touch sensitivity. Different areas of the body reflect different tactile issues. Research literature shows some agreement about areas of the body that are more sensitive, or "charged," in terms of emotion or erotic interpretation. The more emotionally or physically charged a body area is, the more the person may feel insecure, anxious, fearful, threatened, connected emotionally, intimate, or aroused when touched in that area.

Some body areas are considered taboo or "no-touch zones" in terms of professional bodywork touch. Orifices, including the anus, genitals, mouth, ears, and nose, have the highest level of taboo in most societies. The ventral, or front, surfaces of the body, including the breasts, are more charged than the dorsal surfaces. We see this pattern in massage; much of the massage session is devoted to the back of the torso and the legs while the client is lying face

down, with the front of the body "protected" by the massage table.

The trunk of the body is more "charged" than are the limbs. For this reason, a client may feel more comfortable having the legs and arms massaged than the torso. However, this does not always hold true; often the least intrusive form of touch is laying a hand on a person's upper back near the shoulder, whereas having the hands massaged can feel very intimate and connected.

The head also is an area sensitive to touch. Although children often are touched on the head and face, adults

---

1-2

PROFICIENCY EXERCISE

My Touch History

On a separate piece of paper, write a brief touch history and explain the way this history may influence your delivery of professional touch. An example is provided as a model.

Culture
I grew up in the United States in Michigan. I lived in a small town that was primarily Caucasian.

Subculture
My family was blue collar and working class.

Genetic Predisposition
I am most comfortable with a large personal space and plenty of time alone.

Gender
Female.

Age
Mid-40s.

Life Events
I experienced touch trauma from a grandfather and uncles, who would tickle me until I could not stand it.
I gave birth to three children and am a single parent.
I had a special friend who was blind.

Spiritual Path
I initially had an unstructured Protestant focus. I developed a specific fundamentalist path in early adulthood. I embraced many paths as truth in later years as I evolved from the practice of religion to the development of personal spirituality.

How My Touch History May Influence My Delivery of Professional Touch
I had to learn a lot about different cultures because my exposure to a diverse population was limited while I was growing up. I have to be careful to understand a person's culture before I approach to touch him or her. I am most comfortable with blue-collar, working-class people. I am more relaxed and find myself willing to spend more time when I touch someone from this population. I feel overwhelmed if I am touched too much and tend to limit initiated touch from the client. I am a woman and learned during my gender role development to fulfill others' needs before my own. I often overextend myself for a client instead of setting time limits. I am hypersensitive to light

touch and tend to avoid giving light touch when I give a massage. I am understanding of the numerous demands on a single parent and tend to touch one in similar circumstances with sympathy instead of empathy. I have to be careful of boundaries when I touch stressed, overwhelmed, single parents. I am casual when touching someone with a disability. I seek to understand various spiritual paths and deeply wish to respect issues of touch within each discipline. I tend to assume that one must actually make physical contact during spiritual healing and must remind myself that this is not everyone's truth.

Your Turn
Culture

Subculture

Genetic Predisposition

Gender

Age

Life Events

Spiritual Path

How My Touch History May Influence My Delivery of Professional Touch

seldom are touched casually in these areas. Adults often respond emotionally to touching of the face and head.

Areas of a person's body that have undergone trauma, such as through accidents or surgery, carry more emotional charge and therefore are more sensitive to interpretation of the appropriateness of touch.

The appropriateness or inappropriateness of touch, then, is about when, the way, and with what intent we touch.[5]

Forms of Appropriate Touch

Nontherapeutic forms of touch that people often encounter are *inadvertent touch,* such as touch that occurs when people are jostled together in an elevator, and *socially stereotyped touch,* which involves highly ritualized touch that carries a consensual meaning within a culture, such as a handshake.

Therapeutic forms of touch involve *touch that communicates information or expresses feeling as part of the therapeutic relationship.* This form of touch is not so much about creating a specific outcome as it is about delivering information or expressing comfort or understanding.[6] Some examples of this type of touch are touching a client's shoulder to direct him to the massage room or holding a client's hand as she thanks you for the session.

Touch technique. **Touch technique** is the basis of soft tissue forms of bodywork methods. Touch is the tool for massage. Massage consists of various forms of touch to achieve a specific outcome. This type of touch can be thought of as technical touch. In terms of touch technique, a therapeutic intent exists. The intention of touch therapy can be classified in two ways:

- **Mechanical touch** of a specific anatomic or physiologic outcome. Using massage to increase the range of motion of the shoulder is an example of this type of touch.
- **Expressive touch** is touch applied to support and convey awareness and empathy for the client as a whole person. An example of this is using massage for general relaxation and pleasure to comfort a client after a particularly hard day at work.[5]

The professional's choices on the type of therapeutic intention influence the interpretation of touch. A client with a mechanical restriction in the shoulder might find a more expressive form of touch uncomfortable because it might feel too intimate for the circumstances. Stressed, overworked clients may find a mechanical approach distant and impersonal because they are seeking empathy and understanding along with physical changes.

As we develop as professionals, both forms of touch technique must be perfected. Mechanical touch skills increase as we learn anatomy, physiology, language, record keeping, and effective delivery of specific forms of massage, which are presented in Chapters 3 and 6 through 11.

Development of the expressive form of touch technique is more complex and involves the professional's own personal growth, interpersonal and communications skills, and understanding of one's life experiences. This information is explored in this chapter and in Chapters 2, 4, 5, and 12 through 14.

Touch Appropriateness and Consciousness Levels

Another way to consider concepts of touch appropriateness is based on consciousness levels, as represented by the theory of the chakra system. Seven chakra, or energy, centers are located along the trunk of the body (Fig. 1-2).

The base, or first, chakra pertains to survival, security, and safety. The second chakra concerns pleasure experiences of sensuality and sexuality. The third chakra involves power and control. The lower chakras are transcended by the fourth, or heart, chakra, which is the center for nonjudgmental love. The heart chakra is the pivot point between the lower three chakras and the upper, more spiritual chakras. The fifth chakra is the throat center, which is concerned with communication and creativity. The brow, or sixth, chakra concerns the reflection of the total or essential self, and the crown, or seventh, chakra reflects the transcended and spiritual self.

Based on this chakra model, the intention of professional touch does not come from the lower chakra energy and needs because the energy of these chakras can be equated with types of inappropriate touch (hostile, aggressive, and erotic), and the potential for misinterpretation and manipulation is greater. The intention of professional touch projects from the fourth through seventh chakras, which support nonjudgmental love and respect for each person's personal mode of expression of the sense of self and sacredness.[6]

The touch intention of therapeutic massage closely fits with both models except in the area of pleasure. Many seek massage because it feels good, and these pleasure needs project from the second chakra. The importance of this pleasure factor and the interpretation of the meaning of the experience for clients can blur the boundaries of the professional relationship.

It is also important to consider the touch intention projected from the sixth and seventh chakras. Interacting professionally with the essential self (sixth chakra) requires extensive training in mental health, which can provide expertise in the development of the essential self. Touch that influences the transcendent or spiritual self requires the discipline to walk any of the many spiritual paths. Commitment to this training prepares one to provide support that leads to understanding of the transcendent self.

Professional energy focused from these areas can lead to dual roles for the massage professional. Dual or multiple roles occur when a professional operates from many bases of knowledge in interacting with clients therapeutically. The main concern with dual roles is the distribution

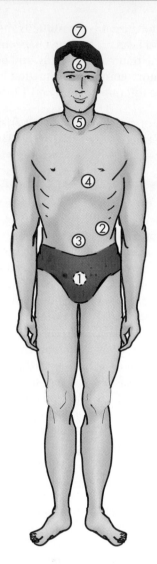

	English Name	Sanskrit Name	Situation
1	Root of basic chakra	Mūlādhāra	At the base of the spine
2	Spleen or splenic chakra	*	Over the spleen
3	Naval or umbilical chakra	Manipūra	At the naval, over the solar plexus
4	Heart or cardiac chakra	Anāhata	Over the heart
5	Throat or laryngeal chakra	Vishudda	At the front of the throat
6	Brow or frontal chakra	Ājnā	In the space between the eyebrows
7	Crown or coronal chakra	Sahasrāra	On the top of the head

fig. 1-2

Names and locations of major chakras. (Modified from Leadbeater CW: *The chakras,* Wheaton, Ill., 1927, Quest Books.)

of power in the therapeutic relationship. The more roles a professional plays with a client, the more power the professional acquires in the therapeutic relationship. It is easy for a client to feel disempowered with professionals who work from dual or multiple roles. This disempowerment can manifest in various forms, including a submissive at-

titude ("the professional knows best") or excessive admiration ("no one is as gifted as you").

In addition, the development of professional expertise in more than one role requires devotion to acquiring the knowledge contained in several areas. As you begin to study massage, you will soon realize that you could study for a lifetime just within the massage knowledge base and not absorb all the information available. It may be unrealistic to expect that one can operate effectively as a professional in several areas, because each of those areas also reflects a lifetime of experience and study.

A generalized knowledge of different areas of expertise and several forms of intervention adds to professional development. It can be helpful in fostering professional relationships with other professionals and in recognizing when a client can best be served by another discipline. However, developing expertise in several areas can become overwhelming. Professional touch provided through therapeutic massage, coupled with an understanding of the various needs and the diversity of the population we serve, is complex enough in itself. I often feel as if there is too much to know and can imagine the feeling of being overwhelmed that frequently besets a beginning student. It is important in professional development to honor personal and professional limits and set appropriate personal and professional boundaries. When touch is the primary treatment method, it is even more important to understand the interpersonal dynamics of the therapeutic relationship. Professional boundaries are discussed further in Chapter 2.

The Uniqueness of Touch

A specific touch experience is difficult to replicate, because it is extremely multifaceted. The interaction between two individuals is unique. Students often ask instructors to demonstrate a method on them so that they know how it feels. Although this is a good learning experience, it is somewhat limited in that the feeling cannot be replicated with a different touching pair.

Students or fellow practitioners may tell an instructor about a client's situation and ask for recommendations. Often this is difficult for the instructor. Although instructors usually can give information about the pathology or technical description of various methodologies, they really do not know in what way they would do a massage until they touch that particular client. If the instructor actually touches the client to whom the student is referring in a professional teaching session, the client's experience of the instructor's touch and the student's touch does not end up being the same, even if both use the same method. The instructor's interaction through touch is no more right than the student's; rather, it is the unique quality of the touch experience that makes the difference.

When an instructor demonstrates a method of massage, this touch often is one developed through experience. The person receiving the massage probably notices the difference in the touch—not the method—when the student attempts to replicate the instructor's actions because the experience level is different. The confidence of experience is displayed not so much in the expert execution of the methods as in the quality of the touch used in delivering those methods.

Subjective and Objective Quality of Touch

Writing a textbook is mostly the dispensing of objective (fact-based) information and is separate from the author's personal, subjective experiences. Each one who reads the information in a textbook incorporates the skills and information as tools and resources in their own experience. Most of this text is written objectively, and that is as it should be; however, ideas on the experience of touch are so subjective in interpretation and experience that it seems impossible to present concepts of touch only through purely objective data. The authors of the books used as references in this section have not been able to accomplish this objectification of touch either. Something expansive and abstract about the simple, concrete experience of touch transcends technical writing. The experience of touching and being touched seems to extend beyond words and verbalization, beyond the skin, nervous system, and endocrine system, to the soul.

As this section concludes and the foundation for using touch in a therapeutic and professional way begins to be built, it seems appropriate to reflect personally on touch needs.

I know that I need to be touched, and I know what happens to me when I am not touched enough or when the touch does not feed me because it is not safe touch or because it is needy touch that requires me to feed someone else. When those with whom I can share or experience safe touch (my close family and friends, my pets, my woods, and my massage therapist) are unavailable, I become out of sorts and moody, my back hurts, I don't sleep as well, and I find myself involved in substitute behavior that attempts to feed my touch hunger.

When I'm alone, on good days I experience my own sense of touch through exercise and the enjoyment of tactile sensation, such as with my flannel sheets, or I listen to music. However, these forms of self-touch lack body contact with another, and often touch longings are not satisfied unless they are shared with another living being.

On not-so-good days, I overeat or use other excessive and detrimental forms of sensory stimulation. The excessiveness of the behavior is somewhat like trying to be satisfied with a carrot stick when you really crave vanilla pudding. It takes lots of carrots to fill me up, but I am still not satisfied. Then, when I finally give in to the vanilla pudding, I eat the whole box instead of the indicated serving. It is because I feel starved, beyond physical need, and I am operating in realms of emotional and maybe spiritual longing. Even more, this substitution behavior never really fulfills the desire. I still feel touch deprived and unsatisfied after the physiologic effects of the behavior (substituting food) wear off. No matter how many times I try to use them as substitutes, neither food nor exercise can replace the real need to be touched by someone who cares.

The desire for physical contact is an instinctive and physiologic need for well-being. What happens to you if your hunger for safe and nurturing (nutritious) touch is not met? Professional therapeutic touch often feeds touch hunger for people in a safe professional environment. Massage professionals serve by providing touch.

It is important for professionals of touch to embrace the expansive, abstract experience of touch. No one really cares how much you know until they know how much you care. The concrete experience of caring most often is conveyed through touch. That knowing, or "felt sense," experienced both by the client and the practitioner often is internalized through professional touch. We must show our willingness as practitioners to be open personally to sharing the experience with the client, at the same time being professional enough to respect the client and maintain the focus of the experience for him. To do this, each of us who uses touch professionally must be aware of self-care, and we must develop resources and support people (as well as pets and plants) who touch us in a safe, respectful, and healing way (Proficiency Exercise 1-3).

HISTORICAL PERSPECTIVES

section objectives

Using the information presented in this section, the student will be able to perform the following:

- **Trace the general progression of massage from ancient times to today**
- **Relate historical information to present-day events**

To understand professional, structured, therapeutic touch, the student must explore historical influences and the evo-

---

1 - 3
PROFICIENCY EXERCISE

In the space provided, answer the following questions.

What do I do when I am touch hungry?

Who and what touches me in a safe, respectful, and healing way?

---

lution of massage from its ancient foundations through projections for the future (Fig. 1-3).

A knowledge of history helps massage therapists develop a sense of professional identity and pride in their profession. Historic perspectives help members of a profession identify the profession's strengths and weaknesses. As students of massage read historic books about massage, they discover that the fundamental body of knowledge has changed little over the centuries. The most prevalent concepts in massage today were in fact written about many years ago. Massage has stood the test of time, proving itself a vital, health-enhancing technique, as well as a rehabilitative discipline. Currently the profession is at a defining moment; it is growing in acceptance and scientific rigor but is still paying for grave mistakes made long ago. As we move forward into the future with success, we will also make mistakes. In the future, beginning massage professionals will learn from us as well.

Many people have played important roles in tracing the historic journey of therapeutic massage and bodywork methods. Many of these books are listed in Appendix D. Specific acknowledgment must be given to Richard van Why, who compiled the *Bodywork Knowledgebase,* a collection of more than 100 historical books and more than 4000 research and journal articles on therapeutic massage and related methods. Much of the information in this chapter comes from this work. If it were not for van Why's diligence, much of the history of massage would be scattered in research libraries and would be unknown to us today. Another who deserves mention is Fran Tappan, a true master of massage. Not only has she written respected textbooks about massage that include a historical perspective, she is a part of that history.

This chapter consolidates the historical information. Because of extensive overlapping between the references used, text citation has been kept to a minimum. With gratitude and respect for those who have devoted their lives to this work, the many who are mentioned and the many more who are not, let us begin the journey forward by looking to the past.

The History of Massage

Identified animal behavior, such as the application of pressure, rubbing, and licking, indicates that massage is used instinctively either to relieve pain or respond to injury. In human beings, massage probably began when cave dwellers rubbed their bruises.[7] Massage has always been one of the most natural and instinctive means of relieving pain and discomfort. When a person has sore, aching muscles, abdominal pains, or a bruise or wound, the instinctive impulse is to touch and rub that part of the body to obtain relief.

Touch as a method of healing appears to have numerous cultural origins (Box 1-1).

MASSAGE

The word *massage* is thought to be derived from several sources. The Latin root *massa* and the Greek roots *massein* or *masso* mean to touch, handle, squeeze, or knead. The French verb *masser* also means to knead. The Arabic root *mass* or *mass'h* and the Sanskrit root *makeh* translate as "press softly."

Therapeutic massage has strong roots in Chinese folk medicine, but it also has many aspects in common with other healing traditions, such as Indian herbal medicine and Persian medicine. It is believed that the art of massage was first mentioned in writing about 2000 B.C.,[7] and it has been written about extensively in books since about 500 B.C. Egyptian, Persian, and Japanese historical medical literature are full of references to massage. The Greek physician Hippocrates advocated massage and gymnastic exercise. Asclepiades, another eminent Greek physician, relied exclusively on massage in his practice.

Throughout history, many different systems and supporting theories for the management of musculoskeletal pain and dysfunction have come and gone. The scientific thinking of the day has provided the validation for massage. Scientific research has changed the philosophy of massage theory. Current research continues to define the physical effects of therapeutic massage.

The endurance of massage through the centuries has been amazing. Current trends suggest an increase in the popularity of massage and body-related therapies used for stress reduction and treatment of chronic musculoskeletal problems (for more information, see Chapter 4).

Manual medicine, which has always been a part of the art of medicine, is the use of the hands in the treatment of injury and disease. Its therapeutic value is gained from changes in soft tissue and structure, rather than from surgery or pharmaceuticals.[3] Massage can be considered a part of manual medicine, although throughout history it has also stood independently to promote health. Manual medicine has grown to become the foundation of osteopathy, chiropractic, and physical therapy.[1]

THINK IT OVER

- If you were going to rename massage, what would you call it?
- If touch is so instinctive, why do you have to go to school to learn to do it?
- Why do you think every culture has had some form of massage?
- What do you think is the difference between massage and manual medicine?

Ancient Times

According to research reports, most ancient cultures practiced some form of healing touch. Often a ceremonial leader, such as a healer, priest, or shaman, was selected to perform the healing rituals. The healing methods often used herbs, oils, and primitive forms of hydrotherapy. Archaeologists have found many prehistoric artifacts depicting the use of massage for healing and cosmetic purposes. Some speculate that massage used for pain relief incorporated concepts of counterirritation, such as scraping, cutting, and burning of the skin, as part of the process. Massage may have been used as a cleansing procedure, along with fasting and bathing, in preparation for many tribal rituals.

In China, massage has been known by two names. *Anmo amma,* the more ancient name, means press-rub; *Tui-na,* of more recent origin, means push-pull. These Chinese methods were administered by kneading or rubbing down the entire body with the hands and using a gentle pressure and traction on all the joints.[8]

The practice of acupuncture involved the stimulation of specific points along the body, usually by the insertion of tiny, solid needles, but massage and other forms of pressure also were used. Such practices were also found in traditional Eskimo and African medicine, in which sharp stones were used to scratch the skin's surface. Today, scientists are able to give physiologic reasons for the value of these ancient practices.

Knowledge of massage and its applications already was well established in Chinese medicine at the time of the Sui Dynasty (A.D. 589-617). The Japanese came to know massage through the writings of the Chinese. Massage has been a part of life in India for almost 3000 years. The Chinese introduced the methods to India during trading forays. Like Chinese acupuncture, Hatha yoga, which was developed in India, has reappeared in modern forms of body therapy, with its energetic concepts of prana, chakras, and humoral balances.

The ancient Egyptians left artwork showing foot massage. Before Greek athletes took part in the Olympic games, they underwent friction treatment, anointing, and rubbing with sand. The use of touch as a mode of healing is recorded in the writings of the Hebrew and Christian traditions. The "laying on of hands" was particularly prominent in first-century Christianity. Full-body massage with oils (anointing) goes back even farther in Jewish practices. The ancient Jews practiced anointing for its ritual, hygienic, and therapeutic benefits. The Jewish culture honored rubbing with oils to such an extent that the root word for rubbing with oils and for the Messiah is the same (*Māshīah*).[8]

The ancient Mayan people of Central America, the Incas of South America, and other native people of the American continent also used methods of joint manipulation and massage.

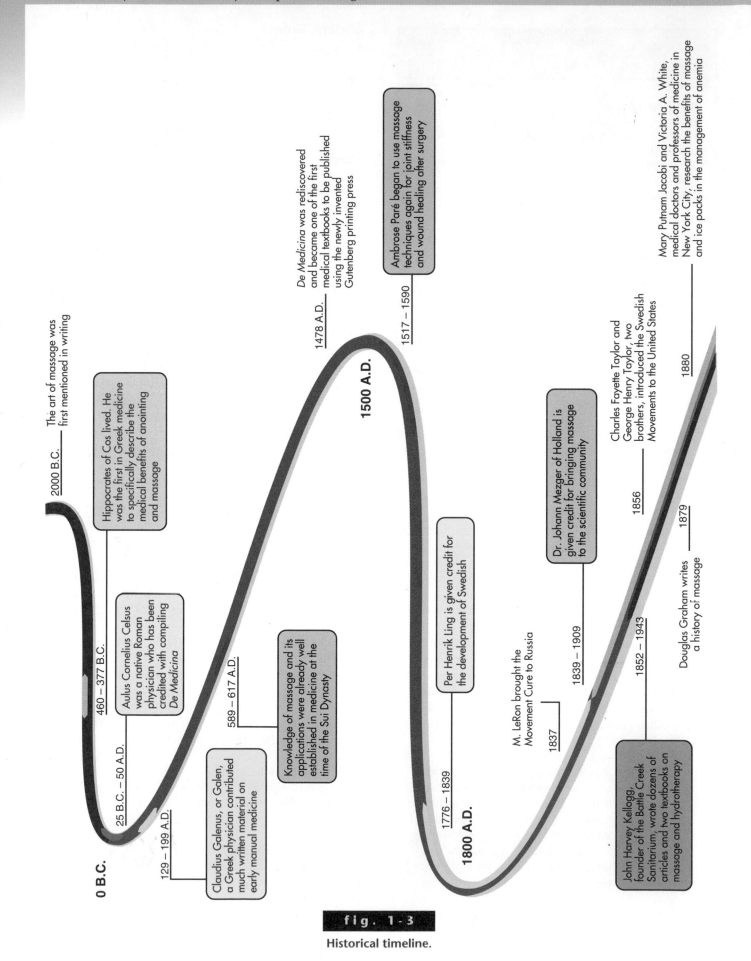

fig. 1-3

Historical timeline.

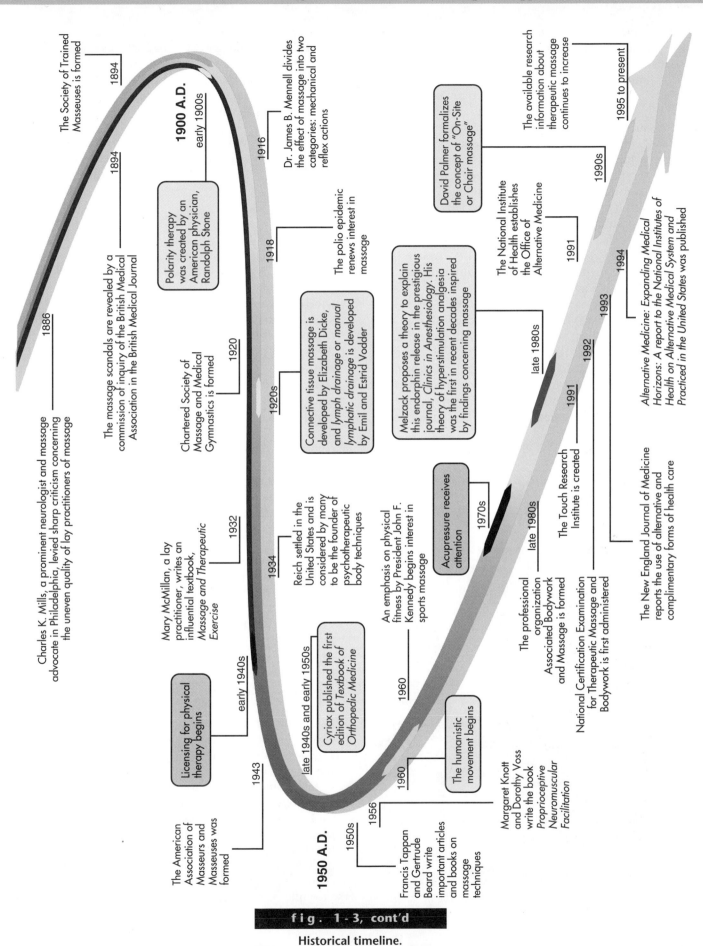

The Society of Trained Masseuses is formed — 1894

1894

1886

The massage scandals are revealed by a commission of inquiry of the British Medical Association in the British Medical Journal

Charles K. Mills, a prominent neurologist and massage advocate in Philadelphia, levied sharp criticism concerning the uneven quality of lay practitioners of massage

1900 A.D.
early 1900s

Polarity therapy was created by an American physician, Randolph Stone

1916

Dr. James B. Mennell divides the effect of massage into two categories: mechanical and reflex actions

1918

The polio epidemic renews interest in massage

1920

Chartered Society of Massage and Medical Gymnastics is formed

1920s

Connective tissue massage is developed by Elizabeth Dicke, and lymph drainage or manual lymphatic drainage is developed by Emil and Estrid Vodder

1932

Mary McMillan, a lay practitioner, writes an influential textbook, *Massage and Therapeutic Exercise*

1934

Reich settled in the United States and is considered by many to be the founder of psychotherapeutic body techniques

early 1940s

Licensing for physical therapy begins

1943

The American Association of Masseurs and Masseuses was formed

late 1940s and early 1950s

Cyriax published the first edition of *Textbook of Orthopedic Medicine*

1950s

Francis Tappan and Gertrude Beard write important articles and books on massage techniques

1950 A.D.

1956

Margaret Knott and Dorothy Voss write the book *Proprioceptive Neuromuscular Facilitation*

1960

The humanistic movement begins

1960

An emphasis on physical fitness by President John F. Kennedy begins interest in sports massage

1970s

Acupressure receives attention

Melzack proposes a theory to explain this endorphin release in the prestigious journal, *Clinics in Anesthesiology*. His theory of hyperstimulation analgesia was the first in recent decades inspired by findings concerning massage

late 1980s

The professional organization Associated Bodywork and Massage is formed

late 1980s

The Touch Research Institute is created

1991

National Certification Examination for Therapeutic Massage and Bodywork is first administered

1991

The National Institute of Health establishes the Office of Alternative Medicine

1992

The New England Journal of Medicine reports the use of alternative and complimentary forms of health care

1993

Alternative Medicine: Expanding Medical Horizons: A report to the National Institutes of Health on Alternative Medical System and Practiced in the United States was published

1994

David Palmer formalizes the concept of "On-Site or Chair massage"

1990s

The available research information about therapeutic massage continues to increase

1995 to present

fig. 1-3, cont'd

Historical timeline.

Hippocrates of Cos (460-377 B.C.) (Fig. 1-4) was the first physician in Greek medicine to describe specifically the medical benefits of anointing and massage, along with the chemical properties of oils used for this purpose. He called his art *anatripsis,* which means to rub up. Of this art he said, "The physician must be acquainted with many things and assuredly with anatripsis, for things that have the same name have not always the same effects, for rubbing can bind a joint that is too loose or loosen a joint that is too hard."[8] Hippocrates' methods survived, virtually unchanged, well into the Middle Ages. Many techniques similar to those methods, especially traction and stretching principles, are still in use today.[1]

Claudius Galenus, or Galen, another Greek physician (A.D. 129-199), contributed much written material on early manual medicine, including many commentaries on Hippocrates' methods.[1]

Massage came to the Romans from the Greeks. Julius Caesar (100-44 B.C.) had himself "pinched all over" daily to relieve his neuralgia and prevent epileptic attacks.[7] Aulus Cornelius Celsus (25 B.C.–A.D. 50), a Roman physician, has been credited with compiling *De Medicina,* a series of eight books covering the body of medical knowledge of the day. Seven of the books deal extensively with prevention and therapeutics using rubbing, exercise,

bathing, and anointing. This work was rediscovered during the late Middle Ages by Pope Nicholas V (1397-1455). In 1478 *De Medicina* was one of the first medical textbooks to be published with the newly invented Gutenberg printing press. It was one of most popular medical textbooks during the Renaissance.

THINK IT OVER   Why do you think ancient people started sticking things into the skin and scratching the skin to produce healing?

The Middle Ages

Massage developed differently in the East and the West. In the East, as part of the Islamic Empire, it represented a continuation of Greco-Roman traditions. In the West, the Greco-Roman traditions disappeared, but massage was kept alive by the common people, to become a part of folk culture. In this form, massage was an important part of the healing tradition of the Slavs, Finns, and Swedes. As massage was integrated into the health practices of the common people, it often was associated with supernatural experiences and observances. This association alienated massage from what little scientific approach there was during this time. Practitioners of folk medicine often were persecuted, with the Church claiming that the practitioner's healing powers came from the devil.[8]

Not until the sixteenth century did massage regain its respectability in Europe. One of the founders of modern surgery, the French physician Ambrose Paré (1517-1590), began to use massage techniques again for joint stiffness and wound healing after surgery. In his work Paré described three types of massage strokes: gentle, medium, and vigorous. His ideas were passed down to other French physicians who believed in the value of manual therapeutics.

The Nineteenth Century

Per Henrik Ling.   Per Henrik Ling (1776-1839) is credited with developing Swedish massage, but he did not invent it. He learned massage from others and through persistent experimentation put the information together in a workable form.

Ling proposed an integrated program for the treatment of disease using active and passive movements and massage. Legend has it that Ling's interest in these methods was sparked by the gout in his own elbow. He developed a system of massage that used many of the positions and movements of Swedish gymnastics. Combining these strokes with exercises, he healed his diseased elbow. Ling's program was based on the newly discovered knowledge of the circulation of the blood and lymph. (It is interesting to note that the Chinese had been using these methods for centuries.)

While teaching fencing, Ling observed that habitual movements interfered with the development of desired

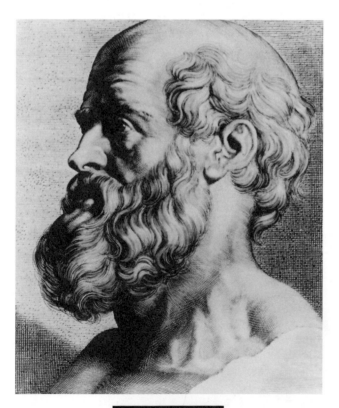

fig. 1-4

Hippocrates. (From Donahue MP: *Nursing, the finest art: an illustrated history,* ed 2, St Louis, 1996, Mosby.)

movements. He determined that the development of a skill depended on the mental mastery of habit; therefore he began teaching bodily movements systematically. He developed his medical gymnastics in 1814, but his methods were bitterly opposed by the Swedish medical establishment for almost 20 years. He was not trained in medicine, and his tendency to use poetic and mystic language in his writings on gymnastics was thought to interfere with wider acceptance of his ideas.[9] Current experts in massage would be wise to take note of Ling's experience; it is essential that massage be explained in the medical and scientific terminology of the day.

With the support of influential clients, Ling was granted a license to practice and teach his method, and he established the Royal Gymnastic Central Institute. The primary focus of Ling's system, especially in his later writings, was on gymnastics applied to the treatment of disease. This position was a change from his earlier educational and military gymnastics, which was intended only for healthy people.

In his system, Ling divided movements into active, duplicated, and passive forms. Active movements are performed by the person's own effort and correspond to what commonly is called *exercise*. Duplicated movements are performed by the person with the cooperation of a gymnast (therapist) and involved active effort by both parties, in which the action of the one was opposed by the action of the other. Duplicated movements correspond to what today is commonly called *resistive exercise*. Passive movements are performed for the person by the active effort of the gymnast alone. They consist of passive movements of the extremities, what we today call *range of motion* and *stretching*. Movement therapy was not separated from massage, and both were considered integral to the system.

Ling taught many physicians from Germany, Austria, Russia, and England, who spread his teachings to their own countries. Ling was recognized by his contemporaries and later followers not so much as a great innovator, but as a keen observer who adopted methods only after testing their effectiveness. He combined many techniques into one coherent system. By the time of Ling's death in 1839, his system had achieved worldwide recognition.[8] Ling's teachings endured because he developed a school to continue teaching medical gymnastics, or the Swedish movement cure, as it became known in the United States in the late nineteenth century.

THINK IT OVER Why do you think that Ling's development of a school was so important?

The Modern Revival of Massage

Per Henrik Ling and others who practiced the Swedish movement cure deserve credit for reviving massage after the Middle Ages. Initially, nonprofessionals spoke to physicians in a language they did not share, making communication difficult. Dr. Johann Mezger of Holland (1839-1909) is credited with bringing massage to the scientific community. He presented massage to fellow physicians as a form of medical treatment. The French terms *effleurage, pétrissage,* and *tapotement* did not come from Ling. Mezger's followers in Holland began to use these names, although historical references do not explain why French terms were chosen. So often history is confused, and the issue of who deserves credit for what becomes clouded.[9]

As physicians talked to one another about massage, its popularity began to grow. They sought common ground between their methods and massage, both to justify their current view of massage and to expand it. Lay magazines and medical journals published manuscripts on massage. The successful experience and testimony of distinguished people, especially monarchs and diplomats, further bolstered the image of massage and increased public and medical acceptance. Many physicians were drawn to study massage because they had a strong scientific interest in its effects. They conducted animal studies and well-designed clinical trials, which further persuaded physicians of the value of the method and increased the interest of the medical community. The same situation has held true for massage in the 1990s; it currently is bolstered by the work of Dr. Tiffany Field at the Touch Research Institute at the University of Miami Medical School and by studies conducted under grants from the National Institutes of Health.

The Swedish movement cure quickly spread to the other countries of Europe; the first institute outside Sweden was established in Denmark. In 1837, 2 years before Ling's death, his disciple, M. LeRon, brought the Movement Cure to Russia, establishing a clinic in St. Petersburg.

Massage in the United States. In the United States the first waves of European immigration came from Northern Europe, which had accepted massage earlier because of its therapeutic benefits. The immigrants provided many great writers and teachers of massage, as well as eager, trusting clients.[8]

Two brothers, Charles F. Taylor and George H. Taylor, introduced the Swedish movement system to the United States in 1856. They had learned the skills from Dr. Mathias Roth, an English physician who studied directly with Ling. Roth, also a leader in the homeopathic movement, felt that massage worked on the same principles as homeopathy: the law of similars and the concept of "like cures like."

Dr. John Harvey Kellogg (1852-1943), founder of the Battle Creek Sanitarium in Michigan, wrote dozens of articles and two textbooks on massage and hydrotherapy and edited and published a popular magazine, *Good Health.*

In 1879 Douglas Graham, in his history of massage, described the Lomi-Lomi of the Hawaiians as a hygienic measure used to relieve fatigue or for the pure pleasure of it. Graham continued to write on massage and its use in almost every area of medicine until his death in the late 1920s.

In 1889 a letter from a physician in Kansas appeared in a New York medical journal, in which the physician said that he had thought massage was but "a novel method of therapeutics" until he had read a passage from Captain James Cook's diary of his third voyage around the world near the end of the eighteenth century. Cook had described how his pseudosciatic pain was relieved in an elegant and generous ritual by a Tahitian chief and his family, using a method called *romee*.

The massage scandals of the late 1800s. In a very real sense, massage was a victim of its own success. In 1886 Dr. Charles K. Mills, a prominent neurologist and advocate of massage in Philadelphia, sharply criticized the uneven quality of lay practitioners of massage and their often unsubstantiated and unethical claims. In 1889 British physicians, who were just beginning to view massage favorably because Queen Victoria supported the methods, became increasingly aware of patterns of abuse, including false claims about lay practitioners' education or skills, client stealing, and the charging of high fees. The massage scandals of 1894, revealed by a commission of inquiry of the British Medical Association in the *British Medical Journal,* eroded the public's and the medical profession's confidence in massage as a legitimate medical art.

An inconsistent system of education, which encompassed private trade schools, hospitals, and physicians who took private students, appeared to be one of the major contributors to the downfall of confidence in massage. Courses in technique, anatomy, physiology, and pathology varied immensely, as did the teachers' experience and capability. Some held that they could teach with minimal training in massage or directly after graduation from programs of questionable quality. Students often were encouraged to have grand expectations of career opportunities, only to find a difficult job market in which many of them were inadequately trained to compete.

Richard van Why provides an example of the problem[8]:

Many schools used improper student recruitment tactics. The worst involved young women from poor neighborhoods, who were approached by recruiters claiming that extraordinary career opportunities awaited masseuses or medical gymnasts upon graduation from schools of professional training. The recruiters offered to defer payment of tuition until a reasonable time had elapsed after their graduation, so that the women could build resources to pay their living expenses and still pay the loans back. They were typically trained in short programs and then were released to a marketplace full of lay practitioners. As they found no work, they could not pay the loans back. Soon the recruiters returned, demanding payment. The women were told that if they did not pay, they would be thrown into debtors prison until they

did. To work off the debt, they would have to work at a clinic attached to the school or for a friend or a colleague of a school administrator. The best of these 'clinics' offered incompetently performed classical massage. The worst of the 'clinics' were pretexts for houses of prostitution. In the scandals that followed in British cities and in Chicago and New York, the 'massage parlor' caught on, and the lay practice of massage became associated with vice.

Another notorious abuse involved "certification," which some physicians who supported massage considered merely a "receipt for money paid."

Still another problem concerned advertising. The medical profession and the well-trained, classical lay practitioners of massage and medical gymnastics did not make false claims in their advertisements. Conversely, many entrepreneurs and poor massage practitioners, seeking publicity to increase enrollment at their schools and attendance at their clinics, did make such claims, which often flew in the face of the principles of anatomy, physiology, and pathology.

In 1894, the same year that the massage scandals were revealed in Britain, eight women who envisioned massage professionals as "well-trained, properly equipped masseuses serving those in need" formed the Society of Trained Masseuses. Before this time, the quality of lay practitioners of massage was inconsistent. Recognizing the need for rigorous standards, the founders modeled theirs after the medical profession. They set academic prerequisites for the study of massage. Training could be given only in recognized schools, which were to be inspected regularly to ensure that standards were maintained. Only qualified instructors could teach classes. Examinations for teachers and graduates of basic massage training were conducted by a board, which included a physician. Examinations were to include both written tests and a demonstration of clinical achievement.

Problems arose within the Society of Trained Masseuses during a period of sustained growth, and another, competing association was established. This weakened both of them. In 1920 the Society assembled an advisory committee to aid reorganization and reconcile with the opposing association. The two groups joined as the Chartered Society of Massage and Medical Gymnastics. In 1909, before the reorganization, the Society had 600 members; by 1939 the membership had grown to 12,000. Certificates of competence were granted to individuals who had passed a rigorous examination. To be admitted to the Chartered Society of Massage and Medical Gymnastics, prospective members had to pledge not to accept clients unless they had been referred by a physician. Members were forbidden to advertise in the lay press. The Society worked to provide a central registry of well-trained massage practitioners and to provide referrals for inquiries from the medical profession or the public, based on location and any special needs. However, membership in the association was voluntary, and many ill-trained, unscrupulous practitioners continued to thrive.

THINK IT OVER

- How is the success of massage today similar to the success of massage in the early and mid-1800s?
- Do you think it is possible that an unfortunate repeat of the darker history of massage could happen today? If so, what factors would contribute to the problem?
- What can members of the profession do today to avoid a downfall similar to that which occurred in the late 1800s?

Massage endures. Even during the difficult time of the late 1800s, massage endured. Institutes of massage appeared in France, Germany, and Austria by the mid-nineteenth century. Between 1854 and 1918, the practice of massage developed from an obscure, unskilled trade to a field of medical health care, from which the profession of physical therapy began. Treatments consisted of massage, mineral baths, and exercise.[8]

Dr. David Gurevich, a Russian physician and instructor of Russian medical massage, believed that the long-standing interest in massage and its continuing development are strong proof of its usefulness and necessity.[4] According to Dr. Gurevich, massage was practiced by ancient Slavic tribes, especially in combination with therapeutic bathing. Beginning in the eighteenth century, many great Russian scientists and doctors (Mudroff, Manasein, Botkin, Zakharin, and others) contributed to the development of the theory and practice of massage. I. Z. Zabludovski wrote more than 100 books, textbooks, and scientific articles devoted to the methods of massage and its physiologic basis in therapy, postsurgical care, and sports.

An institute of massage and exercise was founded in Russia at the end of the nineteenth century, and many courses in massage also were started. Massage gradually progressed from an auxiliary method of therapy to an independent therapeutic method that was used effectively with other types of treatment. The practice of massage has become widespread in Russia. All therapy clinics have a massage room. Massage used with therapeutic exercises has been adapted for the management of the viscera, the nervous system, and gynecologic disorders, as well as in orthopedics, post-trauma care, and postsurgical care. Prospective students of massage must have some medical education. The change in Russia's economy in the late 1980s and early 1990s to a market system has made it possible for private massage clinics, which charge a fee, to open.[4]

The Historical Influence of Women

Women made early and important contributions to the development of massage and medical gymnastics, primarily in the United States. Two women physicians conducted the first controlled clinical trial of the benefits of massage in the management of disease. Drs. Mary P. Jacobi and Victoria A. White were professors of medicine in New York City in 1880. Their research addressed the benefits of massage and ice packs in the management of anemia.

Contemporary massage has been influenced extensively by women, and most practicing massage professionals today are women. Broad licensing for physical therapy began in the early 1940s. Louise L. Despard's *Text-Book of Massage and Remedial Gymnastics* was one of a handful of textbooks on massage recommended in 1940 as essential reading for all students of massage by the Massage Round Table of the American Physical Therapy Association.

Mary McMillan, an English lay practitioner of massage, wrote an influential textbook, *Massage and Therapeutic Exercise*, in 1932. She had extensive experience in the field. From 1911 to 1915 she was in charge of massage and therapeutic exercise at the Greenbank Cripples Home in Liverpool, England, and from 1916 to 1918 she served as director of massage and remedial gymnastics at the Children's Hospital in Portland, Maine. During World War I she served in the military as a rehabilitation aide.[7]

Eunice Ingham formalized the system of reflexology. Dr. Janet Travell's work with myofascial pain and trigger points is unsurpassed. Bonnie Prudden popularized trigger point work. Fran Tappan's outstanding contributions to massage and physical therapy are formalized in her textbook, *Healing Massage Techniques*. Sister Kenny used massage in the treatment of polio. Ida Rolf's massage system grew to become the technique of *Rolfing*. Dr. Dolores Krieger has made major contributions to the more energetic approaches through her system of therapeutic touch. Because of the extensive influence of women in massage today, it is likely that when massage history is written in 20 years, many women will be listed as vital contributors to the continued development of massage.

The Twentieth Century

Sigmund Freud (1856-1939), an Austrian neurologist and theorist who developed the system of psychoanalysis, experimented with the use of massage in the treatment of hysteria, a form of mental illness common in his day. This condition is characterized by a paralysis that has no physiologic basis. Freud's *Studies on Hysteria*, published in 1895, explained his methods.

Wilhelm Reich, an Austrian psychoanalyst who was a clinical assistant to Freud for 6 years, became interested in the physiologic basis of neurosis. In 1934 Reich emigrated to the United States. He is considered by many to be the founder of psychotherapeutic body techniques. Reich gradually moved the emphasis of his therapeutic approach away from the psychologic and toward the realm of the physical, the body. Reich developed many somatic techniques to dissolve the muscular armor. Because of his controversial techniques, he came into conflict with the medical establishment and eventually was investigated by the U.S. Food and Drug Administration. He was convicted of fraudulent medical practices and died in 1957 while serving his sentence in federal prison.

Reich's earlier ideas and therapies have greatly influenced contemporary bodywork. *Bioenergetics,* a popular somatotherapy, evolved directly from his system. Bioenergetics was founded by Alexander Lowen, an American psychiatrist who was Reich's student for 12 years.

1900 to 1960. In the early 1900s Dr. Randolph Stone, an American physician, devised polarity therapy. Stone studied many body systems, both ancient and modern, including acupuncture, hatha yoga, osteopathy, chiropractic techniques, and reflexology. From his investigations he concluded that "magnetic fields" regulated and directed the physiologic systems of the body. Influenced by Eastern philosophy and medicine, Stone believed that all aspects of the universe were expressed in opposite poles (e.g., male and female, positive and negative electric charges); therefore he called his therapeutic method "polarity."

In 1907 Edgar F. Cyriax began a distinguished publishing career that spanned almost 40 years. He was the last great proponent of Ling's Swedish movement cure, which he called *mechanotherapeutics.*

At the turn of the nineteenth century, the United States and England looked to Japan for innovation in the vocational rehabilitation of the blind. The British Institute for Massage by the Blind was established in 1900. Other European nations tried to develop their own models of the Japanese and the British institutions but failed.

A textbook published in 1900 by Albert Hoffa and revised in 1913 by Max Bohm describes the more classical massage techniques such as *effleurage, pétrissage, tapotement,* and vibration. Most therapists learn these methods as standard massage techniques in entry-level programs. However, many massage professionals of the time disregarded this type of massage, considering it too basic to be included in the realm of advanced manual therapy. Others warned against leaving behind traditional massage techniques, believing that fundamentals could not be replaced with more modern forms of bodywork.

In 1916 Dr. James B. Mennell divided the effects of massage into two categories: mechanical actions and reflex actions. Mennell showed that massage exerts a mechanical effect in four ways:

- By aiding venous return of blood to the heart
- By promoting lymph movement out of the tissues
- By stretching the connective tissue (e.g., tendons, scar tissue)
- By mechanical stimulation of the stomach, small intestine, and colon

Mennell also maintained that certain forms of tactile stimulation, such as stroking and light touch, stimulated reflex arcs, causing muscles to relax or contract according to the type of stroke. He theorized that both smooth and skeletal muscles were under the control of such reflexes. Experimental research now supports the theories of Ling, Mennell, and others that massage has mechanical and reflex effects.

The polio epidemic of 1918 sparked a more widespread interest in massage because victims and their families were desperate for any remedy that offered any promise at all. Research on the benefits of massage in preventing the complications of paralysis began at this time.

Connective tissue massage (CTM) was developed in the 1920s by German physiotherapist Elizabeth Dicke; it was later expanded by Maria Ebner. CTM was first used when Dicke herself was suffering from a prolonged illness caused by an "impairment of the circulation" in her right leg. As with Ling, her search for self-healing added much to the development of massage.

During this time Emil Vodder, a Danish physiologist, and his wife, Estrid, developed a technique of light massage along the course of the surface lymphatics; this technique was called *lymph drainage* or *manual lymphatic drainage.* It was and still is used to treat chronic lymphedema and other diseases of the lymphatic and peripheral vascular systems.

The American Association of Masseurs and Masseuses was formed in Chicago in 1943. It subsequently was renamed the American Massage Therapy Association. Another professional organization, the International Myomassetics Federation, was formed later through the efforts of Irene Gauthier, a notable massage instructor, and others.

James H. Cyriax, the son of Edgar Cyriax, became an orthopedic surgeon at St. Thomas Hospital, a prestigious teaching institution in London. The younger Cyriax gained fame through his development of transverse friction massage. In the late 1940s and early 1950s, he published the first edition of his now classic *Textbook of Orthopedic Medicine.* His work is especially significant in the area of massage because of its recognition, categorization, and differential diagnosis of pathology of the body's soft tissues. The fact that pain can be caused by dysfunction of soft tissues, including but not limited to periarticular connective tissue, is the foundation of soft tissue manipulation today. Cyriax also was the first to introduce the concept of "end feel" in the diagnosis of soft tissue lesions.

Dr. Herman Kabat researched neuromuscular concepts based on the work of neurophysiologists and Pavlov's conditioning of reflexes. Sherrington's law of successive induction provided the foundation for the development of rhythmic stabilization and slow reversal techniques. By 1951 research had begun on a new method, which was formalized in 1956 in the book *Proprioceptive Neuromuscular Facilitation,* written by Margaret Knott and Dorothy Voss (for more information, see Chapter 9).

Francis Tappan and Gertrude Beard also wrote important articles and books on massage techniques during the 1950s. Their texts are still available, and serious students of massage would benefit from reading these classic works. As of this writing, Fran Tappan continues to influence the profession of massage in interviews, conferences on the future of massage, and consultation with many leaders in the field. She has been honored by the American Massage Therapy Association for her contributions to massage.

1960 to the present: the most recent revival of massage. The most recent revival of massage began around 1960 and has continued to this day. Recognition of chronic diseases that are resistant to surgical or drug treatment has increased. Neither the acute care concept nor a single solution approach seems to work with these cases. A more complex way of envisioning and treating these diseases has had to be developed, and massage is one approach that has proven effective over time.

The humanistic movement that began during the 1960s spilled over into medicine and allied health. Concerns about "bedside manner," "genuineness," and the benefits of touch again raised the issue of the legitimacy and value of massage for its psychic use alone. Later, the Esalen movement and Gestalt psychology inspired psychologists and psychotherapists to explore massage and other movement therapies. Many controlled clinical studies in medicine, nursing, physical therapy, and psychology inspired more academic and clinical interest in massage.

In 1960 increased medical awareness that lack of exercise contributed to cardiovascular disease and other disorders prompted President John F. Kennedy to emphasize physical fitness, especially for children. This new interest grew into the physical fitness movement of the late 1960s and led the health sciences into a movement toward preventive medicine. The benefits of sports were rediscovered, and as a result historic literature in the field of massage was brought to light, such as Albert Baumgartner's book, *Massage in Athletics,* which discussed the relationship between massage and exercise and the value of massage in conditioning and stress control.

Acupressure received more attention than any other bodywork method during the 1970s and 1980s. The medical, physical therapy, and nursing literature examined it closely on the basis of controlled clinical trials. In writings on nursing and rehabilitation medicine, a body of knowledge arose concerning the benefits of massage in preventing and treating decubitus ulcers and in the overall management of heart rate and blood pressure in people suffering from acute and chronic manifestations of cardiovascular disease.[8]

Richard van Why has said, "It was in the field of pain research and pain management that the greatest gains for massage were made."

Ronald Melzack, a professor of psychology in the anesthesiology department of McGill University Medical School and one of the initial proponents of the gate control theory of pain, published the results of several controlled clinical trials on the value of ice massage and manual massage for the relief of dental pain and low back pain. Melzack not only found these techniques effective in preventing or reducing pain, he also proposed the neural mechanisms by which they operated. Other researchers picked up on this theme and began to examine the role of massage in the liberation of endorphins, pain-killing chemicals more potent than morphine that are produced by the brain in response to certain stimuli, including massage. In the late 1980s Melzack proposed a theory to explain this endorphin release in the prestigious journal *Clinics in Anesthesiology.* His theory of hyperstimulation analgesia was the first in recent decades inspired by findings concerning massage. It argued that certain intense sensory stimuli, such as puncture with a needle or exposure to extreme cold or pressure, when applied near the site of an injury, sent a signal to the brain by a faster channel than that used by the pain signal it was attempting to treat, thereby disrupting the pain.[8] Perhaps this is why ancient men and women scratched themselves with stones.

Recent Trends

In the late 1980s the professional organization Associated Bodywork and Massage Professionals was formed to serve the needs of a growing and diverse group of bodywork therapists. Additional professional organizations are likely to form in the future.

In 1988 the American Massage Therapy Association spearheaded a proposal for the development of a national certification process. The proposal stirred up much controversy and was hotly debated. With the participation of other professional massage and bodywork sources, the National Certification Examination for Therapeutic Massage and Bodywork was devised in 1992. Since its inception, the examination has had a positive influence on the professional development of therapeutic massage.

The trend toward state licensure of massage continues. Educational requirements set through state licensure average 500 to 1000 hours and show signs of increasing in the future. European and Canadian standards range from little or no training to extensive educational requirements (2200 to 3500 hours).

The University of Westminster in England offers bachelor's and master's degrees in massage and bodywork. This program was developed by Dr. Patrick Peitroni, Dr. Leon Chaitow, and others. Schools of massage therapy have begun to work with colleges and universities to develop articulation agreements that allow graduates of their program to complete degrees in massage. The first of these articulation agreements was made in 1995 between the Health Enrichment Center in Lapeer, Michigan, and Sienna Heights College in Adrian, Michigan, to grant both associate's and bachelor's degrees in applied science in massage therapy.

Some private massage schools have increased their educational requirements to enable them to grant associate's degrees. More community colleges are developing certificate programs in therapeutic massage, and some of these programs can lead to an associate's degree in applied or general science.

Those who have experienced the revival of massage from 1960 to the present may wonder if this success carries with it mixed blessings. Before 1985 massage professionals worked primarily in independent settings with little or no supervision. The very best of this situation was the freedom to serve clients' needs without the constraints of regulation. The worst was the lack of consistent training and the confusion among other professionals and the public about what constituted therapeutic massage.

Frustration with massage parlor regulations to control prostitution and the desire of many massage professionals to enter the mainstream of public awareness pushed the massage therapy profession to begin seeking an alliance with the existing heath care structure to justify the validity of massage. In some instances this movement into the existing health care world created turf battles over which profession would provide massage therapy. Questions and concerns, both legitimate and reactionary, were expressed by the physical therapy and nursing professions.

The public's desire for physical fitness had reached its peak during this time, and the concept of "sports massage" provided an avenue for mainstreaming massage therapy. During the 1990s the mainstream approach shifted from sports to corporate America. David Palmer can be given credit for formalizing the concepts of "on site" and "chair" massage. These two trends allowed the public to see massage in a way much different from the preconceived notions of a "feel good" luxury of the wealthy or a front for prostitution.

As research continues to validate massage therapy and as it evolves into a distinct professional course with credible and standardized education, the turf battles in the health care system seem to be quieting down. Multidisciplinary teams are formed in which many different professionals work together. As this process continues, nurses and physical therapists probably will find themselves supervising massage paraprofessionals and working as partners with more comprehensively trained massage therapists who have earned a degree.

In 1991 the Touch Research Institute at the University of Miami opened under the direction of Dr. Tiffany Field. More than any other single development in the 1990s, the research from the institute has moved massage into the mainstream and into accepted health care practice.

In 1991, the National Institutes of Health established the Office of Alternative Medicine. Two years later, the *New England Journal of Medicine* reported on a national survey of the use of alternative and complementary forms of health care. Massage was the third most used treatment. In line with this trend, *Alternative Medicine: Expanding Medical Horizons: A report to the National Institutes of Health on Alternative Medical Systems and Practices in the United States* was published in 1994.

The credibility and acceptance of natural approaches to health and illness are developing, and knowledge bases are beginning to overlap. Three areas in osteopathic medicine

that currently are applicable to massage are muscle energy techniques, positional release and strain/counterstrain techniques, and neuromuscular techniques. The most noteworthy educator and author in these methods is Dr. Leon Chaitow, who, similar to Ling, is a master synthesizer of the best of many concepts. Dr. Chaitow developed a strong foundation in manual medicine working as an assistant to his uncle, Dr. Boris Chaitow, the codeveloper of neuromuscular technique with his cousin, the legendary Stanley Lief, D.C., D.O., N.D.[2] Dr. Leon Chaitow has written many books that have enriched the body of knowledge for soft tissue methods, including therapeutic massage.

Other authors worthy of mention are Ida Rolf, developer of the Rolfing system, Dr. Milton Trager, developer of Trager, and Dr. Janet Travell, coauthor with David Simons of the most comprehensive texts written on the subject of trigger points.* Since 1995 the amount of information available on therapeutic massage has increased dramatically. Many new and exciting books are on the market, and web sites for therapeutic massage have been created on the Internet. All forms of media, including television, magazines, and newspapers, carry supportive stories about the benefits of massage.

Research continues to validate the benefits of massage. After years of struggle for acceptance and validation, massage in the mid-1990s has moved into the mainstream. What the future will bring depends on our commitment to the ideals of massage.

The Future of Massage

The role of massage and related bodywork methods is expanding at an accelerated rate. Massage now has enough validation to justify its use by the public as well as health care professionals. An explosion of information and awareness has occurred. The future will determine the way the profession responds to the needs created by this success.

The massage therapy profession is changing. It is becoming more sophisticated, requiring education not only in technical skill development but also in pathology, medications, record keeping, communications skills, and in the important area of professional ethics. The more massage professionals work with other heath care professionals, the more they need to know to be able to understand the world of health care. As we blend our world of professional touch with theirs, it will be interesting to watch the exchange of information. We hope that the best of both worlds will emerge and that the lessons of the past will temper and soften the process.

More and more employment opportunities are becoming available in the area of health care. Mental health interventions that use massage are becoming commonplace.

---

*The two texts by Travell and Simons are *Myofascial Pain and Dysfunction: the Trigger Point Manual* and *Myofascial Pain and Dysfunction: the Trigger Point Manual: the Lower Extremities*, vol. 2.

Some health care insurance plans and managed care systems are beginning to look at ways to include massage therapy among their covered services.

In the wellness and personal service areas, day spas are bringing the art of pampering to the public. No longer does a person have to travel to some far-off place and spend thousands of dollars to experience the pleasure of a day of luxury. Massage clinics that focus on wellness massage are becoming commonplace, as are massage professionals in the corporate setting.

Research into genetics, stress responses, neuroendocrine influences, and environmental hazards, as well as support for the whole person in coping with a world that seems to be moving too fast, encourages the development of massage as a counterbalance to a stressful lifestyle. The current trends supported by research seem to indicate that manual therapies are gaining recognition. Dr. Field of the Touch Research Institute probably will be recognized as a major contributor to the growth of massage therapy because of her dedication to touch research.

As the world becomes a global community, the ever-increasing exchange of information will enrich the knowledge base of therapeutic massage. Exploration of ancient healing methods will reveal the wisdom and scientific validity of a body/mind/spirit approach to well-being.

Hopefully, the abundance of massage and bodywork methods will combine into a consolidated system of therapeutic massage without losing the rich diversity of professional expression. Terminology and education will standardize, although the integrity of the individual applications of massage and bodywork will be maintained. Two tracks of massage service probably will standardize: wellness massage outside the health care system and medical massage within the heath care system. These trends will allow easy access for all to both types of services.

The future is very bright and promising, especially if we pay attention to our past and remember the words and wisdom of an old Russian physician, who says "massage is massage." We ourselves constitute one of the biggest threats to the future of massage. All bodywork professions must come together to work for the common good. As the massage profession moves forward and reclaims its heritage as an important health service, it is important to look back. In retrospect, we can see the strengths and weaknesses of the professional journey.

It also is important to honor those who have dedicated so much of their lives to developing the body of knowledge of therapeutic massage. Many today are dedicating a significant portion of their lives to the professional advancement of therapeutic massage. When the history of massage is written in the future, these names will appear with the information they have organized and contributed. We are all contributors to the future of massage, and we all will become part of its history.

THINK IT OVER

- **What do you want the future of massage to bring?**
- **How are you going to assist in the development of that future?**

SUMMARY

This chapter began with questions and ended with questions. The importance and nature of touch in the professional setting were discussed. The reader should now be aware of the ways in which culture, gender, age, life events, spirituality, and diversity all influence the experience of touching and being touched. Inappropriate forms of touch were identified, and appropriate forms of professional touch were explored. An understanding of the subjective experience of touch was addressed personally.

The history of massage from ancient times to the present was presented, as were projections for the future. A timeline highlighted many key dates. The foundation has been laid for the study of therapeutic massage.

REFERENCES

1. Cantu RI, Grodin AJ: *Myofascial manipulation: theory and clinical application,* Gaithersburg, Md., 1992, Aspen Publishers.
2. Chaitow L: *Soft tissue manipulation,* Rochester, Vt., 1988, Healing Arts Press.
3. Greenman PE: *Principles of manual medicine,* Baltimore, 1989, Williams & Wilkins.
4. Gurevich D: *Historical perspective,* 1992 (unpublished article).
5. Lederman E: *Fundamentals of manual therapy physiology, neurology, and psychology,* New York, 1997, Churchill Livingstone.
6. Smith EWL, Clance PR, Imes S: *Touch in psychotherapy,* New York, 1998, Guilford Press.
7. Tappan FM, Benjamin PJ: *Tappan's handbook of healing massage techniques: holistic, classic, and emerging methods,* ed 3, Norwalk, Conn., 1998, Appleton & Lange.
8. van Why RP: *History of massage and its relevance to today's practitioner, the Bodywork Knowledgebase,* New York, 1992, self-published.
9. van Why RP: *Notes toward a history of massage,* ed 2, New York, 1992, self-published.

WORKBOOK SECTION

Short Answer

1. What is the skin's significance in touch?

   _____

   _____

   _____

   _____

2. What factors can influence an individual's experience of touch?

   _____

   _____

   _____

   _____

3. What are the forms of inappropriate professional touch?

   _____

   _____

   _____

   _____

4. What are the forms of appropriate professional touch?

   _____

   _____

   _____

   _____

5. In what way and where did massage originate? Why is this answer important?

   _____

   _____

   _____

   _____

6. What has provided the validation for massage?

   _____

   _____

   _____

   _____

7. What methods did the ancient Chinese massage system use? In what ways are the methods of today different?

   _____

   _____

   _____

   _____

8. Why was massage associated with folk medicine and connected with supernatural experiences during the Middle Ages in Europe?

   _____

   _____

   _____

   _____

9. Why is credit given to Per Henrik Ling for the development of the Swedish movement cure and Swedish massage?

   _____

   _____

   _____

   _____

10. In what way did problems with terminology interfere with the acceptance of Ling's work?

    _____

    _____

    _____

    _____

11. Who or what was one of the main contributors to the massage scandals in the late 1800s?

    _____

    _____

    _____

    _____

WORKBOOK SECTION

12. What aspect of massage remained active outside the medical establishment from the 1940s to the present?

_____

_____

_____

_____

13. What research has provided the current validation of massage?

_____

_____

_____

_____

14. In what way has massage brought the best of the East and West together?

_____

_____

_____

Review Questions

Write your personal definition for the following words.

1. Professional

_____

_____

2. Structured

_____

_____

3. Therapeutic

_____

_____

4. Touch

_____

_____

Essay Questions

1. What does "touch intention" mean to you?

_____

_____

_____

_____

2. How would you describe your professional touch intention?

_____

_____

_____

_____

WORKBOOK SECTION

Matching

Match the person or information in the first column with the best response in the second column.

1. Massage in the Eastern world _____

2. Massage in the Western world _____

3. Ambrose Paré _____

4. Per Henrik Ling _____

5. Followers of Johann Mezger _____

6. Duplicated movements _____

7. Active movements _____

8. Passive movements _____

9. Charles F. and George H. Taylor _____

10. Mathias Roth _____

11. Sister Kenny _____

12. Ida Rolf _____

13. Dr. Dolores Krieger _____

14. Dr. John Harvey Kellogg _____

15. Dr. Charles K. Mills _____

16. Wilhelm Reich _____

17. Alexander Lowen _____

18. Elizabeth Dicke _____

19. Margaret Knott and Dorothy Voss _____

20. Esalen and Gestalt _____

21. Autonomic approach _____

22. Mechanical approach _____

23. Movement approach _____

24. Dr. Boris Chaitow and Dr. Stanley Lief _____

25. Dr. Milton Trager _____

a. known as exercise

b. proposed an integrated program of active and passive movements based on Swedish gymnastics

c. an English physician who studied with Ling

d. developed Rolfing

e. a neurologist and massage advocate who criticized uneven quality of practitioners

f. founded bioenergetics

g. inspired psychotherapists to explore massage and movement therapies

h. changes abnormal movement patterns into optimal ones

i. used French terms such as *effleurage* and *pétrissage*

j. a continuation of Greco-Roman traditions

k. commonly called *resistive exercises*

l. cofounders of the neuromuscular technique

m. developed therapeutic touch-energetic approach

n. range of motion and stretching when performed by a therapist

o. a Battle Creek physician who used massage and hydrotherapy

p. attempts mechanical changes in soft tissue

q. introduced Swedish movements in the United States

r. used massage for joint stiffness and wound healing after surgery

s. kept alive as part of folk culture

t. founded psychotherapeutic body techniques

u. developed Trager system

v. developed connective tissue massage

w. wrote the first major book on proprioceptive neuromuscular facilitation

x. used massage in the treatment of polio

y. exerts a therapeutic effect on the autonomic nervous system

WORKBOOK SECTION

Time Line Exercise

Number the following events, activities, and people in chronologic order. For example, (e) is no. 1.

a. _____ The art of massage is first mentioned.

b. _____ Ambrose Paré uses massage to aid postsurgical recovery.

c. _____ M. LeRon introduces the Swedish movement cure in Russia.

d. _____ Julius Caesar has himself pinched all over to relieve pain.

e. _____ A cave dweller stubs his toe and instinctively rubs it.

f. _____ Per Henrik Ling combines massage and Swedish gymnastics into a new system.

g. _____ Dr. Mary P. Jacobi and Dr. Victoria A. White research massage benefits.

h. _____ The massage scandals occur in England.

i. _____ Charles F. and George H. Taylor introduce Swedish movements in the United States.

j. _____ Galen writes on early manual medicine, supporting the methods of Hippocrates.

k. _____ Albert Hoffa publishes a textbook on classic techniques of massage.

l. _____ The polio epidemic sparks widespread interest in massage.

m. _____ Elizabeth Dicke develops connective tissue massage.

n. _____ The Royal Gymnastic Central Institute is established.

o. _____ Celsus compiles *De Medicina*.

p. _____ The American Association of Masseurs and Masseuses is formed.

q. _____ Hippocrates encourages physicians to use massage.

r. _____ Dr. James H. Cyriax writes the classic *Textbook of Orthopedic Medicine*.

s. _____ Dr. Charles K. Mills criticizes the uneven quality of the practice of massage.

t. _____ Margaret Knott and Dorothy Voss write *Proprioceptive Neuromuscular Facilitation*.

u. _____ The National Certification Examination for Therapeutic Massage and Bodywork is developed.

Professional Application Exercise

You are asked to present a brief lecture on the history of massage at a meeting of the local historical society. Develop your presentation outline below.

_____

_____

_____

_____

_____

_____

_____

_____

ANSWER KEY
Short Answer

1. The skin is the largest sensory organ of the body. Many subcutaneous soft tissue structures (e.g., muscles, connective tissue) as well as visceral structures (e.g., the lungs, heart, digestive organs) project sensation to the skin. The autonomic nervous system, which regulates the visceral and chemical homeostasis of the body, is highly responsive to skin stimulation in support of well-being. Mood (the way a person feels) often is reflected in the skin, because we touch ourselves from the inside. We blush with embarrassment, flush with excitement, or grow pale with fear.

2. Personal space, culture, and subculture, including social structure and spiritual discipline, gender, age and life events

3. Hostile or aggressive touch, erotic touch

4. Socially stereotyped touch, touch that communicates information, touch technique

5. Massage or touch as a method of healing developed from many cultural origins. This means that no one culture owns massage and that some sort of underlying, instinctive mechanism spurred the development of a type of massage in most if not all cultures on the planet.

WORKBOOK SECTION

6. Scientific research is the key to validation. Massage has been validated by the science of the day. Today we know that many of the ideas that past scientists had were incorrect. The important thing is that even though the "scientific rationale" for massage was incorrect, the benefits of massage were still real.

7. The ancient Chinese massage system consisted of kneading and rubbing down the entire body with the hands, joint movement, and traction. The ancient Chinese methods are not much different from massage today.

8. The Church was all powerful. Much of the scientific information concerning massage had been lost during this time. Massage reverted from a form of sanctioned medicine to use by the common people, many of whom held to their early traditions of healing. The Church could not explain these healing abilities, so it claimed that the power came from the devil. It is important to remember the value of objective research for validation as opposed to experiential validation, and also that practitioners of massage must not put themselves forth as "healers."

9. Ling began a recognized school to teach the methods. He did a fine job of putting much of the existing knowledge together in a usable form, but it is important to remember that much of what we consider Swedish massage came later from Mezger's work.

10. Because Ling was not trained in medicine, he did not speak the same language as the medical community of his time. Instead, he had a tendency to use poetic and mystical language that was discounted. Eventually, physicians spoke about massage with other doctors in a language that they understood, and by 1839 Ling's system had gained worldwide recognition. The importance of a common terminology is another lesson to remember as modern massage moves toward standardization.

11. Unfortunately, profit-oriented schools and educators were the major contributors to the downfall of massage. It is important to watch for this situation today.

12. Athletic or fitness massage and personal service massage have retained a small but strong following and constitute a growing market. Today, prevention, stress reduction, and health-enhancing methods are the primary avenues pursued. Massage has reasserted itself as a major contributor to personal health programs.

13. Pain research has uncovered many of the physiologic explanations for the benefits of massage.

14. Many of the massage methods currently used are a combination of structural and energetic concepts. History does repeat itself, and massage has reemerged in every age. The best results have occurred when science is advanced enough to figure out why massage works. It will be exciting to move into the future, as long as we keep in mind the lessons of the past.

Matching

1. j	10. c	18. v
2. s	11. x	19. w
3. r	12. d	20. g
4. b	13. m	21. y
5. i	14. o	22. p
6. k	15. e	23. h
7. a	16. t	24. l
8. n	17. f	25. u
9. q		

Time Line Exercise

a. 2	h. 14	o. 5
b. 7	i. 11	p. 18
c. 10	j. 6	q. 3
d. 4	k. 15	r. 19
e. 1	l. 16	s. 13
f. 8	m. 17	t. 20
g. 12	n. 9	u. 21

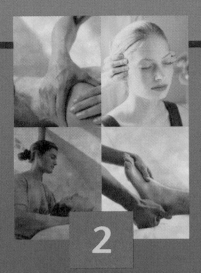

2

PROFESSIONALISM AND LEGAL ISSUES

After completing this chapter, the student will be able to perform the following:

- Define *professionalism*
- Define *therapeutic* massage
- Define a scope of practice for therapeutic massage
- Develop and explain a code of ethics and the standards of practice for therapeutic massage
- Complete an informed consent process
- Take ethics into consideration in maintaining professional boundaries and the therapeutic relationship
- Use basic communication skills to listen effectively and deliver an I-message
- Use a problem-solving approach to enhance ethical decision making
- Identify legal and credentialing concerns of the massage professional
- Identify and report unethical conduct of colleagues

THE student of massage therapy must be able to define therapeutic massage, identify the types of professional services a massage practitioner legally and ethically can provide, and establish guidelines for conduct in the professional setting. The following professional development issues and skills are addressed in this chapter:

- The definition of massage
- The scope of practice for massage professionals
- Ethical conduct and standards of practice for massage professionals
- The therapeutic relationship
- Communication skills to support professional interaction
- Professional record keeping, including informed consent procedures and charting
- Credentialing, licensing, and other legal concerns of the massage professional

This information base provides the structure for professional and ethical decision making. This chapter is intended to encourage the student to develop the level of professionalism essential to the successful practice of therapeutic massage.

First we will explore the name of our profession. What do we call ourselves? The student will discover that this is more complicated than it might at first seem. Then we will look at what we do—the definition of therapeutic massage. Armed with these two pieces of information, we will discuss the scope of practice for therapeutic massage and the appropriate training for the practice of therapeutic massage.

The chapter further describes professional services and the various forms of therapeutic massage services, ranging from wellness massage to medical rehabilitative massage. The following questions are considered:

- What is ethical conduct for the massage professional, and how does one make ethical decisions?
- What communication and record-keeping skills are necessary to support a professional practice and fulfill legal responsibilities?
- What are the legal requirements for practice?
- What professional organizations represent the profession?
- How does one identify and report unethical conduct in peers?

The following definitions clarify some of the terminology used in this chapter:

Countertransference is an inability on the part of the therapist to separate the therapeutic relationship from personal feelings and expectations for the client; it is personalization of the professional relationship by the therapist.

A **dual role** results when scopes of practice overlap, with one professional providing support in more than one area of expertise.

Ethics is the science or study of morals, values, and principles, including the ideals of autonomy, beneficence, and justice. Ethics comprises principles of right and good conduct.

Ethical behavior is right and correct conduct based on moral and cultural standards as defined by the society in which we live.

Ethical decision making is the application of ethical principles and professional skills to determine appropriate behavior and resolve ethical dilemmas.

Informed consent is a consumer protection process; it requires that clients be informed of treatment steps, that their participation be voluntary, and that they be competent to give consent. Informed consent is an educational process that allows clients to make knowledgeable decisions about whether to receive a massage.

A **principle** is a basic truth or rule of conduct.

The **scope of practice** is the knowledge base and practice parameters of a profession.

Standards of practice are principles that serve as specific guidelines for directing professional ethical practice and quality care, including a structure for evaluating the quality of care. They are an attempt to define the parameters of quality care.

A **therapeutic relationship** is created by the interpersonal structure and professional boundaries between professionals and their clients.

Transference is the personalization of the professional relationship by the client.

PROFESSIONALISM AND THERAPEUTIC MASSAGE

section objectives

Using the information presented in this section, the student will be able to perform the following:

- Compare therapeutic massage with professional development criteria
- Describe the two professional development trends for therapeutic massage

The subjects of ethics and professionalism are very important to the bodywork profession. In any professional practice, the ambiguity of ethics and the concreteness of professionalism and standards of practice converge to form a basis for ethical decision making. A profession is different from a job, and a professional does more than go to work. Expanding on the definition of a professional that was presented in Chapter 1, we could say that a professional is one who has the following characteristics:

1. A specialized body of knowledge
2. Extensive training
3. An orientation toward service
4. A commonly accepted code of ethics

5. Legal recognition through certification or licensure by a professional association
6. A professional association

A specialized body of knowledge—Massage therapy and many other bodywork methods are grounded in a specialized body of knowledge (some of this knowledge base is presented in this textbook). Historical foundations and current research validate this knowledge base. As we discussed in Chapter 1, a lifetime of study easily could be devoted to bodywork methods.

Extensive training—Questions have arisen about the duration of massage training and the information and technical skills to be included in that training. The area of professional development for therapeutic massage requires some standardization to allow continued progress toward professionalism. No agreement has been reached on the difference between a wellness orientation to massage and a medical or remedial orientation.

The current standard of 500 contact hours (10 to 12 credit hours) may be sufficient for basic wellness massage methods, but judging from data collected from actual job duties and current trends in licensing requirements, 1000 contact hours (20 to 24 credit hours) probably is more appropriate for supporting professional development in the wellness realm. It does not seem reasonable to expect that programs of 500 to 1000 contact hours provide sufficient time for integration of clinical reasoning methods, extensive physical assessment procedures, and the study of pathophysiology, pharmacology, and psychology, as well as other information the massage professional needs to work effectively with other health care professionals and with complicated, multifaceted health concerns. The same can be said for sports massage or working with athletes. To work effectively with athletes, the professional must have an in-depth education in the dynamics of sports activity.

Current employment trends are toward the development of two professional tracks in therapeutic massage: (1) vocationally trained wellness massage service professionals and paraprofessionals in the health care area and (2) degree-holding professionals in the allied health care system.

The current model for service professionals (such as those found in the field of cosmetology) and paraprofessionals (those trained to assist a professional) in the health care area calls for 300 to 1800 contact hours (7 to 40 credit hours) of vocational training in technically based programs, after which the student is granted a certificate or diploma. A professional usually is considered to be one who has a degree; it may be an associate's degree (usually requiring 64 credits), such as respiratory therapists earn; a bachelor's degree (usually requiring 124 credits); or doctoral or medical degrees, such as those held by teachers, physicians, and mental health professionals.

Most educational models for therapeutic massage and bodywork in the United States fall into the vocational services professional or paraprofessional realm. However, more massage programs have begun offering programs leading to an associate's degree or higher. Many Canadian provinces, as well as England, Poland, Russia, and other countries, require or offer training that meets the current definition of a professional degree. Individuals who already have professional degrees are obtaining massage therapy training and combining the two skills to function effectively in the health and athletic worlds; some examples of these combinations are nurse/massage therapist, athletic trainer/massage therapist, respiratory therapist/massage therapist, physical therapy assistant/massage therapist, occupational therapist/massage therapist, and social worker or psychologist/massage therapist, to name a few. Career options are increasing in the areas of medical and specialty massage (e.g., sports massage).

The level of information in this text supports training programs of 500 to 1500 contact hours (10 to 34 credit hours) in the service and paraprofessional realm. The greatest employment potential for therapeutic massage probably will follow this career orientation. The training level of this text is sufficient to allow those with other degrees to integrate massage therapy into their professional worlds. In longer programs (i.e., those requiring more than 2000 contact hours), the information base in this text can serve as the foundation on which rehabilitative or more specific forms of bodywork approaches are built.

An orientation toward service—The dictionary definition of service that best applies to this discussion is "to meet a need." An additional concept in a service orientation is that, although reimbursement is expected for services rendered, the desire to meet a need takes precedence over financial return. Observation of those who practice massage professionally and the attitudes of current students indicates that providers of therapeutic massage definitely have an orientation toward service, sometimes to the detriment of sound business practices. Although it is important to care for the people we serve, it is just as important to generate the necessary and appropriate income base to support the professional practice and a reasonably comfortable lifestyle for the professional.

A commonly accepted code of ethics—As you study the rest of this chapter, you will see that although general agreement exists about what a code of ethics entails, no agreement has been reached on a specific code of ethics to serve the entire massage and bodywork profession.

Legal recognition through certification or licensure by a pro-

fessional association—This area of professional development for therapeutic massage is not standardized and therefore remains ambiguous. About half the U.S. states and half the Canadian provinces have formal licensing or legislated certification for massage professionals. Legal recognition in various other countries ranges from extensive licensing requirements to no legal control. The United States now has a voluntary national certification process, which eventually may clear up the confusion in the eyes of the public and other professionals over the practice parameters of therapeutic massage and bodywork methods. It will be interesting to watch this whole issue unfold in the next few years.

A professional association—Several organizations attempt to represent the massage therapy profession. In addition, each of the various bodywork methods (e.g., reflexology, shiatsu, polarity) has its own professional organization. Although diversity is good for a profession and supports professional development, the lack of coherence in the field of bodywork confuses the public, ourselves, and other professionals. Developments in this area also will be interesting to watch (Proficiency Exercise 2-1).

---

2 - 1

PROFICIENCY EXERCISE

In the space provided, answer each of the questions with your opinion. Exchange and compare your opinions with others.

How would you rate massage therapy against the six criteria listed previously on pp. 31 and 32?

What areas of the massage profession do you think are well developed, and what areas need development?

What do you think is required to enable the therapeutic massage and bodywork profession to continue to evolve?

What can you do to contribute to this evolution?

FINDING A NAME

section objectives

Using the information presented in this section, the student will be able to perform the following:

- Explain the differences and similarities of various approaches to massage and bodywork
- Clarify the seven basic approaches to therapeutic massage and bodywork
- Classify a massage method according to its fundamental physiologic basis

The therapeutic massage profession has not yet agreed on a professional career name. It is difficult to establish a unique professional identity when we do not know our name. The lack of a single name also makes the creation of standardized textbooks somewhat frustrating. What do we call ourselves? Are we technicians, practitioners, or therapists?

A technician is perceived differently from a therapist, particularly in terms of educational level. A *technician* can be defined as one who has expertise in a technical skill or process. A technician has the least training and the most limited scope of practice in a professional group.

On the next educational level is the practitioner. A *practitioner* can be defined as one who practices an occupation or profession. A practitioner operates from a greater knowledge base and within a larger scope of practice than does a technician.

A *therapist* can be defined as one who treats illness or disability. A therapist requires the highest educational background and has the broadest scope of practice.

The massage profession currently does not use these designations as they are defined in this text, but the public and the health care professions often do. What is the public's perception, then, if *massage therapist* becomes our name? Perhaps the names *technician* and *practitioner* are best suited to therapeutic massage as it currently is practiced outside the health care system. *Massage therapist* might be more fitting when massage is practiced in the health care environment and the person has a more extensive education.

The confusion continues. Are we massage professionals, myomassologists, neuromuscular therapists, or soft tissue practitioners? Are we bodyworkers, and is massage a form of bodywork? Are we massage professionals, with other forms of bodywork becoming subcategories of massage?

For the purposes of this text, as is explained in the Preface on p. xi, the terms *massage technician, practitioner, therapist,* and *professional* are used interchangeably (Proficiency Exercise 2-2).

THE DEFINITION OF THERAPEUTIC MASSAGE

section objectives

Using the information presented in this section, the student will be able to perform the following:

- **Develop a definition of massage**

In Chapter 1 we began the development of the term *massage*. The roots of the word *massage* mean to touch, handle, squeeze, knead, and press softly (see Box 1-1, p. 13); therefore we defined *massage* as professional, structured therapeutic touch. In the past few years, as the popularity of therapeutic massage has grown, the profession has seen an expansion of styles and systems (Box 2-1). The term *bodywork* has been used to cover the scope of these developments. As individual systems have emerged, a difference in styles has developed. However, the overlapping of these methods reveals a fundamental sameness in all the work. These similarities should not detract from the devotion, training, and expertise of the various practitioners in specific disciplines.

Research has shown that application of systematic touching for health purposes (i.e., therapeutic massage and bodywork) has relevance (see Chapter 4). By carefully examining any style or system of massage or bodywork, the student can see that basic methods are used to stimulate sensory receptors. These methods either stimulate a rhythmic order in body functions or disrupt an existing pattern in the central nervous system control centers, which results in a shift in nerve and chemical patterns to reestablish homeostasis (reflexive methods). The very same methods can be applied in a different way to change the consistency or position of connective tissue or shift pressure in the vessels to facilitate blood and lymph circulation (mechanical methods). Although most of the systems have been developed over the centuries, a few new massage approaches have come into their own over the past few years (Fig. 2-1).

Technology and research probably will prove that massage and bodywork methods share the same physiologic basis in their effectiveness. All massage and bodywork approaches have the same basis because the people they serve share the anatomy and physiology of the human form. No one particular style of massage is better than another if the fundamental components are included and the method serves the client's needs and is used purposefully by a trained professional. Clients do not all have the same needs. Variations in applications develop to meet the specific needs of individual clients.

The profession must begin to standardize terminology to avoid confusion about the various styles and systems of massage. The explanations of anatomy and physiology given in Asian styles of bodywork may be different from those of Western science, but the human body is the same, and the effects of these styles are the same as those of systems developed in Polynesia, India, Europe, Africa, the United States, and around the world. Various massage and bodywork systems (Swedish, deep tissue, reflexology, sports massage, and body/mind integration, to name a few) work through the same anatomic and physiologic mechanisms, but each has developed a language unique to that approach. The study of various systems becomes confusing only when so many different names are used for similar methods. A core body of knowledge exists from which massage and bodywork approaches have evolved, and a skilled practitioner should be able to identify and explain any approach based on physiologic effects.

The different systems and styles presented in this text are variations on a theme. To become skilled practitioners, students learn the theme and explore the variations.

2-2

PROFICIENCY EXERCISE

Write the name you prefer for a therapeutic massage professional and justify your choice. An example is provided.

Example

Preferred name: *Bodywork practitioner*

Justification: *Bodywork encompasses more methods than just massage, and because most students of massage also learn other methods, this name is more representative of the professional practice. The name "practitioner" indicates a level of training that meets the definition of professional but does not indicate the function of therapy, which is the treatment of illness or disability.*

Your Turn

Preferred name:

Justification:

box 2-1

POPULAR METHODS IN THE BODYWORK PROFESSION

This list of styles, systems, founders, and developers is not meant to be all-inclusive because the information changes almost daily. Rather, it is meant to show the great variety of bodywork approaches.

Oriental (Asian) Approaches

Amma, acupressure, shiatsu, jin shin do, do-in, hoshino, tui-na, watsu, Tibetan point holding, Thai massage

These methods derive from original Chinese concepts and from offshoots of the Chinese base. These compressive manipulations and stretches, which focus on specific areas of the body, elicit responses in the nervous and circulatory systems. The efficient use of the therapist's body and the performance of these techniques on a clothed client have many benefits. The philosophy of these systems is grounded in ancient concepts that have stood the test of time. The effects are both reflexive and mechanical.

Structural and Postural Integration Approaches

Bindegewebs massage, Rolfing, Hellerwork, Looyen, Pfrimmer, Soma, Bowen therapy

These techniques focus more specifically on the connective tissue structure to influence posture and biomechanics. The approaches are systematic and effective because they are grounded in the fundamentals of physiology and biomechanics. Practitioners of these styles have received an extensive education.

Neuromuscular Approaches

Neuromuscular techniques, muscle energy techniques, strain/counterstrain, orthobionomy, Trager, myotherapy, proprioceptive neuromuscular facilitation, reflexology, trigger points

These are the European approaches based on the work of Dr. Stanley Leif and Dr. Boris Chaitow and the Western methods based on the work of Dr. Janet Travell, Dr. John Mennell, Dr. Raymond Nimmo, Dr. Lawrence Jones, Dr. Milton Trager, Eunice Ingham, William Fitzgerald, Arthur Lincoln Pauls, Bonnie Prudden, and others. Dr. Leon Chaitow has written extensively on these concepts and currently teaches in the United States and Europe. Many of the techniques are similar to those found in Rolfing, Asian methods, and Swedish massage and gymnastics. As the name implies, the approach is a nervous or reflexive method. Observation of the systems reveals that connective tissue also is affected. The common threads running through all the styles are the basic concepts of activation of the tonus receptor mechanism, reflex arc stimulation, positional receptors, and applications of stretching and lengthening.

Manual Lymphatic Drainage

Vodder lymph drainage

Emil Vodder developed an excellent system that uses the anatomy and physiology of lymphatic movement with both mechanical and reflexive techniques to stimulate the flow of lymphatic fluid. The variations of this system sometimes are called *systemic massage.*

Energetic (Biofield) Approaches

Polarity, Therapeutic Touch, Reiki, Zero Balancing

These systems, which are based on ancient concepts of body energy patterns, recently were formalized by Dr. Randolph Stone, Dr. Dolores Krieger, Dr. Fritz Smith, and others. Subtle energy medicine is under study at the Menninger Foundation in Topeka, Kansas, by Dr. Elmer Green, and by other researchers. Polarity and similar energetic approaches use near touch or light touch to initiate reflexive responses, often with highly effective results.

Craniosacral and Myofascial Approaches

Craniosacral therapy, myofascial release, soft tissue mobilization, deep tissue massage, connective tissue massage

These systems focus more specifically on the various aspects of both mechanical and reflexive connective tissue functions. Dr. William Garner Sutherland was the first to formalize the concept of minute movement of the cranium and dura. Dr. John Upledger, and John Barnes, P.T., have expanded and formalized his work. Both light and deep touch are used, depending on the method. Dr. James Cyriax's cross-fiber friction methods fall into this category.

Applied Kinesiology

Touch for Health, Applied Physiology, Educational Kinesiology, Three-in-One Concepts

Dr. George Goodheart formalized the system of applied kinesiology within the chiropractic discipline. The approach blends many techniques but works primarily with the reflexive mechanisms. A specific muscle testing procedure is used for evaluation; this process acts somewhat like a biofeedback mechanism. Some of the corrective measures use Asian meridians and acupressure; others rely on the osteopathic reflex mechanisms defined by Chapman, Bennett, and McKenzie that seem to correspond to traditional Chinese acupuncture points. Dr. John Thie and others modified these techniques for use by massage professionals and the public.

Integrated Approaches

Sports massage, infant massage, equine massage, on-site or seated massage, prenatal massage, geriatric massage, massage for abuse survivors, Russian massage

Many styles of bodywork that focus on a specific type of population are combinations of methods rather than physiologic interventions. Founders and teachers of integrated methods include every massage professional who designs a massage specifically for an individual client and every devoted massage instructor who attempts to combine and explain methods to students.

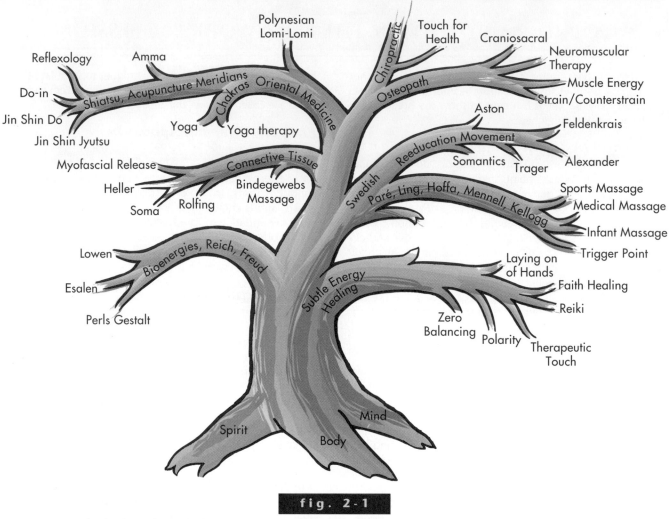

fig. 2-1

The bodywork tree—diversity as represented in the metaphor of a tree. The representation shows that all forms of therapeutic massage and related bodywork methods stem from the same roots.

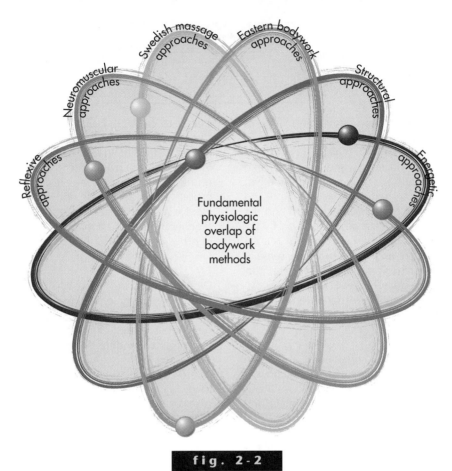

Swedish massage approaches

Eastern bodywork approaches

Neuromuscular approaches

Structural approaches

Reflexive approaches

Energetic approaches

Fundamental physiologic overlap of bodywork methods

fig. 2-2

The fundamental physiologic overlap of bodywork methods.

Any of these systems can be explained in anatomic and physiologic terminology (Fig. 2-2).

Defining Massage

A definition of *massage* (Box 2-2) must encompass all the methods used by various systems. Massage cannot be considered a single skill; a more appropriate concept is that of a collection of skills. In addition, the definition of therapeutic massage depends on individual laws and the definition of massage included in those laws. Those within the profession itself have not agreed on a definition. This text offers a general definition of *massage*. It is difficult to define massage accurately and completely because of the many forms of massage and bodywork currently practiced. An attempt is made to include items from the many definitions found in historical literature, from guidelines provided by state and local laws and professional organizations, and from individual styles and approaches to massage and bodywork.

SCOPE OF PRACTICE

section objectives

Using the information presented in this section, the student will be able to perform the following:

- Understand the scope of practice of various health and service professionals
- Explain what constitutes the "practice of medicine"
- Explain the difference between medical or rehabilitative massage and wellness massage
- Develop a scope of practice for massage that respects the scope of practice of other professionals

A scope of practice defines the knowledge base and practice parameters of a profession. Each health and service profession has a unique information/knowledge base, yet members of many professions share a common knowledge and methodology. Because of this shared base, the lines defining a profession's scope of practice are not always clear and overlap can occur.

Each member of a particular profession acquires a specific knowledge base and must define her personal scope of practice. The individual professional must be able to evaluate her acquired body of knowledge and skills realistically to determine the parameters of ethical practice within the scope of practice. True professionals understand the limits of their technical skills and scopes of practice and choose to work with other professionals for the best possible outcome for the client.

box 2-3

OCCUPATIONAL DEFINITIONS AND SCOPE OF PRACTICE

The following are typical regulations governing scope of practice. Most of these regulations have been taken from the administrative rules of the Michigan Occupational Regulations' Department of Licensing and Regulation and the Occupational Regulations section of the Michigan Public Health Code. The information on acupuncture and Oriental medicine is based on Florida legislation and the book *Planning Your Career in Alternative Medicine,* by Dianne J.B. Lyons. Each state has slightly different regulations, but they are consistent enough to provide a sense of uniformity across the United States. More specific information on occupational regulations and health codes can be obtained from the department responsible for licensing and regulation.

Acupuncture

Acupuncture is a form of primary health care, based on traditional Chinese medical concepts, that uses acupuncture diagnosis and treatment, as well as adjunctive therapies and diagnostic techniques, to promote, maintain, and restore health and prevent disease. Acupuncture includes but is not limited to the insertion of acupuncture needles and the application of moxibustion to specific areas of the human body.

Chiropractic

Chiropractic is the discipline within the healing arts that deals with the nervous system, its relationship to the spinal column, and its interrelationship with the other body systems. Chiropractic uses radiography to detect spinal subluxation and misalignment and adjusts related bones and tissues to establish neural integrity through techniques that use the inherent recuperative powers of the body to restore and maintain health. Examples of these techniques include the use of analytic instruments, the provision of nutritional advice, and the prescribing of rehabilitative exercise. Chiropractic does not include the performance of incisive surgical procedures or any invasive procedure that requires instrumentation, or the dispensing or prescription of drugs or medicine.

Dentistry

Dentistry is the discipline of diagnosis, treatment, prescription, and surgery for disease, pain, deformity, deficiency, injury of human teeth, alveolar processes, gums, jaws, and dependent tissues. Dentistry is also concerned with preventative care and the maintenance of good oral health.

Medicine

Medicine is the diagnosis, treatment, prevention, cure, or relief of human disease, ailment, defect, complaint, or other physical or mental condition by attendance, advice, device, diagnostic test, or other means.

Naturopathy

Naturopathy is the combination of clinical nutrition, herbology, homeopathy, acupuncture, manipulation, hydrotherapy, massage, exercise, and psychologic methods, including hypnotherapy and biofeedback, to maintain health. Naturopathic physicians use radiography, ultrasound, and other forms of diagnostic testing but do not perform major surgery or prescribe synthetic drugs.

Currently much of the literature defines the scope of practice of massage by what cannot be done, to avoid infringing on the scope of practice of other health and service professions (Box 2-3).

The scope of practice authorized by a medical or surgical degree is broad and extensive. It authorizes the physician to use drugs and medical preparations and the surgeon to sever and penetrate human tissue during treatment. It further authorizes them to use other methods to treat disease, injuries, deformities, and other physical and mental conditions. The law grants such a broad authorization to physicians because the education and testing requirements for a physician's license ensure that the individual is qualified to act as a healer.

No one but the physician has the legal right to perform any act that falls within the parameters of a medical license. The principle underlying this is simple: a person may not dispense therapeutic or medicinal advice about the effect of his or her services on a specific disease, ailment, or condition unless that person has adequate training, knowledge, and experience to ensure that the advice given is sound and reliable.

All the professionals listed in Box 2-3 must meet educational standards that far exceed the current accepted requirements for massage in most areas. Professionals with more education are allowed to do more within their specialized fields. Those with less education work under supervision or within a limited scope of practice. The scope of practice for therapeutic massage should complement but not infringe on the boundaries of the work of these professionals. It is to be hoped that the future will allow more flexibility and overlap of professional practice for the benefit of clients.

The Unique Scope of Practice Parameters for Therapeutic Massage

As mentioned previously, therapeutic massage is unique in that it can be used in two distinct professional worlds: wellness and personal services, and health care services.

---

box 2-3

OCCUPATIONAL DEFINITIONS AND SCOPE OF PRACTICE—CONT'D

Nursing

Nursing is the systematic application of substantial specialized knowledge and skill derived from the biologic, physical, and behavioral sciences to the care, treatment, counsel, and health education of individuals who are experiencing changes in the normal health process or who require assistance in the maintenance of health and the prevention or management of illness, injury, and disability.

Osteopathic Medicine

Osteopathic medicine is an independent school of medicine and surgery using full methods of diagnosis and treatment in physical and mental health and disease, including the prescription and administration of drugs and vitamins; operative surgery; obstetrics; and radiologic and electromagnetic diagnostics. Osteopathy emphasizes the interrelationship of the musculoskeletal system with other body systems.

Physical Therapy

Physical therapy is the evaluation or treatment of an individual by the use of effective physical measures, therapeutic exercise, and rehabilitative procedures, with or without devices, to prevent, correct, or alleviate a physical or mental disability. It includes treatment planning, performance of tests and measurements, interpretation of referrals, instruction, consultative services, and supervision of personnel. Physical measures include massage, mobilization, and the application of heat, cold, air, light, water, electricity, and sound.

Podiatric Medicine

Podiatric medicine is the examination, diagnosis, and treatment of abnormal nails and superficial excrescences (abnormal outgrowths or enlargements) on the human hands and feet, including corns, warts, callosities, bunions, and arch troubles. It also includes the medical, surgical, or mechanical treatment and physiotherapy of ailments that affect the condition of the feet. It does not include amputation of the feet or the use or administration of general anesthetics.

Psychology

Psychology is the rendering to individuals, groups, organizations, or the public service involving the application of principles, methods, and procedures of understanding, predicting, and influencing behavior for the purpose of diagnosis, assessment, prevention, amelioration, or treatment of mental or emotional disorders, disabilities, and behavioral adjustment problems. Treatment is by means of psychotherapy, counseling, behavior modification, hypnosis, biofeedback techniques, psychologic tests, and other verbal or behavioral methods. Psychology does not include the prescription of drugs, performance of surgery, or administration of electroconvulsive therapy.

Cosmetology

Cosmetology is a service provided to enhance the health, condition, and appearance of the skin, hair, and nails through the use of external preparations designed to cleanse and beautify. The application of beautification processes, such as makeup and skin grooming, is included.

Massage professionals are involved in various levels of care and support, each requiring more education and a higher level of competence.

Wellness and Personal Services

In the professional world of wellness services, clients seek massage for pleasure, relaxation, and general health maintenance. Wellness approaches enhance and maintain the functioning of the person. They usually focus on education and methods that encourage normal balance and the activation of self-regulating mechanisms of the mind and body. In addition to massage/bodywork skills, a massage professional must be educated and skilled in teaching prevention measures and encouraging a general wellness lifestyle for clients. When presenting this type of information in the educational context, the professional must make general recommendations rather than specifically tell clients what to do, which can be interpreted as diagnosing and prescribing, both of which are out of the scope of practice for massage.

In the service world of wellness massage, the key is enhancing the client's health or providing massage for individuals who already are healthy and who want to maintain or improve their health. It also is important not to infringe on the cosmetology scope of practice by working with cosmetic applications to the skin through the use of oils, wraps, or other preparations.

The service world allows the therapeutic massage professional to work most independently, with the broadest spectrum of people (and in some instances animals), and share the gifts of professional touch with the general population, many of whom need support in managing stress so that they do not become ill and require medical attention. This world of wellness services is a wonderful place for a professional, and it is important that the professional development of therapeutic massage not abandon it.

Taking a wealth of information into account, this textbook determines the scope of practice of wellness massage to be a nonspecific approach to massage that focuses on assessment procedures to detect contraindications to massage and the need for referral to other health care professionals, and on the development of a health-enhancing physical state for the client. The plan for the massage session is developed by combining information, desired results, and directions from the client with the skills of the massage practitioner to provide an individualized massage session aimed at normalizing the body systems. This normalization is accomplished through external manual stimulation of the nervous, circulatory, and respiratory systems, connective tissue, and muscles to achieve generalized stress reduction, decrease in muscle tension, symptomatic relief of pain related to soft tissue dysfunction, increased circulation, and other benefits similar to those of exercise, or through other relaxation responses produced by therapeutic massage to increase the client's well-being.

In 1998 the American Massage Therapy Association released the following scope of practice statement[2]:

Massage or massage therapy is any skilled manipulation of soft tissue, connective tissue, and/or body energy fields with the intention of maintaining or improving health by effecting change in relaxation, circulation, nerve responses, or patterns of energy flow. Massage or massage therapy may be accomplished manually with or without the use of the following: movement, superficial heat or cold, electrical or mechanical devices, water, lubricants, or salts.

Health Care Services

The professional world of health care requires specific training for the skilled application of massage to promote rehabilitation and manage pathologic conditions (sports massage comes under this definition).

Currently, health care professionals do not receive extensive education in massage therapy. The knowledge base and methods of application of massage probably have expanded too greatly for massage to be included as part of currently practiced professions such as physical therapy and nursing. The time and labor intensity of massage makes it difficult for physicians, physical therapists, nurses, occupational therapists, and athletic trainers to include therapeutic massage with their other interventions and responsibilities. These considerations support the development of massage therapy as a distinctive health practice and an adjunct to these other professions.

Physical therapy is the profession most likely to be compared with the practice of rehabilitative massage, and care must be taken to respect the professional boundaries of physical therapy. This is particularly important because as massage training increases, the massage professional is becoming qualified to work with more complicated situations involving rehabilitation and the management of chronic conditions. However, even the most comprehensive massage training programs do not compare with the extensive training of the physical therapist or other professionals such as nurses and athletic trainers.

This does not invalidate the expertise of the therapeutic massage professional. A higher level of education allows the massage professional to work effectively with the physician, physical therapist, or other health professional in the heath care setting. These professionals probably will supervise an overall treatment program of which massage is a part.

The scope of practice for medical or rehabilitative massage, massage delivered within the health care setting, and massage in conjunction with specific athletic training protocols is as follows: Massage therapists develop, maintain, rehabilitate, or augment physical function, relieve or prevent physical dysfunction and pain, and enhance the well-being of the client. Methods include assessment of the soft tissue and joints, as well as treatment by soft tissue manipulation, hydrotherapy, remedial exercise programs, and client self-care programs.

The Canadian provinces of Ontario and British Columbia have this type of scope of practice for therapeutic massage. The educational requirement exceeds 2200 class hours and is rising.

The information in this text will carry the student from the service world of wellness massage into the world of health care services, primarily working to manage dysfunctional conditions such as pain and chronic conditions and support those who may benefit from a generalized approach to massage. This text does not attempt to develop specific protocols for the precise intervention measures needed for serious illness and trauma. As presented here, massage can provide supportive care using stress and pain management for those who are ill, if the massage professional is supervised by qualified medical personnel (Fig. 2-3).

The distinction between wellness massage and medical rehabilitative approaches to massage used for illness and trauma may seem subtle, but the difference is simple. Wellness massage practitioners do not work with sick or injured people unless directly supervised by licensed and qualified professionals, such as physicians, nurses, and physical therapists. Rather, they help most of the population, who are not sick but are stressed and uncomfortable, to feel better and cope with stress. This benefit of massage may help prevent more serious stress-induced illness.

Consider this metaphor: The owner's manual for a car recommends regularly scheduled maintenance. According to this schedule, a technician changes the oil and filter and checks the fluids. A mechanic's assistant performs tune-ups. If the preventive maintenance schedule is followed, the car will be kept running for a long time. It is a good idea to have a qualified mechanic do a complete evaluation of the car annually to catch problems while they are small and can be corrected easily. If this is not done, serious problems may arise, and a skilled mechanic may have to correct them.

The wellness massage technician is similar to the technician who keeps the car in order, changes the oil, and checks the fluids. Complete tune-ups by a qualified mechanic's assistant reflect the increased skill levels of the more comprehensively trained massage practitioner or massage therapist. The skilled mechanic represents the

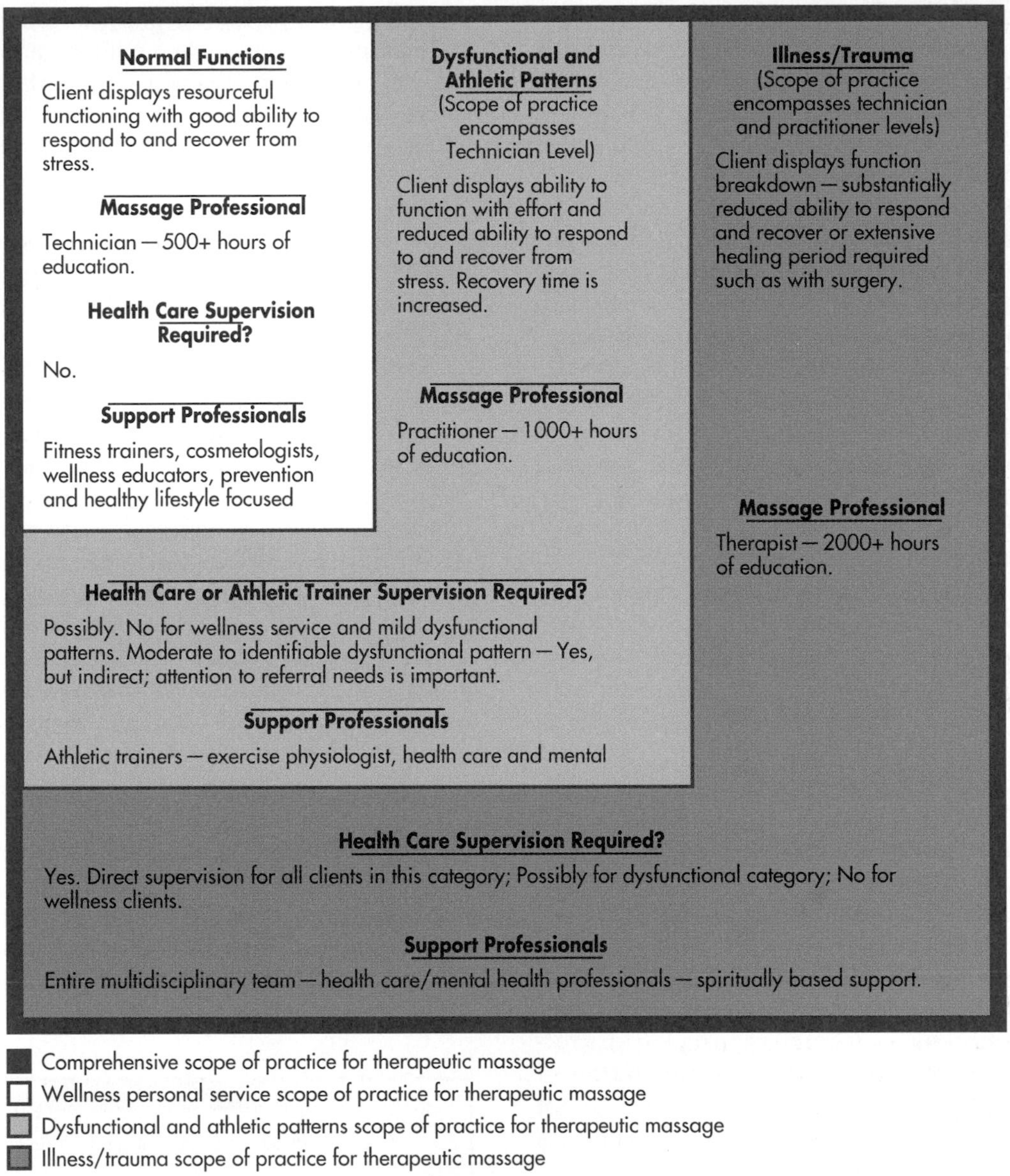

Normal Functions

Client displays resourceful functioning with good ability to respond to and recover from stress.

Massage Professional

Technician — 500+ hours of education.

Health Care Supervision Required?

No.

Support Professionals

Fitness trainers, cosmetologists, wellness educators, prevention and healthy lifestyle focused

Dysfunctional and Athletic Patterns
(Scope of practice encompasses Technician Level)

Client displays ability to function with effort and reduced ability to respond to and recover from stress. Recovery time is increased.

Massage Professional

Practitioner — 1000+ hours of education.

Illness/Trauma
(Scope of practice encompasses technician and practitioner levels)

Client displays function breakdown — substantially reduced ability to respond and recover or extensive healing period required such as with surgery.

Massage Professional

Therapist — 2000+ hours of education.

Health Care or Athletic Trainer Supervision Required?

Possibly. No for wellness service and mild dysfunctional patterns. Moderate to identifiable dysfunctional pattern — Yes, but indirect; attention to referral needs is important.

Support Professionals

Athletic trainers — exercise physiologist, health care and mental

Health Care Supervision Required?

Yes. Direct supervision for all clients in this category; Possibly for dysfunctional category; No for wellness clients.

Support Professionals

Entire multidisciplinary team — health care/mental health professionals — spiritually based support.

■ Comprehensive scope of practice for therapeutic massage
☐ Wellness personal service scope of practice for therapeutic massage
▨ Dysfunctional and athletic patterns scope of practice for therapeutic massage
▨ Illness/trauma scope of practice for therapeutic massage

fig. 2-3

The most expansive scope of practice for therapeutic massage is represented by the entire box *(outlined in dark purple).* Within this scope of practice are levels of professional function based on training and experience. The entry-level position, or technician, for a therapeutic massage scope of practice is found in the Normal Functions box *(white box).* The next higher level of professional practice, the massage practitioner, is depicted in the Dysfunctional and Athletic Patterns box *(light violet box).* The third and highest level of professional practice, massage therapist, requires the most education and experience; it is depicted in the Illness/Trauma box *(light purple box).* Note that each level encompasses the one below it. As the model shows, a massage therapist can work effectively with all groups: normal function, dysfunctional/athletic patterns, and illness/trauma; the practitioner works only with normal function and dysfunctional/athletic patterns groups; and the technician works only with those displaying normal functioning. Most people who seek therapeutic massage services can be served effectively by professionals trained to the practitioner level.

physician or physical therapist. However, lest you think that the technician is the least important person in the chain, remember that if prevention is done well, a serious problem is less likely to develop. If the car is involved in an accident or something breaks down, it certainly goes straight to the mechanic and other specialists for repair, in just the same way that a person who suffers trauma or illness should see a physician for evaluation and treatment.

All professionals have specialized training, certain responsibilities, and positions in which they function best. Remembering and respecting each professional's strengths are the ethical things to do. While therapeutic massage waits for a formalized scope of practice, knowing the definition and scope of practice of other health and service professionals helps the massage practitioner respect these professionals and maintain appropriate boundaries.

Limits of Practice

Each professional has limits to his ability to practice massage. A scope of practice that has been legally adopted through legislation defines as well as limits the ability to practice massage. Respectful practice of therapeutic massage limits the scope of practice so as not to encroach on the scope of practice of other professionals.

Each professional also has personal limits to her scope of practice. These limits involve the type and extent of her education, personal biases, life experiences, specific interests in terms of the type of client served, and any physical limitations, such as size and endurance levels (Proficiency Exercise 2-3).

Professional limits are valid and valuable. They allow us to set and maintain boundaries that support each professional in the most successful professional practice structure. Limits of practice free us from falling into the trap of believing we must be all things to all people; we cannot be, and it is professional to acknowledge limits of practice and work together with other professionals.

Functioning realms also indicate limits on practice. The three functioning realms are normal functioning, dysfunction or complex circumstances, and illness/trauma and breakdown. These functioning realms are related to the scope of practice (see Fig. 2-3).

Normal Functioning

A person who is functioning well is able to be involved with work that is satisfying in both an intrinsic and extrinsic sense. For example, a woman may not love her work but may appreciate that the job supports her family (extrinsic value). Or she may love her work even if it does not financially provide for all wants (intrinsic value). A person responds normally when play balances work in such a way that the result is self-regulation and support for mental and physical functions. Another example of normal functioning is a person who can share with others or who has a passion for a mission, a cause, or a vision—be it as simple as gardening or as complex as an encom-

passing environmental or political cause—and who receives intimacy, support, and fulfillment from the process. A person who can make choices to regulate and cope with exterior influences internally and who can be resourceful and flexible in life situations displays normal functioning. The ability to love and be loved supports normal functioning. The supportive balance of these factors and the ability to exert an internal control to accommodate less than ideal situations, as well as to develop realistic and attainable goals and a plan to alter situations, indicates normal functioning.

Wellness approaches enhance and maintain normal functioning. Professional support can assist in the general maintenance of normal functioning through wellness approaches, education, and preventive care. Therapeutic massage has a definitive role in general health maintenance. The client uses massage/bodywork on a regular basis as part of a health and wellness program, comparable to the daily hygiene activities of bathing or brushing the teeth, or to a daily or weekly house cleaning. These clients want to maintain their current normal functioning status.

Massage technicians who provide services at the level of supportive wellness care require fundamental information about general wellness processes. Massage/bodywork technicians should be able to teach general methods of stress management, including effective breathing, progressive relaxation, quieting responses (meditation-type activities); give general dietary recommendations; and emphasize the importance of appropriate exercise programs. Most people do better with the discipline required to

---

2-3

PROFICIENCY EXERCISE

Write a scope of practice statement for therapeutic massage that fits your level of practice on graduation from your training program. If possible, talk with other professionals about this scope of practice and ask how it compares with their own.

Investigate the scope of practice defined by licensed professionals in your community for the listed health and service professions in this section. This information can be obtained from the state agency that oversees licensing and regulation.

maintain these activities when they have the support of a professional acting as a coach. A well-trained massage technician can provide this type of service.

Massage professionals need not always be supervised directly when working within a wellness scope of practice. A properly trained massage professional can recognize a client who is not functioning effectively, not recovering from the stress of daily activities, and beginning to fall into dysfunctional patterns. As the client's problems become more complicated, the support and expertise of the health or training professional becomes more important, and referral or supervision is indicated.

Dysfunction or Complex Circumstances

People who are functioning with effort and are beginning to break down fall into the dysfunctional category. Physical or emotional strain may indicate the need for more focused and specific inventions. Optimal functioning by persons who rely on fine motor skills and coordinated physical action, such as athletes, musicians, and dancers, requires a more complex massage interaction than that given in wellness and preventive care. Such cases require a level of professional support similar to that for dysfunctional patterns.

A multidisciplinary team approach may be needed, one that uses a defined care and treatment plan to reduce the level of physical stress and reestablish or teach internal coping methods. A massage practitioner who works with dysfunction or deals with the complexities of fine motor functioning needs a broader base of education and the supportive supervision of other health care or training professionals, such as coaches and athletic trainers. The broader-based education should encompass stress response, the origin of physical and mental difficulties, methods of improving functioning, standard health care interventions, and training protocols.

These clients benefit from a specifically designed treatment or care plan that includes a means of measuring the outcomes of care objectively. Realistic and attainable short- and long-term goals are developed, and time frames are set for the achievement of these goals.

The general goal of the bodywork professional is to help the client move toward normal functioning, regain personal control of the body/mind/spirit systems, and achieve and maintain optimal functioning. This approach is different from that of massage used for wellness or preventive care. The methods and information provided may be the same or similar, but the focus and goals are different. Clients dealing with dysfunction and complex circumstances want to change where they are in life, not maintain the status quo.

Because massage temporarily helps take the edge off physical discomfort and reduces arousal levels, allowing people to feel better where they are, massage intervention may or may not be appropriate in these circumstances. People tend to be less motivated to change if their cir- cumstances seem tolerable. Massage may diminish the client's motivation to change, interfering with the process being worked through with other health care or training professionals.

Massage can help support stress management in clients who find themselves faced with extraordinary stress loads. If the person cannot alter the situation causing the dysfunctional stress, massage can be a way to ease physical stress and a beneficial coping measure when combined with other medical, behavioral, and emotional coping techniques. Massage does not deal directly with the physical, emotional, or spiritual state contributing to the stress; rather, it supports the physical system so that the person can better withstand stress.

Illness/Trauma and Breakdown

A person experiencing a breakdown or illness requires a comprehensive intervention process. Often little distinction can be made between dysfunction and breakdown or illness. During acute illness or breakdown, massage/bodywork is not likely to be a part of therapy, at least initially. The client cannot handle any additional demand to respond. Even the most subtle forms of bodywork involve a controlled physiologic stress to the system that requires a physical response. These individuals may need very specific professional intervention to reestablish some level of functioning before they can cope with the "stress" of massage.

A massage therapist working with a person in this situation must be monitored carefully and supervised by a health care professional, especially if the client is taking medications (see Appendix C). In such cases massage intervention supports health care approaches; a comprehensive treatment and care plan is developed with massage as one of the treatment approaches. Often massage is used primarily for palliative (comfort) care, and supervision by the primary health care professional is necessary. The massage professional needs additional training in pathology, pharmacology, psychology, and clinical reasoning skills to be able to help integrate massage into an overall health care plan.

Body/Mind/Spirit

The body, mind, and spirit of a person share a definite link. The physical biologic (body) functions involve all the anatomy and physiology, including the body's chemical responses. Feelings are body functions.

The cognitive process (mind) interprets physical sensations and sets physical responses in motion. Emotions seem to be the result of the interplay between body and mind. Behavior is the action that results from the physical, emotional, and cognitive combination.

The spirit provides the strength, hope, faith, and love that create a reason for being. Each of these areas of functioning influences and interacts with the others.

In reality the body, mind, and spirit cannot be separated, yet together they involve too much information to allow a person to become an expert in all areas of human function. Professional skill levels, the parameters of the scope of practice, and avoidance of dual and multiple roles in the professional relationship artificially divide the functioning of the person seeking assistance. This is undesirable, yet many times unavoidable. An excellent solution is for professionals to work together. A multidisciplinary approach to care is best, with each professional showing a cooperative spirit and supporting a comprehensive care plan that addresses all the client's needs. Most hospice programs are excellent models for multidisciplinary teams.

Determining the Limits of Practice

As a massage/bodywork professional, you can determine if you are within your scope of practice by making sure your responses to the client are from a body and massage perspective. When a client expresses distress, shares personal information, or requests specific information, first determine whether the issue is most specifically a body, mind, or spirit issue. If it is a mental or spiritual issue, use listening skills and acknowledge the situation but do not attempt to problem solve or provide professional intervention. If the situation presented is physical, decide whether the information falls within the scope of therapeutic bodywork and respond accordingly.

The severity or complexity of a situation determines whether simple listening, without advice being given, is sufficient or whether a professional referral is indicated. Often the physical stress of the circumstances can be managed by massage/bodywork approaches while the client seeks additional help from supportive resources and professionals who can deal more specifically with the source of the problem.

Health care, training, coaching, and cosmetology professionals have committed a significant part of their lives to formal schooling, licensing procedures, and continual experiential and formal education. The information they possess is specific to their professional discipline yet is also quite broad. Although massage techniques are not common knowledge among many professionals, the importance and power of touch is. Many of these professionals understand that we bring touch skills that they may be unable to provide because of the nature of their therapeutic relationship with the client. To develop and support a cooperative, multidisciplinary philosophy of care, massage professionals must respect the dedication of the professionals with whom they work by maintaining the appropriate scope of practice for massage and bodywork.

Massage/bodywork professionals benefit from being able to adapt massage therapy to various health care, training, and personal service needs; in doing so they are best able to serve both the professionals with whom they work and the clients they serve. In a multidisciplinary setting it is important to be able to communicate effectively with any professional with whom you work; this requires you to be familiar with the language and terminology used in that profession. It is important to be able to explain massage therapy intervention in terms familiar to the professionals on the team and also to be able to explain the ways you, as a massage professional, intend to support health or training professionals in providing appropriate care.

Understanding the functioning realms of people and the scope of practice of massage and bodywork helps the professional establish an ethical practice and begin the discovery of the therapeutic process.

ETHICS AND STANDARDS OF PRACTICE

section objectives

Using the information presented in this section, the student will be able to perform the following:

- **Develop a personal and professional code of ethics using the eight ethical principles**
- **Explain the standards of practice for therapeutic massage**

Ethics

Culture, time, location, events, politics, religion, scientific knowledge, and many other factors affect the way we interpret behavior. Ethics defines the behavior we expect of ourselves and others and society's expectations of a profession. A simplified definition of *ethics* is "what is right." Our society determines that a person has acted ethically when the right thing has been done. But what is the right thing? No one individual or group has the answer. Often the best that can be offered in discussions of ethics are questions and guidelines based on principles of conduct established by a group.

Ethics has social, professional, and personal dimensions. It is not easy, in theory or in practice, to separate these elements. We behave according to a complex and continually changing set of rules, customs, and expectations. Because of this, ethical behavior must be a dynamic process of reflection and revision.

Ethics is not just a varied collection of do's and don'ts; rather, it is a system of values and principles that tie together in a reasonable, coherent way to make our society and our lives as civilized and happy as possible. Conflicts and uncertainties are inevitable. For this reason, in applying ethics we must learn more than a list of guidelines or principles, more than just what to do in this or that particular case; we must also develop a set of priorities and a way of thinking about them. To use ethics in decision making, we must be able to reason about what we have learned in order to capture the spirit of being ethical. Although ethics is ultimately a personal concern, it also is a reflection of one's professional and social character.

The purpose of practicing our profession ethically is to promote and maintain the welfare of the client. Laws often reflect the minimal standards necessary to protect the safety and welfare of the public, whereas codes of ethics represent the ideal standards set by a profession. Through their behavior professionals can comply both with the law and with professional codes. If compliance with the law is the only motivation in ethical behavior, the person is said to be practicing "mandatory ethics." If, however, the professional strives for the highest possible benefit and welfare for the client, the professional behaves with "aspirational ethics."[1]

As professionals we must constantly be alert not only to gross violations of ethical principles, but also to the more subtle ethical violations that occur when the client's welfare is not the primary determining factor of professional behavior. An example of the latter is hesitating to refer a client to a more qualified massage professional because referral means the loss of a paying client. Often this type of unethical conduct goes unnoticed, yet the client's welfare is compromised. This situation is further complicated because the professional often does not recognize the breach in ethical behavior. **Supervision** (monitoring by one with more expertise), **peer support** (interaction and exchange of information among fellow professionals), and meticulous objective personal reflection on professional behavior can bring to light these more subtle types of ethical violations. Professionals can monitor their own behavior by asking themselves often if they are doing what is best for the client and if their behavior is ethical.

Professional growth involves change in our knowledge, skills, attitudes, values, and beliefs. A professional code of ethics is a set of moral norms adopted by a professional group to direct value-laden choices in a manner consistent with professional responsibility. Many elements in the profession of massage enhance the lives of its practitioners, such as respect, authority, and prestige. In return, professionals must therefore be willing to adjust their personal behavior for the professional good. We have to gauge our personal and professional behavior not only by what is right and good for us as individuals, but also by what is appropriate for the client and the profession as a whole.

Ethical Principles

The following eight principles guide professional ethical behavior:

1. *Respect*—Esteem and regard for clients, other professionals, and oneself
2. *Client autonomy and self-determination*—The freedom to decide and the right to sufficient information to make the decision
3. *Veracity*—The right to the objective truth
4. *Proportionality*—The principle that benefit must outweigh the burden of treatment

5. *Nonmaleficence*—The principle that the profession shall do no harm and prevent harm from happening
6. *Beneficence*—The principle that treatment should contribute to the client's well-being
7. **Confidentiality**—Respect for privacy of information
8. *Justice*—Equality

These broad concepts direct the development of standards of practice.

Standards of Practice

Standards of practice provide specific guidelines and rules that form a concrete professional structure. For example, in standards of practice, the ethical principle of respect translates into professional behavior, such as maintaining the client's privacy and modesty, providing a safe environment, and being on time for appointments. Client autonomy and self-determination requires informed consent and ready access to files.

Standards of practice guidelines direct quality care and provide a means of measuring the quality of care. They usually are more specific than ethical principles.

Code of Ethics and Standards of Practice for Therapeutic Massage

Because the massage therapy and bodywork profession is not yet united in terms of professional affiliation and techniques, it is difficult to present a code of ethics or provide agreed standards of practice for the massage professional (Proficiency Exercise 2-4). Because each professional group within the massage and bodywork profession has developed its own code of ethics and standards of practice, this text offers a comprehensive compilation of many ethical codes and standards of practice, developed through professional organizations, licensing requirements, and the standards of practice of other health professions (Box 2-4). An attempt has been made to include all points presented in the various ethical conduct codes and standards of practice statements.

INFORMED CONSENT

section objectives

Using the information presented in this section, the student will be able to perform the following:

- List and explain the nine components of informed consent (Box 2-5)
- Determine if a client can provide informed consent for a massage
- Prepare written client information materials to support the informed consent process
- Complete two different types of informed consent forms

2 - 4

PROFICIENCY EXERCISE

Given each point of the code of ethics and standards of practice statement presented in Box 2-4, consider this question: "How will I implement this ethical principle or standard of practice in my professional practice?" Then, in the space provided, develop a personal code of ethics and standards of practice statement.

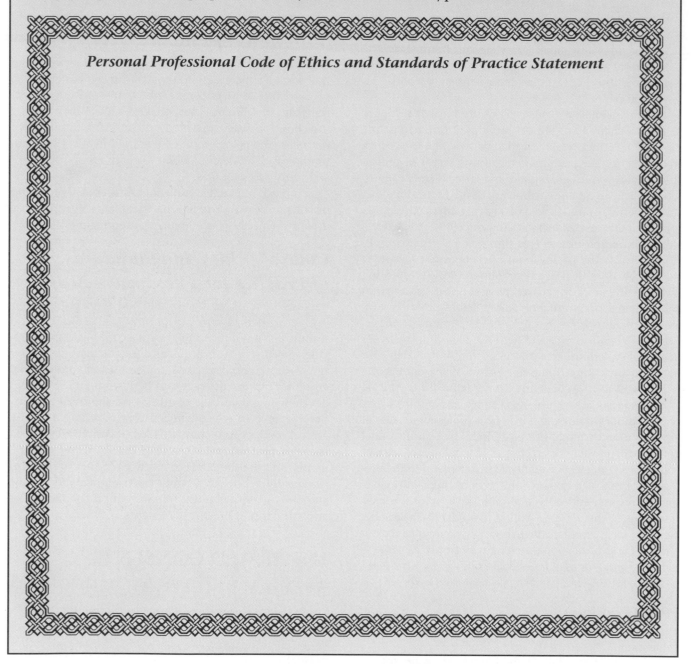

Personal Professional Code of Ethics and Standards of Practice Statement

---

box 2-4

CODE OF ETHICS AND STANDARDS OF PRACTICE

Ethical Principles

- *Respect for the dignity of people*—Massage professionals will maintain respect for the interests, dignity, rights, and needs of all clients, staff, and colleagues.
- *Responsible caring*—Competent, quality client care will be provided at the highest standard possible.
- *Integrity in relationships*—At all times the professional will behave with integrity, honesty, and diligence in practice and duties.
- *Responsibility to society*—Massage professionals are responsible and accountable to society and shall conduct themselves in a manner that maintains high ethical standards.

Standards of Practice Based on Ethical Principles

In compliance with the principles of the code of ethics, massage professionals will perform the following:

1. Respect all clients, colleagues, and health professionals through nondiscrimination regardless of age, gender, race, national origin, sexual orientation, religion, socioeconomic status, body type, political affiliation, state of health, personal habits, and life-coping skills.
2. Perform only those services for which they are qualified and honestly represent their education, certification, professional affiliations, and other qualifications. The massage professional will apply treatment only when a reasonable expectation exists that it will be advantageous to the client's condition. The massage professional, in consultation with the client, will continually evaluate the effectiveness of treatment.
3. Respect the scope of practice of other health care and service professionals, including physicians, chiropractors, physical therapists, podiatrists, orthopedists, psychotherapists, counselors, acupuncturists, nurses, exercise physiologists, athletic trainers, nutritionists, spiritual advisors, and cosmetologists.
4. Respect all ethical health care practitioners and work with them to promote heath and healing.
5. Acknowledge the limitations of their personal skills and, when necessary, refer clients to an appropriately qualified professional. The massage professional will require consultation with other knowledgeable professionals when:
   - A client requires diagnosis and opinion beyond a therapist's capabilities of assessment
   - A client's condition is beyond the scope of practice
   - A combined health care team is required

If referral to another health care provider is necessary, it will be done with the informed consent of the client.

6. Not work with any individual who has a specific disease process without supervision by a licensed medical professional.
7. Be adequately educated and understand the physiologic effects of the specific massage bodywork techniques used to determine if any application is contraindicated and to ensure that the most beneficial techniques are applied to a given individual.
8. Not make false claims about the potential benefits of the techniques rendered, and educate the public about the actual benefits of massage and bodywork.
9. Acknowledge the importance and individuality of each person, including colleagues, peers, and clients.
10. Work only with the informed consent of a client, and professionally disclose to the client any situation that may interfere with the massage professional's ability to provide the best care to serve the client's best interest.
11. Display respect for the client by honoring a client's process and following all recommendations by being present, listening, asking only pertinent questions, keeping agreements, being on time, draping properly, and customizing the massage to address the client's needs.

    Note: Draping is covered in Chapter 8. Ontario guidelines[3] give these requirements for draping:
    - It is the responsibility of the massage professional to ensure the privacy and dignity of the client and to determine if the client feels comfortable, safe, and secure with the draping provided.
    - The client may choose to be fully draped or clothed throughout the treatment.
    - The female client's breasts are not undraped unless specified by referral from a qualified health care professional, and the massage professional is working under the supervision of such a health care professional.
    - The genitals, perineum, and anus are never undraped.

    The consent of the client is required for work on any part of the body, regardless of whether the client is fully clothed, fully draped, or partly draped.
12. Provide a safe, comfortable, and clean environment.
13. Maintain clear and honest communication with clients and keep client communications confidential. Confidentiality is of the utmost importance. The massage professional must inform the client that the referring physician may be eligible to review the client's records, and records may be subpoenaed by the courts.

Continued.

box 2-4

CODE OF ETHICS AND STANDARDS OF PRACTICE—CONT'D

14. Conduct business in a professional and ethical manner in relation to clientele, business associates, acquaintances, governmental bodies, and the public.
15. Follow city, county, state, national, and international requirements.
16. Charge a fair price for the session. A gift, gratuity, or benefit that is intended to influence a referral, decision, or treatment may not be accepted and must be returned to the giver immediately.
17. Keep accurate records and review the records with the client.
18. Never engage in any sexual conduct, sexual conversation, or any other sexual activities involving clients.
19. Not affiliate with any business that uses any form of sexual suggestiveness or explicit sexuality in advertising or promoting services or in the actual practice of service.
20. Practice honesty in advertising, promoting services ethically and in good taste and advertising only techniques for which the professional is certified or adequately trained.
21. Strive for professional excellence through regular assessment of personal strengths, limitations, and effectiveness and through continuing education and training.

22. Accept the responsibility to oneself, one's clients, and the profession to maintain physical, mental, and emotional well-being and to inform clients when the professional is not functioning at best capacity.
23. Refrain from using any mind-altering drugs, alcohol, or intoxicants before or during professional massage bodywork sessions.
24. Maintain a professional appearance and demeanor by practicing good hygiene and dressing in a professional, modest, and nonsexual manner.
25. Undergo periodic peer review.
26. Respect all pertinent reporting requirements outlined by legislation regarding abuse.
27. Report to the proper authorities any accurate knowledge and its supportive documentation regarding violations by massage professionals and other health or service professionals.
28. Avoid interests, activities, or influences that might conflict with the obligation to act in the best interest of clients and the massage therapy profession, and safeguard professional integrity by recognizing potential conflicts of interest and avoiding them.

box 2-5

INFORMED CONSENT

The following questions should be answered at the outset of the professional relationship:

What are the goals of the therapeutic program?
What services will be provided?
What behavior is expected of the client?
What are the risks and benefits of the process?

What are the practitioner's qualifications?
What are the financial considerations?
How long is the therapy expected to last?
What are the limitations of confidentiality?
　　In what areas does the professional have mandatory reporting requirements?

From Corey G, Corey MS, Callanan P: *Issues and ethics in the helping professions,* ed 4, Pacific Grove Calif., 1993, Brooks/Cole Publishing.

Informed consent is a protection process for the consumer. It requires that clients understand what will occur, that they participate voluntarily, and that they be competent to give consent. Informed consent is an educational procedure that allows clients to decide knowledgeably whether they want to receive a massage, whether they want a particular therapist to work with them, and whether the professional structure, including client rules and regulations, is acceptable to them. Informed consent supports professional ethical behavior. It reflects the ethical principle of client participation and self-determination in a client-centered approach.

Clients must be able to provide informed consent and demonstrate that they understand the information presented to them (Proficiency Exercise 2-5). Parents or guardians must provide informed consent for minors. Guardians must provide informed consent for those unable to do so. Ethical decision making becomes important in "gray areas," such as when a language barrier exists and the massage professional is not sure the client understands her or if any form of intoxication or prescription drug use is involved, altering the client's judgment.

True informed consent entails the opportunity to evaluate the options available and risks involved in each method and requires the massage professional to include information about the inherent and potential hazards of the proposed treatment, the alternatives available, and the probable results if treatment is not given. Clients have the legal right to choose from a range of suggested options and receive enough information to allow them to pick the most appropriate approach for them. Credentials and personal and professional limitations that may affect the client-therapist relationship must be disclosed and validated. As professionals we are ethically bound to ensure that the client makes choices based on a solid understanding of the information presented. The professional is responsible for providing the client with this information.

---

2 - 5

PROFICIENCY EXERCISE

Gather in groups of three and write about a specific situation in which informed consent is difficult to obtain from a client. The groups should then exchange responses and role play some of the situations, with one student acting as the massage practitioner, one being the client, and the third evaluating the way the situation was handled. Try different situations until each student has had a chance to play each role.

Intake Procedures

A comprehensive intake procedure, including an informed consent process, is necessary for the client when defined outcomes span a series of sessions. A **needs assessment,** based on the client's history and a physical assessment, is used to devise an **initial treatment plan.** The initial treatment plan states the therapeutic goals, duration of the sessions, number of appointments needed to meet the agreed goals, cost, general classification of intervention to be used, and an objective progress measurement for identifying goals that have been reached. (The forms used for these procedures are presented in Chapter 3.)

Single or random massage sessions usually do not require a full needs assessment or a treatment plan. Instead, possible contraindications to massage are identified. The informed consent process informs the client of the limitations of a single massage session and describes the approaches used in the single-session massage/bodywork experience.

A form with all the pertinent information is signed by the client and kept in the massage practitioner's files. Maintaining a record of signed informed consent forms is an important legal issue; in many jurisdictions, touching a person without his consent can be prosecuted as assault.

The following is a possible sequence for obtaining informed consent:

1. The massage professional provides a general explanation of massage, supported by written information (often in the form of a brochure) about indications, benefits, contraindications, and alternative approaches that provide benefits similar to those of massage/bodywork.
2. The massage professional informs the client about the scope of practice for massage; reporting measures for therapist misconduct; the professional's training, experience, and credentials; and any limiting factors that may affect the professional relationship, including lack of training in a particular area and special circumstances of the massage professional (such as hearing or vision difficulty) that may need to be considered. The client is given written information covering these topics, often in the form of a brochure, to enhance her understanding of this discussion.
3. The massage professional then discusses business and professional policies and procedures, including the logical consequences of noncompliance on the part of the client. These policies include handling of payment, returned checks, additional charges, gratuities, late arrival, scheduling, sexual impropriety, draping, hygiene, sanitation, and confidentiality and limits of confidentiality. The client also is given pertinent written information about these topics, such as a professional policy statement (Box 2-6).

The client signs an informed consent form (see sample in Box 2-8 on pp. 52-53) after these procedures have taken

box 2-6

DEVELOPING A CLIENT BROCHURE AND POLICY STATEMENT

A massage professional should cover the following important points in developing a client brochure and policy statement.

Type of Service

Explain the type of work you provide.

Explain the benefits and limitations of this particular style of bodywork.

Specify whether you specialize in working with a particular group, such as elderly persons, athletes, or people with specific problems such as headaches or back pain.

Indicate any situations or conditions with which you do not care to work, such as pregnancy or certain medical conditions.

Develop a referral network of related professionals.

Training and Experience

If your state requires licensing, have documents available confirming that you are licensed.

State how long you have been in practice, what school you attended, whether the school was approved by any professional organization, and how many classroom hours were required for graduation.

Provide information about continuing education you have pursued.

Provide information about any additional education; for example, that you are also an athletic trainer.

Provide the names of any professional organizations of which you are an active member.

Appointment Policies

Define the length of an average session.

Inform the client of the days you work and your hours and if you do on-site residential or business work.

Inform the client that the first appointment for intake will be longer than subsequent appointments; also state whether you take emergency appointments, and how often you suggest that clients come for massage sessions.

Be clear about the cancellation policy and your policy for late appointments.

Explain to the client any change in or restriction on physical activity before or after the session.

Client/Practitioner Expectations

Explain in detail what happens at the first bodywork session (i.e., paperwork, medical history, other preliminaries).

Make sure that clients know they can partly undress or undress down to their underclothes, and that they are always covered and draped during the session.

Explain the order in which you massage (face up or face down to begin), the parts of the body on which you work and in what order, if you use oils or creams, if a shower is available before or after the massage, and if bathing at home before the massage appointment is expected.

Make sure the client understands whether talking is appropriate during the session and that you should be informed if anything feels uncomfortable.

If you have low lighting and music during the session, be sure the client is comfortable with that atmosphere.

Make sure the client understands when a reaction might be expected, such as tenderness over a trigger point when direct pressure methods were used.

Tell clients that before the session you will discuss with them the goals for the massage, as well as the proposed styles and methods of massage, and that consent must be given for all massage procedures.

Inform the client that your profession has a code of ethics and indicate your policy on confidentiality.

Let clients know that if they are uncomfortable in any way, a friend or relative may accompany them.

Fees

Make sure your fee structure is clearly defined regarding the following:

How often you raise your fees

If you have a sliding fee scale

If you take only cash or will accept money orders, checks, or credit cards

If you bill

If you accept insurance

How often insurance covers your services

Different fees for variations in the length of a session

If a series of sessions can be bought at a discount

If you pay any referral fees for new clients

Sexual Appropriateness

Sexual behavior by the therapist toward the client or by the client toward the therapist is always unethical and inappropriate. It is always the responsibility of the therapist or health professional to ensure that sexual misconduct does not occur.

Recourse Policy

If a client is unhappy or dissatisfied, do you offer a refund or a free session? Let the client know that if the matter is not handled satisfactorily, a professional organization or licensing board is available where complaints can be registered.

Note: Some professionals send out client policy and procedure booklets before the scheduled appointment. If this is done, include a personalized cover letter asking the client to read the booklet carefully and stating that you will discuss it with him or her at the first appointment.

box 2-7

NEEDS ASSESSMENT AND DEVELOPMENT OF THE INITIAL TREATMENT PLAN

The client's goals and desired outcomes for the massage sessions are determined. The client agrees to proceed with the next part of the session, which consists of history taking, using a client information form, and a physical assessment, using an assessment form. The information is evaluated to develop a care plan for the client; this is called a *needs assessment*. Care plans usually envision a series of sessions.

A care/treatment plan is developed that spells out the following:

Specific outcomes (i.e., the therapeutic goals)

Frequency of visits (number of appointments per week or month) and duration of visits (e.g., 30, 45, 60 minutes)

Number of appointments needed to achieve the therapeutic goals (e.g., 10 sessions, 15 sessions, ongoing with no time limit)

General methods to be used (e.g., Swedish, relaxation, deep tissue, neuromuscular, trigger point)

Objective progress measurements (e.g., pain decreased on a scale of 1 to 10, 50% increase in range of motion, sleep improved by increasing 1 hour per night, episodes of tension headache reduced from four per week to one per week, feelings of relaxation maintained for 24 hours)

The client provides (informed) consent for the care/treatment plan by signing the appropriate form.

place. The client should not be overwhelmed with extensive, detailed information, but it is important to provide enough information for the client to make an informed choice. Informed consent is a continual process, and client education and involvement in the therapeutic approach are always supported and encouraged.

Needs Assessment and Initial Treatment Plan

If the client is working toward specific goals that will require several appointments, a needs assessment and an initial treatment plan are completed (Box 2-7). Specific details on completing this process are provided in Chapters 3 and 11.

The process of assessing needs and developing a treatment plan takes 30 minutes to an hour and constitutes

the initial intake procedure. In complex circumstances this process can extend over the first two or three sessions. It is appropriate to charge for the intake session, which is an important part of the professional interaction. The treatment plan may evolve or change during subsequent sessions as the client's needs change during the therapeutic process. The initial treatment plan is the massage practitioner's best educated guess of the way the therapeutic relationship will proceed.

When massage is used in a very nonspecific way, especially if the client is seen only once or a series of massage sessions is not appropriate, it is not necessary to provide an extensive needs assessment or develop a comprehensive treatment plan. Instead the massage professional predetermines the outcome of the session by informing the client that in these circumstances no specific work can be done and that massage can provide a general normalizing of the body. A short history and physical assessment are done to detect any contraindications to massage. A condensed version of the client policy statement is prepared and provided in written form. The client always provides formal written consent for the massage. An example of an informed consent process is presented in Box 2-8.

CONFIDENTIALITY

section objectives

Using the information presented in this section, the student will be able to perform the following:

- Establish and maintain client confidentiality
- Complete a release of information form

Confidentiality is the principle that the client's information is private and belongs to the client. It is built on respect and trust. In professional terms, confidentiality concerns client information and files. Client information is never discussed with anyone other than the client without his written permission. During peer counseling or supervision, client confidentiality extends to the professionals we consult. Even when the client's name is withheld, the situational uniqueness often is enough to breach confidentiality requirements.

Client files must represent information accurately and only as it relates to the service offered. Personal information about a situation surrounding a muscle or skeletal complaint need not be recorded. For example, a client describes her headache and says that a coworker is disruptive and the manager does nothing about it, which she feels contributes to the tension aggravating her headache. The only part recorded in the client's record is her belief that emotional tension is contributing to the headache. To include more of the story is considered a breach of confidentiality because it makes a permanent record of an

box 2-8

INFORMED CONSENT PROCESS

A new client arrives for a massage.

The massage professional shows the client an informational brochure explaining massage, why it works, the procedures and process of massage, the benefits of massage, and the general contraindications. The client is asked to read the information. The massage professional then discusses the information with the client. In general terms the massage professional explains alternatives to massage, such as exercise and self-hypnosis, that provide benefits similar to massage.

The massage professional then tells the client about his or her professional background: that he or she graduated from a state-licensed massage therapy school 2 years ago, after a training program of 1000 hours; that he or she has been nationally certified by the National Certification Board for Therapeutic Massage and Bodywork; that he or she has been in professional practice part time for 2 years and averages eight massages a week; and that he or she has taken additional training in myofascial approaches and massage for elderly persons (approximately 100 hours for each). The client also is given information on methods of reporting misconduct of the massage therapist to state agencies, national professional organizations, and the police.

The client is given the policy and procedures booklet or statement and asked to read it. After he or she has done so, the massage professional goes over the booklet with the client, point by point, so that he or she understands the rules and requirements of the massage therapist. The massage professional makes sure that the requirements to report abuse and threat of deadly harm, as well as the release of files by court order, are discussed.

The massage professional hands the client a form that states the following:

I, (client's name)_____, have received a copy of the rules and regulations for Massage Works operated by Sue and John Grey. I have read the rules and regulations, and I understand them. The massage procedures, information about massage in general, general benefits of massage, contraindications for massage, and possible alternatives have been explained to me. The qualifications of the massage professional and reporting measures for misconduct have been disclosed to me.

I understand that the massage/bodywork I receive is for the purpose of stress reduction and relief from muscular tension, spasm, or pain, and to increase circulation. If I experience any pain or discomfort, I will immediately inform the massage/bodywork practitioner so that the pressure or methods can be adjusted to my comfort level. I understand that massage/bodywork professionals do not diagnose illness or disease or perform any spinal manipulations, nor do they prescribe any medical treatments, and nothing said or done during the session should be construed as such. I acknowledge that massage is not a substitute for medical examination or diagnosis and that I should see a health care provider for those services. Because massage/bodywork should not be performed under certain circumstances, I agree to keep the massage practitioner updated as to any changes in my health profile, and I release the massage professional from any liability if I fail to do so.

Client's signature_____ Date_____

Therapist's signature_____ Date_____

Consent to Treat a Minor

By my signature I authorize _____ to provide massage/bodywork to my child or dependent.

Signature of Parent or Guardian_____ Date_____

box 2-8

INFORMED CONSENT PROCESS—CONT'D

For clients who will have several sessions, the next step is completion of the needs assessment and initial treatment plan (presented in detail in Chapter 3).

Modified Informed Consent Form for Single Session

For clients who will be seen only once (such as might occur if the professional is working on a cruise ship, doing sports massage at an event, or doing promotional chair massage at a health fair), the following modification in informed consent can be made.

I, (client's name)_____, have received a copy of the rules and regulations for (name

of business)_____, operated by (owner)_____. I have read the rules and regulations, and I understand them. The general benefits of massage and contraindications for massage have been explained to me. I have disclosed to the therapist any condition I have that would contraindicate massage. Other than to determine contraindications, I understand that no specific needs assessment has been performed. The qualifications of the massage professional and reporting measures for misconduct have been disclosed to me.

I understand that the massage/bodywork I receive is for the purpose of stress reduction and relief from muscular tension, spasm, or pain, and to increase circulation. If I experience any pain or discomfort, I will immediately inform the massage/bodywork practitioner so that the pressure or methods can be adjusted to my comfort level. I understand that massage/bodywork professionals do not diagnose illness or disease or perform any spinal manipulations, nor do they prescribe any medical treatments. I acknowledge that massage is not a substitute for medical examination or diagnosis and that I should see a health care provider for those services.

I understand that a single massage session or massage used on a random basis is limited to providing a general, nonspecific massage approach using standard massage methods and does not include any methods to address soft tissue structure or function specifically.

Client's signature_____ Date_____

Therapist's signature_____ Date_____

Consent to Treat a Minor

By my signature I authorize _____ to provide massage/bodywork to my child or dependent.

Signature of Parent or Guardian_____ Date_____

---

box 2-9

RELEASE OF INFORMATION FORM

I, (client's name)_____, grant permission for _____, a massage

practitioner, to provide or exchange information with (other professional's name) _____

about the following conditions_____ for the time

frame beginning _____ and ending _____. This permission may be revoked at any

time either verbally or in writing.

Client's signature_____ Date_____

---

event that may be made public if the client's files are ordered released to the court.

Clients must be told during initial informed consent procedures that files may be ordered released to the court. Massage and bodywork therapists have no professional exemptions. Clients must be made to understand these limits to confidentiality during informed consent procedures.

Confidentiality also refers to public recognition. Clients should not be acknowledged in public unless they recognize and greet the professional first. To do so puts clients in a position of having it revealed that they were seeking professional services that they may want kept private.

Clients also must be informed that confidentiality will be breached under laws that require professionals to report abuses and threat of deadly harm. If information is disclosed to you that a child, an elderly person, or a person who may be physically or mentally unable to report abuse or to protect herself is being harmed, as a professional you must report this alleged abuse to the appropriate government agencies. If a client threatens deadly harm to another person or to himself, a professional must report this information to the police or other appropriate agency. Because the massage and bodywork professional is not specifically trained to identify or diagnose those who may harm themselves or others, all threats must be taken seriously. In these most difficult situations, the bodywork professional should seek legal counsel on ways to proceed.

To allow professionals to exchange information, the client must sign a release of information form (a sample is provided in Box 2-9).

A copy of the information release form is kept in the client's file, and the original is sent to the consulting professional. Use of the words *exchange information* in the form allows each professional involved to share pertinent information; otherwise each professional must obtain a release of information form from the client to share information about that client.

PROFESSIONAL BOUNDARIES

section objectives

Using the information presented in this section, the student will be able to perform the following:

- **Develop strategies for maintaining professional boundaries with clients**
- **Explore personal prejudices, fears, and limitations that may interfere with the ability to provide the best care for a client**
- **Help a client recognize personal boundaries in the massage process**

Needs and Wants

People have needs and wants. Needs sustain life; when needs are not met, people become ill and die. Needs include air, water, food, shelter, and sensory stimulation. Wants lead to a sense of satisfaction. Some examples of wants are a certain type of car or home, a particular job, chocolate cake, or a relationship with a particular person. We all need shelter, but I want a cabin in the woods. We all need food, but I want home-baked, whole grain bread hot from the oven. We all need to be touched, but I want to be hugged by my children. Massage provides sensory stimulation in the form of touch. It can be argued, then, that bodywork meets a need for clients and that a client may want only a particular professional to provide the massage to meet the need of sensory stimulation.

When a need or perceived need is met for someone by another, it is very easy to feel bonded to that other person. Needs and wants often become confused in the mind of the client; thus the more unsettled or dysfunctional a client is, the more important it becomes to maintain boundaries in the professional relationship. This type of

box 2-10

DETERMINING A CLIENT'S BOUNDARIES

An effective way to learn what a client's boundaries are is to ask. For example, the massage professional might ask the client the following questions:

Is there any part of your body that you would rather not have massaged?

Do you prefer any particular kind of music?

I am a smoker, and I know the smell lingers. Will that bother you? (What will you do if the client says "Yes"?)

I have three different massage lubricants. Which would you prefer?

---

connection and interaction can lead to transference or countertransference (see pp. 57-58), and it can happen with therapeutic massage and bodywork. The massage professional should have a clear understanding of personal motivation in the therapy setting and should carefully maintain professional boundaries.

A *boundary* can be defined as the personal space within an arm's-length perimeter. It also can be thought of as the personal emotional space designated by morals, values, and experience. Some people are not very good at defining personal boundaries or respecting others' boundaries. Certainly boundaries are defined by more than physical space, but for our purposes, a respect for personal boundaries simply begins with staying an arm's length away from another until invited to come closer. Personal space can be defined by extending the arm directly in front of the body and turning in a circle; the area within that space is that individual's personal space. Cultural differences may change this boundary, but for therapeutic massage we will consider this a person's personal space range (see Touch in Chapter 1, p. 4). No one should ever enter this space uninvited (without informed consent). It is important that students practice this policy while in school. They should ask whether another person may be approached, wait for the response, and act accordingly. This practice may seem silly at first, but it teaches an awareness of boundaries.

Sometimes people who have been emotionally, physically, or sexually abused have not had the chance to define or recognize personal boundaries. Practitioners should be especially respectful in their approach and explain professional therapeutic boundaries carefully to the client (Box 2-10). It is just as important for those who have boundary difficulties to learn to define their own personal boundaries. Setting limits during a massage session may be a safe way to begin this process.

What is acceptable for us may be offensive for someone else. We may offend someone unintentionally because of differences in our value systems. It is important for the massage therapist to help the client define a personal boundary. Once a client's boundaries are defined, we must respect them. If a professional cannot respect a client's boundary needs, she should refer him to a massage practitioner better able to deal with those needs.

The massage professional should tell the client, "I will not be offended if you share with me things that you do not like about the massage. I will be happy to refer you to someone else if a different massage approach will better serve you. There are as many different ways to give a massage as there are people giving massage. I am here to serve your needs, as long as those needs do not conflict with my professional and personal standards."

It is equally important that the client understand the therapist's personal and professional boundaries; therefore the therapist must be honest in creating a personal code of ethics and must clearly communicate the professional boundaries to the client. Boundaries are discussed with the client during the initial informed consent procedures and are included in writing in the client policy statement. (Communication skills are presented later in this chapter.) Even when a massage professional is conscientious about establishing boundaries with the client during the initial intake procedure, those boundaries can become blurred as the professional interaction progresses, or something may occur that the professional had not considered. When this happens, the situation must be dealt with immediately; waiting only allows the problem to escalate.

Boundaries are difficult to define; they are an individual value concept. We bring to our adulthood varying experiences that shape what we feel is correct and define our personal boundaries. As professionals we are responsible for finding the client's comfort zone. This responsibility begins with learning our personal comfort zones.

Anything that prevents us from being able to touch a person in a respectful, nonjudgmental way must be considered so that we can decide whom we may best serve as massage professionals. Hindrances include personal prejudices regarding body size, color, gender, and attitude. For example, some people do not relate well to children. It is ethical for such professionals to refer children to someone else for professional care. Others may be uncomfortable with those of the opposite gender, and again, it is best to refer such clients elsewhere. We may be uncomfortable with the prospect of working with people who have certain types of diseases. If this is the case, our touch may be uncomfortable for these people. A potential client may have a behavior that drives us crazy (i.e., snorting). The behavior interferes with our ability to be the best massage professional for that particular client.

It therefore is important to explore professional boundaries by looking honestly at our fears, frustrations, prejudices, biases, and value systems (Proficiency Exercise 2-6).

These emotions and beliefs are very personal and often deeply held. The anchors for many of these beliefs may not be understood easily at a conscious level. Acknowledging factors that define and limit our personal and professional boundaries does not necessarily involve changing or even understanding why we feel a certain way. It is important to recognize when our personal boundaries will affect the professional relationship because massage professionals work very closely with their clients. We touch our clients. (The essential quality of touch communication was explored in Chapter 1.) We must be honest with ourselves and about ourselves to be able to respect the individual needs and space of our clients.

Right of Refusal

Clients have the right to refuse the massage practitioner's services; this is called the **right of refusal**. It is a client's right to refuse or stop treatment at anytime. When this request is made during treatment, the therapist must comply despite prior consent.

Professionals also have right of refusal. Massage professionals may refuse to massage or otherwise treat any person if a just and reasonable cause exists. The next few paragraphs give some direction for determining what constitutes "just and reasonable cause" for refusing to provide professional massage services to a client. At the same time, massage professionals are bound by a nondiscrimination code of conduct. You may refuse to work with anyone, as long as you explain the reasons why; this is called *disclosure*.

For example, a person with multiple sclerosis wishes to be your client. Your mother had multiple sclerosis, and you have bitter feelings about how her illness interfered with your childhood. It is difficult for you to be with anyone who has this condition because of your memories. Here are your choices:

- Tell the prospective client that you have personal issues that prevent you from effectively working with that particular condition, and offer to refer her to a therapist who can provide the work needed. Make sure that at least three different qualified individuals are given as referrals so that the client has a choice.
- Be very honest with the client. Explain that you are uncomfortable working with a particular condition and that you are concerned that the way you feel may interfere with doing what is best for her. Leave out all personal details. Knowing this up front, if the client still wants to work with you, you may decide to give it a try.

Either way, the massage practitioner has taken responsibility for personal attitudes, and the client has the information necessary to make an informed choice. Remember, touch tells the truth. It is difficult to touch someone with whom you are uneasy, whatever the reasons. By honestly telling the person about the situation, the client can make the decision. If the professional's touch seems strained, the client may realize that it is the practitioner's issue.

A massage professional has the right to refuse to treat any area of the body of a client and terminate the profes-

---

2 - 6

PROFICIENCY EXERCISE

The following exercise may be the most difficult one you will have to do. On a separate piece of paper, write at least one page about your personal prejudices and fears about people, and honestly list the physical and behavioral aspects of others that are difficult for you to deal with.

Here are some examples:

Old people frustrate me. I cannot make myself listen to the same stories over and over.

I hate ragged toenails. I do not know if I can rub anyone's feet if the nails are not well trimmed.

People who are fat are undisciplined. They should exercise more.

People who are skinny are obsessed with their appearance and are exercise addicts.

When someone sniffs all the time, it makes me crazy.

I am afraid of men with mustaches because of something that happened to me when I was young.

I am afraid of people with the human immunodeficiency virus (HIV). I do not understand much about the ways it is transmitted, and I do not want to catch it.

Women are so bossy; I hate it when they tell me what to do.

As a man, I am uncomfortable with giving another man a massage.

I am uncomfortable working with someone who is physically disabled. I especially feel squeamish with amputations.

It is important that you be very honest with yourself. Only by accepting that we have these areas of challenge will we be able to best serve potential clients.

sional relationship if she feels the client is sexualizing the relationship or if the professional feels adversely influenced in any way by the client.

Refusal becomes more difficult when clearly defined discrimination issues are involved. This might occur if a professional limits his practice to a particular ethnic group or refuses to provide services to someone with a legally classified disability. In these cases the professional is wise to seek legal counsel to determine the extent of professional liability.

Blurred boundaries create an environment conducive to the development of ethical dilemmas. Although it is true that professional boundaries are situational and must be identified and established with each client, clear professional boundaries support an effective therapeutic process for both the client and the professional.

THE THERAPEUTIC RELATIONSHIP

section objectives

Using the information presented in this section, the student will be able to perform the following:

- **Define and recognize potential transference and countertransference issues**
- **Explain the professional power differential**
- **List factors that create dual or multiple roles**
- **Explain to clients feelings of intimacy between them and the massage professional**
- **Defuse sexual feelings during the massage session**
- **Recognize and avoid sexual misconduct activities**

In the therapeutic setting, specific parameters define the professional relationship between the client and massage professional. As was explained in Chapter 1, the therapeutic relationship has an inherent power differential, which stems from the difference in knowledge and skills between the client and professional. Even when services are exchanged between peer professionals, the power differential exists because one is placed in the position of controlling the situation. This power imbalance must be minimized as much as possible without denying its existence (Proficiency Exercise 2-7).

Transference

Issues of transference and countertransference diminish the effectiveness of the therapeutic relationship. Transference is the personalization of the professional relationship by the client. When a person seeks out a professional, very important issues of power, trust, and control in the thera-

peutic relationship become the professional's responsibility. The more disorganized a person is, the stronger is the feeling of disempowerment. Clients often seek a sense of control outside themselves to help reestablish or replace their internal sense of control. The client is in a vulnerable state when doing this.

This situation is more common with people who are ill or under considerable stress, but even the well client is vulnerable in the therapeutic setting. The reality of today's

---

2 - 7

PROFICIENCY EXERCISE

Working with a partner, follow the directions provided so that each of you plays the role of strength and of vulnerability.

The person playing the role of strength stands up. The person playing the role of vulnerability sits on the floor. The person who is standing looks down at the person sitting on the floor and says in a robust voice, "I am so strong, I am as strong as I have ever been. I am very strong." The person sitting on the floor looks up at the one standing and replies in a fragile voice, "I am so vulnerable. I have never been this vulnerable before. I am very vulnerable."

Remain in the standing and seated positions, but this time the person sitting on the floor says, "I am so strong, I am as strong as I have ever been. I am very strong." The person standing says, "I am so vulnerable. I have never been this vulnerable before. I am very vulnerable."

Change positions so that the one standing now sits on the floor, and the one sitting on the floor now stands. Repeat the exercise.

Now, discuss what occurred. Possible experiences to explore include:

Did a particular role cause discomfort?
What was it like to be strong or vulnerable?
How did the position influence the feelings?
Which statement did you prefer to make?
What position was most comfortable?
In what way does this exercise relate to the therapeutic relationship?

In the space provided, describe what you learned about power differentials in the therapeutic relationship.

society is that although most people cannot be diagnosed as sick, most have not achieved true wellness either. Although we ideally speak of wellness massage to help a client maintain or achieve optimal wellness, the truth is somewhat different. Unfortunately, very few people seek massage for pure pleasure and to enhance their health. Most of the clients we serve, even outside the health care setting, are not optimally well. They just are not sick yet. Most seek massage services because they do not feel good and want to feel better.

The more disorganized, disempowered, and lacking in internal resources clients are, the more susceptible they will be to transference. Manifestations of transference include demands for more of the therapist's time, bringing the therapist personal gifts, attempting to engage the professional in personal conversation, proposals of friendship or sexual activity, and expressions of anger and blame. Transference occurs when the client sees the therapist in a personal light instead of a professional manner. This usually is a distorted view, because the professional is displaying a specific role and not letting her whole self be involved with the client. It is easy for the client to see the professional as all knowing. If the client becomes dependent on the professional, instead of reestablishing his personal functioning, unrealistic expectations may develop. If the client's expectations are not met, he may blame the professional. If the client's expectations are met, he may project the credit to the therapist instead of acknowledging his own efforts. In both cases the professional takes on a superhuman image that sooner or later crumbles, often leaving the client disillusioned and disempowered.

The bodywork professional must understand and separate the client's appropriate, genuine feelings from the transference issues. For example, a client may be angry if the therapist continually arrives late for the appointment; this is a justified feeling, not transference. Also, the client may truly appreciate the massage therapist's skill and may express that appreciation, but this does not constitute transference unless it interferes with the boundaries of the therapeutic relationship.

The professional has the ultimate responsibility for the therapeutic relationship and the direction of the therapeutic process.

Countertransference

Countertransference is the inability of the professional to separate the therapeutic relationship from personal feelings and expectations for the client; it is the professional's personalization of the therapeutic relationship. Countertransference presents itself in feelings of attachment to the client such as sexual feelings, excessive thinking about a client between visits, a feeling of professional inadequacy if the client does not make anticipated progress, or a sense of the client as being special; it also can manifest as favoritism, anger, or revulsion toward a client. Counter-

transference often is fed by the following personal needs of the therapist (Proficiency Exercise 2-8):

- The need to fix people
- The need to remove pain and discomfort
- The need to be perfect
- The need to have the answer
- The need to be loved

The client's problems may serve as a reflection of the professional's personal life experiences. The massage professional is wise to consider her own personal needs and develop a reliable sense of self-awareness. Without a high level of self-awareness on the part of the professional, it is possible for the focus of the massage session to shift from meeting the goals of the client to meeting the needs of the therapist. The massage therapist may begin to treat herself while treating the client and lose objectivity and empathy in the therapeutic relationship.

Another way this can be stated is that the massage professional gives the client the kind of massage the professional would like to receive instead of the massage appropriate for the client. This situation actually occurs quite often. For example, the massage professional prefers to lie on his stomach when he receives a massage and enjoys deep work on his back. Because this position and level of pressure feels good to the massage practitioner, he may have a tendency to keep clients in the face-down position

---

2-8

PROFICIENCY EXERCISE

Work with a partner. Face each other and look at each other. Decide who is "A" and who is "B." A asks B the following questions, and B quickly answers. Then reverse roles.

When do you need to fix people?
When do you need to remove pain and discomfort?
When do you need to be involved in a dual role?
When do you need to be perfect?
When do you need to have the answer?
When do you need to be loved?

Now talk for a moment with your partner about the experience, and in the space provided write down the areas in which you feel you may have the most difficulty with countertransference.

Go through the exercise again and substitute the word *want* for *need*. Discuss the feelings that arise with the word *want* and the ways they may be different from those produced by the word *need*.

and use deep pressure on the back, even if this is not what the client would choose. The massage professional also may avoid using a method he does not enjoy but that the client may like.

If the client's personal situation is similar to that of the massage practitioner, especially with regard to life challenges, the practitioner may give subconsciously based advice to the client in an attempt to solve the massage practitioner's personal problem. For example, both the professional and the client may be facing difficult marital issues, or struggling with managing menopause, or dealing with the recent loss of a parent or relocation to a new city. This dynamic can be detrimental to the client because it breaches the professional relationship and fosters psychologically unhealthy behaviors between the massage practitioner and the client. An environment of sympathetic dependence often results. This dynamic is a basis for countertransference.

The goal is not for the bodywork professional to be faultless before beginning practice; rather, the goal is for the therapist to be aware of personal challenges that could interfere with the therapeutic relationship and thus her ability to maintain professional boundaries.

Practitioners personalize the professional relationship when they assume too much responsibility for the outcome of the session for the client or they project a personal situation into the client process. Countertransference issues often reflect unresolved issues on the part of the professional. Identifying countertransference in the therapeutic relationship can point out areas the practitioner may wish to explore and resolve with a qualified professional in order to remain objective and increase effectiveness as a bodywork professional.

Managing Transference and Countertransference

Transference can be expected in some form in the therapeutic relationship. As it arises, it is the professional's responsibility to reinforce the boundaries of the professional relationship. The practitioner should explain to clients why these feelings may occur and help them redirect the transference activity to the appropriate people or situations in the client's life. This becomes difficult when the client does not move through the transference stage toward more self-directed resources and coping structures or when the client has extremely limited resources and coping mechanisms. It may be necessary to refer such clients to another professional, with appropriate disclosure for the reason for referral, to help them understand that the boundaries of the professional relationship are being breached and that the existing situation is inappropriate.

It is always the professional's responsibility to self-monitor for the development of countertransference issues and to seek supervision or professional support, if necessary, to resolve personal issues. When the professional faces the realization that countertransference has occurred, the first step in resolving these issues has been taken. It is a breach of professional boundaries to allow countertransference issues to develop and linger or be acted on. In extreme cases the client may need to be referred to a different therapeutic massage professional, with the appropriate disclosure on the part of the therapist, so that the client does not take the need for referral personally.

Peer support and supervision are important for the massage professional dealing with transference and countertransference. Seeking information from more experienced professionals, which supervision encourages, supports professional development. The supervising professional does not necessarily need to be a massage therapist. Various health care professionals grapple with similar issues. Mental health professionals in particular must consider transference and countertransference issues frequently. If supervision is not part of your professional practice, it may be helpful to seek out a qualified mental health professional and establish a professional relationship with her to sort out these particular issues.

Peer support is important as well. Interacting regularly with other massage practitioners creates an environment that promotes healthy work practices through both technical information and guidance on solving interpersonal dilemmas. When sharing with peers, be attentive to the confidentiality of your clients. It is important not to allow yourself to become isolated, with no regular sources of fresh information and perspectives.

Dual or Multiple Roles

Dual or multiple roles develop when professionals assume more than one role in their relationship with their clients. These roles develop in many different ways. Providing bodywork in the professional environment with family members is a classic example of a dual role, as is providing professional services for a personal friend. A dual role exists when scopes of practice overlap and one professional provides support in more that one area of expertise.

Dual and multiple roles are difficult to manage in the professional relationship and can be a breeding ground for ethical dilemmas. As soon as one professional assumes professional authority with the body and the mind, the body and the spirit, or the spirit and the mind, the therapist can be said to be assuming a dual role (or multiple roles if the authority is assumed in all three areas). In this situation the professional holds more power in the relationship than is appropriate, and the client begins to become disempowered. This allows a very dangerous power shift that supports the development of transference and countertransference. It often leads to enmeshment and dependence on the part of the client and burnout on the part of the therapist. It is difficult enough to manage the inherent power differential of the therapeutic relationship without increasing the likelihood of transference and countertransference or breach of professional boundaries by assuming dual and multiple roles.

In the professional bodywork relationship, it is not necessary to deal with mental and spiritual issues directly. The focus of massage/bodywork is the body. When interacting with your client, maintain the focus of the work on the body while using attentive listening, acknowledging the client's circumstances, and always being alert to the possible need for referral. Interacting professionally in the area of the mind or spirit may breach the professional contract for services, which focuses on the body. Always recognize and appreciate the wholeness of the person while staying within the scope of massage/bodywork therapy, and work with other professionals to deal with other areas so that the client remains empowered in the process of achieving wellness.

A dual role can arise in more subtle situations as well. The sale of products to a client, bartering of services, excessive personal disclosure by the therapist to the client, shared social interaction, or shared professional services all create situations in which the power balance of the therapeutic relationship can become problematic. As in all ethical dilemmas, decisions about conduct are gauged against the welfare of the client.

Massage Therapy and Intimacy

To dispel in advance any sexual innuendo associated with many of the terms used in the following paragraphs, definitions[4] are included at this point for clarification.

The dictionary defines *intimacy* as "the state or fact of being intimate"; *intimate* is defined as "inmost, essential, internal, most private or personal; closely acquainted or associated; very familiar." *Essential* means "intrinsic, fundamental, basic, and inherently primary." *Sensory* is defined as "connected with the reception and transmission of sense impressions" through the nervous system. *Stimulation* is defined as the act of exciting or increasing activity.

The work of a massage practitioner is sensory stimulation; therefore by its very definition body stimulation is sensual and may become intimate.

The massage professional must understand the physiologic aspects of therapeutic massage and recognize that the same massage techniques that alleviate stress and promote relaxation also stimulate the entire sensory mechanism, which may include a sexual arousal response. A more thorough knowledge of the physiologic and psychologic network leads to a better understanding of the responses by both client and practitioner. The practitioner then is better able to alter the session to maintain a proper professional relationship.

Within the parameters of professional ethics, it is always considered unethical for the client or the practitioner to interact on a sexual level, whether verbally or physically. However, it is essential that both client and practitioner understand why the urges and sensations of sexuality may present themselves.

The lumbar nerve plexus and the sacral nerve plexus conduct sensory information to and from the abdominal area, the lower extremities, and the buttocks, as well as to and from the genital area. Stimulation of a nerve plexus area is not confined to local perception, but rather is diffused throughout the area. For example, when the lower abdominal area is stroked, the nerve signals of the genital area are influenced as well. The entire sexual arousal response is part of the relaxation response via the output from the parasympathetic autonomic nervous system. Therefore each time a client relaxes out of the "fight or flight" responses of the sympathetic autonomic nervous system into the more relaxed response, the predisposing physiologic factors are present for sexual arousal. This reaction is possible not only for clients but also for practitioners as they begin to relax and entrain with the massage.

On a physiologic level, parasympathetic stimulation activates most of the benefits of massage for stress reduction. This neuralgic state also is favorable to sexual arousal. These physical responses are all connected, but it seems that the sexual response is short lived and quickly replaced by feelings of deep relaxation as the massage continues. Responses vary with each client, and the sexual response may be totally bypassed. However, sexual arousal may occur, and the massage practitioner needs to understand both the physiology of this situation and the way to deal with it ethically should it present itself.

It is the practitioner's responsibility to put the whole issue of sexuality into perspective, understand it clearly, and explain the "feelings" to the client on a physiologic level. It also becomes the practitioner's responsibility to monitor the client's responses and act appropriately to adjust the physiology and change the pattern of the massage to diffuse the sexual energy (Box 2-11). This is easily accomplished by altering the approach of the session. It is

---

DIFFUSING FEELINGS OF SEXUAL AROUSAL

1. Recognize the physiology and interrupt it; change what you are doing.
2. Be aware of your own psychologic state.
3. Adjust the intent of the session to stimulate a more sympathetic output response by using stretching, compression, joint movement, and active participation by the client.
4. Change the music, lighting, and conversation and the client's position.
5. Stop working with your hands and use your forearms.
6. Explain the feelings in a professional manner using clinical terminology.

common knowledge that sexual arousal is not purely physical and depends on both psychologic and tactile responses. It is here that the practitioner can modulate the client-practitioner responses.

Intercourse is defined as "connection or reciprocal action between persons or nations; the interchange of thought, feelings, products, services, communication, commerce, and association."[4] Massage becomes an intercourse in the purest sense. Essential intimacy is the circle that begins to develop between practitioner and client. People want this type of intimacy; it is the type of interaction that promotes survival and health. Essential touch is vital, fundamental, and crucial to well-being. It is the touch of a litter of puppies, sleeping in one big pile. It is the caring, understanding look of a friend, and it can be combined with the sexual interchange between lovers. But it does not have to have sexual expression to be essential intimacy.

When a person encounters the essential touch that a sensitive and confident massage practitioner provides, that person's whole system responds. For many, the closest thing to essential touch ever experienced is sexual interaction. Because our bodies constantly react to new situations through comparison to past experience, it is understandable why a client's response system might interpret these feelings as sexual arousal. Furthermore, for

many people the only familiar routine they have for expressing these feelings is a sexual one. It is easy to see why the client would confuse the sensations and perceive the interaction of the feelings associated with massage in sexual responses and terms.

Remember, as massage professionals, when we touch we are also being touched. The exchange is unavoidable, and we need to monitor our own feelings and expressions of intimacy as well.

If we do not deal effectively with these responses, the feelings associated with them could become very uncomfortable. The client may react by discontinuing the massage sessions, or the therapist may effectively detach from the client and possibly stop seeing the client altogether. In the latter case, the client may feel abandoned.

As the therapist closes the session and leaves the client's space, it is important to change both physiology and body language. When greeting a client and providing the massage, the body language is open, inviting, connecting, and moving toward the client (Fig. 2-4). When it is time to close the session, the body language moves away from the client, pulls in toward the massage therapist, separates, and indicates that the session is finished (Fig. 2-5). Separating well from the client is a skill that gives both the client and the massage therapist a sense of closure. It often helps to establish a "time to go" ritual by

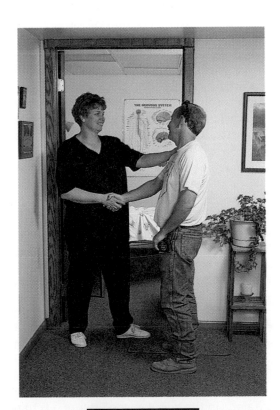

fig. 2-4

Greeting body language. When greeting a client, the massage professional leans toward the client and gently draws him into the space of the massage session.

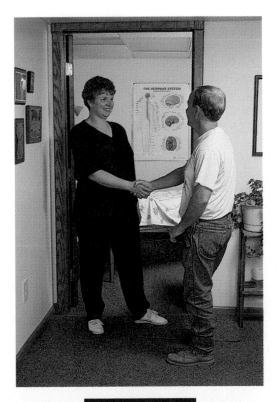

fig. 2-5

Closure body language. When the massage is complete, the massage professional gently withdraws from the client by using body language that moves away from him.

always saying good-bye the same way. Clients who linger at the door may not know how to leave or may not recognize that it is time to leave. A "time to go" ritual helps considerably.

One example of a leaving ritual is to keep a box labeled "A thought to take with me" that contains fun, empowering quotes on note cards. Have the client pick a card from the box. Put the information for the next appointment on the back of the card, hand it to the client with a warm handshake, and say good-bye. When the session is finished, let the client go physically and emotionally as the room is prepared for the next person.

Remember, as was explained in Chapter 1, the *intention* of the touch is a determining factor in the *interpretation* of the touch. The touch of the massage professional is not focused on sexual arousal and release. The psychologic aspect of this topic is another matter. Here the practitioner can set the stage and monitor responses. Keep discussions light. Change the topic. This is where the interpersonal communication skills of the practitioner come into play.

The moments of intimacy must be dealt with very carefully. Misunderstanding the psychologic or physiologic responses, the client may interpret this response as an indication of feelings of love or that the therapist is a new best friend. Clients manifest this response in different ways. Usually clients want to bring the professional into their lives, perhaps through invitations to lunch, a desire for more frequent sessions, or a proposal for a relationship. Do not allow this to happen. The practitioner must maintain professional space and monitor personal feelings. Keep the balance by confining the intimacy of massage to the therapy room.

Having no understanding of all these subtle interactions, the client cannot be blamed for wanting more attention from the massage practitioner. The moments of togetherness that are shared are special and can range from a great deal of laughter to sharing work-related experiences. The session can accomplish something as simple as relieving the day's tension or as complex as overcoming years of pain. Make no more and no less of the interaction.

Clients may look to the professional for emotional support beyond the ethical scope of practice for massage. Encourage them to find the support they require from another source. If a client needs assistance with coping skills, refer him to someone who is qualified to help. Credit counselors, ministers, rape crisis counselors, marriage counselors, counselors for sexual dysfunction, chiropractors, therapists, physicians, and many other caregivers can provide the help clients may need. The massage practitioner's job is to support and accept the client in a nonjudgmental manner, listen, and blend touch skills to benefit the client.

Sexual Misconduct

Although sexual misconduct has been relatively well defined (Box 2-12), what is invasive remains a gray area. A joke told between friends may be totally inappropriate in the professional setting. A statement about appearance may be taken as a compliment or could be interpreted as a sexual remark. What is appropriate with one client may not be acceptable with another. It can be overwhelming to try to second-guess what is appropriate for clients. The best defense against confusion is communication. Ask questions and provide clients with information about acceptable behavior in the professional setting (Proficiency Exercise 2-9).

Managing Intimacy Issues

Do not be afraid of the special professional intimacy of therapeutic massage. Instead, educate clients by answering their questions intelligently, basing your answers on the facts of physiology, and encourage them to use this information to interact more resourcefully with others. If you begin to feel physically and emotionally receptive to a client, take steps to diffuse the response (see Box 2-11, p. 60). Later, review the session to evaluate your personal feelings. Was it a fleeting warm feeling? Is there just something about this particular person? Could it have been a hormonal response? (Therapists should be aware that some women become more sexually responsive during certain times of their monthly cycle.) Were you feeling alone and needing to be connected? If the problem arises from something lacking in life, empower yourself to search out the cause and change circumstances so that personal reactions are kept out of the therapy room.

If a professional relationship cannot be maintained with a client, stop providing therapeutic massage and refer the client to someone else. Give an honest, simple explanation so that the client understands it was not something he or she said or did that prompted the referral. Professional ethics cannot safeguard us from being human; however, behavior becomes unethical when the problem is not acknowledged and resourceful action is not taken to solve it.

If a client refuses or is unable to change an inappropriate response to the massage, the client must be refused further treatment. Explain to the client that the situation is uncomfortable and massage therapy can no longer be provided. The dismissal must be done gently but firmly, and the client must be told the decision is final.

A client who immediately asks for sexual release is a different case. If this occurs, the massage professional explains succinctly that neither sexual release nor any other kind of sexual interaction is provided, and then dismisses the person immediately.

Care must be taken in situations that could become difficult, and any situation in which behavior could be questioned must be avoided. One such situation concerns male therapists who wish to do home calls for women who are alone in the house. A good solution is to pair up with a woman practitioner and do these massages as a team. It is important that a parent or legal guardian be in the room when massage services are given to a child under

---

box 2-12

GUIDELINES ON SEXUAL MISCONDUCT

The guidelines developed in Ontario, Canada, provide the following criteria for determining what is sexual misconduct[3]:

Sexual Impropriety and Sexual Abuse

1. The therapist will respect the integrity of each person and therefore not engage in any sexual conduct or sexual activities involving clients.
2. The therapist will not date a client.
3. The therapist will not commit any form of sexual impropriety or sexual abuse with a client.
4. Whatever the behavior of the client, it is always the responsibility of the massage therapist not to engage in sexual behavior.

Sexual impropriety includes the following:

Any behavior, gestures, or expressions that are seductive or sexually demeaning to a client
Inappropriate procedures, including but not limited to the following:
- Disrobing or draping practices that reflect a lack of respect for the client's privacy
- Deliberately watching a client dress or undress
- Inappropriate comments about or to the client, including but not limited to the following:
  Sexual comments about a client's body or underclothing

Sexualized or sexually demeaning comments to a client
Criticism of the client's sexual orientation
Discussion of potential sexual performance
Conversations about the sexual preferences or fantasies of the client or the massage therapist
Requests to date
- Kissing of a sexual nature

Sexual abuse includes the following:

- Therapist-client sex, whether initiated by the client or not.
- Engaging in any conduct with a client that is sexual or reasonably may be interpreted as sexual, including but not limited to the following:
  Genital to genital contact
  Oral to genital contact
  Oral to anal contact
  Oral to oral contact (except CPR)
  Oral to breast contact
  Touching or undraping the genitals, perineum, or anus
  Touching or undraping the breasts
  Encouraging the client to masturbate in the presence of the massage therapist
  Masturbation by the massage therapist while the client is present
  Masturbation of the client by the massage therapist

2-9

PROFICIENCY EXERCISE

Working in groups of three, write down specific situations in which sexual misconduct or feelings of intimacy may develop. Exchange responses with other groups and role play a situation, with one student acting as the massage practitioner, one playing the client, and the third evaluating the way the situation was handled. Try different situations until each student has had a chance to play each role.

Develop a "time to go" ritual and write it down in the space below.

---

18 years of age. A practitioner should never work behind a locked door because this may be construed as entrapment. Instead, a sign should be posted indicating that a massage is in session, and the room should not be entered without knocking.

Maintaining the delicate professional balance between client and practitioner is especially difficult with long-term clients. The nurturing approach of the massage prac-

titioner fosters an environment in which friendships can form. Regular clients do become important as people, as well as in their roles as clients. Massage practitioners must always be honest with themselves about the development of personal feelings for a client. Remember, this is a relationship, and professional relationships can last a very long time. These people become important to us. When clients move away, we miss them. When a client dies, we

box 2-13

MAINTAINING PROFESSIONAL SPACE

1. At the beginning of a professional relationship, a formal informed consent process must be completed.
2. In most instances the time frame for working with a client should not exceed 90 minutes, with 45 to 60 minutes being the norm. If more time is spent with the client, it becomes difficult for both the professional and the client to maintain the original intent and focus of the session, and the result is an environment that fosters transference and countertransference.
3. Professionals should wear clothing that sets them apart from clients; this is one of the benefits of a uniform. A name tag that identifies one as a massage therapist also is helpful. Wearing a uniform or maintaining a professional style of dress that is different from casual clothing gives visual stimulation that reflects professionalism. The clothes do not have to be white but must be nonrevealing and present an understated appearance. Therapists must be conscious of their appearance and make sure it is kept as nonsexual as possible.
4. The therapist should avoid assuming a dual role and multiple scopes of practice. The professional contract is for a specific type of intervention. General information about lifestyle, health, or spiritual issues can be provided, but the contract is for massage/bodywork. This is a consideration even if the professional is credentialed in more than one area or discipline. Often the therapist needs to decide which professional hat to wear.
5. The professional environment should be neutral and must not indirectly imply any content other than bodywork. Choices made in decorating the space or in reading material can be seen as creating an environment that fosters a dual role by promoting a specific mental, spiritual, nutritional, or exercise approach.
6. Selling products to clients can become an issue because of the perceived authority influence of the professional. Closely related products, such as self-massage tools that are made available for the client's convenience, as opposed to products sold for profit making, often present less of a problem than something like nutritional products. The client may like the services of the massage therapist but does not want to feel pressured into buying products. These situations must be managed with careful reflection, because ethical dilemmas often result from the sale of products.
7. Privacy can be preserved by using an answering machine or service and returning calls within set hours. If it is financially possible, have a receptionist or secretary monitor phone calls.
8. Maintain regular appointment hours. Begin and end sessions on time.
9. If you go to clients' homes, be extra cautious about entering a home alone. It is important to screen your clients carefully. The initial intake interview is a good opportunity to do this. Have the client come to your location, where you have more professional control over the screening process. Individual circumstances will dictate when the following recommendations are necessary, but remember, it is better to be safe than sorry.

   An on-site massage session for a bedridden elderly person will have a different level of concern than a female massage therapist providing on-site massage to a single male client. At the very least, make sure someone always knows where you are and check in with someone periodically throughout the day. If you are anxious about doing an on-site massage session, consider referring the client to someone else.

   Hire someone to go with you to the client's home. This person does not need to be a massage professional but should be able-bodied in case there is a need to leave the home in a hurry. This person remains within hearing distance of the place where the massage is given and can act as a witness should the client claim inappropriate behavior by the massage professional. This person also provides protection from any type of entrapment or illicit advances against the massage practitioner. It is appropriate to charge for this protection, and it is reflected in the fee structure.

   It is also important to use the phone when entering a home or other location where less control is available to the massage practitioner. Call a pre-arranged number and give an associate the name, address, and phone number of the client, the time of arrival, and the expected time of departure. Tell this person that you will call just before you leave. Leave instructions to call the authorities should you not call at the agreed time. Make sure that your client hears this conversation.
10. Do not spend personal time, such as lunch, with clients. In rare situations the professional may choose to forgo the professional relationship to develop a personal relationship. This decision can be considered a breach of professional ethics and is almost always a professional and personal mistake. The initial relationship structure was built on the basis of one who serves and one who is served. It is very rare that an effective transition is made to a relationship of mutual support. Both people usually end up hurt.
11. Think carefully before setting rules about client conduct, rescheduling, and payment methods. Make sure you are willing to enforce your policies. If you are not, don't make them. Record this information clearly and concisely, and make sure the client reads it. Posting it on the wall provides additional reinforcement.

grieve. When clients rejoice, so do we. And when clients do not need us anymore, we celebrate. Clients touch our lives. They are our best teachers. How can we not care about them?

Consider all the dynamics of the therapeutic relationship, but if an error in judgment is to be made, err on the side of compassion, connection, and caring, which is no error at all. Learn from the experience. Do not become so "professionally detached" that the client does not connect with you, the person.

The touch of a massage professional is safe touch. What does it mean to be safe? According to the dictionary definition, *safe* means not apt to cause danger, harm, or hurt, to be free of risk.[4] Physiologically, *safe* means a state of homeostasis rather than the alarm of the "fight or flight" responses of the sympathetic autonomic nervous system or the intense retreat and withdrawal responses of the parasympathetic autonomic nervous system (see Chapter 4). Being *safe* means having the ability to maintain well-being in a situation and alter responses easily to cope resourcefully with the inevitable change and demands of everyday life. The therapeutic massage professional must consider everything, including personal beliefs and fears, that may make touch unsafe for clients.

By using this educational experience to explore these issues, more safe places can be found for the practitioner, which will influence professional touch and make the massage environment a safe place. The essence of this work is human touch. By dealing with personal intimacy issues, not only can the massage professional provide essential touch for the client, the client also learns to establish proper boundaries. It must always be kept in mind that each individual massage practitioner represents the entire massage therapy profession. Demonstrating respect for the self demonstrates respect for the profession as a whole.

Maintaining the Professional Environment

The therapeutic relationship is a unidirectional focus in which the knowledge and skills of the professional are used to assist the client in achieving therapeutic outcomes. To preserve the unidirectional focus, certain crucial professional boundaries must be maintained. For example, it is important to maintain professional space (Proficiency Exercise 2-10). Some simple ways to accomplish this are presented in Box 2-13.

ETHICAL DECISION MAKING

section objectives

Using the information presented in this section, the student will be able to perform the following:

■ **Implement an eight-step decision-making process**

When ethical dilemmas are difficult to resolve, massage professionals are expected to engage in a conscientious decision-making process that is explicit enough to bear public scrutiny.

Decisions are thought-out responses based on principles, information, and the complexities of the situation. Decision making requires a person to consider the facts, possibilities, logical consequences of cause and effect (pros and cons), and impact on people. Each decision is unique. A few rules are absolutes: A professional does not breach sexual boundaries with a client; clients are to be referred when the skills required are out of the scope of practice or training of the professional; all care must focus on giving help and avoiding harm; and clients are to be given complete information about the treatment. However, most ethical dilemmas revolve around more ambiguous situations and require a thoughtful approach to decision making. These situations often are difficult to identify, and solutions may require objective input. Where does a professional go for help?

As stated previously, supervision and peer support are very helpful to a professional grappling with ethical dilemmas that fall into the more common situational gray areas. Supervision involves periodic review of a professional's actions by a practitioner more experienced in the profession. This can be direct supervision, in which the supervising professional actually observes the professional at work, or reflective supervision, in which the supervisor discusses the professional practice with the practitioner. Regardless of the approach, the more experienced professional is able to guide, coach, and mentor the one being supervised, as well as help identify potential ethical concerns and assist in ethical decision making.

Peer support provides a format for discussion, brainstorming, and reflection on the professional practice. Two or three heads are better than one when working with ethical decision making.

Ethics is not just about answers; it is also the willingness to ask the questions. It is said that professionals do not let personal judgments interfere with professional care, but what do we do, for example, when we can't keep our mind on our work because of a client's body odor? What do we do when a client schedules appointments

---

2-10

PROFICIENCY EXERCISE

In the space provided, list three things you will do to maintain professional space. Choose from the list in Box 2-13 or make up your own.

1.
2.
3.

box 2-14

PROBLEM-SOLVING MODEL FOR DECISION MAKING

Step 1: Gather the Facts to Identify and Define the Situation

Key questions: What is the problem? What happened in factual terms?

What are the facts?

What has happened?

What caused the situation?

What was done or is being done?

What has worked or not worked?

Who is involved and what responsibilities do they have?

Step 2: Brainstorm Possible Solutions

Key question: What might I do? or What if?

What are the possibilities?

What does my intuition suggest?

What are the possible contributing factors?

What are possible approaches for corrective action?

What might work?

What are other ways to look at the situation?

What do the data suggest?

Step 3: Logically and Objectively Evaluate Each Possible Solution Identified in Step 2; Look at Both Sides and the Pros and Cons

Note: This objective analysis of the possible solutions generated in Step 2 is very important. It has been my experience that most people drawn to learn massage therapy are not naturally attuned to this type of analysis and therefore tend to bypass this vital step in evaluating information to arrive at the most appropriate decision. The ability to analyze objectively is an essential skill for effective professional practice. In addition, this area of processing becomes important in dealing with conflict situations that may arise from ethical dilemmas because the focus of this information is a process. Processes can be evaluated and altered; people's feelings usually cannot. A professional who has not developed the ability to evaluate a situation logically and objectively will have difficulty identifying where processes have broken down. Remember, change an action and people's feelings change.

Key question: What would happen if I... (insert each brainstormed idea from step 2)

What are the costs, resources needed, and time involved?

What is the logical progression of the pattern, contributing factors, and current behaviors?

What are the logical causes and effects of each solution identified?

What are the pros and cons of each solution suggested?

What are the consequences of not acting?

What are the consequences of acting?

Step 4: Evaluate the Effect of Each Possible Solution on the People Involved

Key question: How would each person involved feel if I . . . . (insert each brainstormed idea from step 2)

In terms of each possible solution being considered, what is the impact on the people involved: client, practitioner, and other professionals working with the client?

How does each person involved feel about the possible interventions?

Does the practitioner feel qualified to work with such situations?

Does a feeling of cooperation and agreement exist among all parties involved?

Step 5: Choose a Solution and Develop an Implementation Plan after Carefully Processing Steps 1 through 4

Implementation plans are step-by-step procedures that detail what must be done to carry out the solution. For example, a solution arrived at using the previous steps is: I will learn more about asthma so that I can work with my client better. The implementation plan is as follows:

Use the Internet to research asthma

Look up asthma at the library

Contact the local asthma support group for information

Contact the client's physician for specific recommendations

Talk with my friend who is a respiratory therapist

Compile the information into a massage and benefit report to develop the massage approach

Discuss the report with my client

Step 6: Implement the Plan and Set a Date for Reevaluation; This is Sometimes the Hardest Part—Doing It

Step 7: Determine the Logical Consequences If the Plan is not Followed

It is important to determine what will happen if one of the parties in a decision that affects more that one person does not perform to his or her commitment. For example, a decision is made between a massage therapist and a chronic "no show" client that the client will be charged for the full session unless she calls 24 hours in advance to cancel the appointment. Both parties agree, but the very next session, the client does not show and does not call. Because the consequence has been agreed on in advance—the client will be charged for the full session—the possibility of escalation of the conflict is diminished.

Step 8: Reevaluate and Make Necessary Adjustments; Then Implement the Refined Plan

Remember, decisions are not static. Reevaluation procedures can alter, refine, or change them.

PROFICIENCY EXERCISE

Decision Making Using the Problem-Solving Model with Peer Support

Identify an ethical dilemma with which you are dealing, or make up a dilemma that you believe you will deal with in the future. Describe the dilemma by answering the questions posted in Step 1 of the problem-solving model from Box 2-14.

Identify and Define the Situation
What are the facts?

What has happened?

What caused the situation?

What was done or is being done?

What has worked or not worked?

Who is involved and what responsibilities do they have?

Next, divide into groups of four. Choose who will present the facts of his or her dilemma to the group. This presentation should not take more than 5 minutes. Each of the other three group members will play a role in the decision-making process.

One of the three remaining group members now provides input from Step 2 of the problem-solving model by suggesting possible solutions, using the following questions as a guide. For the purpose of this exercise, limit the possibilities to three or four. Spend 3 to 5 minutes on this portion of the exercise, and remember to stay within your role; it confuses the process when you bounce between Steps 3 and 4.

What are the possibilities?
What does my intuition suggest?
What are the possible contributing factors?
What are possible approaches for corrective action?
What might work?
What are other ways to look at the situation?
What do the data suggest?

The next person uses logic to evaluate each of the possible solutions presented in Step 2, using the following questions as a guide. Spend 3 to 5 minutes on this part of the exercise. Again, stay in your role; do not work with Steps 2 or 4.

What are the costs, resources needed, and time involved?
What is the logical progression of the pattern, contributing factors, and current behaviors?
What are the logical causes and effects of each solution identified?
What are the pros and cons of each solution suggested?
What are the consequences of not acting?
What are the consequences of acting?

The last person evaluates each of the possible solutions generated in Step 2 in terms of the people involved, using the following questions as a guide. Spend 3 to 5 minutes on this part of the exercise. Stay with the process; do not become chatty or conversational.

In terms of each possible solution being considered, what is the impact on the people involved: client, practitioner, and other professionals working with the client?

How does each person involved feel about the possible interventions?

Does the practitioner feel qualified to work with such situations?

Does a feeling of cooperation and agreement exist among all parties involved?

Now, the person who originally presented the ethical problem chooses a solution and develops an implementation plan. Again, spend 3 to 5 minutes on this part of the exercise. Write the solution here with the implementation plan.

Continued.

2-11

PROFICIENCY EXERCISE—CONT'D

Rotate the roles so that each member of the group plays all four roles. It will take 1 hour to complete the entire exercise with all participants playing all four roles. After the entire process has been completed, answer the following questions.

What was the easiest part of the process for me?

What was the hardest part of the process for me and what made it difficult?

What was the most difficult part of the process for the group?

What might help the group problem solve more effectively?

How would I implement the process by myself without a peer support group?

---

more frequently than necessary because the client likes being with us? How do we handle a client who refuses to seek medical intervention when indicated? And the questions continue . . .

The professional may wish to ask himself the following questions:

- Can I handle the professional power differential from a position of respect and empowerment for the client?
- Do I have the knowledge and skills to respond effectively to the situation?
- Am I avoiding dual or multiple roles with the client?
- Am I maintaining the boundaries of the therapeutic relationship?
- Am I within the established scope of practice for therapeutic massage and bodywork?
- Am I respecting the scope of practice of other professionals?
- Do I have the highest good of the client in mind?
- Is what I am doing supporting the highest good of the profession?
- Are my professional and communication skills effective?
- Would I want anyone else to know what I am doing?

A problem may be developing if the answers to these questions become ambiguous or inconsistent. When openly answered, these questions help us recognize the need to use a problem-solving approach to make ethical decisions.

Problem-Solving Approach to Ethical Decision Making

Problem solving to reach an effective decision is not an easy task. A generic model created from many different problem-solving methods is presented here for the purpose of ethical decision making. This model is expounded

on throughout the text in regard to what may be called *clinical reasoning,* which involves taking the client's health history, performing a physical assessment, developing a treatment plan, choosing methods to implement the treatment plan, and charting. Most of this information is presented in Chapter 3, with additional refinement of the process presented in Chapter 5.

We are most comfortable believing that our decision-making abilities are comprehensive, objective, intuitive, and workable. For some this actually may be the case, but years of teaching and self-exploration have shown that most people have never learned comprehensive decision-making skills.

To complicate matters, different people, when gathering information, are naturally attracted to certain types of information and are influenced by certain types of criteria when evaluating possible solutions. Some experts believe that this attention focus is a genetic predisposition, and others believe that it is learned behavior. Regardless, most people, unless specifically trained, effectively consider only about half of the relevant and available information when making a decision. No wonder many of the decisions we make do not serve us well.

A problem-solving model not only leads us through the steps we more naturally would take, but also reminds us to look at important information we might tend to overlook when making a decision (Proficiency Exercise 2-11). When this process is followed diligently, it eventually becomes a habit. In the beginning the process may feel cumbersome and uncomfortable. The parts of the process that we do not understand or with which we become impatient or frustrated often are the areas on which we do not naturally focus. These are the areas, then, that need the most practice.

The decision-making process presented in Box 2-14 acknowledges the importance of factual data, intuitive insight, concrete and objective cause and effect, and the feelings, experiences, and influences of the people involved.

COMMUNICATION SKILLS

section objectives

Using the information presented in this section, the student will be able to perform the following:

- ■ **Identify a person's preferred communication pattern**
- ■ **Develop and use an I-message to deliver information and listen reflectively**
- ■ **Follow a suggested communication pattern for resolving ethical dilemmas and conflict**
- ■ **Identify three barriers to effective communication**

Effective communication often is a difficult process for both the professional and the client. Without a direct communication approach, ethical dilemmas tend to escalate, and both parties suffer in the process. Professionals seek to establish genuine positive regard for all clients and to relate to each with sensitivity to that person's uniqueness. Professional ethics demands that when a feeling of criticism and negative judgment of a client occurs, we must be aware of it and work to prevent it from interfering with our commitment to compassionate, quality care. Direct, honest communication, focusing on the situation rather than the person and delivered in a gentle, respectful way, opens the door for resolution.

Communication is the act of exchanging thoughts, feelings, and behavior. Many ethical and professional dilemmas result from communication difficulties. To make ethical decisions and resolve ethical dilemmas, it is necessary to communicate effectively. As was described in Chapter 1, touch is a powerful mode of communication. The intent of professional touch may be influenced by many factors, including countertransference and the thought process of the therapist at the moment of the touch. The way touch is interpreted by the client often is determined by the unspoken intent of the therapist; therefore it is important to monitor thoughts and feelings while professionally communicating through touch.

Putting ethical principles into action requires some basic communication skills. Communication skills are required to retrieve information, maintain charting and client records, and provide information effectively so that the client can give informed consent. Using the following communication skills will assist the professional in maintaining ethical practices in the therapeutic relationship.

The strongest message is delivered through the kinesthetic mode, or body language. As we express ourselves through our bodies, others visually receive the messages and feel our touch. It is important that congruence exist between what is heard, what is seen, and what is felt.

When lack of continuity is a problem, the kinesthetic message seems to have the strongest effect.

The tone of voice is more important than the words spoken. Tone is kinesthetic and auditory because of the pressure waves emitted. We hear and feel the sound waves from the tone of voice.

The words are the least effective part of the communication pattern. Words can have mixed meanings, depending on each person's definition of a particular word (Proficiency Exercise 2-12). It is important to make sure that each of the people communicating is working from the same definition of a word. For example, the massage technician's definition of the word *disrobe* may be different from the client's definition. To a massage professional *disrobe* may mean to remove external clothing but keep underwear on; the client interprets the same word as meaning to take off all clothing. During the informed consent process, the massage technician may say, "It is out of my scope of practice to diagnose or treat any specific condition." The technician defines the word *treat* as meaning to provide remedial or rehabilitation procedures. The client interprets the word *treat* as any type of method used. The potential for misunderstanding is greater.

Preferred Communication Patterns

Each person has a preferred method of delivering and receiving information in a style that is most comfortable for

---

2-12

PROFICIENCY EXERCISE

Write what each of the words below means to you and in what way you would behave if you were experiencing these words.

Joy

Love

Peace

Competence

Compare your list with three other students and identify the similarities and differences. What did you learn about the interpretation of a word?

that individual. This is determined by genetic predisposition and conditioning (learning).

Those who prefer the visual mode make pictures in their mind and use many descriptive words as they paint word pictures during conversation. They tend to use "see" words and want to make eye contact when conversing.

Others prefer the auditory mode. These people use "hear" words during conversation and are very attentive to the tone and rhythm of speech. They often hum, talk to themselves, and listen with their eyes closed.

Almost everyone processes visual and auditory messages through the kinesthetic mode. The most common pattern is visual/kinesthetic, and the second most common is auditory/kinesthetic. People see and feel or hear and feel.

Some operate primarily from the feeling, or kinesthetic, mode of communication. These people may find talking and listening fatiguing. When speaking they use a lot of body language and "feel" words. Often they find that they have to touch something or someone to understand.

The way information is delivered and received also depends on fundamental processing styles. Some people prefer facts and sequence, whereas others prefer concepts and ideas. Some people make decisions based primarily on processes of cause and effect, and others structure decisions in terms of people and social structure. No one way is better than another, only different.

When providing information, it is important to deliver the message in the style the person receiving it prefers to process information.

Listening

Effective listening involves the development of focusing skills. You cannot listen effectively if you are planning what you will say next or in what way you will respond. Reflective listening involves restating the information to indicate that you have received and understood the message. Active listening may clarify a feeling attached to the message but does not add to or change the message. Listening does not involve giving advice, resolving the problem presented, or in any other way interjecting information about what was said. Effective listening occurs when we listen to understand instead of to respond. Understanding the message and agreeing with the content of the message are not the same thing; the basis for this confusion most likely evolved from our feeling of being most understood when someone agrees with us. Understanding can occur regardless of whether agreement exists. Much time is wasted and conflict encouraged when people equate understanding with agreement.

For example, while studying this chapter, the student may not agree with the position on wearing a uniform in the professional setting. Because the student has a different position does not mean that the textbook is wrong or that the student is wrong; the two positions are simply dif-

ferent. The student can understand that the author is basing her information on the existing standards of professionalism and her prior experience but can choose not to follow the recommendation. I, as the author of the text, can understand that a valid case can be made for not visually creating distinction (a uniform) between the professional and the client, but I do not agree with the student's decision not to wear a uniform. Sometimes this is called "agreeing to disagree," but this approach still seems to hold to the context of right or wrong, whereas being understood feels nonjudgmental and essential.

Delivering Information with I-messages

I-messages share feelings and concerns. You-messages put a person down, blame, criticize, and provoke anger, hurt, embarrassment, and feelings of worthlessness. I-message patterns require the four components of information used in effective decision making (Box 2-15).

It takes practice to use the simple I-message communication pattern well (Proficiency Exercise 2-13). Just as in problem solving, each individual attends to certain parts of the information and ignores other parts. If you are a person who naturally attends to people's feelings and you attempt to deliver a message to someone who views the world through logical outcomes, it is as if the two of you are on different wavelengths or speaking different languages. If a message is to be understood, it must be delivered on the wavelength most easily received by the person attempting to understand.

The following metaphor may help you understand the importance of delivering information the way the receiver (listener) is most apt to understand.

---

box 2-15

I-MESSAGE PATTERN

Describe the behavior or problem you find bothersome (Facts)
State your feelings about the situation (Impact on people)
State the consequence (Logical cause and effect)
Request the preferred behavior or action (Possibilities)

The pattern is:

When _____ happens, I feel _____.
The result is _____, and what I would prefer is _____.

When delivering I-messages, remain pleasant, respectful, and honest. Be aware of your body language, tone of voice, and quality of touch.

A father enjoys country music and keeps the car radio tuned to a country station. His daughter, a teenager, likes contemporary rock. Whenever the teenager drives her dad's car, she changes the radio station. On the few occasions the two find themselves in the car at the same time, a battle begins over which station will be on, country or rock. Now, if the father has something important to say to his daughter or wants to connect with her, he would be wise to put the radio on the rock station, even though he prefers country music and may even find rock difficult to listen to. It may be that the father can have the radio on rock only for a short period before it becomes too difficult for him and he changes to the country station. If he insists on country music to begin with, his daughter will tune him right out, and the opportunity for connection is lost.

To encourage effective communication, begin by identifying a person's communication pattern, that is, the words used, tone of voice, and body language. Use neutral topics to generate general discussion. During this time adjust your communication pattern to meet the person's communication style. Shift your body language, word choice, and tone to match the client's before attempting to deliver a message.

When communicating feelings, be specific. Words such as *upset* are too ambiguous. Instead, use words such as *afraid, angry, annoyed, discouraged, embarrassed, irritated, rejected, accepted, appreciated, capable, determined, compassionate, glad, grateful, proud, loved,* and *trusted*. Define the words you use. Do not assume that what you mean by a word is what your listener understands it to mean.

After an I-message has been delivered, request a response using open-ended questions. Open-ended questions encourage the sharing of information and cannot be easily answered in one word. Open-ended questions begin with *where, when, what, how,* and *which*. Avoid *why* questions because they encourage defensive reactions. When listening to the response, use active and reflective listening.

The I-message format also can be an effective listening tool. While listening, organize the information using the following questions:

What happened or what are the facts?

What feelings are being expressed?

What was the logical outcome?

What are the possibilities?

When listening reflectively, repeat the information as follows:

What I heard you say was: When _____ happened, you felt _____. The result was _____, and what you prefer is _____. Did I understand correctly?

If a person leaves out information (as commonly occurs), you will not be able to fill in that blank. In that case a clarifying question can be formed such as, "What would you prefer?" or "What was the logical outcome of the situation?"

Construct an I-message about a piece of information in this chapter that you feel is important.

Example: *When I read about I-messages to enhance communication, I felt relieved. The result is that I will practice this pattern with my family, and I prefer that the communication between my family members improves.*

Sit in a circle with at least three other people (more is better). Turn to your left and deliver your I-message to the person sitting next to you. That person repeats the I-message to you using the same format. Note what pieces are left out or how the pieces of the message become confused; or, on the other hand, note the clarity of the I-message when it is understood. Also note the preferred communication.

Now the person who just listened and repeated the message turns to the person on her left and delivers an I-message, which he repeats to her. Continue this way around the circle.

Communicating during Dilemmas

The following is a suggested pattern for resolving ethical dilemmas:

1. Carefully examine the facts, possibilities, logical causes and effects, and your feelings about the situation. Speak with a peer about the situation in a peer review or support context.
2. Plan a time to talk about the situation with the other person or people involved.
3. Begin the conversation by identifying the problem as you see it.
4. Use the standard I-message format to provide information and professional disclosure about your inability to work with or be comfortable with the situation.

In the following example a massage professional uses an I-message to talk with a client about the client's body odor:

When a client seems to have a distinctive body odor that I am aware of (facts), I feel distracted from my work (impact on people). As a result, because of my inability to focus, the client does not receive the best massage (logical cause and effect). I would like to see if we can resolve this difficulty, and if I can't deal with the situation better, I may find it to your benefit to refer you to someone who is not as sensitive to odors as I am (possibilities).

The client's body language and tone of voice may indicate embarrassment. The therapist then uses another I-message, "When I find it necessary to speak with someone about issues as personal as this (facts), I feel uncomfortable and embarrassed because I am afraid I will embarrass or hurt the person (impact on people). It is very difficult for me, but I truly want you to have the best possible care (logical cause and effect). What information do you have that can help me (possibilities and open-ended question)?"

Ending with an open-ended question encourages a problem-solving discussion.

It is essential to determine who has the problem. This can be done easily by deciding who will have to implement the solution to resolve the problem. Sometimes both parties own a part of the problem, with each needing to implement a portion of the solution for total resolution.

Continuing with the example of body odor, the therapist identifies and owns the problem by saying, "The difficulty is in my sensitivity to odors."

Next, information is gathered and possible solutions are devised. The client continues to express embarrassment through body language and states that he was aware of the problem. He tells you that body odor has been a problem since he began taking medication for a health problem but that he had just showered before he came to the session and thought the odor was gone.

The massage practitioner responds using reflective listening: "If I understand correctly, you are taking a medication that causes the body odor (facts), but you felt the odor was gone (impact on people) since you showered before coming to the session (logical cause and effect). Can I assume you would prefer that you did not have this situation (possibilities)?" The client nods.

The therapist asks, "Do you have any suggestions?" The client replies, "Could you use a scented oil or a room scent?" The client also says that he can speak to his physician and continue to shower just before coming for the session (generating possible solutions).

The therapist explains that using a scented oil may be a problem because she has sensitive skin and that using a room scent bothers other clients. The therapist asks, "Would it bother you if I wore a mask treated with a scented oil?" The client indicates that would be fine (evaluating possible solutions in terms of logical outcomes and pros and cons, as well as people's feelings).

The therapist says, "How about if I try the mask next time you are here, and we will talk about it after the massage? If this doesn't work, we will see if we can come up with some other solution. If nothing works, I will help you find a good therapist who can better serve your needs." The client agrees (deciding on and implementing a plan, setting a date for reevaluation, and agreeing on logical consequences).

After a decision has been made and agreed, it should be well defined, and all parties should be in agreement about what will happen if the solution to the problem is not implemented effectively. The plan and the agreed consequences should be written down.

The therapist closes with an I-message, "When I am able to work so well with a client about my sensitivity to odors (facts), I feel relieved (impact on people). This conversation has encouraged me to be more honest with myself and my clients (logical cause and effect). I hope that I will be able to continue to communicate effectively with you (possibilities). Thank you for being open with me."

A week later the plan is carried out, and the therapist finds that using the mask is distracting but effective. A sense of humor and understanding on the part of both the therapist and the client continue to support an effective solution (reevaluate and make the necessary adjustments).

Barriers to Effective Communication

Time

It takes time to communicate effectively. This is why writing is sometimes a more effective form of communication. When writing we make time to consider the words and reflect on what is being said. The person responding to the written message also has time to reread and reflect on the message.

Old Patterns

Falling into old patterns and old conditioning limits effective communication. It is important to "know thyself," and we must recognize personal triggers to old reactionary patterns in communication (Proficiency Exercise 2-14).

2-14

PROFICIENCY EXERCISE

In the space provided, evaluate your communication skills against the criteria presented in this section. Identify at least one area in which your communication skills currently are effective and one area that needs improvement. An example is provided.

Example: *My communication skills generally are effective when I am not stressed. I remember to listen in a focused way and use the I-message pattern often. However, when I have many things on my mind, I become distracted, do not listen effectively, and tend to interrupt people.*

Your Turn

Sometimes we need to leave a situation and come back to it so that we can respond instead of react.

Avoidance

People generally avoid conflict until it is unavoidable, and they avoid people who display strong emotion because it makes them feel uncomfortable.

Effective communication is a skill. It can be learned. Effective communication is essential in the therapeutic relationship. A professional diligently seeks to improve his communication skills.

CREDENTIALING AND LICENSING

section objectives

Using the information presented in this section, the student will be able to perform the following:

- **Describe the difference between governmental and private credentials**
- **Determine whether a credentialing program is valid**
- **Explain the basic roles of local and state laws and legislation and their influence on therapeutic massage**
- **Describe the two levels of practice for therapeutic massage**
- **Contact local, state, or provincial governments to obtain information about laws pertinent to the practice of therapeutic massage**

Credentials

Credentials are a form of official verification, earned by completing an educational or examination process, that confirms a certain level of expertise in a given skill. Governmental and private professional credentialing processes are being developed in the massage profession. Standardization of the profession has resulted in different methods of proving one's skills in order to practice therapeutic massage. The massage professional should understand the various credentialing processes and the requirements of practicing legally.

The only credentials required for the practice of therapeutic massage are those specified by governmental bodies (Box 2-16). All others are voluntary. Because of some confusing and difficult local laws, special legislative concerns need to be addressed by the massage professional.

Many massage and bodywork organizations and training programs have developed their own types of credentials. These credentials are valid only insofar as they indicate a level of professional achievement. A school diploma, which is granted on completion of a course of study, is an example. This is a very important document for a massage professional, but it is not a legally required credential unless stipulated by the law. For instance, a massage professional may need a diploma from a state-regulated school to take licensing examinations in states that license massage therapists.

Anyone can offer private certification. Given this fact, it is important to make sure that any educational program or examination you take is sanctioned and administered by a reputable, regulated provider. As an example, state-licensed schools, recognized national and state professional organizations, and classes approved for continuing education credits have had to undergo a review process that validates their educational offerings. Approval by the

---

box 2-16

GOVERNMENTAL CREDENTIALS AND REGULATIONS

Licensing
Requires a state or provincial board of examiners
Requires all constituents who practice the profession to be licensed
Legally defines and limits the scope of practice for a profession
Requires specific educational courses or an examination
Protects title usage (e.g., only those licensed can use the title *massage therapist*)

Governmental Certification
Administered by an independent board
Voluntary, but required for anyone using the protected title (e.g., *massage therapist*); others can provide the service but cannot call themselves massage therapists
Requires specific educational courses and an examination

Governmental Registration
(Not to be confused with private registration processes)
Administered by the state Department of Registry or other appropriate state agency
Voluntary
Does not necessarily require a specific education, such as a school diploma; often other forms of verification of professional standards, such as years in practice, are acceptable
Does not provide title protection

Exemptions
Means that a practitioner is not required to comply with an existing local or state regulation
Excuses practitioners who meet specified educational requirements from meeting current regulatory requirements
Does not provide title protection

National Commission for Certifying Agencies (NCCA) validates certification processes.

Since 1992 the National Certification Examination for Therapeutic Massage and Bodywork has been available. The examination covers human anatomy, physiology, kinesiology, clinical pathology, massage and bodywork theory, assessment, adjunct techniques, business practices, and professionalism. It was originally developed by a professional team through the Psychological Corporation, a recognized test development firm, and it continues to be refined to reflect the skills and knowledge base needed to meet the current job market for massage professionals. Periodically a job analysis survey is used to upgrade and improve the examination. The examination is meant to evaluate the entry level knowledge base and skills. The educational requirement for taking the examination is equivalent to 500 hours, which must cover the information base and competencies required as indicated by the most recent job survey. The examination is computer generated and is administered regularly in convenient locations. It does not include a practical demonstration of skills. The questions are multiple choice. Most of the questions are not answered with a regurgitation of factual data but rather require effective decision-making skills to identify the best answer.

This examination is not a government-regulated test. It is a voluntary, privately administered examination unless an individual state decides to use it for a licensing examination. Some states have done this, and some have also required additional test components such as a practical demonstration of skills.

Passing the National Certification Examination for Therapeutic Massage and Bodywork is a concrete means of validating professional achievement. Appendix D provides additional information on finding out more about the examination.

Laws and Legislation
State and Local Regulation

The types of legislative controls most often encountered are state or provincial controls and local controls. A province is a political unit of some countries, such as Canada. It typically is a large area made up of many small local units of government. In the United States, states are the equivalent of provinces. States are further subdivided into counties, local townships, and cities.

The main purpose of a law or an ordinance is to protect the safety and welfare of the public. When a governing body decides to enact regulations, the regulations must meet this criterion. Laws and ordinances are not passed to protect the interests of a small group, also known as a special interest group.

Many but not all health professionals are regulated at the state level through licensing (Proficiency Exercise 2-15). If the government feels that a particular activity could cause harm to the public, it seeks to control and limit the

individuals who can participate in the activity. (For example, physicians, nurses, chiropractors, physical therapists, dentists, builders, electricians, cosmetologists, and plumbers are all licensed.) Requirements for a knowledge base and the amount and type of education are determined. Tests, often called *boards*, are given. The scope of practice is described in the law that governs the licensed professional.

If the state does not choose to license a particular profession (occupational licensing), local governments (usually townships and cities) can choose to regulate activities within their jurisdiction. Again, local laws, usually called *ordinances*, are in place to protect the public's safety and welfare. Local governments are most concerned with what types of activities go on in their region and the way the land is used (zoning).

If the state licenses a professional, the local government does not feel the need to regulate the actual practice of the professional by setting educational standards and administering competency tests. The local government does regulate where the professional may work. This is done through zoning ordinances. Professionals such as physicians, lawyers, and accountants often are required to locate their place of business in a particular zone or area of land use. Land use usually is determined on a master plan that directs the way the local government wants to see the area grow and develop. It is important to designate areas as residential (living), industrial (manufacturing), retail business districts (commercial), professional offices, and farming (agriculture). Without such zoning, a loud industrial operation could disturb the quiet living in a residential area. Local governments are also concerned with the safety of the buildings in their area. Monitoring the safety of buildings is the responsibility of the building inspector.

Medical massage should be supervised by licensed medical professionals, and the responsibility for public safety falls to the supervising personnel. If proper supervision is in place, states have no reason to license massage professionals unless they feel that wellness massage is a threat to the public's safety and welfare. Medical massage usually is provided as part of a multidisciplinary practice. Because the massage professional is working in an estab-

2-15
PROFICIENCY EXERCISE

1. Investigate the legal requirements to practice massage in your area.
2. Collect information to create an educational packet about massage for government officials and the public.
3. Attend a local government board meeting and observe the process.

lished medical setting and the massage is part of the medical treatment plan, local regulation is seldom an issue.

The inherent problems include wellness massage businesses being classified with massage parlors and medical rehabilitative massage being practiced outside an established medical setting without direct medical supervision.

A more serious difficulty arises when other health professionals feel that massage practitioners are doing medical or rehabilitative massage, which is more in line with the other health professionals' scope of practice. This difficulty may also arise with athletic trainers and exercise physiologists, who may not be state licensed but who usually have at least a bachelor's degree in their chosen field. The level of education becomes an important factor. A legitimate concern of these professionals is a lack of adequate education of the massage professional in procedures and the effects of massage in relation to a total treatment plan. Massage therapy educators must address the issue of appropriate education to accommodate those who want to work in the medical setting.

A case could be made for licensing massage therapists as a means of protecting the public, with the profession's need for formal training in sanitation, contraindications, and necessary referrals to licensed medical personnel for suspected health problems. A case also could be made for enacting massage laws to protect the massage professional from discrimination and provide the ability to practice a professional livelihood.

Currently therapeutic massage is not consistently regulated by law. Each state in the United States, each province in Canada, and each country in Europe has different ways of dealing with massage regulation. Because of this inconsistency, massage professionals must carefully research the governmental controls and the laws that apply in the areas where they plan to open their business.

Many old laws and local massage ordinances were written to control prostitution by preventing the practice of massage. This type of ordinance is easy to recognize because it specifies finger printing, medical examinations for sexually transmitted disease, and other degrading requirements. Although the situation is improving, local ordinances of this type are still found in states where the profession of massage has not yet been licensed.

Currently about 40% of the United States has some type of state licensing for the professional practice of therapeutic massage. The trend continues in this direction. Licensing requirements in the European countries, Canada, and other countries vary to such an extent that it is impossible to cover all of that information in this chapter. Overall, licensing requirements are changing quickly. Educational requirements that allow a person to sit for a licensing examination are increasing, and the competencies reflected in the examinations are becoming more sophisticated, reflecting the evolving professionalism of therapeutic massage. To obtain the most current information on licensing requirements, contact licensed massage therapy schools or governmental licensing offices in your specific area.

In states where massage professionals must be licensed, the practitioner still must comply with local zoning ordinances and building requirements when setting up a professional practice. If the state licenses massage, the local government usually treats the massage professional like any other licensed health or service professional. The business is classified as a service, and it must be set up in the proper zoning location, usually an area of office or commercial zoning.

Local governments often discourage any type of business operation in residential areas but with special restriction will designate what types of businesses can be operated from a home. These home occupations usually are service orientated rather than retail (the sale of goods) and limit traffic to and from the home. To establish a home office, the home may need to have a special and separate area, including a separate entrance. Another requirement might be that no employees other than the family in the home may be hired. Sometimes only those with a special need, such as a disability that prevents working outside the home, are eligible for a home office permit. Usually a special permit is required for a home office; each local government is different. Many massage practitioners choose to work from a home office. The "cottage industry," or home business, is growing rapidly. A massage practice is a business that fits well within these special requirements.

It is true that written tests and practical demonstrations cannot measure the massage professional's gentleness, care, nonjudgmental behavior, intuition, and touch. This does not mean that formal tests are not valid; they are. Unfortunately, most governmental bodies are not concerned with these attributes. Local governments need to establish that the massage business is legitimate therapeutic massage and not a front for prostitution. State governments must protect the public's health, safety, and welfare from the unregulated practice of massage. Both units of government must protect the public from potentially dangerous acts by defining performance criteria based on education or the ability to pass a test.

Licensing, compliance with ordinances (Box 2-17), and passing any of the nationally recognized certification examinations are important in the professional practice of massage. The bottom line is, the massage professional must comply with the existing standards of practice, both required and voluntary. If a difficult state law or local ordinance is encountered, massage therapists must work together to change the regulation. The staff at a licensed massage school is the best resource on procedures for working with local governments to change a nonsupportive massage ordinance.

Reciprocity

Reciprocity is the right of exchange of privileges between governing bodies. Some states have similar licensing requirements for professionals. When this is the case, a state may accept a different state's license. This is not common for many professionals, and it is even less common for

box 2-17

STEPS FOR COMPLYING WITH LICENSING REQUIREMENTS

1. Find out whether your state or province requires licensing. Contact the Department of Licensing and Regulation, Occupational Licensing Division, for this information. If state licensing is required, find out what educational requirements must be met to take the examination.
2. If your state does not have licensing, contact the local government where you intend to work to inquire about local ordinances. Obtain a copy of the ordinances and read them carefully. Look especially for the educational, zoning, and facility requirements. Whether you live in a city, township, or similar government unit, the clerk's office is the department that usually has this information.

Note: Even if there is no state or local regulation, it is a good idea to attend only a licensed school or an approved training program. Other states or local governments may require this type of education, and without it you cannot practice in their areas.

3. Shop carefully for your school of massage training. Contact the state Department of Education, and confirm that the school is licensed and in compliance with state regulations.
4. Before renting, buying, or setting up the actual massage practice, contact the local government concerning zoning requirements and building codes. If you are considering a home office, check the zoning ordinances to make sure you will be in compliance. Again, your city or township officials (usually the clerk) are your best sources of information.

   Zoning permits require a public hearing. Your neighbors are notified by mail, and the hearing is advertised in the newspaper. Contact the zoning department to find out what action is required. Whether you are establishing your business in a home office or a business zone, contact the neighbors to explain your business and find out their response. Without their approval, or at least lack of opposition, you are unlikely to obtain a permit. Attend the hearing at all costs. Remember: **no permit = no business.** Zoning permits may require 6 to 8 weeks to complete. If you start your business without proper permits, you could be shut down at any time by government authorities.
5. Before you actually rent space or begin your business, contact the local government and apply for any necessary permits or business licenses. Make sure you meet all regulations. Fees can run anywhere from $25 to $500.

massage therapists. Individual state licensing or any type of certification does not secure the right to practice massage in any location other than that of the government issuing the license.

Regulations, standards of practice, codes of conduct, scopes of practice, and so forth are methods of setting the rules for cooperative professional relationships. All organized groups have rules that permit effective interaction between members. Respect is important, and working together as a team is essential in professional practice. Let us hope that the massage therapy profession is an example of cooperation, respect for other professions, and ethical standards of practice that provide for internal professional regulation and compliance with external government control.

DEALING WITH SUSPECTED UNETHICAL OR ILLEGAL BEHAVIOR OF FELLOW BODYWORK PROFESSIONALS

section objectives

Using the information presented in this section, the student will be able to perform the following:

■ **List and explain the four steps involved in reporting unethical behavior.**

What is the appropriate way to address unethical behavior and violations of standards of practice by colleagues? This is a difficult dilemma. Everything covered in this chapter is an important consideration when dealing with inappropriate behavior of others (Proficiency Exercise 2-16). When concern develops about the conduct of a colleague,

2-16

PROFICIENCY EXERCISE

Working in groups of three, make up and then develop a specific situation in which a colleague has acted in an unethical manner. Exchange responses with a different group and role play to resolve the situation. One student acts as the massage practitioner, one plays the colleague, and the other evaluates the way the situation was handled. Role play different situations until each student has had a chance to play each role. Use the problem-solving model and communication skills during the role play.

an approach that combines self-reflection, peer support, supervision, and effective communication skills is the best way to deal with these situations.

Self-Reflection

Carefully reflect on the personal motivation causing the concern. It is important that motives for confronting a fellow professional be based on a genuine concern for the person and her clients, as well as the higher good of the profession as a whole. It is necessary to make sure that the situation is purely one of professional ethical concern and not a reaction based on personal values or beliefs.

Peer Support and Supervision

Discuss the situation with a colleague in a peer support situation, maintaining the confidentiality of the suspected party. Explore the motives supporting the concern with a supervisor.

Talking with Those Involved

If others share your concern, speak directly to the colleague. Often the person is not consciously aware of the breach of standards of practice or that the behavior appears to be unethical. Peer support and bringing the concern to his attention can help resolve the problem.

Formal Reporting

Depending on the seriousness of the infraction and the colleague's response, it may be necessary to file a formal complaint through the professional organization or the legal system in your area.

It is unprofessional to ignore unethical behavior in colleagues. A willingness to be involved with profession-wide ethical concerns supports professional integrity as a whole.[1] Carefully document the concerns and the process of intervention. Follow all ethical principles in these types of situations.

SUMMARY

A tremendous amount of information has been covered in this chapter. Years of experience confirm that when a professional encounters difficulty in the professional setting, it is seldom a problem with a technical skill and almost always an ethical dilemma. Wise students will review this chapter time and again during the course of study and probably will find support in reviewing the information periodically as they mature in their professional practice after graduation.

Decision-making skills garnered using the problem-solving model and developing effective communication skills probably will prove to be some of the most valuable information in this text. Both decision making and communication are skills to be learned. Massage professionals must practice these skills to gain proficiency in the process. And as with any skill, when you first begin to use them, you will feel awkward and uncomfortable. That's okay. You probably will have the same feeling as you practice all the new skills in this text, such as body mechanics, draping procedures, and all the massage manipulations and techniques. It is not okay to avoid the practice needed to perfect the skills required of a massage professional.

Ethical behavior is professional behavior. It revolves around a high regard and respect for our clients, for other health, training, and service professionals, and for ourselves. Being a professional is a compassionate and caring responsibility that requires a commitment to continued learning, self-reflection, and the highest good for all concerned. For massage and bodywork professionals, it is a privilege to serve others in such an important way and watch as the respect we give our clients evolves into a respect for ourselves.

REFERENCES

1. Corey G, Corey MS, Callanan P: *Issues and ethics in the helping professions,* ed 4, Pacific Grove, Calif, 1993, Brooks/Cole Publishing.
2. *Hands On* 14(3): 1998 (newsletter of the American Massage Therapy Association).
3. *Regulated Health Professions Act and the Massage Therapy Act,* Ontario, Canada, 1992, Ontario.
4. *Webster's new universal unabridged dictionary deluxe,* ed 2, New York, 1983, Simon & Schuster.

WORKBOOK SECTION

Short Answer

1. Define *ethics*.

   _____

   _____

   _____

   _____

2. Why is it difficult to develop a definition for therapeutic massage?

   _____

   _____

   _____

   _____

3. Why does the massage professional need to understand the scope of practice for other professionals?

   _____

   _____

   _____

   _____

4. In what ways do massage practitioners avoid falling
into a situation that could allow them to be accused
of practicing medicine?

   _____

   _____

   _____

   _____

5. Why is it unethical to provide massage services to a
client the practitioner does not like or with whom the
practitioner is uncomfortable?

   _____

   _____

   _____

   _____

6. What is the importance of disclosure in the right of
refusal?

   _____

   _____

   _____

   _____

7. Why is informed consent so important?

   _____

   _____

   _____

   _____

8. In what way does the word *respect* relate to boundaries?

   _____

   _____

   _____

   _____

9. It is easy to determine the acts that constitute sexual
misconduct, but how do you decide if more subtle activities and feelings are a breach of the trust between
client and practitioner?

   _____

   _____

   _____

   _____

10. Why might a client interpret the experience of massage as a sexual one?

   _____

   _____

   _____

   _____

WORKBOOK SECTION

11. Why is it ethical to establish rules of conduct for the client and massage therapist and maintain professional space in the client-practitioner relationship?

_____

_____

_____

_____

12. What are the important aspects of credentialing for the massage practitioner?

_____

_____

_____

_____

13. Why does the massage professional need to understand legislative issues, local ordinances, and zoning regulations?

_____

_____

_____

_____

14. What is the main purpose of a law?

_____

_____

_____

_____

15. What are the two types of massage therapy practice?

_____

_____

_____

_____

WORKBOOK SECTION

Matching

Match the term to the best definition.

1. Applied kinesiology _____

2. Bodywork _____

3. Boundary _____

4. Certification _____

5. Coalition _____

6. Craniosacral and myofascial _____

7. Credential _____

8. Disclosure _____

9. Energetic approaches _____

10. Essential touch _____

11. Ethics _____

12. Exemption _____

13. Informed consent _____

14. Integrated approaches _____

15. Intimacy _____

16. License _____

17. Manual lymph drainage _____

18. Medical rehabilitative massage _____

19. Neuromuscular approaches _____

20. Oriental approaches _____

21. Right of refusal _____

22. Safe touch _____

23. Sexual misconduct _____

24. Scope of practice _____

25. Structural and postural integration approaches _____

26. Therapeutic massage _____

27. Wellness personal service massage _____

a. A term describing all the various forms of massage, movement, and touch therapy

b. Methods of bodywork that focus on subtle body responses

c. Vital, fundamental, primary touch that is crucial to well-being

d. A voluntary credentialing process that usually requires education and training, as well as testing administered privately or by governmental regulatory bodies

e. A tender, familiar, and understanding experience between human beings

f. A designation earned by completing a process that verifies a certain level of expertise in a given skill

g. Standards, ideals, morals, values, and principles of honorable, decent, fair, responsible, and proper conduct

h. Methods of bodywork that influence lymphatic movement

i. Methods of bodywork that evolved from the ancient Chinese systems

j. Methods of bodywork that influence the reflexive responses of the nervous system and its link to muscular function

k. Any sexually oriented behavior that occurs in the professional setting

l. The where, when, and how a professional may provide a service or function as a professional

m. Methods of bodywork derived from biomechanics, postural alignment, and the importance of the connective tissue structures

n. Personal space located within an arm's-length perimeter; Personal emotional space designated by morals, values, and experience

o. Combined methods of various forms of massage and bodywork

p. A case in which a professional is not required to comply with an existing law because of educational or professional standing

WORKBOOK SECTION

q. Acknowledging any situation that interferes with or affects the professional relationship and informing the client of that situation

r. A scientific art and discipline involving assessment and the systematic, external application of touch to the superficial soft tissue of the skin, muscles, tendons, ligaments, and fascia and to the structures that lie in the superficial tissue, methods of touch include stroking (effleurage), friction, vibration, percussion, kneading (pétrissage), stretching, compression, passive and active joint movements within the normal physiologic range of motion, and adjunctive applications of water, heat, and cold

s. Methods of evaluation and adaptation that use an application of muscle testing, along with various forms of massage and bodywork, for corrective procedures

t. Secure, respectful, considerate, sensitive, responsive, sympathetic, understanding, supportive, and empathetic contact

u. The level of professional responsibility based on extensive education that prepares the massage therapist to develop, maintain, rehabilitate, or augment physical function, to relieve or prevent physical dysfunction and pain, and to enhance the client's well-being; methods include assessment of the soft tissue and joints and treatment by soft tissue manipulation, hydrotherapy, remedial exercise programs, acinotherapy (light therapy), and client self-care programs

v. A type of credential required by law as a means of regulating the practice of a profession to protect the public health, safety, and welfare

w. Client authorization for any service from a professional, based on the premise that the massage professional has provided adequate information to enable the client to make an educated choice

x. A nonspecific approach to massage that focuses on assessment for the purposes of detecting contraindications to massage or a need for referral to other health care professionals and also for developing a health-enhancing physical state for the client

y. A group formed for a particular purpose

z. Methods of bodywork that work both reflexively and mechanically with the fascial network

aa. The entitlement of both the client and the professional to stop the session

Standards of Practice Activity

Put an X on the line by the situations that indicate a person is not able to provide informed consent.

a. _____ Elderly client living alone

b. _____ 50-year-old man taking high blood pressure medication

c. _____ Freshman high school student

d. _____ 30-year-old woman, victim of a closed head injury, who communicates with a computer

e. _____ 24-year-old developmentally disabled client

f. _____ Client who does not speak English, with no interpreter present

g. _____ Client who seems to be under the influence of alcohol

h. _____ 21-year-old woman in the third trimester of pregnancy

i. _____ Severely depressed client

j. _____ Elderly client with dementia

k. _____ Client who insists that you cure her sore knee

l. _____ Terminally ill hospice client

Determining Licensing Needs Activity

List five steps in determining licensing needs.

_____

_____

_____

_____

_____

WORKBOOK SECTION

Problem-Solving Exercises

1. A new client tells you about treatment he received during a massage in another community. Some of the information seems to conflict with the principles of the code of ethics presented in this text. The client explains that the massage professional told him he needed to lose weight; did not stop working on his feet when he asked her to; did not explain that a trigger point area could be sore the next day; gave him a hug at the end of the session without first asking permission; told a joke containing sexual innuendo; let the drape slip while massaging his buttocks; talked about difficulties with her own children; walked in to get a chart without knocking first while he was dressing after the session; and said that physical therapists were bad at dealing with neck pain and that she could fix his neck problem. He also indicated that the massage professional did not give him a receipt when he paid for the massage.

    Which of the 28 standards of practice presented in Box 2-4 did the massage professional breach, and in what way would you explain that you practice differently?

    _____

    _____

    _____

    _____

    _____

    _____

The following cases are situations in which intimacy issues must be explained. After reading each case, write three ways to deal with the issue. Use the clinical reasoning model to develop your answers.

2. Kathy has been a massage professional for 3 years. She has been seeing Mr. Adams for a monthly massage for 2 years. He is in the process of a divorce and begins to schedule a massage every week because of the stress. Last week he mentioned to Kathy how important the massage is for him and lightly touched her hand. Should Kathy be concerned?

    _____

    _____

    _____

    _____

    _____

3. Matt has been a massage therapist for 10 years. Recently he has been seeing a client, Jeff, who attended the same high school as Matt. Although they were only acquaintances during high school, Jeff speaks often of the good old school days. At the last appointment Jeff offered Matt an extra hockey ticket and asked if he would like to go to the game with him. How should Matt respond?

    _____

    _____

    _____

    _____

    _____

4. Mary is new to the massage therapy profession and has had only a few clients. She finds a new client very attractive and notices that she is spending extra time with that client each session. She recognizes that she is attracted to the client physically and emotionally. How should she handle the situation?

    _____

    _____

    _____

    _____

    _____

ANSWER KEY
Short Answer

1. Ethics is the system of rules, based on morals, values, and standards of accepted conduct, that guide correct behavior.
2. The variety of massage/bodywork methods makes it difficult to please all practitioners of specific approaches. It is hard to encompass all these approaches to develop a concise definition for our profession.
3. The scope of practice for therapeutic massage, when formally developed, must fit into the spaces left by these other professionals. Fortunately, the area left unfilled by other professionals is a very important space for personalized supportive wellness care. With additional training, massage therapists can become important team players and work within the scope of practice of other health care professionals to assist them in providing the best care for their clients.

WORKBOOK SECTION

4. To avoid such situations massage professionals must not focus on specific treatment for specific problems, but rather provide a service that helps the client maintain or enhance good health. The massage professional also must refer the client to other health care professionals when appropriate.

5. The massage therapist's touch is to be safe, nonjudgmental touch. How could we ethically say that we are providing this service for a client for whom we feel dislike, disapproval, or fear?

6. If a massage professional wishes to maintain a nondiscriminatory approach but cannot best serve a particular client, simple disclosure to the client of the massage practitioner's problem allows the massage professional to best serve the needs of the client without discrimination.

7. The relationship between the massage professional and client is based on professional trust and safety. If the client is unable to make an informed choice, the trust is broken and the touch is not safe.

8. All boundary concerns could be resolved through respect for clients that equally serves our needs and theirs. We invade a person's boundaries when our needs are put above their needs.

9. If each massage professional establishes professional boundaries, and these are respected by equal consideration of each person's needs in a situation, the massage professional's respect for the client and the client's understanding of professional ethics will support decision making in most such vague situations.

10. Short-lived feelings of sexual arousal that occur when a person relaxes have a physiologic basis. If the client has experienced essential touch only in a sexual situation, the client logically connects the two experiences. Education and explanation help clients understand the difference.

11. In the professional relationship, in which expectations and rules are understood clearly, clients can make an informed choice about their behavior. If the situation is vague and the rules change from week to week, the expectations between client and practitioner become unclear.

12. Massage practitioners must know what credentialing is required by law to practice massage therapy and what types of credentialing are voluntary. They also must know that credentials must be issued by verifiable sources.

13. Depending on where the massage therapist wants to practice, these legal issues to a large extent determine the requirements for starting a business.

14. The main purpose of a law is to protect the public's health, safety, and welfare.

15. Massage seems to be subdividing into wellness personal service massage and medical rehabilitative massage. Wellness personal service massage has an entry level educational requirement of 500 to 1000 clock hours. This is the standard in much of the United States. The medical rehabilitative type of massage is most typified by the educational requirement set by the Canadian provinces of Ontario and British Columbia, which is approximately 2200 clock hours of training. This is the equivalent of the associate's degree required for medical technicians such as respiratory therapists and physical therapy assistants. Practitioners involved in medical rehabilitative massage are supervised by a highly trained medical professional.

Matching

1. s	8. q	15. e	22. t
2. a	9. b	16. v	23. k
3. n	10. c	17. h	24. l
4. d	11. g	18. u	25. m
5. y	12. p	19. j	26. r
6. z	13. w	20. i	27. x
7. f	14. o	21. aa	

Standards of Practice Activity

c, e, f, g, i, j, k

Determining Licensing Needs Activity

1. Find out if your state or province requires licensing.
2. If a licensing program exists, find out the educational requirements for sitting for the boards. If your state does not have licensing, contact the local government where you intend to work to see if a local ordinance applies.
3. Contact the state Department of Education and confirm that the school you plan to attend is licensed and in compliance with state regulations.
4. Contact the local government about zoning requirements and building codes.
5. Contact the local government and apply for any permits or business licenses required.

WORKBOOK SECTION

Problem-Solving Exercises

(The numbers shown in parentheses in the answers below refer to the standards of practice list presented in Box 2-4, pp. 47-48.)

1. The client says that the massage professional told him he needed to lose weight (1), did not stop working on his feet when asked to (11), did not explain that a trigger point area could be sore the next day (10), gave him a hug at the end of the session without asking first (9), told a joke that had a sexual innuendo (18), let the drape slip while massaging the buttocks (11), talked about difficulties with her children (22), walked in to get a chart without knocking first and interrupted him getting dressed after the massage (1), said that physical therapists were bad at dealing with neck pain and that she could fix it (3, 8), and gave him no receipt for his payment (14).

2. Kathy can do any of the following:

    She can ignore the situation and see if it occurs again.

    After the massage, when she and Mr. Adams are in the office area, she can explain that she understands the extra stress he is under, but that it is important to remember the boundaries of the therapeutic relationship. During times of loss, it is easy to personalize a professional relationship (i.e., transference).

    She can acknowledge the touch when it happens and gently explain that although she understands that the massage helps with the stress and provides for professional companionship, it is important for both to remember the ethical standards of massage and the professional relationship.

3. Matt's choices are as follows:

    He can thank Jeff for the offer but decline, explaining the importance of not spending time with clients outside the professional setting, even when a past acquaintance exists.

    He can talk with Jeff after the massage and explain that although it's pleasant to remember school days, being a professional who provides massage services and spending social time together don't mix. He should thank Jeff for the offer but refuse it.

    He can let Jeff know that if he accepts the ticket, their professional relationship will have to end, and Jeff would have to see another therapist at the same office from now on.

4. Mary's choices are as follows:

    She can acknowledge to herself that her feelings are a form of countertransference and have nothing to do with the client; she then can restore the professional boundaries and time limits of the massage and continue to see the client.

    She can speak with the client about her feelings in a very brief way, explaining the difficulty with maintaining the professional relationship, and refer the client to another therapist.

    She can initiate peer review by talking to an experienced therapist. Another massage professional can understand the interactions that take place in the therapy room and may be able to give her some good advice on ways to handle such a situation. This peer support system is an excellent means of preserving our professional integrity and providing encouragement and guidance for each other.

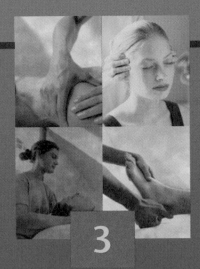

3

MEDICAL TERMINOLOGY FOR PROFESSIONAL RECORD KEEPING

objectives

After completing this chapter, the student will be able to perform the following:

- Identify the three word elements used in medical terms
- Combine word elements into medical terms
- Comprehend unfamiliar medical terms
- Identify pertinent abbreviations used in health care and their meanings
- Relay relevant anatomy and physiology terminology
- Combine this information to be used for effective professional record keeping

THE study of medical terminology provides a key to understanding the accepted language of the sciences. As massage therapy again moves into the position of a medically valid service, it is becoming increasingly important for the massage professional to be able to speak, write, and understand scientific language. In addition, the massage professional must be able to maintain client records effectively. The ability to record written information accurately and concisely depends on the correct use of terminology and an organized approach to charting procedures. This chapter provides an outline of the medical terminology most often encountered by the massage professional, particularly as it relates to charting and record-keeping procedures.

This chapter consolidates the vast array of medical terminology, focusing on that of specific use to the massage professional. Success in mastering the information in this chapter depends on the use of both a medical terminology textbook and a medical dictionary. Developing skills in using medical dictionaries, medication reference books, and other reference materials is important. The expanding and changing knowledge base makes it almost impossible to remember all the details required for professional practice. The chapter frequently includes a list of the terms most often encountered by the massage professional. Definitions for these words are available in a medical terminology text or medical dictionary.

Exploring medical terminology automatically provides an overview of anatomy and physiology. This section is not meant to replace an anatomy and physiology text. The purpose of this information is to provide a quick reference as the student develops record-keeping and charting skills. Used with a standard anatomy and physiology textbook and class instruction, this section can help the professional focus on information specific to the field of massage. The recommended anatomy and physiology text is Fritz's *Mosby's Basic Science for Soft Tissue and Movement Therapies* because it has been developed specifically for massage and bodywork students. However, the information in this chapter is relevant for use with any comprehensive anatomy and physiology book.

The information in this chapter is significant for understanding massage as it relates to anatomy, physiology, pathophysiology, and client records. Because the basis for medical terminology is scientific language, understanding this information helps the massage student understand massage therapy research as well as articles and books on subjects related to massage.

Learning the names of muscles, bones, joints, and other anatomic structures serves as a firm foundation for understanding and correct use of medical terminology.

It is important to have agreement across different medical fields regarding terminology. Without a common language we cannot communicate. Massage professionals must be able to communicate with their clients in a common language both can understand. It is just as important to understand the communications of other health professionals.

Currently, the terminology used in massage therapy is inconsistent. Although similar words are used, the meanings of those words do not always coincide. The definitions for the massage therapy vocabulary in this textbook are based on traditional Swedish definitions, Canadian resources, available books, and common knowledge. This chapter offers a basis for agreement for terminology for the massage profession. This must occur before others in the health profession can communicate with us as a group. As is mentioned in Chapter 1, Ling had difficulty in communicating with the established authorities of his time because he did not speak their language. To receive the respect and understanding of other health professionals, we as massage professionals must explain ourselves in terms other health professionals understand and patiently educate them in our language.

MEDICAL TERMINOLOGY

section objectives

Using the information presented in this section, the student will be able to perform the following:

- **Define words by breaking them down into their word elements**
- **Use Appendix A to identify indications and contraindications to massage**
- **List and define anatomy and physiology terminology by body system**
- **List and identify common abbreviations**

Fundamental Word Elements

Medical terms are made up of a combination of word elements. A term can be interpreted easily by separating the word into its elements. These word elements include prefixes, roots, and suffixes.

Prefixes

A **prefix** is placed at the beginning of a word to alter its meaning. A prefix cannot stand alone; it must be combined with another word element. See Table 3-1 for a list of common prefixes.

Root Words

Root words provide the fundamental meanings of words. Combined roots, prefixes, and suffixes form medical and scientific terms. A vowel, called a *combining vowel,* is often added when two roots are combined, or when a suffix is added to a root. The vowel used is usually an *o* and occasionally an *i.* See Table 3-2 for a list of common root words.

t a b l e   3 - 1
COMMON PREFIXES

Prefix	Meaning	Prefix	Meaning
a-, an-	Without or not	intro-	Into, within
ab-	Away from	leuk-	White
ad-	Toward	macro-	Large
ante-	Before, forward	mal-	Bad, illness, disease
anti-	Against	mega-	Large
auto-	Self	micro-	Small
bi-	Double, two	mono-	One, single
circum-	Around	neo-	New
contra-	Against, opposite	non-	Not
de-	Down, from, away from, not	para-	Abnormal
dia-	Across, through, apart	per-	By, through
dis-	Separation, away from	peri-	Around
dys-	Bad, difficult, abnormal	poly-	Many, much
ecto-	Outer, outside	post-	After, behind
en-	In, into, within	pre-	Before, in front of, prior to
endo-	Inner, inside	pro-	Before, in front of
epi-	Over, on	re-	Again
eryth-	Red	retro-	Backward
ex-	Out, out of, from, away from	semi-	Half
hemi-	Half	sub-	Under
hyper-	Excessive, too much, high	super-	Above, over, excess
hypo-	Under, decreased, less than normal	supra-	Above, over
in-	In, into, within, not	trans-	Across
inter-	Between	uni-	One
intra-	Within		

Suffixes

A **suffix** is a word element that is placed at the end of a root to alter the meaning of the word. Suffixes cannot stand alone; like prefixes, they must accompany a root to form a word. The suffix should be the starting point when interpreting medical terms.

Roots ending with a consonant require a combining vowel. If the root ends with a vowel and the suffix begins with a vowel, the vowel at the end of the root is deleted. See Table 3-3 for a list of common suffixes.

Combining Word Elements

Word elements are the building blocks that are combined to create medical and scientific terminology. Prefixes al-ways precede roots and suffixes always follow roots (Proficiency Exercise 3-1).

Abbreviations

Abbreviations are shortened forms of words or phrases. They are used primarily in written communication to save time and space. Table 3-4 is a list of common abbreviations. A more complete list of acceptable abbreviations can be found in most medical dictionaries.

When you use abbreviations in any record keeping, including charting, provide an abbreviation key either on the forms or in a conspicuous place in the file. This is especially important if you generate a specialized list of ab-

table 3-2
COMMON ROOT WORDS

Root (combining vowel)	Meaning	Root (combining vowel)	Meaning
abdomin (o)	Abdomen	neur (o)	Nerve
aden (o)	Gland	ocul (o)	Eye
adren (o)	Adrenal gland	orth (o)	Straight, normal, correct
angi (o)	Vessel	oste (o)	Bone
arterio (o)	Artery	ot (o)	Ear
arthr (o)	Joint	ped (o)	Child, foot
broncho (o)	Bronchus, bronchi	pharyng (o)	Pharynx
card, cardi (o)	Heart	phleb (o)	Vein
cephal (o)	Head	pnea	Breathing, respiration
chondr (o)	Cartilage	pneum (o)	Lung, air, gas
colo	Colon	proct (o)	Rectum
cost (o)	Rib	psych (o)	Mind
crani (o)	Skull	pulmo	Lung
cyan (o)	Blue	py (o)	Pus
cyst (o)	Bladder, cyst	rect (o)	Rectum
cyt (o)	Cell	rhin (o)	Nose
derma	Skin	sten (o)	Narrow, constriction
duoden (o)	Duodenum	stern (o)	Sternum
encephal (o)	Brain	stomat (o)	Mouth
enter (o)	Intestines	therm (o)	Heat
fibro (o)	Fiber, fibrous	thorac (o)	Chest
gastr (o)	Stomach	thromb (o)	Clot, thrombus
gyn, gyne, gyneco	Woman	thyr (o)	Thyroid
hem, hema, hemo, hemat (o)	Blood	toxic (o)	Poison, poisonous
hepat (o)	Liver	trache (o)	Trachea
hydr (o)	Water	ur (o)	Urine, urinary tract, urination
hyster (o)	Uterus	urethr (o)	Urethra
ile (o), ili (o)	Ileum	urin (o)	Urine
laryng (o)	Larynx	uter (o)	Uterus
mamm (o)	Breast, mammary gland	vas (o)	Blood vessel, vas deferens
my (o)	Muscle	ven (o)	Vein
myel (o)	Spinal cord, bone marrow	vertebr (o)	Spine, vertebrae
nephr (o)	Kidney		

table 3-3 COMMON SUFFIXES	
Suffix	**Meaning**
-algia	Pain
-asis	Condition, usually abnormal
-cele	Hernia, herniation, pouching
-cyte	Cell
-ectasis	Dilation, stretching
-ectomy	Excision, removal of
-emia	Blood condition
-genesis	Development, production, creation
-genic	Producing, causing
-gram	Record
-graph	Diagram, recording instrument
-graphy	Making a recording
-iasis	Condition of
-ism	Condition
-itis	Inflammation
-logy	Study of
-lysis	Destruction of, decomposition
-megaly	Enlargement
-oma	Tumor
-osis	Condition
-pathy	Disease
-penia	Lack, deficiency
-phasia	Speaking
-phobia	Exaggerated fear
-plasty	Surgical repair or reshaping
-plegia	Paralysis
-rrhage, -rrhagia	Excessive flow
-rrhea	Profuse flow, discharge
-scope	Examination instrument
-scopy	Examination using a scope
-stasis	Maintenance, maintaining a constant level
-stomy, -ostomy	Creation of an opening
-tomy, -otomy	Incision, cutting into
-uria	Condition of the urine

3-1 PROFICIENCY EXERCISE

Combine five words using the prefixes, root words, and suffixes listed in Tables 3-1 to 3-3. Define the words created. Look up each word in a medical dictionary to verify that it exists and you have the correct meaning and spelling.

Example: *Fibromyalgia*

Divided into elements: *Fibro- fiber, my- muscle, algia- pain*

My definition: *Pain in muscle fibers*
Dictionary definition: *Diffuse muscle pain*

1.

2.

3.

4.

5.

table 3-4
COMMON ABBREVIATIONS

Abbreviation	Meaning	Abbreviation	Meaning
ABD	Abdomen	IBW	Ideal body weight
ADL	Activities of daily living	ICT	Inflammation of connective tissue
ad lib	As desired	Id.	The same
alt. dieb	Every other day	L	Left, length, lumbar
alt. hor	Alternate hours	lig	Ligament
alt. noct	Alternate nights	M	Muscle, meter, myopia
AM (am, AM)	Morning	ML	midline
a.m.a.	Against medical advice	meds	Medications
ANS	Autonomic nervous system	n	Normal
approx	Approximately	NA	Nonapplicable
as tol	As tolerated	OB	Obstetrics
BM	Bowel movement	OTC	Over-the-counter
BP	Blood pressure	P	Pulse
Ca	Cancer	PA	Postural analysis
CC	Chief complaint	PM (pm)	Afternoon
c/o	Complains of	PT	Physical therapy
CPR	Cardiopulmonary resuscitation	Px	Prognosis
CSF	Cerebrospinal fluid	R	Respiration, right
CVA	Cerebrovascular accident, stroke	R/O	Rule out
DM	Diabetes mellitus	ROM	Range of motion
DJD	Degenerative joint disease	Rx	Prescription
Dx	Diagnosis	SOB	Shortness of breath
ext	Extract	SP, spir	Spirit
ft	Foot or feet	Sym.	Symmetric
fx	Fracture	T	Temperature
GI	Gastrointestinal	TLC	Tender loving care
GU	Genitourinary	Tx	Treatment
h (hr)	Hour	URI	Upper respiratory infection
H_2O	Water	WD	Well-developed
Hx	History	WN	Well-nourished

breviations, such as *SWM* for *Swedish massage* or *CTM* for *connective tissue method.*

Excessive use of abbreviations is discouraged. An overabundance of abbreviations results in a passage that is difficult to read and that requires interpretation. If you are unsure whether an abbreviation is acceptable, write the term out to communicate accurately.

Avoid using jargon. Jargon consists of word forms specially developed within a system or the use of existing words that have other definitions besides the dictionary meaning. The word *mouse* is a computer jargon word, for example. Many forms of jargon exist in the bodywork world, which continues to confuse communication. In general, the words used in record keeping should be found in either a standard comprehensive dictionary or a medical dictionary and represent the definition as listed.

On occasion jargon becomes understandable within the general community. Referring to the previous example of "mouse," many readers would have thought immediately of the computer hand controller instead of a brown furry creature. This is an example of the way language can change. As massage becomes more generally accepted, much of our language will be standardized and lose its jargon quality. Until then clarity and concise expression is crucial when choosing the words used for written records.

Terms Related to Diagnosis and Diseases

The massage practitioner must be able to understand medical terms related to diagnosis and various diseases. Two terms often encountered by the massage professional related to the diagnosis of a disease are **indication** and **contraindication.**

An indication is a situation in which an approach would be beneficial for health enhancement, treatment of a particular condition, or support of a treatment modality other than massage.

A contraindication exists when an approach may be harmful (Proficiency Exercise 3-2). Contraindications may be further subdivided by severity:

- General avoidance of application—do not massage
- Regional avoidance of application—do massage but avoid a particular area
- Application with caution usually requiring supervision from appropriate medical or supervising personnel—do

---

3 - 2

PROFICIENCY EXERCISE

1. *In a medical dictionary, look up and define each of the following terms related to the diagnosis of disease conditions of the body:*

acute	diagnosis
ambulatory	malignant
anomaly	metastatic
atrophy	prognosis
benign	sign
chronic	symptom
clinic	syndrome
clinical	systemic

massage but carefully select the type of methods to be used, duration of the massage, and frequency

Terminology of Location and Position

Directional Terms

Directional terms are used to describe the way one body part relates to another. The massage professional must be able to use directional terminology to describe a location of an area of the body accurately.

The directional terms in Fig. 3-1 are used most often (Proficiency Exercise 3-3).

The abdomen is divided into four quadrants, and the location of abdominal organs and contents is described in terms of the quadrants in which they are located (Fig. 3-2).

Positional Terms

Positional terms are used to describe the relationship of the body to the different planes (Proficiency Exercise 3-4):

1. *Anatomic position*—The stance of the body when it is erect, with the arms hanging to the side, palms facing forward
2. *Erect position*—The body in a standing position
3. *Supine position*—The body lying in a horizontal position with the face up
4. *Prone position*—The body lying with the face down in a horizontal position

---

3 - 2

PROFICIENCY EXERCISE—CONT'D

2. *In a medical dictionary, look up and define each of the following terms related to diseases:*

bacterial

cancer

congenital

degenerative

epidemic

exacerbation

fungal

idiopathic

infectious

trauma

viral

3. **Write a descriptive statement about a fictional client. Use at least five terms listed in this section.**

Example: *Mr. X reveals during the client history procedure that he is suffering from an <u>acute exacerbation</u> of a <u>chronic viral infectious</u> process.*

Your Turn

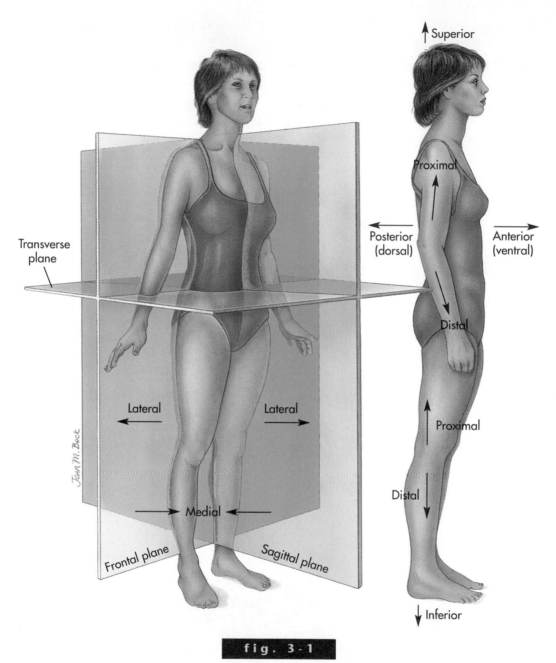

fig. 3-1

Directions and planes of the body. (From Thibodeau GA, Patton KT: *Structure and function of the body,* ed 10, St Louis, 1997, Mosby.)

PROFICIENCY EXERCISE

Consult your medical dictionary or medical terminology text to define the following terms:

anterior   medial

cephalad   peripheral

caudad   plantar

deep   posterior

distal   proximal

dorsal   superior

external   superficial

inferior   valgus

internal   varus

lateral   volar

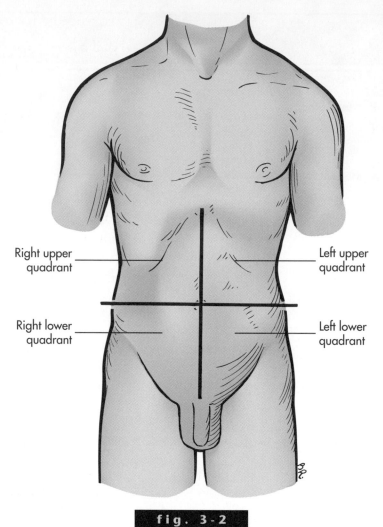

fig. 3-2

Quadrants of the abdomen. (From Fritz S, Paholsky KM, Grosenbach MJ: *Mosby's basic science for soft tissue and movement therapies,* St Louis, 1999, Mosby.)

3-4
PROFICIENCY EXERCISE

1. *Act out each directional and positional term by creating a movement or a pantomime or by assuming the position.*
2. *With a partner, place each other in the positions listed above. Say each term as you position your partner.*

---

5. *Laterally recumbent position*—The body lying horizontally on either the right or left side

Structure of the Body
Tissues

The structure of the body consists of tissues. A *tissue* is a collection of specialized cells that perform a special function. *Histo* is a root word meaning tissue. *Histology* is the study of tissue.

The primary tissues of the body are epithelial, connective, muscular, and nervous (Proficiency Exercise 3-5).

Organs and Systems

An *organ* is a collection of specialized tissues. An organ has specific functions, but it does not act independently of other organs.

Organs make up systems. The body as a whole is made

table 3-5	
SYSTEMS OF THE BODY AND THEIR IMPORTANT ORGANS	
System	*Organs in the system*
Musculoskeletal (can be classified separately as the skeletal, articular [joints], and muscular systems)	Bones, ligaments, skeletal muscles, tendons, joints
Nervous	Brain, spinal cord, nerves, special sense organs
Cardiovascular	Heart, arteries, veins, capillaries
Lymphatic	Lymphatic vessels, lymph nodes, spleen, tonsils, thymus gland
Digestive	Mouth, tongue, teeth, salivary glands, esophagus, stomach, small and large intestines, liver, gallbladder, pancreas
Respiratory	Nasal cavity, larynx, trachea, bronchi, lungs, diaphragm, pharynx
Urinary	Kidneys, ureters, urinary bladder, urethra
Endocrine	Endocrine glands: hypothalamus, hypophysis (pituitary), thyroid, thymus, parathyroid, pineal, adrenal, pancreas, gonads (ovary or testis)
Reproductive	Female: ovaries, uterine tubes (oviducts), uterus, vagina; male: testes, penis, prostate gland, seminal vesicles, spermatic ducts
Integumentary	Skin, hair, nails, sebaceous glands, sweat glands, breasts

up of several systems. Some of the systems are concentrated in a particular part of the body (e.g., the urinary system), whereas others reach out to all parts of the body, as the circulatory system does. The body comprises ten general systems (Table 3-5). Each system comprises organs that collectively perform specific functions. Consult an anatomy and physiology textbook for additional information.

Body Cavities

The body cavities contain the organs and are divided into ventral and dorsal regions (Fig. 3-3). The two dorsal cavities are the cranial cavity and the vertebral cavity. The three ventral cavities are the thoracic, abdominal, and pelvic cavities. Sometimes the abdominal and pelvic cavities are considered as one (Proficiency Exercise 3-6).

Posterior Regions of the Trunk

The back or posterior surface of the trunk is also divided into regions. The terms used to describe these regions are related to the names of the vertebrae in the spinal column (Fig. 3-4). In descending order they are as follows:

Cervical region: the neck (seven cervical vertebrae)
Thoracic region: the chest (twelve thoracic vertebrae)
Lumbar region: the loin (five lumbar vertebrae)
Sacral region: the sacrum (five sacral vertebrae that are fused into one bone)
Coccyx: the tailbone (four coccygeal vertebrae that are fused into one bone)

3-5

PROFICIENCY EXERCISE

Look up each of these tissues in a medical terminology book, anatomy and physiology textbook, or medical dictionary, and list the function of each tissue type.

Epithelial

Connective

Muscular

Nervous

The Skeletal System

The skeletal system consists of three elements: bone, cartilage, and ligaments.

Bone

Bone is a dense connective tissue comprising primarily calcium and phosphate; *os-, ossa-, oste-,* and *osteo-* are all combining forms that mean "bone."

The human skeleton comprises approximately 206 bones. The massage professional must be familiar with most of them. The following terms are commonly used:

skull or *cranium, cervical vertebrae, thoracic vertebrae, lumbar vertebrae, sacral vertebrae, coccygeal vertebrae, ribs, sternum, manubrium, body, xiphoid process, clavicle, scapula, humerus, ulna, radius, carpal bones, metacarpal bones, phalanges, pelvis, ilium, ischium, pubis, femur, patella, tibia, fibula, tarsal bones,* and *metatarsal bones* (Figs. 3-4 and 3-5). Other terms related to bones and landmarks on bones are *malleolus, process, crest, insertion, joint, olecranon, origin, spine, trochanter,* and *tuberosity.*

Cartilage

The skeletal system includes two types of cartilage. *Hyaline cartilage,* which is very elastic, cushiony, and slippery, makes up the articular surfaces at the joints, the cartilage between the ribs and at the nose, larynx, and trachea, and the fetal skeleton. It has a pearly, bluish color. *Hyaline* means glass. *White fibrocartilage,* which is elastic, flexible, and tough, is interarticular fibrocartilage found in joints such as the knee. The connecting fibrocartilage is cartilage

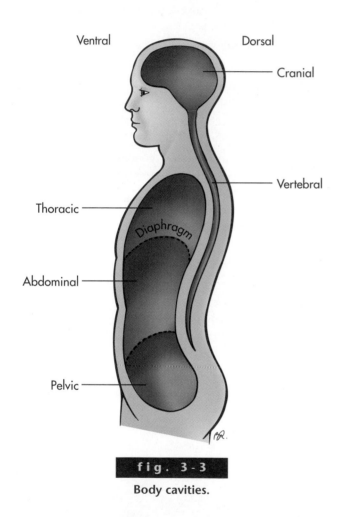

Ventral · Dorsal · Cranial · Vertebral · Thoracic · Diaphragm · Abdominal · Pelvic

fig. 3-3

Body cavities.

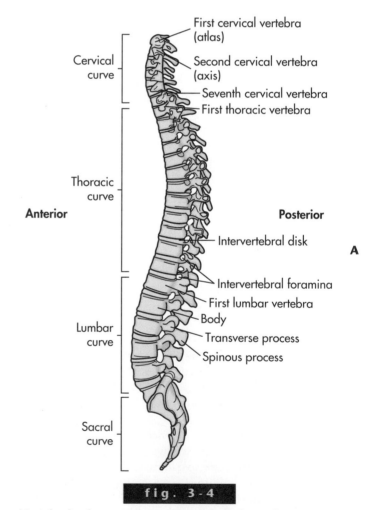

First cervical vertebra (atlas)
Cervical curve
Second cervical vertebra (axis)
Seventh cervical vertebra
First thoracic vertebra

Thoracic curve

Anterior   **Posterior**

Intervertebral disk

A

Intervertebral foramina
First lumbar vertebra
Body
Transverse process
Spinous process

Lumbar curve

Sacral curve

fig. 3-4

Vertebral column and common types of vertebrae (two views of T7 and L4 vertebrae). A, Vertebral column.

3-6

PROFICIENCY EXERCISE

Using clay or some other modeling compound, build the body cavities and the organs and structures they contain.

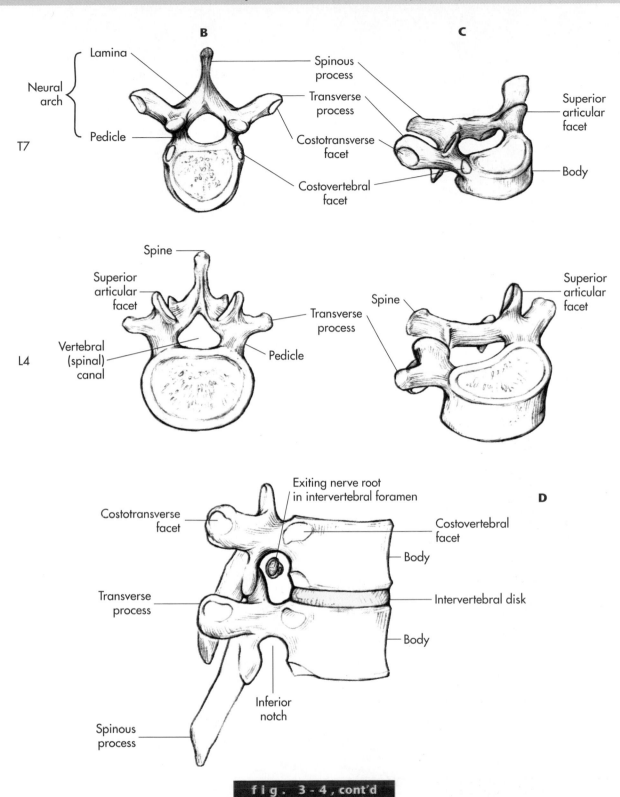

B, Superoinferior views. **C,** Right anterior oblique views. **D,** Intervertebral foramen. Vertebrae T5 and T6 have been articulated, and the resultant intervertebral foramen is shown with a segmental nerve in place. Blood vessels (not shown) enter and leave the interior of the vertebral canal through the intervertebral foramen. (**A** from Fritz S, Paholsky KM, Grosenbach MJ: *Mosby's basic science for soft tissue and movement therapies,* St Louis, 1999, Mosby; **B-D** from Mathers LH et al: *Clinical anatomy principles,* St Louis, 1996, Mosby.)

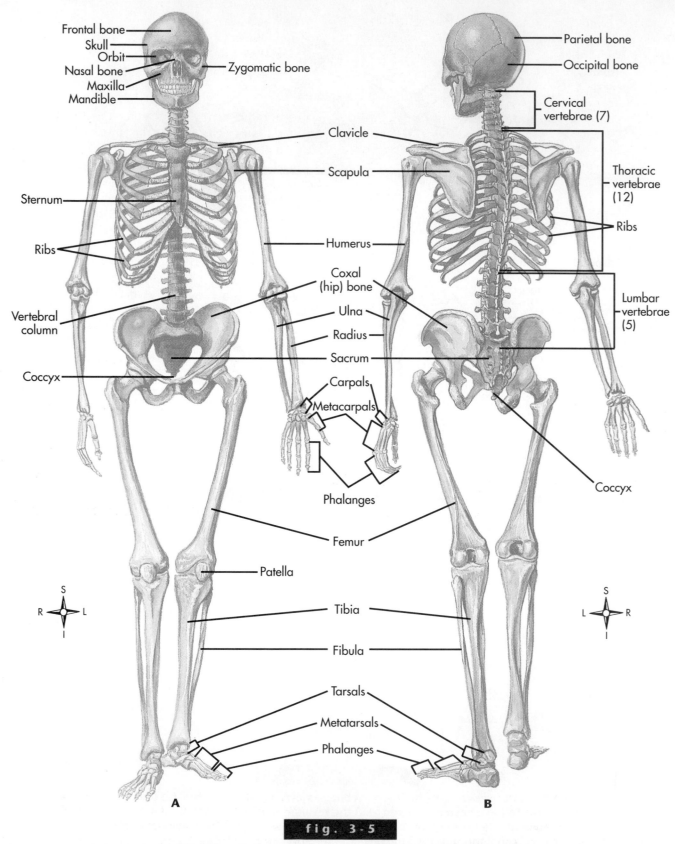

fig. 3-5

Skeleton. A, Anterior view. B, Posterior view. (From Thibodeau GA, Patton KT: *Anatomy and physiology,* ed 3, St Louis, 1996, Mosby.)

that is only slightly mobile. It is found between the vertebrae (referred to as *disks*) and between the pubic bones (the symphysis pubis).

Ligaments

A *joint* or *articulation* is the point at which the bones of the skeleton meet. Movable joints are covered by cartilage and are held together by ligaments. Ligaments are made of white fibrous tissue. They are pliant, flexible, strong, and tough (Proficiency Exercise 3-7).

The Articular System

Articulations are joints at which two or more bones meet. The articular system concerns all of the anatomic and functional aspects of the joints.

Joints

Joints are places where bones come together, where limbs are attached, and where the motion of the skeletal system occurs. Some joints are rigid, and some allow a great degree of flexibility.

The joints function to allow motion of the musculoskeletal system, bear weight, and hold the skeleton together.

Terms related to the articular system include the following: *articulation, flexibility, synarthrodial, amphiarthrodial, diarthrodial, symphysis pubis, sacroiliac, symphysis, articular cartilage, articular disks, ligaments, synovial fluid,* and *tendon.*

Types of movement permitted by diarthrodial joints. The types of movement permitted by diarthrodial joints are as follows (Fig. 3-6):

Flexion: bending that reduces the angle of a joint
Extension: straightening or stretching that increases the angle of a joint
Abduction: movement away *(ab-)* from the midline
Adduction: movement toward *(ad-)* the midline
Pronation: turning of the palm downward
Supination: turning of the palm upward (you can hold a bowl of soup in a supinated hand)
Eversion: turning *(version)* of the sole of the foot away from *(e-)* the midline (when you evert your foot you move your little toe toward your ear)
Inversion: turning *(version)* of the sole of the foot inward *(in-)*
Plantar flexion: bending of the plantar surface of the sole of the foot downward (plant your toes in the ground)

---

3 - 7

PROFICIENCY EXERCISE

1. *Consult your medical dictionary or medical terminology text to define the following terms:*

Fracture

Osteoarthritis

Osteochondritis

Osteochondrosis

Osteoporosis

Ankylosing spondylitis

2. *Using Appendix A choose one condition from the previous list and note any indications or contraindications involved.*

Condition:
Indications or contraindications:

3. *Palpate each bone listed in this section of text and say its name.*
4. *With a group of fellow students, assign each person to be a particular bone. By lying on the floor, build the skeleton by having each person assume the proper bone position. Be prepared to laugh and learn.*

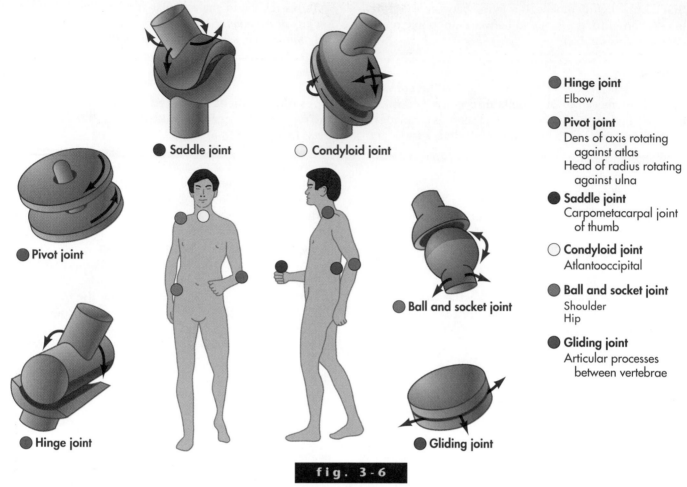

Saddle joint

Condyloid joint

Pivot joint

Hinge joint

Ball and socket joint

Gliding joint

● **Hinge joint**
Elbow

● **Pivot joint**
Dens of axis rotating
against atlas
Head of radius rotating
against ulna

● **Saddle joint**
Carpometacarpal joint
of thumb

○ **Condyloid joint**
Atlantooccipital

● **Ball and socket joint**
Shoulder
Hip

● **Gliding joint**
Articular processes
between vertebrae

fig. 3-6

Types of diarthrotic joints. Notice that the structure of each type dictates its function (movement). (Modified from Thibodeau GA, Patton KT: *Anatomy and physiology,* ed 3, St Louis, 1996, Mosby.)

Dorsiflexion: bending of the top or dorsal surface of foot toward shin

Rotation: rolling to the side (internal rotation: rolling toward the midline, external rotation: rolling away from the midline)

Circumduction: making a cone; the ability to move the limb in a circular manner

Protraction: thrusting a part of the body forward *(pro-)*

Retraction: pulling a part of the body backward *(re-)*

Elevation: raising a part of the body

Depression: lowering a part of the body

Opposition: the act of placing part of the body opposite another, as in placing the tip of the thumb opposite the tips of the fingers

Bursae. *Bursae* are closed sacs or saclike structures (bursa) usually close to the joint cavities, with a lining similar to the synovial membrane lining of a true joint. Some bursae are continuous with the lining of a joint. The function of a bursa is to lubricate an area between skin, tendons, ligaments, or other structures and bones where friction would otherwise develop (Proficiency Exercise 3-8).

The Muscular System

Tissues that are contractile make up the muscular system. Muscle is made up of three different types of tissue: cardiac muscle, smooth muscle, and skeletal muscle.

Muscle tissue is found in many organs of the body. Muscle tissue also makes up muscles, which are themselves organs. These muscles give the body shape and produce movement.

Skeletal Muscle

Each skeletal muscle is made up of sections. Most muscles have two ends, which are attached to other structures, and a belly.

Muscles cause and permit motion by the actions of contraction and relaxation. See Table 3-6 for terms used to describe movement.

Contraction refers to the reduction in size or the shortening of a muscle. When one muscle contracts, another opposite muscle is stretched and put into a state of tension. *Relaxation* occurs when tension is reduced, and thus the muscle returns to its resting size.

Muscles work in pairs of agonists and antagonists. *Ago-*

3 - 8
PROFICIENCY EXERCISE

1. Consult your medical dictionary or medical terminology text to define the following terms:

Ankylosis

Arthritis

Bursitis

Degenerative joint disease

Diastasis

Dislocation

Ganglion cyst

Genu valgum

Genu varum

Gout

Hallux malleus

Kyphosis

Lordosis

Rheumatoid arthritis

Scoliosis

Slipped disk

Spinal curvature

Spondylolisthesis

Sprain

Subluxation

Tendinitis

Tenosynovitis

2. Using Appendix A, choose one condition from the previous list and note any indications or contraindications involved.

Condition:
Indications or contraindications:

3. Do a dance that incorporates each of the joint movements listed in this section.

table 3-6

TERMS TO DESCRIBE MUSCLE MOVEMENT

Term	Definition
Adductor	Muscle moving a part toward the midline
Abductor	Muscle moving a part away from the midline
Flexor	Muscle that bends a part
Extensor	Muscle that straightens a part
Levator	Muscle that raises a part
Depressor	Muscle that lowers a part
Tensor	Muscle that tightens a part

nists are muscles responsible for the primary desired movement. The agonist is the prime mover. *Antagonists* are the muscles that oppose the action of the agonist.

Synergists are muscles that assist the agonists by holding a part of the body steady and thus giving leverage. Sometimes synergists also do the same action as the prime mover. The agonist-antagonist-synergist relationship permits the skeletal muscles to work in a purposeful manner and gives fluidity to motion. This fluid movement is referred to as *coordination*. See Fig. 3-7 for an anterior and posterior view of the muscular system.

Terms related to the muscular system include the following: *aponeurosis, asthenia, atrophy, belly, clonus, contracture, cramp, fascia, fascicle, fasciculation, hyperkinesia, hypertrophy, insertion, musculotendinous junction, myalgia, origin, proximal attachment, insertion, distal attachment, spasm, tendon,* and *tone.*

Names of muscles can be broken down into medical terminology word elements. Muscles are named for a variety of reasons, including where they are located, what they do, and the way they are shaped. Having a basic understanding of medical terminology can assist the student in both remembering and understanding muscle names (Table 3-7) (Proficiency Exercise 3-9).

The Nervous System

The nervous system is the most complex system in the body. The information included here on the workings of this system is very general but is expanded in the text where needed. Study of the nervous system is very important for the massage professional. Serious students of massage will challenge themselves to study the nervous system in comprehensive depth.

For purposes of study, terms related to the nervous system are presented in the following three groups:

1. Central nervous system (CNS)
2. Peripheral nervous system (PNS)
3. Autonomic nervous system (ANS)

Central Nervous System

The CNS is the center *(central)* of all nervous control. It consists of the brain and spinal cord, which are located in the dorsal cavity (cranial and vertebral).

Peripheral Nervous System

The PNS is composed of cranial and spinal nerves. The term *nerve* refers to a bundle of nerve fibers consisting of individual nerve cells outside the spinal cord or brain. The PNS consists of the nerves that carry impulses between the CNS and muscles, glands, skin, and other organs that are located outside (peripheral) the CNS. The part of the PNS that has nervous control over smooth muscle, heart muscle, and glands is called the *ANS.* Individual nerve cells are called *neurons.* Two types of nerve cells exist: sensory neurons and motor neurons.

Spinal nerves. The 31 pairs of spinal nerves are attached to the spinal cord along almost its entire length. They are named for the region of the spinal column through which they exit. Many of the spinal nerves are located in groups called *somatic nerve plexuses.* The term *somatic* refers to the body wall. Thus these nerve plexuses contain nerves that are involved with the wall of the body as opposed to the organs within the body. A *plexus* is a network of intertwined (plexus) nerves. The major plexuses of spinal nerves are the cervical plexus, brachial plexus, lumbar plexus, and sacral plexus.

Autonomic Nervous System

The ANS is the part of the PNS that is an automatic or self-governing (self *[auto]*, governing *[nomic]*) system. It is also called the *involuntary system* because the effects of this system are not usually under voluntary control. The ANS is divided in two parts: the sympathetic division and the parasympathetic division.

The sympathetic division controls the body's response to feelings *(sympath).* The nerves in this division come off the thoracic and lumbar segments of the spinal cord; thus this division is sometimes referred to as the *thoracolumbar division.* Actions resulting from these nerves include the fight or flight and fear responses. The reaction of some organs includes an increase in the heart rate, dilation of the pupils, and increase in adrenaline secretion. A person may sometimes exhibit great strength as a result of a sympathetic response.

The nerves in the parasympathetic division come off the cranial nerves and sacral segments of the spinal cord; thus it is sometimes called the *craniosacral division.* The

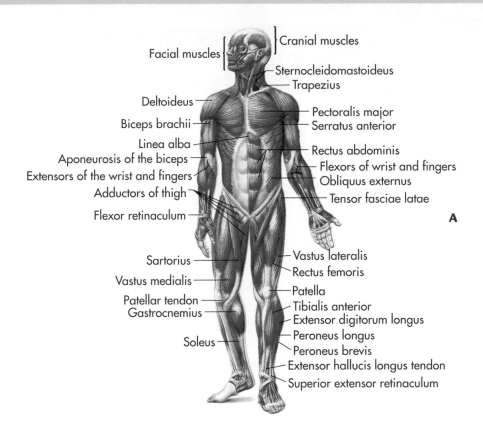

Cranial muscles
Facial muscles
Sternocleidomastoideus
Trapezius
Deltoideus
Pectoralis major
Biceps brachii
Serratus anterior
Linea alba
Rectus abdominis
Aponeurosis of the biceps
Flexors of wrist and fingers
Extensors of the wrist and fingers
Obliquus externus
Adductors of thigh
Tensor fasciae latae
Flexor retinaculum
A
Sartorius
Vastus lateralis
Rectus femoris
Vastus medialis
Patella
Patellar tendon
Tibialis anterior
Gastrocnemius
Extensor digitorum longus
Peroneus longus
Peroneus brevis
Soleus
Extensor hallucis longus tendon
Superior extensor retinaculum

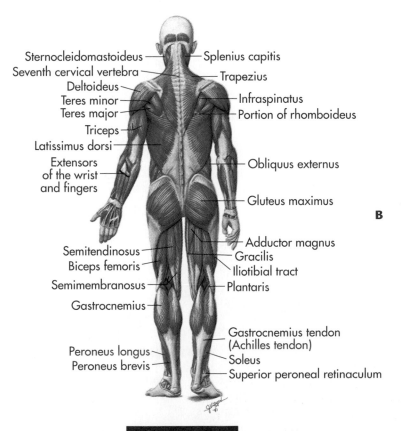

Sternocleidomastoideus
Splenius capitis
Seventh cervical vertebra
Trapezius
Deltoideus
Teres minor
Infraspinatus
Teres major
Portion of rhomboideus
Triceps
Latissimus dorsi
Extensors of the wrist and fingers
Obliquus externus
B
Gluteus maximus
Semitendinosus
Adductor magnus
Biceps femoris
Gracilis
Iliotibial tract
Semimembranosus
Plantaris
Gastrocnemius
Gastrocnemius tendon (Achilles tendon)
Peroneus longus
Soleus
Peroneus brevis
Superior peroneal retinaculum

fig. 3-7

Muscular system. A, Anterior view. B, Posterior view. (From LaFleur Brooks M: *Exploring medical language: a student-directed approach,* ed 3, St Louis, 1994, Mosby.)

table 3-7

MUSCLE DESCRIPTIONS USING MEDICAL TERMINOLOGY WORD ELEMENTS

The muscles listed have been chosen because they are made of common word elements. After learning this list, the student should be able to figure out the meaning of muscles not listed.

Muscle	Description
Abductor digiti minimi pedis	Little (*minimi*) muscle that moves the little toe (*digit*) away from (*abductor*) the midline of the foot (*pedis*)
Adductor longus	Long muscle that moves the leg toward (*adductor*) the midline
Adductor magnus	Large (*magnus*) muscle that moves the leg toward (*adductor*) the midline
Biceps brachii	Muscle with two (*bi-*) heads (*ceps*) in the arm (*brachii*)
Deltoid	Triangular (*deltoid*) muscle of the shoulder
Dilatator naris posterior	Muscle of the nose (*naris*) that opens (*dilate*) the back (*posterior*) portion of the nostril
External oblique	Outermost (*external*) muscle that is at an angle (*oblique*) from the ribs to the hip
Extensor hallucis longus	Long (*longus*) muscle that extends (*extensor*) the great toe (*hallucis*)
Extensor pollicis brevis	Short (*brevis*) muscle that extends (*extensor*) the thumb (*pollicis*)
Flexor carpi radialis	Muscle that flexes (*flexor*) the wrist (*carpi*) toward the radius (*radialis*)
Flexor carpi ulnaris	Muscle attached to the ulna (*ulnaris*) that flexes (*flexor*) the wrist (*carpi*) and hand
Frontalis	Muscle over the frontal bone
Gastrocnemius	Muscle that makes up the belly (*gastroc*) of the lower leg (*nemius*)
Gluteus maximus	Largest (*maximus*) muscle of the buttocks (*gluteus*)
Gluteus medius	Muscle of the buttocks (*gluteus*) that lies in the middle (*medius*) between the other gluteal muscles
Gracilis	Slender (*gracilis*) muscle of the thigh
Iliopsoas	Muscle that is formed from the iliacus and psoas major muscles; the iliacus extends from the iliac bone (*iliacus*), and the psoas major is the large (*major*) muscle of the loin (*psoas*)
Latissimus dorsi	Broadest (*latissimus*) muscle of the back (*dorsi*)
Masseter	Muscle of chewing (*masseter*) or mastication

parasympathetic division generally causes effects opposite (*para-*) those caused by the sympathetic system. These effects include constriction of the pupils, the return of the heart rate to normal, and the stimulation of the lacrimal glands to produce tears.

Intertwined nerves (plexus) of the ANS are called the *autonomic plexuses.* Some examples of these plexuses are the cardiac plexus, or the intertwined nerves of the heart (cardiac) and the celiac plexus, or the intertwined nerves of the organs of the abdomen (celiac). The latter plexus is sometimes called the *solar plexus* because of the sun ray (solar) fashion in which the nerves exit the plexus.

Proprioception. Proprioception is the kinesthetic sense. Sensory receptors receive information about position, rate of movement, contraction, tension, and stretch of tissues through the distortion and pressure on the sensory receptor. After proprioceptive sensory information is processed in the central nervous system, motor impulses carry the response message back to muscles. Muscle then contracts or relaxes to restore or change posture, movement, or position.

Terms related to proprioception include the following: *kinesthetic, muscle spindle cells, Golgi tendon organ,* and *joint kinesthetic receptors.*

table 3-7
MUSCLE DESCRIPTIONS USING MEDICAL TERMINOLOGY WORD ELEMENTS—CONT'D

Muscle	*Description*
Orbicularis oculi and oris	Muscles circling *(orbicularis)* the eye *(oculi)* or mouth *(oris)*
Palmaris longus	Long *(longus)* muscle of the palm *(palmaris)*
Pectineus	Muscle from the pubic *(pectineus)* bone
Pectoralis major	Large *(major)* muscle of the chest *(pectoralis)*
Peroneus longus	Long *(longus)* muscle attached to the fibula *(peroneus)*
Plantaris	Muscle that flexes the foot *(plantaris)* and leg
Pronator teres	Long round *(teres)* muscle that turns the palm downward into a prone *(pronator)* position
Rectus abdominis	Muscle that extends in a straight *(rectus)* line upward across the abdomen *(abdominis);* the center border of the left and right rectus abdominis muscles in the linea alba or the white *(alba)* line *(linea)* at the midline of the abdomen
Rectus femoris	Part of the quadriceps muscle that is straight *(rectus)* and lies near the femur *(femoris)*
Sartorius	Muscle of the leg that enables a person to sit in a cross-legged tailor's *(sartorial)* position
Semitendinosus	Muscle made up partly *(semi-)* of tendinous tissue; this is one of the hamstring muscles
Semimembranosus	Muscle made up partly *(semi-)* of membranous tissue; part of the hamstring group
Serratus anterior	Sawtooth-shaped *(serratus)* muscle in front of *(anterior)* the shoulder and ribcage
Soleus	Muscle that resembles a flat fish *(sole)* located in the calf of the leg
Sternocleidomastoid	Muscle attached to the breastbone *(sterno),* the collarbone *(cleido),* and the mastoid *(mastoid)* process of the temporal bone
Temporalis	Muscle over the temporal *(temporalis)* bone
Tensor fascia lata	Muscle that tenses *(tensor)* the fascia of the thigh *(lata)*
Teres minor	Small *(minor)* round *(teres)* muscle that moves the arm
Tibialis anterior	Muscle in front *(anterior)* of the tibia *(tibialis)*
Trapezius	Four-sided, trapezoid-shaped *(trapezius)* muscle of the shoulder
Triceps brachii	Three- *(tri-)* headed *(ceps)* muscle of the arm *(brachii)*
Vastus lateralis, medialis, intermedialis	Large *(vastus)* lateral *(lateralis),* toward the midline *(medialis),* and middle *(intermedius)* muscles of the quadriceps muscle group; the quadriceps has four *(quadri-)* heads *(ceps)*

Reflex

A *reflex* is an involuntary body response to a stimulus. Important reflexes stimulated by massage are crossed, extensor thrust, flexor withdrawal, intersegmental, monosynaptic, nociceptive, optical righting, pilomotor, psychogalvanic, postural, proprioceptive, righting, startle, stretch, tendon, vasomotor, and visceromotor reflexes.

Function of the Nervous System

The function of the nervous system is to receive impressions from the external environment, organize the information, and provide appropriate responses. In other words, the nervous system allows the body to react to outside influences (environment). Outside information enters the nervous system through nerve endings in the skin and in special sense organs. These nerve endings are referred to as *receptors.*

Nerve endings in the skin are sensitive to pain, touch, pressure, vibration, and temperature. Special sense nerve endings are responsible for taste, smell, vision, hearing, and sense of position and movement. Sensations from the environment are picked up by these receptors and sent to the CNS by way of the PNS. The CNS sorts out the information and sends back a message, again by way of the PNS.

The nervous system and neurotransmitters, along with the endocrine system, also maintain the internal environment, or the balance of the many activities within the body (homeostasis). Although the divisions of the nervous system may be treated independently, they do not function independently (Fig. 3-8).

Terms Related To Nerves

Afferent nerves are nerves that carry *(ferent)* messages to *(af-,* variation of *ad-)* the CNS; they are also known as *sensory nerves* because they pick up and transmit sensation *(sen)* (Proficiency Exercise 3-10).

Efferent nerves are nerves that carry *(ferent)* messages away *(ef-,* variation of *ex-)* from the brain, resulting in motion (motor). They are also known as *motor nerves.*

Cranial nerves are the 12 pairs of nerves that arise from the brainstem in the cranium or skull *(cranial).*

Spinal nerves are the 31 pairs of nerves that branch off the spinal cord.

A ganglion is a mass of nerve cell bodies located outside the CNS; ganglia is the *plural* form.

Neuro is the root word meaning "nerve."

The Cardiovascular System

The cardiovascular system consists of two parts, the heart and the blood vessels (Fig. 3-9). The heart is a four-chambered pump. *Arteries* are tubes (vessels) that deliver oxygenated blood to the body. They carry blood under pressure and are located relatively deep within the body.

---

3 - 9

PROFICIENCY EXERCISE

1. *Locate a more complete list of muscles in your anatomy and physiology textbook or medical dictionary. Break down five muscle names not listed in this section into their word elements. You will need a medical terminology book and medical dictionary to complete this exercise.*

   Example: *Auricularis Superior:* Aur- *means ear,* ar- *means pertaining to,* superior *means above or upward.*

   1.

   2.

   3.

   4.

5.

2. *An excellent way to remember the names of muscles is to make up ridiculous sentences that explain listed muscle names. The crazier these sentences are, the better you will remember them. Use this memory aid as you study muscles in your anatomy and physiology classes.*

   Examples:

   Rectus femoris: part of the quadriceps muscle that is straight (rectus) *and lies near the femur* (femoris)
   Attention rectus! Straighten up and the other three of you in the quads head out to the femur.
   Flexor carpi ulnaris: muscle that flexes (flexor) *the wrist* (carpi) *and hand and is attached to the ulna* (ulnaris)
   Help! There is a big carp pulling my wrist into flexion. It has my ulna in its mouth and my hand has it around the gills.

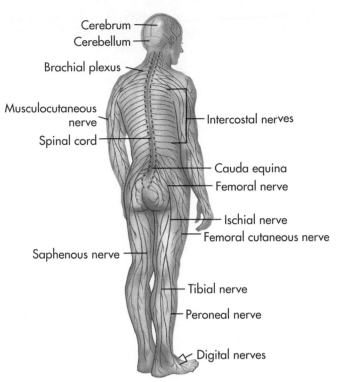

Cerebrum
Cerebellum
Brachial plexus
Musculocutaneous nerve
Spinal cord
Intercostal nerves
Cauda equina
Femoral nerve
Ischial nerve
Femoral cutaneous nerve
Saphenous nerve
Tibial nerve
Peroneal nerve
Digital nerves

fig. 3-8

Simplified view of the nervous system. (From LaFleur Brooks M: *Exploring medical language: a student-directed approach,* ed 3, St Louis, 1994, Mosby.)

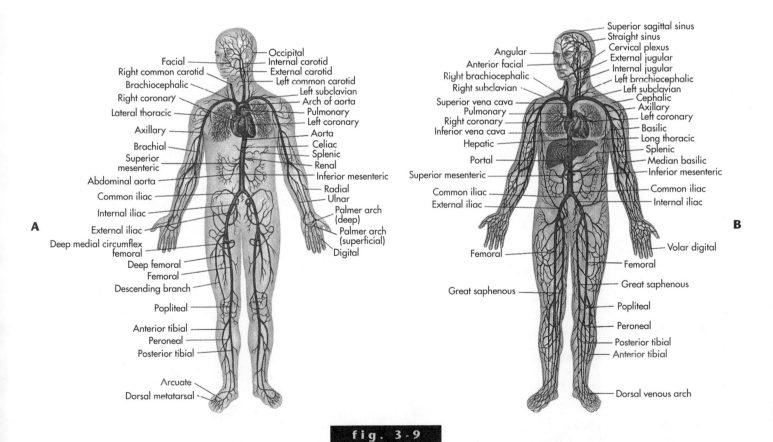

A

Facial
Right common carotid
Brachiocephalic
Right coronary
Lateral thoracic
Axillary
Brachial
Superior mesenteric
Abdominal aorta
Common iliac
Internal iliac
External iliac
Deep medial circumflex femoral
Deep femoral
Femoral
Descending branch
Popliteal
Anterior tibial
Peroneal
Posterior tibial
Arcuate
Dorsal metatarsal

Occipital
Internal carotid
External carotid
Left common carotid
Left subclavian
Arch of aorta
Pulmonary
Left coronary
Aorta
Celiac
Splenic
Renal
Inferior mesenteric
Radial
Ulnar
Palmer arch (deep)
Palmer arch (superficial)
Digital

B

Angular
Anterior facial
Right brachiocephalic
Right subclavian
Superior vena cava
Pulmonary
Right coronary
Inferior vena cava
Hepatic
Portal
Superior mesenteric
Common iliac
External iliac
Femoral
Great saphenous

Superior sagittal sinus
Straight sinus
Cervical plexus
External jugular
Internal jugular
Left brachiocephalic
Left subclavian
Cephalic
Axillary
Left coronary
Basilic
Long thoracic
Splenic
Median basilic
Inferior mesenteric
Common iliac
Internal iliac
Volar digital
Femoral
Great saphenous
Popliteal
Peroneal
Posterior tibial
Anterior tibial
Dorsal venous arch

fig. 3-9

Systemic circulation. A, Arteries. B, Veins. (From Seidel HM et al: *Mosby's guide to physical examination,* ed 3, St Louis, 1995, Mosby.)

Veins are vessels that return the blood to the heart and are located in more surface areas; therefore veins are easier to palpate. Veins have a valve system that prevents backflow of blood. A breakdown of a valve may result in a varicose vein. Capillaries are very small, thin (usually one cell thick) vessels that allow for the exchange of blood gasses and nutrients. Blood vessels vasoconstrict, or become smaller inside, and vasodilate, or become larger inside.

Blood pressure is a measurement of the pressure exerted by the circulating volume of blood on the walls of the arteries, veins, and heart chambers. Blood pressure is maintained by the complex interaction of the homeostatic mechanisms of the body. Normal blood pressure varies based on age, size, and gender but averages approximately 120 mm Hg during systole and 70 mm Hg in diastole. High blood pressure is called *hypertension* and low blood pressure is called *hypotension.*

Blood is composed of a clear, yellow fluid called *plasma,* blood cells, and *platelets.* The main function of blood is to transport oxygen and nutrients to the cells and remove carbon dioxide and other waste products.

Terms that relate to the cardiovascular system include the following: *angio-, artery, arteriole, blood pressure, bruise, capillary, edema, phleb-, vasoconstriction, vasodilation, vein,* and *venule* (Proficiency Exercise 3-11).

The Lymphatic System

The lymphatic system is responsible for several functions and operates in the following ways:

1. It returns vital substances, such as plasma protein, to the bloodstream from the tissues of the body.
2. It assists in the maintenance of fluid balance by draining fluid from the body tissues.
3. It helps in the body's defense against disease-producing substances.
4. It helps in the absorption of fats from the digestive system.

The lymphatic system is a network of channels and nodes in which a substance called *lymph* travels (Fig. 3-10). Lymph is a clear, watery fluid similar to plasma. The system collects and drains lymph from different areas of the body and carries it through the lymphatic channels back

---

3-10

PROFICIENCY EXERCISE

1. List five of the disease conditions of the nervous system described in the indications and contraindications section in Appendix A.

1.

2.

3.

4.

5.

2. Using Appendix A, choose one condition from your list and note any indications or contraindications involved.

Condition:
Indications or contraindications:

3. Choose one of the reflexes listed on p. 107 of the text and look it up in a medical dictionary. Define the term and then write down how you think the reflex is implicated during massage.

Example:

Reflex: psychogalvanic
Definition: psycho- *relates to the mind and* galvanic *pertains to electricity*
Implication: This reflex involves changes in electrical activity in the body connected with mind processes or thoughts. With the galvanic skin response, changes in electrical activity are related to activity of the sweat glands. Massage stimulates the skin as well as electrical activity in the body, which in turn may influence the mind.

Your Turn
Reflex:
Definition:

Implication:

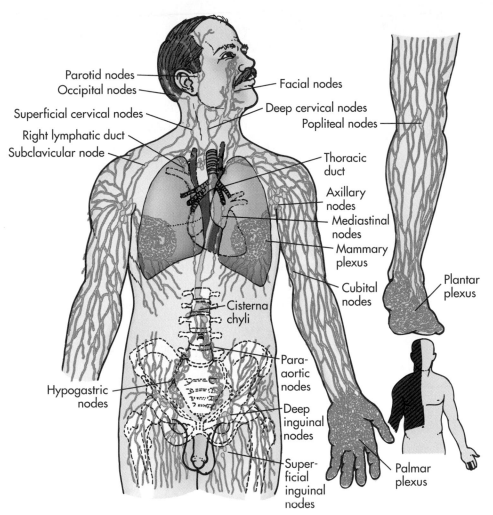

Parotid nodes
Occipital nodes
Facial nodes
Superficial cervical nodes
Deep cervical nodes
Right lymphatic duct
Popliteal nodes
Subclavicular node
Thoracic duct
Axillary nodes
Mediastinal nodes
Mammary plexus
Cubital nodes
Plantar plexus
Cisterna chyli
Para-aortic nodes
Hypogastric nodes
Deep inguinal nodes
Superficial inguinal nodes
Palmar plexus

fig. 3-10

Principal lymph vessels and nodes. (From Birmingham JJ: *Medical terminology: a self-learning text,* ed 2, St Louis, 1990, Mosby.)

3-11

PROFICIENCY EXERCISE

1. *List five of the disease conditions of the cardiovascular system described in the indications and contraindications section in Appendix A.*

   1.

   2.

   3.

   4.

   5.

2. *Using your list, choose one condition and indicate any indications or contraindications involved.*

   Condition:
   Indications or contraindications:

3. *Look up the medication classification "anticoagulant" in Appendix C and in a pharmacology reference text. In the space provided, list contraindications and side effects of these medications. Also describe contraindications to massage that may exist if someone is taking anticoagulant medication.*

4. *Choose a partner and draw the major arteries and veins on the body with washable markers. Use red for arteries and blue for veins. Notice that you can almost trace the veins because they are located near the surface of the body.*

table 3-8
DESCRIPTION OF THE LYMPH NODES

Nodes	Description
Parotid	Nodes around *(para-)* or in front of the ear *(otid)*
Occipital	Nodes over the occipital bone at the back of the head
Superficial cervical	Nodes close to the surface *(superficial)* of the neck *(cervic)*
Subclavicular	Nodes under *(sub-)* the collarbone *(clavicular)*
Hypogastric	Nodes in the area beneath *(hypo-)* the stomach *(gastric)*
Facial	Nodes draining the tissue in the face
Deep cervical	Deeply *(deep)* situated nodes in the neck *(cervic)*
Axillary (superficial)	Nodes in the armpit *(axilla)*
Mediastinal	Nodes in the mediastinal section of the thoracic cavity
Cubital	Nodes of the elbow *(cubit)*
Para-aortic	Nodes around *(para-)* the aorta *(aortic)*
Deep inguinal	Deeply *(deep)* situated nodes in the groin *(inguin)*
Superficial inguinal	Nodes in the groin *(inguin)* close to the surface *(superficial)*
Popliteal	Nodes in back of the knee *(popliteal)*

to the venous system. There it is deposited, mixed with venous blood, and recirculated.

Lymph capillaries are found close to and parallel with the veins that carry blood to the heart. The ends of the lymphatic capillaries meet to form larger lymph vessels. The lymph vessels in the right chest and right arm join the right lymphatic duct, which drains into the right subclavian vein. The lymph vessels from all other parts of the body join to meet the thoracic duct, which drains into the left subclavian vein.

Throughout the lymph system are lymph nodes. *Lymph nodes* are small bodies present in the path of the lymph channels that act as filters for lymph before it returns to the bloodstream. The main locations for the more superficial lymph node are the cervical area, axillary region, and groin or inguinal area. See Table 3-8 for a description of types of lymph nodes.

Plexuses of lymph channels exist throughout the body. These intertwined channels are found in the following areas:

- Mammary plexus: lymphatic vessels around the breasts
- Palmar plexus: lymphatic vessels in the palm *(palmar)* of the hand
- Plantar plexus: lymphatic vessels in the sole *(plantar)* of the foot

The Immune System

The human body has the ability to resist organisms or toxins that tend to damage its tissues and organs. This ability is called *immunity*. As a massage professional, explore the immune system in much greater depth (see Table 3-9 for a list of terms related to immunology). Use your anatomy and physiology textbook as a place to begin, but do not stop there. Exciting new research is being published in professional journals (Proficiency Exercise 3-12).

The Respiratory System

The respiratory system functions supplies oxygen to and removes carbon dioxide from the cells of the body (Fig. 3-11). Respiration is divided into two phases: external and internal. *External respiration* involves the absorption of oxygen from the air by the lungs and the transport of carbon dioxide from the lungs back into the air. *Internal respiration* involves the exchange of oxygen and carbon dioxide in the cells of the body. The mechanisms of breathing and their relationship to massage are discussed in future chapters.

Terms related to the respiratory system include the following: *alveoli, lungs, nares, nostrils, olfactory cells, pneumo-, rhino-,* and *trachea* (Proficiency Exercise 3-13).

table 3-9

SELECTED TERMS RELATED TO IMMUNOLOGY

Nodes	Description
Acquired immunity	Resistance *(immunity)* to a particular disease developed by people who have acquired the disease
Acquired immunodeficiency	Group of symptoms *(syndrome)* caused by the transmission (AIDS) *(acquired)* of a virus that causes a breakdown *(deficiency)* of the immune system
Active immunity	Resistance *(immunity)* in which the antibodies that have been produced by a person currently exist
Allergy	State of hypersensitivity to a particular substance; the immune system overreacts (over *[hyper-]*, reacts *[sensitive]*) to foreign substances and physical changes occur
Antigen	Substance that stimulates the immune response
Susceptible	Said of a person who is capable *(-ible)* of acquiring *(suscept)* a particular disease

3-12

PROFICIENCY EXERCISE

1. List five of the disease conditions of the lymphatic and immune system described in the indications and contraindications section in Appendix A.

1.

2.

3.

4.

5.

2. Using Appendix A, choose one condition from your list and indicate any indications or contraindications involved.

Condition:
Indications or contraindications:

3-13

PROFICIENCY EXERCISE

1. List five of the disease conditions of the respiratory system described in the indications and contraindications section in Appendix A.

1.

2.

3.

4.

5.

2. Using Appendix A, choose one condition from your list and indicate any indications or contraindications involved.

Condition:
Indications or contraindications:

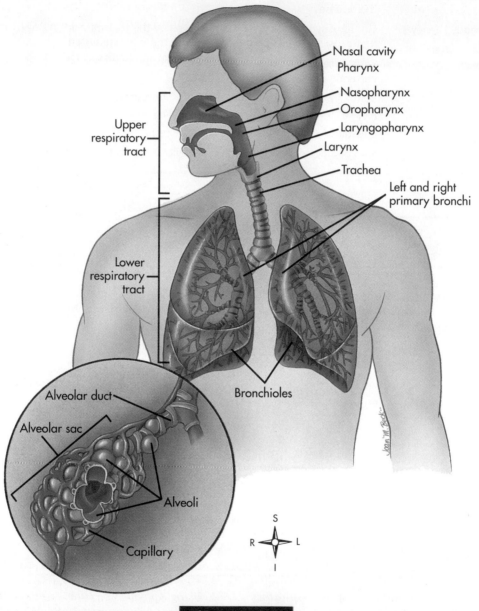

fig. 3-11

Structural plan of the respiratory system. The inset shows the alveolar sacs where the interchange of oxygen and carbon dioxide takes place through the walls of the grapelike alveoli. Capillaries surround the alveoli. (From Thibodeau GA, Patton KT: *Anatomy and physiology,* ed 3, St Louis, 1996, Mosby.)

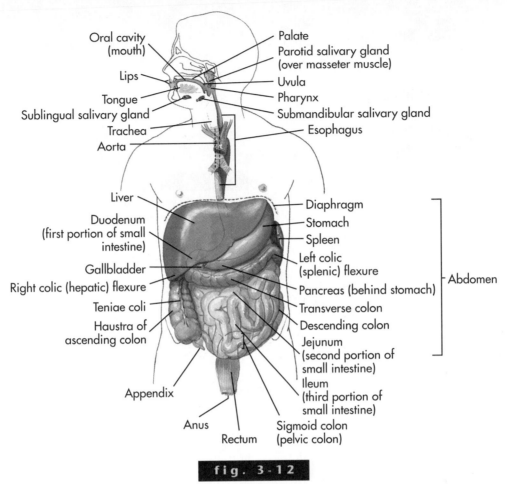

Oral cavity (mouth)
Palate
Parotid salivary gland (over masseter muscle)
Lips
Uvula
Tongue
Pharynx
Sublingual salivary gland
Submandibular salivary gland
Trachea
Esophagus
Aorta

Liver
Diaphragm
Duodenum (first portion of small intestine)
Stomach
Spleen
Left colic (splenic) flexure
Gallbladder
Right colic (hepatic) flexure
Pancreas (behind stomach)
Teniae coli
Transverse colon
Haustra of ascending colon
Descending colon
Jejunum (second portion of small intestine)
Appendix
Ileum (third portion of small intestine)
Anus
Sigmoid colon (pelvic colon)
Rectum
Abdomen

fig. 3-12

Organs of the digestive system and some associated structures. (From LaFleur Brooks M: *Exploring medical language: a student-directed approach,* ed 3, St Louis, 1994, Mosby.)

The Digestive System

The anatomy of the digestive system can be compared with that of a long muscular tube that travels a path through the body (Fig. 3-12). The organs of the digestive system transport food though this muscular tube. The wavelike contraction of the smooth muscles of the digestive tube is called *peristalsis.* Accessory organs carry out functions directly related to digestion and are connected to the system by way of ducts. Understanding the flow of contents through the large intestine is important for the massage professional because methods of massage can be used to enhance this process. Investigate this process further by referring to your anatomy and physiology textbook (Proficiency Exercise 3-14).

The Endocrine System

The endocrine system is composed of glands that produce hormones, which are secreted directly into the bloodstream to stimulate cells in a specific way or to set a body function into action (Fig. 3-13). The endocrine system is complex and important because it serves as a control and regulation system for the body. As with the nervous system, you will want to commit to an in-depth study of the endocrine system, its relationship to the nervous system, and the connection to the mind/body processes. Information from research on the mind/body phenomenon is being released too quickly to be current in any textbook. The massage professional must read medical and scientific journals to remain current. The implications for massage are very important because the effects of massage are connected with the nervous system and endocrine body control functions (Proficiency Exercise 3-15).

The Integumentary System

The integumentary system consists of the skin and its appendages, including hair and nails.

Skin

The skin is the largest organ in the body. It is composed of three layers of tissue (Fig. 3-14): the epidermis, dermis,

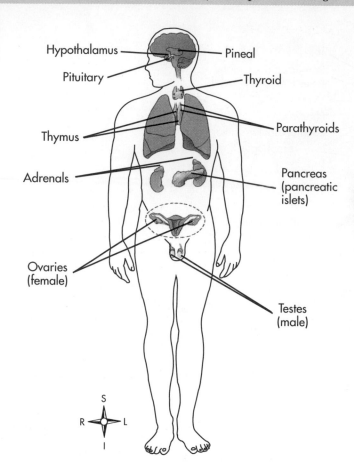

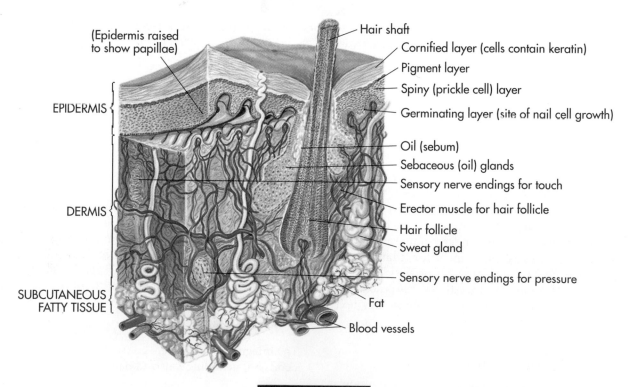

fig. 3-13

Locations of the major endocrine glands. (From Thibodeau GA, Patton KT: *Anatomy and physiology,* ed 3, St Louis, 1996, Mosby.)

fig. 3-14

Structure of skin. (From LaFleur Brooks M: *Exploring medical language: a student-directed approach,* ed 3, St Louis, 1994, Mosby.)

and subcutaneous tissue. The *epidermis* is the outer layer of skin, which contains many layers of tissue and melanocytes, the cells that give skin color. The *dermis,* or dermal layer, lies directly under the epidermis and is often called the *true skin.* It is made of connective tissue. Embedded in the dermis are the blood vessels, lymphatic vessels, hair follicles, and sweat glands. *Subcutaneous tissue* attaches the dermis to the underlying structure. This fatty tissue contains varying amounts of adipose tissue and acts as insulation for the body.

The functions of the skin are protection; control and maintenance of body temperature; detection of the sensations of touch, temperature, pain, and pressure; secretion of sweat and sebum; and production of vitamin D when the skin is exposed to the sun.

Many disease signs (particularly color changes) may be first noticed in the skin. Terms relating to skin color changes include the following: *cyanosis* (bluish), *pallor* (decrease in color), *jaundice* (yellow-orange), and *erythema* (red).

Sebaceous Glands

Sebaceous glands are located in the skin and secrete an oily substance that gives skin and hair its glossy appearance. The oily substance is called *sebum.* Most of these glands open into the walls of hair follicles. Other sebaceous glands are located at the corners of the mouth and around the external sex organs that open directly on the surface of the skin.

Sweat Glands

Sweat glands are found in most areas of the body. They function to cool the body. The most abundant type is the eccrine sweat gland. The palms of the hands and soles of the feet contain large numbers of these glands. Sweat from these glands is odorless. Another type of sweat gland is the apocrine sweat gland, which is connected to hair follicles in the armpits and the pubic area and is found at the navel and nipples. The secretions from these sweat glands increase in response to sexual stimulation. They

---

3-14

PROFICIENCY EXERCISE

1. List five of the disease conditions of the digestive system described in the indications and contraindications section in Appendix A.

1.

2.

3.

4.

5.

2. Using Appendix A, choose one condition from your list and indicate any indications or contraindications involved.

Condition:
Indications or contraindications:

3-15

PROFICIENCY EXERCISE

1. List three of the disease conditions of the endocrine system described in the indications and contraindications section in Appendix A.

1.

2.

3.

2. Using Appendix A, choose one condition from your list and indicate any indications or contraindications involved.

Condition:
Indications or contraindications:

function to lubricate the genital area and play a part in sexual arousal as a result of the mild odor (Proficiency Exercise 3-16).

Terminology as an Ongoing Study

The study of medical terminology, anatomy, physiology, and pathology must be an ongoing process for the massage professional. The massage professional needs this base to understand the research, books, and journal articles that relate to massage, record keeping, and charting. This base is also required to communicate effectively with other health care professionals.

Many clients are not familiar with these terms, so it is important to use the language patterns of the people with whom you speak. Often the use of technical terms with a client is not appropriate; using big words and technical language is not necessary when presenting yourself to the general public. The massage professional must speak two languages and be able to translate effectively back and forth between each.

When speaking with health care professionals and researchers who use this special language of the sciences, it is important to ask questions about any term you do not understand. Acting as though you understand what is being said when you do not is unprofessional. The development of this language base has prepared the student to begin the process of maintaining records and charting.

RECORD KEEPING

section objectives

Using the information presented in this section, the student will be able to perform the following:

- **Complete a client intake process using sample forms**
- **Implement the clinical reasoning problem/ decision-making model for charting purposes**
- **Use a problem- or goal-oriented charting process**
- **Chart using a SOAP note format**

The maintenance of a written record of the professional relationship with clients is essential. In Chapter 2 the informed consent procedure and the legal implications of documentation were presented. In this section the student will learn the procedures for writing records and the ways to use various forms.

The student will also continue to develop the decision-making skills as presented in Chapter 2. Ethical decisions are only one type of decision made in professional practice. Clinical decisions about what might be involved with a client's concerns and what methods to use to achieve clients' **goals** and business decisions are necessary as well. This section focuses on clinical decision making and the records necessary for maintaining a written account of the professional interaction. The topic of clinical decision making is expanded in future chapters as well. Chapter 14 more thoroughly discusses business records.

Record keeping for clients involves the written record of intake procedures, including informed consent, needs assessments (including history and physical assessment), obtaining release of information, and the ongoing process of recording each session, which is called *charting*.

NOTE: It is difficult at this time for you as students to complete a needs assessment and develop an initial treatment plan because you are still developing the assessment skills and technical skills required to complete these procedures. The same is true of charting. Despite this, it is important to understand the mechanics of the record keeping and charting process so that as the technical skills improve, the written record-keeping procedures will develop as well.

Clinical Reasoning and Charting

As the volume of knowledge increases, and as soft tissue modalities such as massage are integrated into the health

---

3-16

PROFICIENCY EXERCISE

1. Using Appendix A, list at least three skin conditions that could be contagious.

1.

2.

3.

2. Using Appendix A, choose one condition from your list and indicate any indications or contraindications involved.

Condition:
Indications or contraindications:

care systems, it is becoming increasingly important to be able to think or reason through an intervention process and justify the effectiveness of a therapeutic intervention. Therapeutic massage practitioners must be able to gather information effectively, analyze that information to make decisions about the type and appropriateness of a therapeutic intervention, and evaluate and justify the benefits derived from the intervention. Charting is the process of keeping a written record of these professional interactions. Effective charting is more than writing down what happens during a session. It represents a clinical reasoning methodology emphasizing a problem-solving approach to client care.

As noted at the beginning of this chapter, a practitioner needs a comprehensive knowledge base of medical terms, abbreviations, and anatomy and physiology in both normal and diseased states of functioning to be able to reason clinically and chart effectively.

Effective assessment, analysis, and decision making are essential to meet the needs of each client. Routines or a recipe-type application of therapeutic massage is often limited and ineffective because each person's set of presenting circumstances and outcome goals are so varied. The mark of an experienced professional is effective clinical reasoning skills. As with all skills, clinical reasoning can be learned.

Functionally Oriented Goals

Sessions with massage professionals are goal oriented. Goals describe desired outcomes. Decisions need to be made as to what goals are obtainable and the way the goals will be reached. Problems indicate limits in functions. Goals reclaim a support function:

Description of a problem: Client has disturbed sleep pattern due to multiple stressors.
Setting of a goal: Reduce stress to support more effective sleep.

Two of the primary reasons for developing treatment and care plans are to set achievable goals and outline a general plan for the way the goals will be reached. Achievable goals often relate to day-to-day activities (functional goals), either personal or work related. It is important to develop measurable activity-based goals that are meaningful to the client.

Goals must be able to be **quantified.** This means that they are measured in terms of objective criteria such as time, frequency, 1-10 scales, measurable increase or decrease in the ability to perform an activity, or measurable increase or decrease in a sensation such as relaxation or pain.

Goals also need to be **qualified.** How will we know when the goal is achieved? What will the client be able to do after the goal is reached that he is not able to do now? For example: How fast will the client be able to run? How will the client behave when relaxed?

Examples of functional goals include the following (Proficiency Exercise 3-17):

- Client will be able to manage independently (qualified) daily hygiene activities of bathing and dressing with a pain level of 5 on a scale of 1 to10 (quantified), with 10 being unable to function without severe pain.
- Client will be able to work at the computer for 1 hour (quantified) without pain (qualified).
- Client will be able to incorporate a 30-minute walking program (quantified) without stiffness in left knee (qualified).
- Client will be able to fall asleep within 15 minutes (quantified) and sleep uninterrupted for 7 hours (qualified).
- Client will be able to reduce anxiety sufficiently (quantified) to drive car to and from market (qualified).
- Client will be able to meditate for 15 minutes (quantified) without racing thoughts (qualified).
- Client will be able to use massage to relax for 1 hour each week (quantified) to enjoy family more by being able to participate in a family outing after each massage (qualified).

Intake Procedures

Before beginning work with a client it is important to gather information on which to build the professional interaction, establish client goals, and develop a plan for achieving them. This is called a **database.**

Database. A database consists of all the information available that contributes to therapeutic interaction. It is

---

3 - 17

PROFICIENCY EXERCISE

Following the examples given in this section of the text, write three quantifiable and qualifiable functional goals that you might set for yourself using therapeutic massage.

1.

2.

3.

created with information obtained from a history-taking interview with the client and other pertinent people, a physical assessment, prior records, and health care treatment orders. Information obtained during the history and assessment process becomes the needs assessment and provides the basis for the development of a treatment or care plan, identification of contraindications to therapy, and assessment of need for referral.

To gather the information, the professional must have effective communication skills. The same communication skills learned for ethical decision making in Chapter 2 are applied in this process also. The I-message pattern can be altered slightly to develop effective open-ended questions that support data collection.

The four basic questions are the following:

1. Will you please explain the situation or tell me what happened?
2. How did/do you feel about the situation?
3. What has been the result of the situation in terms of costs, limitations, and changes in activity or performance?
4. How would you prefer the situation to be or what would you like to occur?

NOTE: The answer to the last question can easily become the basis for the functionally oriented treatment goal.

History. The history interview provides information pertaining to the client's health history, reason for contact, a descriptive profile of the person, a history of the current condition, a history of past illness and health, and a history of any family illnesses. It also contains an account of the client's current health practices (Box 3-1).

Assessment. The physical assessment makes up the second part of the database. Assessment procedures identify deviations from the norm as well as identify effective functioning. The extent and depth of this assessment varies from setting to setting, practitioner to practitioner, and the situation of the client. Practitioners of therapeutic massage generally use some sort of visual assessment process that looks for bilateral symmetry and deviations. Functional assessment looks for restricted, exaggerated, painful or otherwise altered movement patterns. Palpation is used to identify changes in tissue texture and temperature, locate energy changes, and identify areas of tenderness. Various manual tests may be used to differentiate soft tissue problems from such other problems as joint dysfunction and muscle function (Box 3-2).

Analysis of data. After the information is collected, it is analyzed. This is a very important process and follows the same model as found in decision making. Effective decision making depends on both the thorough collection of data and the effective analysis of that data.

Steps of the analysis process are as follows:
1. Review the facts and information collected
   Questions that help with this process are the following:
   • What are the facts?
   • What is considered normal or balanced function?
   • What has happened? *(Spell out events)*
   • What caused the imbalance? *(Can it be identified?)*
   • What was done or is being done?
   • What has worked or not worked?
2. Brainstorm the possibilities
   Questions that help with this process are the following:
   • What are the possibilities? *(What could it all mean?)*
   • What is my intuition suggesting?
   • What are the possible patterns of dysfunction?
   • What are the possible contributing factors?
   • What are possible interventions?
   • What might work?
   • What are other ways to look at the situation?
   • What do the data suggest?
3. Consider the logical outcome of each possibility.
   Questions that help determine this are the following:
   • What is the logical progression of the symptom pattern, contributing factors, and current behaviors?
   • What is the logical cause and effect of each intervention identified?
   • What are the pros and cons of each intervention suggested?
   • What are the consequences of not acting?
   • What are the consequences of acting?
4. Consider how people would be affected by each possibility.
   Questions that help identify this area are the following:
   • In terms of each intervention being considered, what is the impact on the people involved; client, practitioner, and other professionals working with the client?
   • How does each person involved feel about the possible interventions?
   • Is the practitioner within his/her scope of practice to work with such situations?
   • Is the practitioner qualified to work with such situations?
   • Does the practitioner feel qualified to work with such situations?
   • Is there a feeling of cooperation and agreement between all parties involved?

Problems and goals identified. Problems are then identified, based on a conclusion or decision resulting from examination, investigation, and analysis of the data collected. A *problem* is defined as anything that causes concern to the client or caregiver, including physical abnormalities, physiologic disturbances, and socioeconomic or spiritually based problems. Realistic and attainable functional outcome goals are established. A *decision* is then made about an intervention or care/treatment plan.

box 3-1
SAMPLE HISTORY FORM

Name: _____

Today's Date: _____

Address: _____

City, State, Zip: _____

Phone: (day) _____ (eve) _____

Date of Birth: _____

Occupation: _____

Employer: _____

Referred By: _____

Physician: _____

Previous Experience with Massage: _____

_____

Primary Reason for Appointment/Areas of Pain or Tension: _____

_____

Please mark (**X**) all conditions that apply now. Put a **P** for past conditions. Put an **F** for family history of illness:

___ headaches, migraines	___ chronic pain	___ fatigue
___ vision problems, contact lenses	___ muscle or joint pain	___ tension, stress
___ hearing problems, deafness	___ muscle, bone injuries	___ depression
___ injuries to face or head	___ numbness or tingling	___ sleep difficulties
___ sinus problems	___ sprains, strains	___ allergies, sensitivity
___ dental bridges, braces	___ arthritis, tendonitis	___ rash, athletes foot
___ jaw pain, TMJ problems	___ cancer, tumors	___ infectious disease
___ asthma or lung conditions	___ spinal column disorders	___ blood clots
___ constipation, diarrhea	___ diabetes	___ varicose veins
___ hernia	___ pregnancy	___ high/low blood pressure
___ birth control, IUD	___ heart, circulatory problems	
___ abdominal or digestive problems	___ other medical conditions not listed	

Explain Any Areas Noted Above: _____

_____

_____

Current Medications, Including Aspirin, Ibuprofen, Herbs, Vitamins, Etc.:_____

_____

Surgeries:_____

Accidents:_____

Please list all forms and frequency of stress-reduction activities, hobbies, exercise, or sports participation:

_____

_____

box 3-2

SAMPLE PHYSICAL ASSESSMENT FORM

Client Name:_____

Date: _____

PHYSICAL

ALIGNMENT:

___ Chin in line with nose, sternal notch, navel   ___ Other _____

HEAD:

___ Tilted left   ___ Tilted right   ___ Rotated left   ___ Rotated right

EYES:

___ Level   ___ Equally set in socket   ___ Other _____

EARS:

___ Level   ___ Other _____

SHOULDERS:

___ Level   ___ Right high/Left low   ___ Left high/ Right low

___ Left rounded forward   ___ Right rounded forward   ___ Muscle development even

___ Other_____

CLAVICLES:

___ Level   ___ Other_____

ARMS:

___ Hang evenly   ___ Left rotated: ___ medial   ___ lateral   ___ Right rotated: ___ medial   ___ lateral

___ Other_____

ELBOWS:

___ Even   ___ Other _____

WRISTS:

___ Even   ___ Other_____

FINGERTIPS:

___ Even   ___ Other _____

RIBS:

___ Even   ___ Other _____

___ Springy   ___ Other _____

SCAPULA:

___ Even   ___ Other _____

___ Move freely   ___ Other_____

box 3-2

SAMPLE PHYSICAL ASSESSMENT FORM—CONT'D

ABDOMEN:

___ Firm   ___ Other _____

___ Hard areas: Describe _____

WAIST:

___ Level   ___ Other _____

SPINE CURVES:

___ Normal   ___ Other _____

GLUTEAL MUSCLE MASS:

___ Even   ___ Other _____

ILAIC CREST:

___ Even   ___ Other_____

KNEES:

___ Even   ___ Other_____

PATELLA:

___ Left movable   ___ rigid

___ Right movable   ___ rigid

ANKLES:

___ Even   ___ Other _____

FEET:

___ Relaxed   ___ Other_____

ARCHES:

___ Even   ___ High   ___ Flat   ___ Other_____

TOES:

___ Straight   ___ Other_____

SKIN:

___ Moves freely   ___ Pulls   ___ Puffy   ___ Other _____

SOFT TISSUE:

___ Normal   ___ Tender   ___ Restricted   ___ Flaccid   ___ Hot   ___ Cold

___ Other _____

Location(s) of Tissue Change(s): _____

FUNCTIONAL MOBILITY:

___ Normal   ___ Restricted   ___ Exaggerated   ___ Painful

___ Other _____

Location(s) of Mobility Change(s): _____

Continued.

box 3-2

SAMPLE PHYSICAL ASSESSMENT FORM—CONT'D

GAIT

HEAD:

___ Remains steady   ___Other_____

TRUNK:

___ Remains vertical   ___Other_____

SHOULDERS:

___ Remain level   ___ Other _____

ARMS:

___ Motion is opposite leg swing   ___ Motion is even left and right

___ Other _____

___ Left swings freely   ___ Right swings freely   ___ Other _____

HIPS:

___ Remain level   ___ Twist during walking   ___ Other _____

LEGS:

___ Swing freely at hip ___ Other _____

KNEES:

___ Flex and extend freely through stance and swing   ___ Other _____

FEET:

___ Heel strikes first at start of stance   ___ Plantar flexed at push-off   ___ Foot clears floor during swing phase

___ Other _____

STEP:

___ Length is even   ___ Timing is even   ___ Other _____

OVERALL:

___ Rhythmic motion ___ Other_____

Not all therapeutic goals are in relation to problems. It is common for clients to use massage for health maintenance, stress management, and fulfillment of pleasure needs. The same analysis process is used to best determine the methods and approach to meet the client's goals.

Care or treatment plan. After the analysis is complete and problems and goals identified, a *decision* needs to be made about the **care or treatment plan.** Any time a decision must be made, return to the problem-solving model, which includes consideration of the facts, possibilities, logical outcomes, and impact on people.

The plan is not an exact protocol set in stone, but rather a guideline that has fluidity (the best professional educated guess). The care/treatment plan may evolve over the first three or four sessions and be altered with changes in the therapeutic goals. The development of the care/treatment plan is the end of the intake process (Box 3-3).

As the plan is implemented, it is recorded sequentially session by session in some form of charting process such as **SOAP notes.** The plan is reevaluated and adjusted as necessary.

SOAP Charting

Charting is the ongoing record of each client session. Commonly used methods of charting involve the problem-oriented medical record (POMR) and SOAP charting (*subjective, objective, assessment [analysis],* and *plan*), which is another type of problem-oriented medical record.

POMRs are based on a problem-solving and clinical reasoning analysis process. Therefore after one method is

box 3-3

SAMPLE TREATMENT PLAN FORM

Client Name: _____

Date: _____

Choose One: Original plan   Reassessment (original dated _____)

Short-Term Client Goals:

_____

_____

Long-Term Client Goals:

_____

_____

Therapist Objectives:

_____

_____

Frequency, Length, and Duration of Visits:

_____

Progress Measurements To Be Used:

_____

Dates of Reassessment:

_____

Massage Methods To Be Used:

_____

_____

Additional Notes:

_____

_____

_____

_____

Client Signature: _____

Date: _____

Therapist Signature: _____

Date: _____

learned, it is relatively easy to adapt to any of the other charting methods available. The most important skill involved is the ability to reason rationally and comprehensively through a therapeutic interaction. A charting process can provide the structure necessary to think through a process effectively and develop a written record of the process.

During charting any therapeutic action taken, its effectiveness and its outcome is recorded progressively from session to session. Effective charting requires an organized approach to recording the information that relates to the facts, possibilities, logical consequences of cause and effect, and impact on people—an approach similar to that used for the development of the initial treatment/care plan. This process again is a direct application of the decision-making model. While charting, a practitioner gathers and records subjective and objective information, records methods used, and analyzes effectiveness of the process. The plan for further sessions is then indicated and noted.

Although many different forms of charting processes exist, the massage therapy community seems to be using the standardized SOAP model. This is a helpful choice in terms of learning because the four-part model correlates with the clinical reasoning/decision-making model.

SOAP notes or similar charting methods are used to chart all massage sessions. After the initial intake and treatment/care plan development, subsequent visits require a modified and shortened subjective and objective assessment process to determine goals for each individual massage session. When a massage is given to the client after the intake session, specific treatment goals for the particular session are developed. Information from the history pertinent to the first session is transferred to *S* in SOAP notes. Physical assessment information pertinent to this session is transferred to *O* in SOAP notes.

When using SOAP note charting, the practitioner should use the following pattern[1]: *S* stands for subjective data recorded from the client's point of view. Subjective information usually includes the following:

- Key symptoms that are quantified and qualified
- Activities that are affected by the situation; often stated as what can no longer be done or what increase in performance is desired
- What methods or activities are currently being used in treatment

O stands for objective data acquired from inspection and palpation. A list of assessment procedures and interventions used during the session is recorded. Objective information usually includes the following:

- Significant physical assessment findings
- Intervention modalities and locations used (Limit specifics to interventions used to work toward treatment goals)

- General approach used, such as connective tissue, Swedish massage, or neuromuscular
- If not recorded elsewhere, the duration of the session

A stands for analysis or assessment of the subjective and objective data. It includes an analysis of the effectiveness of the intervention and action taken, with a summary of the most pertinent data recorded.

NOTE: Traditionally in SOAP charting the *A* stands for assessment. Observation of many students indicates they confuse physical assessment information that is recorded in the objective data with assessment in the SOAP model, which is actually an analysis of the data and effectiveness of the interventions. Therefore this text uses the idea of analysis for the *A* section of SOAP charting.

Analysis information includes the following:

- Changes, whether *subjective,* relating to the client's experience, such as "pain reduced" or "feel relaxed," or *objective,* which are measurable, such as "flexion of elbow increased by 15 degrees"—If no change occurs or the condition worsens, record this also.
- Analysis of which methods were effective or not effective, such as "Trigger point methods most effective in increase of flexion of elbow," "Client indicated she responded best to rhythmic rocking for relaxation," "Tense-and-relax methods not effective in reducing pain in shoulder"—Also indicate if it is unclear which methods were effective: "Range of motion in neck increased 25%, but it is unclear which methods brought about the change."

The *A* (analysis/assessment) section of the SOAP charting process is very important. It is, in fact, the most important area terms of determining future intervention procedures as well as communicating process information to other caregivers and insurance companies.

The *A* portion of the SOAP note is where the actual process of decision making is recorded. Decision making occurs during in every step of the charting process, but during the other charting areas only the decision is recorded, not the way the decision was made. Obviously a condensed and concise version of the more detailed process is written down in the chart, but the components of the process (facts, possibilities, logical outcomes, impact on people) are evident in the *A* portion of the SOAP note.

P stands for plan, including the methodology for future intervention. The progress of the sessions is developed and recorded. Plan information usually includes the following:

- Frequency of appointments
- Continuation of step-by-step process as it unfolds session by session to achieve treatment plan goals
- Client self-care
- Referrals

A sample SOAP chart form is provided in Box 3-4, and an example of SOAP charting is presented in Box 3-5.

box 3-4
SAMPLE SOAP CHART FORM

Client Name:_____

Date: _____

S: SUBJECTIVE
Client States:

_____

_____

_____

_____

_____

O: OBJECTIVE
I Observed from Assessment Procedures:

_____

_____

_____

_____

_____

What I Did This Session:

_____

_____

_____

_____

A: ANALYSIS (ASSESSMENT OF EFFECTIVENESS)
The Results: What Worked/What Didn't:

_____

_____

_____

_____

_____

_____

_____

_____

Continued.

---

box 3-4

SAMPLE SOAP CHART FORM—CONT'D

P: PLAN
Plans for Next Session, What Client Will Work On:

_____

_____

_____

_____

---

box 3-5

EXAMPLE OF SOAP CHARTING

S: Client reports tension headache and indicates with hand placement that the major concentration of pain is at the occiput and upper cervical area with secondary pain pattern at the temples. Client reports that on a pain scale of 1-10, headache is at a 7.

O: Observation suggests that both shoulders are elevated, with increased elevation on the right. It appears that range of motion of the neck is generally limited to the left. Palpation of upper back muscles elicited some pain behaviors, including pulling away, grimacing, and verbally indicating pain. Upper trapezius muscles seem to be warm without indication of inflammation, suggesting tension in muscles.

Approach Used (What I Did): General massage focus: stress reduction with specific focus to shoulder and neck tension using positional release and lengthening. Basic methods used: effleurage, compression, rocking, and passive joint movement.

Post-Assessment

After the session a post-assessment is done. The client is asked how he or she feels and what is different now than before the session. The client is asked what methods used seemed to be most beneficial. One or two of the methods identified are then modified for client self-care and taught to the client.

After the massage and the post-assessment, the *A,* or analysis/assessment, portion of the chart is recorded.

A: Client indicates a reduction in headache by 50% (pain scale 3), less tension in the shoulders, and increased range of motion of the neck to the left. Pain behaviors in the upper back are not observable, but the client still indicates tenderness in the area during palpation. Upper trapezius area still warm with exaggerated vasomotor response (reddening) and itching after massage, indicating possible connective tissue involvement in this area. Client can now look over her left shoulder; she couldn't do that before the massage without a catch. Observation indicates shoulders are level within 1 inch, indicating change in right shoulder tension pattern. Methods most effective were compression and positional release. Rocking methods ineffective and client reported increase in head pain when rocking was used. Note: Make sure client's feet stay warm.

P: Client selected self-help consisting of towel compression to the head and flexion/extension range of motion of the arms and shoulders. Client scheduled appointment for 2 weeks and will monitor response to massage. Expect three to four sessions before beginning specific connective tissue work on shoulder tension. Client advised to contact personal physician and report that she has begun to receive massage.

NOTE: The interventions used and the plan recorded in the SOAP charting need to reflect the original treatment plan developed during the intake procedure.

Individual session goals need to be in line with the initial care/treatment plan agreed to in the informed consent process. If the goals are radically different, the client needs to sign an addendum to the informed consent form. Minor changes can be reflected in the SOAP notes or session charting procedure.

To maintain the integrity of client charts, make sure that any abbreviations used are universally understood or write out the word. Use a black pen or type the notes. Make sure handwritten notes are readable. Never erase or white-out a correction. Draw a single line through any error, and make the correction above or next to the error. It is important to share and explain the charting notes to the client regularly.

Additional Client File Information

Additional information found in client files includes fee and payment record, and, if applicable, the following: signed release of information form(s), authorized communication with client's health care provider(s), and massage therapy treatment orders. Clients have the right to see their files, receive a copy of their files, and have any information contained in the file explained to them.

SUMMARY

Record-keeping skills, and the necessary language base to keep records effectively, are important parts of professional development. The ability to communicate clearly through writing and when speaking fosters understanding and the accurate exchange of information.

Paperwork is often not the professional's favorite task. However, think of record keeping as writing the client's professional interaction story. Realize that reflection on the healing journey provided by reading this story allows both you and your client, as well as any other authorized individuals, to appreciate the process and remember and replicate the steps toward the achievement of goals that honor the effort put forth by all concerned.

REFERENCE

1. Thompson DL: *Hands heal, documentation for massage therapy: a guide for SOAP charging,* Seattle, 1993, Thompson.

WORKBOOK SECTION

Short Answer

1. What are the three word elements, and how are they used?

_____

_____

_____

_____

_____

2. Define abbreviations and provide guidelines for their use.

_____

_____

_____

_____

_____

3. Describe quantified and qualified functional goals.

_____

_____

_____

_____

_____

4. What is the difference between an intake procedure and charting?

_____

_____

_____

_____

_____

5. What are the four steps of the analysis of data acquired during the intake process, and how does analysis relate to the development of a care/treatment plan?

_____

_____

_____

_____

_____

6. Explain the four parts of the SOAP charting process.

_____

_____

_____

_____

_____

7. What is required to maintain integrity of the charts when writing them?

_____

_____

_____

_____

_____

WORKBOOK SECTION

Matching

Match the term to the best definition.

1. Abbreviation _____

2. Combining vowel _____

3. Prefix _____

4. Root _____

5. Suffix _____

6. Word element _____

a. A vowel added between two roots or a root and a suffix to facilitate pronunciation

b. Word element comprising the fundamental meaning of the word

c. A word element placed at the beginning of a word to alter the meaning of the word

d. A reduced form of a word or phrase

e. A part of a word

f. A word element placed at the end of a root to alter the meaning of the word

Match each of the following word elements to its proper meaning, then designate whether it is a prefix (p), root word (r), or suffix (s). Remember that some of the root words may not have a vowel at the end because vowels are added only when combined with a suffix.

1. ab _____

2. ad _____

3. algia _____

4. arthro _____

5. chondr _____

6. circum _____

7. contra _____

8. cost _____

9. de _____

10. dia _____

11. dis _____

12. dys _____

13. epi _____

14. fibr _____

15. genesis _____

16. genic _____

17. gram _____

18. graph _____

19. graphy _____

20. hyper _____

a. toward

b. over, on, upon

c. producing, causing

d. a diagram, a recording instrument

e. excessive, too much, high

f. around

g. against, opposite

h. joint

i. record

j. a condition

k. away from

l. nerve

m. condition

n. making a recording

o. paralysis

p. maintenance, maintaining a constant level

q. development, production, creation

r. pain

s. above, over

t. disease

WORKBOOK SECTION

21. inter _____
22. intra _____
23. intro _____
24. ism _____
25. itis _____
26. myo _____
27. myel _____
28. neuro _____
29. orth _____
30. osis _____
31. osteo _____
32. pathy _____
33. plegia _____
34. post _____
35. stasis _____
36. sterno _____
37. sub _____
38. supra _____
39. therm _____
40. thoraco _____

u. chest
v. fiber, fibrous
w. cartilage
x. uner
y. heat
z. rib
aa. bad, difficult, abnormal
bb. within
cc. down, from, away from, not
dd. across, through, apart
ee. inflammation
ff. spinal cord, bone marrow
gg. separation, away from
hh. between
ii. into, within
jj. straight, normal, correct
kk. bone
ll. after, behind
mm. sternum
nn. muscle

Match the lymph nodes and plexuses to their correct description.

1. Parotid _____
2. Occipital _____
3. Superficial cervical _____
4. Subclavicular _____
5. Hypogastric _____
6. Facial _____
7. Deep cervical _____
8. Axillary _____
9. Mediastinal _____
10. Cubital _____
11. Para-aortic _____

a. deeply situated nodes in the groin
b. nodes in the groin close to the surface
c. nodes under the collarbone
d. nodes draining the tissue in the face
e. lymphatic vessels in the sole (plantar) of the foot
f. lymphatic vessels in the palm (palmar) of the hands
g. nodes around or in front of the ear
h. nodes over the bone at the back of the head
i. nodes in the area beneath the stomach
j. nodes around the aorta
k. deeply situated nodes in the neck

WORKBOOK SECTION

12. Deep inguinal _____

13. Superficial inguinal _____

14. Popliteal _____

15. Mammary plexus _____

16. Palmar plexus _____

17. Plantar plexus _____

l. lymphatic vessels around the breasts

m. nodes in the armpit

n. nodes of the elbow

o. nodes close to the surface of the neck

p. nodes in back of the knee

q. nodes in the mediastinal section of the thoracic cavity

Problem-Solving Exercise

This week, six new clients come to your office. Each of them has filled out a client history form ahead of time, providing you with the following information on medical conditions that have been diagnosed and treated by their physicians. Take each of the italicized medical terms and break it down into its word parts to define the various conditions.

Dermatitis of the hands

_____

_____

Neuropathy in the left leg

_____

_____

Hypothyroidism

_____

_____

Dyspnea

_____

_____

Hemangioma

_____

_____

Polyarthritis

_____

_____

Myocarditis

_____

_____

Hydronephrosis

_____

_____

Research for Further Study

List three resource books you could use for further study of medical terminology. Include title, publisher, and type of reference.

_____

_____

_____

_____

_____

_____

Record-Keeping Exercise

Complete the forms in Boxes 3-6 through 3-9, using yourself as your client and using the clinical reasoning process. When you complete the SOAP form, make up a massage session that would be applicable to your personal situation as reflected on the intake forms.

NOTE: Before you complete this exercise, you might want to make copies of the blank forms to use during practice sessions. Also remember that these are sample forms and are presented as a guide for learning and for the development of your own professional forms.

WORKBOOK SECTION

box 3-6

SAMPLE HISTORY FORM

Name: _____ Today's Date: _____

Address: _____

City, State, Zip: _____

Phone: (day) _____ (eve) _____

Date of Birth: _____

Occupation: _____

Employer: _____

Referred By: _____

Physician: _____

Previous Experience with Massage: _____

_____

Primary Reason for Appointment/Areas of Pain or Tension: _____

_____

Please mark (**X**) all conditions that apply now. Put a **P** for past conditions. Put an **F** for family history of illness:

___ headaches, migraines　　　___ chronic pain　　　___ fatigue
___ vision problems, contact lenses　___ muscle or joint pain　___ tension, stress
___ hearing problems, deafness　___ muscle, bone injuries　___ depression
___ injuries to face or head　　___ numbness or tingling　___ sleep difficulties
___ sinus problems　　　　___ sprains, strains　　___ allergies, sensitivity
___ dental bridges, braces　　___ arthritis, tendonitis　___ rash, athletes foot
___ jaw pain, TMJ problems　　___ cancer, tumors　　___ infectious disease
___ asthma or lung conditions　___ spinal column disorders　___ blood clots
___ constipation, diarrhea　　___ diabetes　　　___ varicose veins
___ hernia　　　　　　___ pregnancy　　　___ high/low blood pressure
___ birth control, IUD　　　___ heart, circulatory problems
___ abdominal or digestive problems　___ other medical conditions not listed

Explain Any Areas Noted Above: _____

_____

_____

Current Medications, Including Aspirin, Ibuprofen, Herbs, Vitamins, Etc.: ____

_____

Surgeries: _____

Accidents: _____

Please list all forms and frequency of stress-reduction activities, hobbies, exercise, or sports participation:

_____

_____

WORKBOOK SECTION

SAMPLE PHYSICAL ASSESSMENT FORM

NOTE: It is helpful to stand and walk in front of a full-length mirror in a swimsuit or similar clothing while completing this form.

Client Name:_____

Date: _____

PHYSICAL

ALIGNMENT:

___ Chin in line with nose, sternal notch, navel   ___ Other _____

HEAD:

___ Tilted left   ___ Tilted right   ___ Rotated left   ___ Rotated right

EYES:

___ Level   ___ Equally set in socket   ___ Other _____

EARS:

___ Level   ___ Other _____

SHOULDERS:

___ Level   ___ Right high/Left low   ___ Left high/ Right low

___ Left rounded forward   ___ Right rounded forward   ___ Muscle development even

___ Other_____

CLAVICLES:

___ Level   ___ Other_____

ARMS:

___ Hang evenly   ___ Left rotated: ___ medial   ___ lateral   ___ Right rotated: ___ medial   ___ lateral

___ Other _____

ELBOWS:

___ Even   ___ Other _____

WRISTS:

___ Even   ___ Other_____

FINGERTIPS:

___ Even   ___ Other _____

RIBS:

___ Even   ___ Other _____

___ Springy   ___ Other _____

Continued.

WORKBOOK SECTION

box 3-7

SAMPLE PHYSICAL ASSESSMENT FORM—CONT'D

SCAPULA:

___ Even   ___ Other _____

___ Move freely   ___ Other_____

ABDOMEN:

___ Firm   ___ Other _____

___ Hard areas: Describe _____

WAIST:

___ Level   ___ Other _____

SPINE CURVES:

___ Normal   ___ Other _____

GLUTEAL MUSCLE MASS:

___ Even   ___ Other _____

ILAIC CREST:

___ Even   ___ Other_____

KNEES:

___ Even   ___ Other_____

PATELLA:

___ Left movable   ___ rigid

___ Right movable   ___ rigid

ANKLES:

___ Even   ___ Other _____

FEET:

___ Relaxed   ___ Other_____

ARCHES:

___ Even   ___ High   ___ Flat   ___ Other_____

TOES:

___ Straight   ___ Other_____

SKIN:

___ Moves freely   ___ Pulls   ___ Puffy   ___ Other _____

WORKBOOK SECTION

box 3-7

SAMPLE PHYSICAL ASSESSMENT FORM—CONT'D

SOFT TISSUE:

___ Normal   ___ Tender   ___ Restricted   ___ Flaccid   ___ Hot   ___ Cold

___ Other _____

Location(s) of Tissue Change(s): _____

FUNCTIONAL MOBILITY:

___ Normal   ___ Restricted   ___ Exaggerated   ___ Painful

___ Other _____

Location(s) of Mobility Change(s): _____

GAIT

HEAD:

___ Remains steady   ___ Other_____

TRUNK:

___ Remains vertical   ___ Other_____

SHOULDERS:

___ Remain level   ___ Other _____

ARMS:

___ Motion is opposite leg swing   ___ Motion is even left and right

___ Other _____

___ Left swings freely   ___ Right swings freely   ___ Other _____

HIPS:

___ Remain level   ___ Twist during walking   ___ Other _____

LEGS:

___ Swing freely at hip ___ Other _____

KNEES:

___ Flex and extend freely through stance and swing   ___ Other _____

FEET:

___ Heel strikes first at start of stance   ___ Plantar flexed at push-off   ___ Foot clears floor during swing phase

___ Other _____

STEP:

___ Length is even   ___ Timing is even   ___ Other _____

OVERALL:

___ Rhythmic motion   ___ Other_____

WORKBOOK SECTION

box 3-8

SAMPLE TREATMENT PLAN FORM

NOTE: Remember, completion of this form reflects the best professional educated guess as to how a series of massage session would achieve client goals.

Client Name:_____

Date: _____

Choose One: Original plan   Reassessment (original dated _____)

Short-Term Client Goals:

_____

_____

Long-Term Client Goals:

_____

Therapist Objectives:

_____

_____

Frequency, Length, and Duration of Visits:

_____

Progress Measurements To Be Used:

_____

Dates of Reassessment:

_____

Massage Methods To Be Used:

_____

_____

Additional Notes:

_____

_____

_____

_____

Client Signature: _____

Date: _____

Therapist Signature:_____

Date: _____

WORKBOOK SECTION

box 3-9

SAMPLE SOAP CHART FORM

NOTE: Complete this form as if you gave yourself a massage that would reflect work toward achievement of a goal as outlined in the treatment plan. Make it up and use your imagination. Remember, this is a learning exercise. Spend sufficient time to develop the *A,* analysis/assessment, portion of the chart.

Client Name:_____

Date: _____

S: SUBJECTIVE
Client States:

_____

_____

_____

_____

O: OBJECTIVE
I Observed from Assessment Procedures:

_____

_____

_____

_____

_____

What I Did This Session:

_____

_____

_____

_____

Continued.

WORKBOOK SECTION

box 3-9
SAMPLE SOAP CHART FORM—CONT'D

A: ANALYSIS (ASSESSMENT OF EFFECTIVENESS)
The Results: What Worked/What Didn't:

_____
_____
_____
_____
_____
_____
_____
_____
_____

P: PLAN
Plans for Next Session, What Client Will Work On:

_____
_____
_____
_____

WORKBOOK SECTION

ANSWER KEY
Short Answer

1. Prefixes are placed at the beginning of the root word to change the meaning of the word. Root words contain the basic meaning of the word. A suffix is placed at the end of a word to change the meaning of the word. When translating medical terms, begin with the suffix.

2. Abbreviations are shortened forms of words or phrases. When you use abbreviations in any record keeping, including charting, provide an abbreviation key either on the forms or included in a conspicuous place in the file. Excessive use of abbreviations is discouraged.

3. Goals must be able to be *quantified*. This means that they are measured in terms of objective criteria. Goals need to be *qualified*. The question to be answered is "How will we know when the goal is achieved?" What will the client be able to do after the goal is reached that he or she is not able to do now?

4. Intake procedures are done once and updated periodically. Charting is ongoing after each session.

5. The four steps are the following: 1) review the facts and information collected, 2) brainstorm the possibilities, 3) consider the logical outcome of each possibility, 4) consider the ways in which people are affected by each possibility. Decisions made from this process are reflected and recorded in the care treatment plan.

6. **S:** Subjective data is recorded from the client's point of view. **O:** Objective data acquired from inspection, palpation, and a list of assessment procedures and interventions used during the session is recorded. **A:** Analysis or assessment of the subjective and objective data and an analysis of effectiveness of the intervention and action taken is made with a summary of the most pertinent data recorded. **P:** Plan, including the methodology for intervention and progress of the sessions, is developed and recorded.

7. To maintain the integrity of client charts make sure that any abbreviations used are universally understood or write out the word. Use black pen or type the notes. Make sure handwritten notes are readable. Never erase or white out a correction. Draw a single line through any error, and make the correction above or next to the error. It is important to share and explain the charting notes to the client regularly.

Matching

1. d	3. c	5. f			
2. a	4. b	6. e			

The first letter is the definition, and the second letter indicates whether it is a prefix (p), root word (r), or suffix (s).

1. k, p	12. aa, p	23. ii, p	34. ll, p
2. a, p	13. b, p	24. j, s	35. p, s
3. r, s	14. v, r	25. ee, s	36. mm, r
4. h, r	15. q, s	26. nn, r	37. x, p
5. w, r	16. c, s	27. ff, r	38. s, p
6. f, p	17. i, s	28. l, r	39. y, r
7. g, p	18. d, s	29. jj, r	40. u, r
8. z, r	19. n, s	30. m, s	
9. cc, p	20. e, p	31. kk, p	
10. dd, p	21. hh, p	32. t, s	
11. gg, p	22. pp, p	33. o, s	

1. g	6. d	10. n	14. p
2. h	7. k	11. j	15. l
3. o	8. m	12. a	16. f
4. c	9. q	13. b	17. e
5. l			

Problem-Solving Exercise

dermatitis: *derma*-skin, *itis*-inflammation

neuropathy: *neuro*-nerve, *pathy*-disease

hypothyroidism: *hypo*-less than normal, *thyroidism*-condition

dyspnea: *dys*-difficult, *pnea*-breathing

hemangioma: *hemi*-half, *angi*-vessel, *oma*-tumor (tumor made up of a mass of blood vessels)

polyarthritis: *poly*-many, *arthr*-joint, *itis*-inflammation

myocarditis: *myo*-muscle, *card*-heart, *itis*-inflammation

hydronephrosis: *hydro*-water, *nephr*-kidney, *osis*-condition

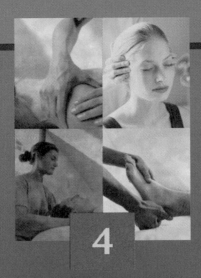

4

THE SCIENTIFIC ART OF THERAPEUTIC MASSAGE

objectives

After completing this chapter, the student will be able to perform the following:

- Cite current research that validates therapeutic massage
- Classify massage methods into basic concepts
- Explain the effects of therapeutic massage in physiologic terms

Student note: Students will find it helpful to keep a medical dictionary and an anatomy and physiology textbook at hand to use as references while reading this chapter. Many technical terms are used, and more in-depth reading may be needed to achieve the best understanding of the information presented. See Appendix D for recommended texts.

THE *American Heritage Dictionary* defines **science** as "the intellectual process of using all mental and physical resources available to better understand, explain, and predict both normal and unusual natural phenomena." The scientific approach to understanding anything involves observation, measurement of things that can be tested, accumulation of data, and analysis of the findings. The scientific approach is different from an intuitive approach.

Intuition is knowing something without going through a conscious process of thinking. Other terms for intuition are *feelings, inspiration, instinct, revelation, impulse,* and *idea.* The term *intuition* is not used in this textbook to mean a psychic or extrasensory experience; rather, it means the ability to act purposefully on subconsciously perceived information. Intuition is the ability to bring subconscious information into conscious awareness. Biofeedback works on a similar principle. Using equipment that detects the heart rate, blood pressure, and skin temperature, a person can monitor and adjust involuntary, or subconscious, responses.

Centering is the ability to pay attention to a specific area. Centering skills allow us to screen sensation and concentrate. It takes practice to learn to pay attention to quiet, subtle information amid all the loud and exaggerated stimulation that blasts our sensory receptors every day. When we are centered, intuition is more apparent.

Art is craft, skill, technique, and talent. When massage professionals work with clients, they must trust their intuition. It is important to maintain the art of the profession by recognizing the validity of intuitional expression.

It is equally important to validate massage therapy on a scientific basis to separate that which is known scientifically from mere speculation about massage and related bodywork methods. In a taped lecture titled "Stress without Distress: Evolution of the Concept,"[19] world-renowned researcher Hans Selye talked about the importance of both science and intuition. He said that if there is not first an idea (intuition), there is nothing to research, and without research (science), an idea does not develop form and usefulness (Proficiency Exercise 4-1). One does not function without the other. The scientific art of therapeutic massage depends on the development of a concept or idea, the testing of the idea through research, and the use of skill and talent in applying the craft through its various techniques.

The beginning student of massage may find scientific justification intimidating. However, without this knowledge, the massage professional cannot make intelligent use of the simple methods of massage presented in this text. It is important to develop an understanding of this body of knowledge at the beginning of the educational process because it is the foundation of the profession. Therefore the purpose of this chapter is to help the student understand the strong physiologic basis for the effectiveness of therapeutic massage. Students must build a firm foundation in the anatomic and physiologic explanations of why massage works so that they can trust their intuition and design a massage based on the information they receive from the client during assessment procedures.

VALID RESEARCH

Effective bodywork is achieved when massage methods interact with physiologic processes. Because massage has demonstrable physiologic effects, those effects can be studied through the scientific method. The scientific method is a way of *objectively* researching a concept to see if it is valid. Research begins with a **hypothesis** (i.e., "if this happens, then that will happen"). The hypothesis must then be tested; this usually is accomplished through an **experiment.** The experiment must follow accepted design measures so that others can replicate the experiment. The results of the experiment should either prove or disprove the hypothesis. Often the results of the research generate more questions, leading to more research.

The subjective (experiential) quality of massage complicates the research issue because of the complexity of human beings and the interaction dynamic between the client and the practitioner, which affects the results of massage. Because of technologic advances, science is able to see more deeply into the human experience than ever before. We are on the edge of being able to see the more mysterious and hidden workings of the body. Only a growing body of research and data replication that establishes the positive biochemical and behavioral reaction to touch will convince the medical profession that massage is therapeutic. Fortunately, this type of research is now being done, and the health care professions and the public are responding by seeking massage therapy services. Validation through scientific research has opened these doors.

---

4 - 1

PROFICIENCY EXERCISE

Give your explanation of Dr. Selye's statement: If there is not first an idea, there is nothing to research. Without research, an idea does not develop form and usefulness. One does not function without the other.

CURRENT RESEARCH

Research is underway at the University of Miami School of Medicine Touch Research Institute (TRI) (Box 4-1). This program is funded by Johnson & Johnson and other corporations and is directed by Tiffany Field, PhD. Dr. Field believes that the clinical health care system will incorporate touch therapy in the same way it incorporated the approaches of relaxation therapy, exercise, and diet.[8]

More than 60 studies have been published or are underway at the Touch Research Institute. These studies, covering a broad range of subjects and conditions, show that massage affects many aspects of human physiology and experience.[13] Other research sites include the following:

- A TRI affiliate, Nova Southeastern University Medical School in Ft. Lauderdale, Florida, is conducting research on the ways massage is related to prevention.
- The International Society for the Study of Subtle Energies and Energy Medicine in Golden, Colorado, sponsors and promotes massage-related research.

- Dr. Norman Shealy of the National Institute of Clinical and Behavior Medicine is conducting other studies. Dr. Dolores Krieger, the developer of therapeutic touch, and Dr. Robert Becker (author of *The Body Electric*) have been researching the electrical component of the body for years.

Many other universities, medical schools, and research facilities are conducting studies, and the National Institutes of Health also has funded research in this field. Studies underway in Europe and Asia will add to the validation of massage as a therapeutic intervention.

Research is proving that massage in beneficial, but why? By what mechanisms are the benefits of bodywork derived? These questions are answered in the next section.

THINK IT OVER   **What type of research study would you like to develop?**

RESEARCH FINDINGS ON THE BENEFITS OF MASSAGE

Studies done at the University of Miami School of Medicine Touch Research Institute have shown that massage has the following benefits:

- Facilitates growth
- Increases attentiveness and learning, which has positive implications for those with attention deficit disorder, hyperactivity, or learning disabilities
- Reduces stereotypical and off-task behavior in autistic individuals while normalizing social behaviors
- Alleviates pain
- Improves immune function (massage increases the number of natural killer cells, which has implications for those with acquired immunodeficiency syndrome [AIDS], cancer, and viral diseases)
- Reduces stress
- Promotes healing of psychiatric problems (Child and adolescent psychiatric patients showed more open verbal communication, improved sleep, less depression, and lower anxiety levels. Clinical progress increased. Similar results were achieved with depressed adolescent mothers and patients with eating disorders.)
- Assists in overcoming addictions such as cigarette smoking
- Supports effective digestion and breathing through stimulation of the vagus nerve
- Diminishes premenstrual symptoms
- Encourages dietary compliance in diabetics, leading to more normal glucose levels

- Lowers blood pressure, anxiety, and hostility levels in individuals with hypertension
- Increases job performance (After a 15-minute chair massage, computation time with figures was cut in half and accuracy almost doubled.)
- Reduces the number of headache days in migraine headaches
- Reduces pain and increases range of motion in individuals with low back pain
- Improves all clinical measures in pediatric eczema
- Improves grip strength, functional activities, positive mood, self-esteem, and body image in multiple sclerosis
- Improves caregiver-child relationships for abused and neglected children
- Has a therapeutic effect on the massage practitioner (administering massage reduces stress and improves sleep patterns in those giving massages)

Research is underway on the effects of massage in cystic fibrosis; childhood irritable bowel syndrome; arthritis in the elderly; sickle cell anemia (to mitigate pain); coma and spinal cord injuries (to upgrade circulation and retard muscle atrophy); mental depression and failure to thrive in the elderly; reduction of the formation of scar tissue from breast surgery, as well as reduction of anxiety, depression, and the cortisol level; Down syndrome (to improve muscle tone and cognitive skills); and cerebral palsy (to help infants gain more muscle flexibility).

WHY MASSAGE IS EFFECTIVE

section objectives

Using the information presented in this section, the student will be able to perform the following:

- Identify and categorize massage methods as reflexive or mechanical
- Explain the anatomic and physiologic influences of massage on the neuroendocrine system, connective tissue, body circulation, and energy systems

The manual techniques of massage are physiologically specific and well defined by (1) the mode of application (rubbing, pulling, pressing, and touching); (2) the speed and depth of pressure (sustained or slow, rhythmic, staccato, or fast); (3) the intensity of touch (light touch, deep touch, and a combination of the two); and (4) the part of the therapist's body used to apply the techniques (fingers, hand, forearm, or knee). The techniques of therapeutic massage and other types and styles of bodywork are merely variations of the fundamental application of manual manipulations that provide external sensory stimulation. The benefits of the techniques are simply the result of basic physiologic effects.

Physiologic Effects

The fundamental concepts that explain the effects of therapeutic massage can be divided into two categories: reflexive methods and mechanical methods:

- **Reflexive methods** stimulate the nervous system, endocrine system, and the chemicals of the body. A **reflex** is an involuntary response to a stimulus, which can be provided by massage. Reflexes are specific and predictable. They are also purposeful and adaptive, and they explain most of the benefits of massage.
- **Mechanical methods** directly affect the soft tissue through techniques that normalize the connective tissue or move body fluids and intestinal contents.

The problem with this simple categorization is that the mechanism by which massage produces an effect cannot always be clearly identified. Dr. Philip E. Greenman has said that the effects of massage occur through the interrelationships of the peripheral and central nervous systems (and their reflex patterns and multiple pathways), the autonomic nervous system (ANS), and the neuroendocrine control.[9] According to Dr. John Yates, "It appears far more reasonable just to recognize that massage produces effects that are due to a combination of mechanical, neural, chemical, and psychological factors and to identify these wherever possible rather than to attempt to use them as a basis for classifying those effects."[25]

To understand the basis of research findings, it is necessary to understand the mechanisms by which massage applications achieve benefits. The anatomic and physiologic areas affected by massage are as follows:

- The neuroendocrine system (the central, autonomic, and somatic nervous systems, as well as neurochemicals and hormones)
- Connective tissue
- Circulation
- Energy systems

The Nervous System

The Effects of Massage on the Nervous System

The responses to massage and its effects on the nervous system are primarily reflexive.

Briefly, the nervous system is divided into the central nervous system (CNS), consisting of the brain and the spinal cord and its coverings, and the peripheral nervous system, which consists of nerves and ganglions (Fig. 4-1). The peripheral nervous system is further divided into the autonomic and somatic divisions. The autonomic division is subdivided into the sympathetic and parasympathetic systems. The sympathetic ANS is responsible for functions that expend energy in response to emergency situations. The parasympathetic division is more restorative and normalizing and returns the body to a non-alarm state. The somatic division of the peripheral nervous system is made up of the peripheral nerve fiber innervation of the body wall (e.g., muscles, joints, other structures).

The nervous system responds to therapeutic massage methods through stimulation of sensory receptors. The sensory stimulation from massage disrupts an existing pattern in the CNS control centers, resulting in a shift of motor impulses, most often in the peripheral nervous system, that reestablishes homeostasis. Usually both the somatic and autonomic divisions of the peripheral nervous system are influenced as balance is restored.

Neuroendocrine Interactions

To understand the benefits of massage as defined in the most current research, it is important to understand the functions of some of the neuroendocrine chemicals.

The endocrine system is regulated through the influence of the nervous system, and the endocrine system in turn influences the nervous system. It is a feedback loop, similar to a thermostat on a furnace. The feedback system and autoregulation (maintenance of internal homeostasis) are interlinked with all body functions. The controls for initiation of a reaction come through the nervous system and the endocrine system. Neuroendocrine chemicals are the communication transmitters of these control systems. A neuroendocrine chemical in the synapse of the nerve is called a **neurotransmitter.** A neuroendocrine chemical carried in the bloodstream is called a **hormone.** *Neuropeptide* also is a term used to describe these substances.

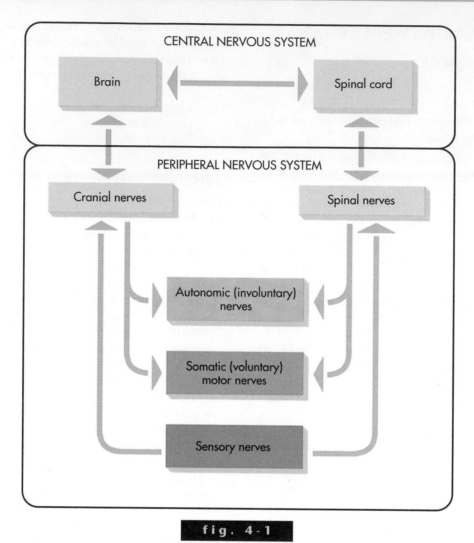

fig. 4-1

Divisions of the nervous system. (From Thibodeau GA, Patton KT: *The human body in health and disease,* ed 2, St Louis, 1997, Mosby.)

The neuroendocrine substances carry messages that regulate physiologic functions. Neuroendocrine regulation is a continuous, ever-changing chemical mix that fluctuates with each external and internal demand on the body to respond, adapt, or maintain a functional degree of homeostasis. The immune system also produces and responds to these communication substances. The substances that make up this "chemical soup" remain the same, but the proportion and ratio change with each regulating function or message transmission. The "flavor" of the soup, which is determined by the ratio of the chemical mix, affects such factors as mood, attentiveness, arousal, passiveness, vigilance, calm, ability to sleep, receptivity to touch, response to touch, anger, pessimism, optimism, connectedness, loneliness, depression, desire, hunger, love, and commitment.

Research now indicates that most problems in behavior, mood, and perception of stress and pain, as well as other so-called mental/emotional disorders, are caused by dysregulation or failure of the biochemicals. These behaviors, symptoms, and emotional and physical states often are normal chemical mixes that occur at inappropriate times.[12] For example, anxiety indicated by increased unresolvable stress is an appropriate chemical soup to have on the burner in a hostage situation because the hypervigilance accompanying such states may allow the hostage to see an opportunity for escape. However, this same soup bubbling away at the mall during holiday shopping is not productive.

Early endorphin research. In 1969 researchers observed that pain could be eliminated in rats without the use of anesthesia by stimulating the periaqueductal gray matter in the brainstem.[3] Other important discoveries soon confirmed this finding. The dedicated work of Dr. Candice Pert and others led to the discovery of the endogenous (made in the body) endorphin and nonendorphin pain-inhibiting systems of the CNS. The body produces several endogenous, opiate-like compounds, including enkephalin and beta endorphins (beta endorphin is a fragment of the pituitary hormone beta lipotropin). These peptides attach to opiate receptors (as does morphine) and, in most cases relieve pain, especially chronic pain, and produce euphoria. This finding supports the validity of acupuncture.

Acupuncture studies and implications for massage.

Acupuncture is an ancient healing art that involves much more than the insertion of needles into the body. Only the most fundamental concepts of acupuncture have been studied scientifically, but that research has revealed physiologic mechanisms affected by the method. Agreement has not been reached on what acupuncture points are, but the points used in acupuncture have an anatomic component. The traditional acupuncture points correspond to nerves that are close to the surface of the body. Most of the points fall over neurovascular bundles (areas of nerves and vessels), motor points (places where nerves innervate muscles), the focal meeting of superficial nerves in the sagittal plane, superficial nerves or nerve plexuses, and muscle-tendon junctions at the Golgi tendons (Fig. 4-2, *A* and *B*).[10]

Rather than needles, acupressure uses specific pinpoint compression over the same points. Some evidence indicates that acupuncture exerts its analgesic effect by causing the release of enkephalins, and the analgesia is said to be blocked by the morphine antagonist naloxone. In addition, a component of stress analgesia seems to arise from endogenous opiates, because in experimental animals some forms of stress analgesia are blocked by naloxone.

Acupuncture and acupressure seem to work by taking advantage of the body's natural inhibitory influences, which normally can block pain pathways. For example, it has been established that sensory pain fibers release a neurotransmitter called *substance P*, which increases the transmission of pain impulses. Enkephalin blocks the release of substance P, thereby inhibiting pain transmission to the brain. The effects of these and other neurotransmitters released during massage may explain and validate the use of sensory stimulation methods for treating chronic pain, anxiety, and depression.[15]

The effect of acupuncture or acupressure is delayed until the enkephalin level rises to inhibitory levels. It usually takes about 15 minutes for the blood level of enkephalin to begin to rise. The implication for massage is that the pain-inhibiting effects do not occur immediately. Massage practitioners should keep this in mind in regard to the intensity and duration of applications as they work. Similarly, the effect of acupuncture lingers after the twirling or vibration of the needles stops. The implication for massage is that the client should experience a prolonged effect from the massage, typically lasting about 48 hours.

The Influence of Massage on Neuroendocrine Substances

Much of the research on massage, especially that done at the Touch Research Institute, revolves around shifts in the proportion and ratio of the composition of the body's "chemical soup" brought about by massage.

Some of the main neuroendocrine chemicals influenced by massage are as follows:
- Dopamine
- Serotonin
- Epinephrine/adrenaline
- Norepinephrine/noradrenaline
- Enkephalins/endorphins
- Oxytocin
- Cortisol
- Growth hormone

Dopamine. Dopamine influences motor activity that involves movement (especially learned, fine movement such as handwriting), conscious selection (the ability to focus attention), and mood in terms of inspiration, possibility intuition, joy, and enthusiasm. Low levels of dopamine result in the opposite effects, such as lack of motor control, clumsiness, inability to focus attention, and boredom. Massage seems to increase the available level of dopamine in the body.

Serotonin. Serotonin allows a person to maintain context-appropriate behavior; that is, to do the appropriate thing at the appropriate time. It regulates mood in terms of appropriate emotions, attention to thoughts, and calming, quieting, comforting effects; it also subdues irritability and regulates drive states so that we can suppress the urge to talk, touch, and be involved in power struggles. For example, when someone tells you to "get a grip," they are saying that you could use a good boost in serotonin. Serotonin also is involved in satiety; adequate levels reduce the sense of hunger and craving, such as for food or sex. It also modulates the sleep/wake cycle. A low serotonin level has been implicated in depression, eating disorders, pain disorders, and obsessive-compulsive disorders. Massage seems to increase the available level of serotonin.

Epinephrine/adrenaline and norepinephrine/noradrenaline. The terms **epinephrine/adrenaline** and **norepinephrine/noradrenaline** are used interchangeably in scientific texts. Epinephrine activates arousal mechanisms in the body, whereas norepinephrine functions more in the brain. These are the activation, arousal, alertness, and alarm chemicals of the fight-or-flight response and of all sympathetic arousal functions and behaviors. If the levels of these chemicals are too high or if they are released at an inappropriate time, a person feels as though something very important is demanding his attention or reacts with the basic survival drives of fight or flight (hypervigilance and hyperactivity). The person might have a disturbed sleep pattern, particularly in a lack of rapid eye movement (REM) sleep, which is restorative sleep. With low levels of epinephrine and norepinephrine, the individual is sluggish, drowsy, fatigued, and underaroused.

Massage seems to have a regulating effect on epinephrine and norepinephrine through stimulation or inhibition of the sympathetic nervous system or stimulation or inhibition of the parasympathetic nervous system. This generalized balancing function of massage seems to recalibrate the appropriate adrenaline and noradrenaline levels. Depending on the response of the ANS, then, massage can just as easily wake a person up and relieve fatigue as it can calm down a person who is angry and pacing the floor. It should be noted that initially touch stimulates the sympathetic nervous system, whereas it seems to take 15 minutes or so of sustained stimulation to begin to engage the parasympathetic functions. Therefore it makes sense that a 15-minute chair massage tends to increase production of epinephrine and norepinephrine, which can help cor-

porate workers become more attentive, whereas a 1-hour slow, rhythmic massage engages the parasympathetic functions, reducing epinephrine and norepinephrine levels and encouraging a good night's sleep.

Enkephalins/endorphins. **Enkephalins/endorphins** are mood lifters that support satiety and modulate pain. Massage increases the available levels of enkephalins and endorphins.

Oxytocin. **Oxytocin** is a hormone that has been implicated in pair or couple bonding, parental bonding, feelings of attachment, and care taking, along with its more clinical functions during pregnancy, delivery, and lactation. Massage tends to increase the available level of oxytocin, which could explain the connected and intimate feeling of massage.

Cortisol. **Cortisol** and other glucocorticoids are stress hormones produced by the adrenal glands during prolonged

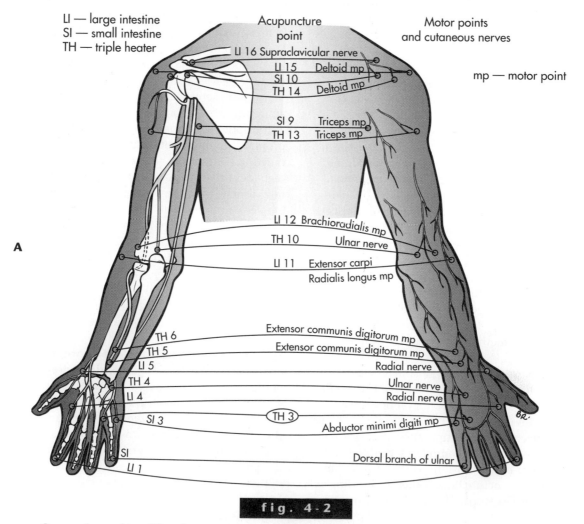

fig. 4-2

Comparison of traditional acupuncture points, motor points, and cutaneous nerves of the arms (**A**) and legs (**B**).

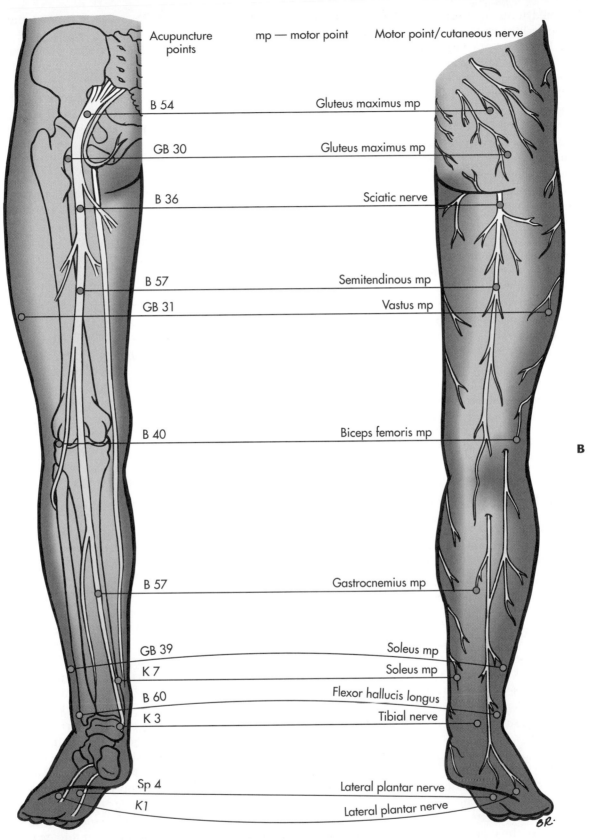

Acupuncture points   mp — motor point   Motor point/cutaneous nerve

B 54 — Gluteus maximus mp

GB 30 — Gluteus maximus mp

B 36 — Sciatic nerve

B 57 — Semitendinous mp

GB 31 — Vastus mp

B 40 — Biceps femoris mp

B 57 — Gastrocnemius mp

GB 39 — Soleus mp

K 7 — Soleus mp

B 60 — Flexor hallucis longus

K 3 — Tibial nerve

Sp 4 — Lateral plantar nerve

K 1 — Lateral plantar nerve

B

BR.

B — bladder
GB — gallbladder
K — kidney
Sp — spleen

fig. 4-2, cont'd

For legend, see opposite page.

stress. Elevated levels of these hormones indicate increased sympathetic arousal. Cortisol and other glucocorticoids have been implicated in many stress-related symptoms and diseases, including suppressed immunity states, sleep disturbances, and increases in the level of substance P. Massage has been shown to reduce levels of cortisol and substance P.

Growth hormone. **Growth hormone** promotes cell division and in adults has been implicated in the functions of tissue repair and regeneration. This hormone is necessary for healing and is most active during sleep. Massage increases the availability of growth hormone indirectly by encouraging sleep and reducing the level of cortisol.

Combined neuroendocrine influences. Massage increases the blood levels of serotonin, dopamine, and endorphins, which in turn facilitates the production of natural killer cells in the immune system. This response indicates that it would be beneficial to include massage as part of the total treatment program for viral conditions and some forms of cancer. Oxytocin tends to increase supporting feelings of connectedness. At the same time, massage reduces cortisol and regulates epinephrine and norepinephrine, which facilitates the action of growth hormone.

It is easy to see why massage is beneficial for so many conditions and indirectly influences many others. Consider the following examples:

- A lonely, depressed person feels more alive after a massage (increase in serotonin and oxytocin; decrease in cortisol).
- A child with attention deficit/hyperactivity disorder (ADHD) can do her homework after a 15-minute massage (increase in dopamine and noradrenaline).
- A person suffering from chronic pain functions better after a massage (increase in endorphin, serotonin, and oxytocin).
- A smoker trying to quit can forestall a craving for a cigarette after a massage (increase in noradrenaline, serotonin, and endorphin).
- A person who has had surgery heals faster with massage (decrease in cortisol and adrenaline; increase in restorative sleep through pain reduction; increase in endorphin and serotonin, resulting in greater availability of growth hormone).
- An individual infected with the human immunodeficiency virus (HIV) may have a stronger immune response after massage (increase in serotonin, dopamine, and endorphin, decrease in cortisol).
- A couple may relate better to their newborn child after learning to give the infant a massage (increase in serotonin and oxytocin; decrease in cortisol).
- People just feel better, cope more easily, and have more joy when massaged (neuroendocrine chemical processes give rise to higher levels of integrated thought, such as

beliefs and values, interpreting context and meaning, forming intuition, making plans, and predicting, choosing, and carrying through with dreams).

Indications are explored in greater depth in Chapter 5. This chapter is intended to help the student understand the research findings that point toward neuroendocrine chemicals as a big piece of the "why massage works" puzzle.

Autonomic Influences

The effects of massage can be processed through the ANS. These effects, which are primarily reflexive, are as follows:

- Sympathetic activation and stress
- Parasympathetic patterns and conservation withdrawal
- Entrainment
- Body/mind effect
- Toughening/hardening
- Placebo effect

The Autonomic Nervous System

The ANS is best known for its regulation of the sympathetic "fight/flight/fear" response and the parasympathetic "relaxation and restorative" response (Table 4-1). The sympathetic and parasympathetic systems work together to maintain homeostasis through a feedback loop system. These systems both affect and are affected by the endocrine glands. Specific muscle patterns are associated with both systems. Arm and leg muscles may be tight with sympathetic response and postural muscles tight with parasympathetic response (Fig. 4-3).

Excessive sympathetic output causes most of the stress-related diseases that physicians see. Examples of such diseases include headaches, gastrointestinal difficulties, high blood pressure, anxiety, muscle tension and aches, and sexual dysfunction.

The ANS is regulated by several centers in the brain, particularly the cerebral cortex, hypothalamus, and medulla oblongata. The hypothalamus largely controls the ANS. It receives impulses from the visceral (organ) sensory fibers and from some somatic (muscle and joint) sensory fibers. The hypothalamus plays an important role in the body/mind connection.[11] It is one of the main components of the limbic system.

The *limbic system* is a group of brain structures, activated by emotional behavior and arousal, that influence the endocrine and autonomic systems. Limbic responses are reflected in a general alteration of mood and in feelings of well-being or distress. A property of limbic neural circuits is their prolonged afterdischarge following stimulation; this may explain why emotional responses generally are extended and outlast the stimuli that initiate them.

Research indicates that the cerebellum, the limbic pain and pleasure centers, and the various relay centers are all part of one circuit.[11] The cerebellum controls both conscious and subconscious movements of skeletal muscle,

table 4-1

FUNCTIONS OF THE AUTONOMIC NERVOUS SYSTEM

Viscera	Sympathetic control	Parasympathetic control
Heart	Accelerates heartbeat	Slows heartbeat
Smooth Muscle		
Most blood vessels	Constricts blood vessels	None
Blood vessels of skeletal muscle	Dilates blood vessels	None
Digestive tract	Decreases peristalsis; inhibits defecation	Increases peristalsis
Anal sphincter	Stimulates (closes sphincter)	Inhibits (opens sphincter for defecation)
Urinary bladder	Inhibits (relaxes bladder)	Stimulates (contracts bladder)
Urinary sphincters	Stimulates (closes sphincter)	Inhibits (opens sphincter for urination)
Iris	Stimulates radial fibers (dilation of pupil)	Stimulates circular fibers (constriction of pupil)
Ciliary muscles	Inhibits (accommodates for far vision; flattening of lens)	Stimulates (accommodates for near vision; bulging of lens)
Hair (pilomotor muscles)	Stimulates ("goose pimples")	None
Glands		
Adrenal medulla	Increases secretion of epinephrine	None
Sweat glands	Increases secretion of sweat	None
Digestive glands	Decreases secretion of digestive juices	Increases secretion of digestive juices

input from proprioceptors, feedback loops, posture, future positioning, and sensations of anger and pleasure.

Sympathetic Activation and Stress

Hans Selye called the body's response to **stress** the **general adaptation syndrome,** which he suggested can be divided into three stages:

- The first stage is the *alarm reaction,* also called the *fight-or-flight response,* which is the body's initial reaction to the perceived stressor.
- The second stage is the *resistance reaction,* which, through the secretion of regulating hormones, allows the body to continue fighting a stressor long after the effects of the alarm reaction have dissipated.
- The third stage is the *exhaustion reaction,* which takes place if the stress response continues without relief.

Selye's general adaptation syndrome responses are commonly called **sympathetic** activations. Activation of the sympathetic nervous system usually results in sensations that people call *stress.* Excessive stress can cause bodywide distress.

Which comes first, the emotion or the release of the hormones? Science has discovered that it is rather like the chicken and the egg problem. Intense emotion, such as fear, rage, and anxiety, plays a part in activating the fight-or-flight response. The hormones epinephrine and norepinephrine are released in response to stimulation, and the alarm reaction begins. The alarm reaction lasts 15 to 30 minutes. When this fight-or-flight response occurs, blood pressure increases, muscles tense, digestion and elimination shut down, circulation patterns shift, and glycogen is mobilized.

Long-term stress (i.e., stress that can't be resolved by fleeing or fighting) may also trigger the release of cortisol, a cortisone manufactured by the body. Long-term high blood levels of cortisol cause side effects similar to those of the drug cortisone, including fluid retention, hypertension, muscle weakness, osteoporosis, breakdown of connective tissue, peptic ulcer, impaired wound healing, vertigo, headache, reduced ability to deal with stress, hypersensitivity, weight gain, nausea, fatigue, and psychic disturbances.

When the body can no longer tolerate the effects of stress, the exhaustion phase begins. In long-term sympathetic stress, tension builds until the body basically wears

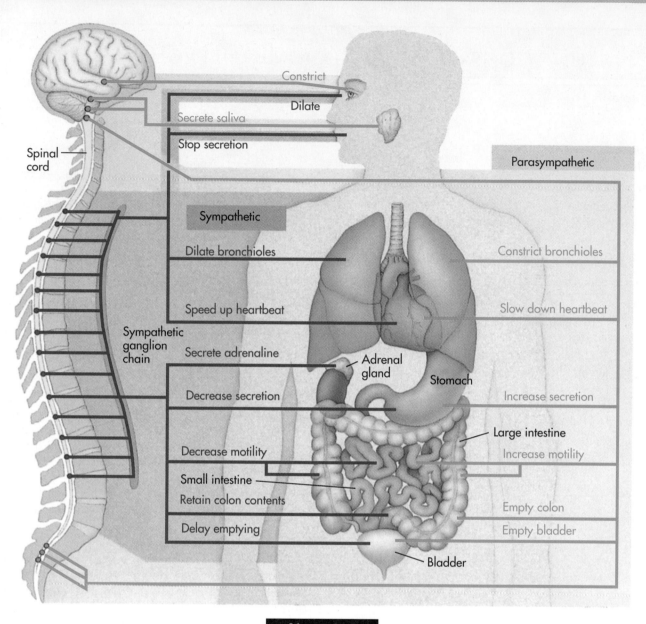

fig. 4-3

Innervation of the major target organs by the ANS. (From Thibodeau GA, Patton KT: *The human body in health and disease,* ed 2, St Louis, 1997, Mosby.)

out. Cardiovascular, upper respiratory, and gastrointestinal problems tend to develop. The body begins to break down.

In our society most of us do not physically fight or flee from stressors, although the chemical reactions commanding these actions may be activated several times a day. So what happens to the chemicals? We each find our own way to dissipate them, such as yelling at our family or driving aggressively. Most of us would like to find more appropriate ways to release the chemicals. Moderate exercise is one of the best ways to burn up fight-or-flight chemicals.

Studies done with slow-stroke back massage suggest a complex interaction among the autonomic, somatic, emotional, and cognitive elements in response to massage.[15]

The results suggest that stroking the back with slow, long strokes causes reflex inhibition of the muscle spindle. If the massage is continued for at least 6 minutes, slow-stroke back massage lowers the autonomic arousal. The long-term effect of slow-stroke back massage is a decrease in psychoemotional and somatic arousal.[15] Simply put, slow-stroke back massage calms people.

Parasympathetic Patterns and Conservation Withdrawal

Because **parasympathetic** patterns are restorative, physical activity is curtailed and digestion and elimination increase. Peace and calmness are results of parasympathetic influence. When we become fatigued, parasympathetic functions signal the body to rest. Chronic fatigue syndrome is a good example of a parasympathetic reaction to stress. More drastically, depression can manifest with parasympathetic dysfunction.

Conservation withdrawal is another factor to be considered in a discussion of the parasympathetic patterns. In animals, conservation withdrawal is similar to "playing possum" or hibernation; in human beings it may arise as a result of intense negative experiences such as abuse, neglect, or starvation. To a lesser degree, conservation withdrawal patterns play a part in depression.

A massage that is more stimulating may help draw a client out of withdrawal patterns. All sensations, including touch, initially stimulate, whether they are received through visual, audio, or kinesthetic processes. Stimulation that is quick and unexpected arouses. More commonly, massage encourages parasympathetic activation to counter the effects of sympathetic overarousal.

Entrainment

Entrainment is an important reflexive effect that seems to be processed through the ANS.

Entrain means "to drag with." **Entrainment** is the coordination of or synchronization to a rhythm. In the body, biologic oscillators such as the heart and thalamus set the rhythm pattern. Research done at the Institute of HeartMath and other facilities indicates that the heart rhythm tends to be the guide for other body rhythms.[16] The heart rate/respiratory rate/thalamus synchronization combines to support the entrainment process, and the other, more subtle body rhythms follow. The synchronization of the rhythms of our heart, respiration, and digestion promotes this balance, or homeostasis, to support a healthy body. A balance between the sympathetic and parasympathetic divisions of the ANS influences the sinus node of the heart and the vascular systems, which in turn modulates heart rate and blood pressure. Our nasal reflexes, stimulated by the movement of air through the nose, rhythmically interact with the heart, lungs, and diaphragm.[23] Thus the entire body is affected because biologic rhythms are interconnected.

The CNS includes a rhythm known as the *craniosacral impulse,* which can be observed and palpated. The effects of bodywork on this particular rhythm currently are being researched, but entrainment methods that synchronize the motions and rhythms of the body are credited with providing the most benefit.[17]

The body also entrains to external rhythms. Any activity that uses a repetitive motion or sound quiets or excites the nervous system (depending on the speed and pace of the rhythm) through entrainment and thereby alters the physiologic process of the body. Sometimes the body rhythms are disrupted. Music with disharmony and discord can be disruptive, as can multiple rhythms out of sync in the same environment, such as a shopping mall with flashing lights, many different types of music being played at one time, and the humming of machinery. People often become fatigued or "out of sorts" in these disharmonic environments.

The body most easily entrains to natural rhythms, such as the sounds of a babbling brook, ocean waves, or the rustling of leaves in the breeze. Studies have shown that the rhythmic physiologic patterns of a dog's or cat's breathing or heart rate can be beneficial to the elderly. Music with a regular 4/4 beat at 60 beats per minute or less tends to order rhythms and calm the body. A tempo faster than 60 beats per minute seems to excite physiologically, but if the rhythm is even, the body can achieve a focused alert state. Many forms of classical music provide resourceful entrainment rhythms. Music therapy is one of the main sources of entrainment research. Music is a common addition to massage and provides an external entrainment rhythm for the practitioner and client.

When a person experiences positive emotional states, the biologic rhythms naturally tend to begin to oscillate together or entrain. Body entrainment processes also can be enhanced by techniques that shift our consciousness to our breathing patterns and heart rate. Most meditation processes or relaxation methods create an environment for entrainment by reducing external influences and focusing on internal rhythms such as breathing. Many disciplines quiet the mind and body during mediation; yoga, for examples, focuses attention on breathing, whereas Qigong focuses on the point below the navel. These systems center attention on body areas with known biologic oscillators. The location of the chakra system correlates with biologic oscillators. The rhythmic patterns of singing, chanting, and movement in our religious and social rituals interact with biologic patterns, resulting in a calming or exciting organization or disruption of body rhythms.

Many years of research will be required before we will understand the magnitude of the influences that affect our body rhythms. Current research focuses on the possibility that disease processes might result from disruptions in body rhythms, and on the effects of work environments that directly disturb or alter natural body rhythms.

The influence of massage on entrainment. To encourage entrainment, massage is provided in a quiet, rhythmic manner. The rhythmic application of massage and the proximity of a centered and compassionate professional's breathing rate and heart rate can support restorative entrainment if body rhythms are out of sync. The focused, centered professional introduces his own ordered rhythms as part of the environment; they serve as an additional external influence that enables the client's body rhythms to synchronize. When synchronization occurs, homeostatic mechanisms seem to work more efficiently.

THINK IT OVER

Rhythms tend to entrain to the rhythm that is strongest. What might happen if the practitioner is tired or a bit out of sorts while working with a client who is strongly out of sync? Who might entrain to whom? How might the professional and the client each feel? On the other hand, if the client is very focused and together, in what way might the entrainment be different?

The Body/Mind Effect

The ANS association is where the body/mind link is best understood. An *altered state of consciousness* is any state of awareness that differs from the normal awareness of a conscious person. Altered states of consciousness are a factor in body/mind interactions. Consciousness can be altered in many ways; for example, by medications or foods that change chemical processes, by repetitive activities or sounds (entrainment), and by a trance state. For centuries many cultures and religions have explored altered states of consciousness and have used them readily in defensive actions, in healing, and in controlling pain. Meditation, tai chi, and yoga are examples of ancient methods used to achieve altered states of consciousness. We can achieve a similar result by gardening, drawing, knitting, or playing a musical instrument.

Both the practitioner and the client can achieve an altered state of consciousness during a bodywork session. After the altered state has been achieved, it must be maintained for at least 15 minutes to reap the most therapeutic benefit.

State-dependent memory. Another aspect of the body/mind connection that interacts with the ANS is state-dependent memory. The triggering of a pattern of movement or a particular pressure sensation caused by trauma or learned habit sometimes is enough to enable the individual to achieve a particular altered state of consciousness. This results in a second release of the chemical codes of the emotions involved. Emotional input registers in the body through the ANS and the endocrine system. As described previously, a definite chemical factor is involved in the arousal of emotions based on the body's production of endorphins, enkephalins, epinephrine, norepinephrine, other hormones, and neurotransmitters. If these chemicals are released into the bloodstream during bodywork, the individual may once again feel the chemical arousal of an emotion, perhaps triggering a memory.

The adrenal hormones that interplay with the sympathetic responses are intimately involved with short-term memory. Norepinephrine depletion reduces memory storage, and elevation increases it. The "state" in state-dependent memory is either a sympathetic or a parasympathetic nervous system function coupled with a unique neuroendocrine chemical mix. If a person has an experience while in one of these states, the memory is encoded (stored in that state). Research shows that memory is accessible to an individual only when the particular body chemistry and function are similar to those of the experience as it first happened.[20]

Because of its effects on the ANS, massage can stimulate these state-dependent memory patterns. This can be useful in allowing the client to resolve a past experience that was unresolvable when it occurred. Often counseling is necessary to help the person sort the memory pattern

---

4-2

PROFICIENCY EXERCISE

In what way do you think the day-to-day activities listed below depend on the ANS?

A person eats when tired, but not hungry.

The driver of a car does not have to stop to use the restroom, although the children in the back seat do.

When the driver of the car tells the children that they are not going to stop to use the restroom and that they have to wait, the children start fighting.

A person's stomach starts growling half an hour after a boring lecture begins.

Watching a scary movie makes you feel like doing something exciting and active.

Give two other daily experiences that are influenced by the ANS.

and develop strategies for resolution, integration, and coping. Although these activities are outside the scope of practice of therapeutic massage, combined with effective counseling by trained professionals, massage can be a very beneficial part of an overall treatment plan. Exciting research currently is underway on state-dependent learning in sympathetic and parasympathetic patterns of function. See Chapter 12 for additional information (Proficiency Exercise 4-2).

Toughening/Hardening

The autonomic reaction to massage can be explained by a concept known as *toughening*, or *hardening*. **Toughening/ hardening** is the reaction to repeated exposure to stimuli that elicit arousal responses. The planned presentation of stimuli teaches the body to manage more efficiently with sympathetic stress responses. Forms of passive toughening/hardening, such as repeated exposure to cold shock, have been found to increase an individual's tolerance to stress. During exposure to the cold, two hormones of the adrenal medulla, epinephrine and norepinephrine, are released into the bloodstream.

Although massage is not as severe as cold shock, the increase in autonomic functioning and its passive nature may indeed be characterized as a form of passive toughening/hardening.[14] As with exercise, massage methods that require the client's active participation help to dissipate sympathetic stress hormones (sympathoadrenal response), allowing the system to reestablish homeostasis (Proficiency Exercise 4-3).

The Placebo Effect

Throughout history people have known that treatment in itself influences the course of a disease, even if the treatment is not specific. This **placebo** effect probably is caused by several mechanisms, most of which are not yet clearly understood. The environment, suggestions from and the attitude of the person giving the placebo, and the patient's confidence in its effectiveness act together to produce a placebo effect. Some studies have reported a success rate of 70% to 90% using placebos. The gentle, caring attention focused on the client during therapeutic massage may work with the powerful placebo effect.

The Influence of Massage on the ANS

Because of its generalized effect on the ANS and associated functions, massage can cause changes in mood and excitement levels and can induce the relaxation/restorative response. Massage seems to be a gentle modulator, producing feelings of general well-being and comfort. However, this does not always mean that the client responds to the massage by becoming very relaxed. The most common response is a sense that "the edge is off" or a less urgent or intense emotional state.

The client may be better able to function in a self-regulating fashion, controlling the emotional state rather than being controlled by it. This ability to self-regulate is very important in the physiologic process. Another name for self-regulation is *internal control*. We tend to feel more at ease when we feel a sense of internal control.

Initially massage stimulates sympathetic functions. This really surprises students who think that they are giving a relaxation massage. The increase in autonomic function is followed by a decrease if the massage is slowed or terminated. To encourage more of a sympathetic response, participation in muscle energy techniques is helpful (see Chapter 9). Compression and a fast-paced massage style, similar to pre-event sports massage, stimulate sympathetic responses and may lift depression temporarily.

Repetitive stroking, broad-based compression, or movement initiates relaxation responses. It is the old "follow the watch" hypnosis induction trick. Rhythmic bodywork creates a trancelike effect. People are very open to suggestion at this time, and the therapist should be attentive to any type of leading discussion or suggestions.

Simple active muscle energy techniques (see Chapter 9) can replace some exercise, dissipate sympathetic stress, and help to alleviate depression.

Point holding, such as acupressure or reflexology (see Chapter 11), and the dry needling of acupuncture release the body's own painkillers and mood-altering chemicals from the entire endorphin class. These chemicals stimulate the parasympathetic responses of relaxation, restoration, and contentment.

Acupressure causes sympathetic inhibition.[7] These methods of massage depend on the creation of a moderate, controlled pain to relieve pain. It takes a larger pain or stress stimulus to generate the endorphin response than the perception of the existing pain. When the release of substance P triggers pain, enkephalins are released, which suppress the pain signal. A negative feedback system activates the release of serotonin and opiates, which inhibit pain.[3] Therapeutic massage methods can be used to create a controlled, noxious (pain) stimulation that triggers this cycle. Clients often refer to this noxious stimulation as *good pain*.

---

4 - 3

PROFICIENCY EXERCISE

In what way is exercise a form of "hardening"?

Breathing is a powerful way to interact with the ANS. Chest breathing and hyperventilation are common components of increased sympathetic stimulation. In order for the body to deal with stress, the muscular patterns of breathing must be normalized (see Chapter 13 for additional information on breathing). Most meditation breathing patterns, singing, and chanting are ways to normalize those patterns through entrainment.

Altering the muscles so that they are more or less tense or changing the consistency of the connective tissue affects the ANS through the feedback loop, which in turn affects the powerful body/mind phenomenon.

Somatic Influences

The effects of massage can be processed through the somatic division of the peripheral nervous system; the somatic division controls movement and muscle contraction and relaxation patterns, as well as muscle tone. The effects are primarily reflexive.

Somatic effects are produced by means of the following:
- Neuromuscular mechanisms
- Hyperstimulation analgesia
- Counterirritation
- Reduction of impingement (entrapment and compression)

Neuromuscular Mechanisms

The prefix *neuro* refers to the nervous system; *muscular* refers to the muscles. The *neuromuscular effect* is the control of the muscles through signals from the nervous system and the response of the muscles to those signals.

Nerve cells stimulate muscles to contract or relax (release a contraction). Specialized nerve receptors called *proprioceptors* (or *mechanoreceptors*) provide a constant monitoring and protective function. Proprioceptors receive and transmit information about muscle tension, static tone, degree of stretch, joint position, and speed of movement.

Dysfunction of soft tissue (muscle and connective tissue) without proprioceptive hyperactivity or hypoactivity is uncommon. Proprioceptive hyperactivity causes tense or spastic muscles and hypoactivity of opposing muscle groups. Put simply, a tight muscle area results in or from a weakened muscle area and vice versa.

Proprioceptors provide the body with information about position, movement, muscle tension, joint activity, and equilibrium. The three main types of proprioceptors are muscle spindles, tendon organs, and joint kinesthetic receptors:

- **Muscle spindles** are found primarily in the belly of the muscle; they respond to both sudden and prolonged stretches.
- **Tendon organs** are found in the tendon and musculotendinous junction; they respond to tension at the tendon. Articular (joint) ligaments, which contain receptors similar to tendon organs, adjust reflex in-

hibition of the adjacent muscle when excessive strain is placed on the joints.
- **Joint kinesthetic receptors** are found in the capsules of joints; they respond to pressure and to acceleration and deceleration of joint movement. The two main types of joint kinesthetic receptors are *type II cutaneous mechanoreceptors* and *pacinian (lamellated) corpuscles.*

Somatic Reflexes

Stimulation of nervous system receptors is interpreted and processed through the somatic reflex arcs. Reflexes are fast, predictable, automatic responses to a change in the environment that help maintain homeostasis (Fig. 4-4). The stimulation of therapeutic massage constitutes a change in the environment. When the body is called on to restore homeostasis, nonproductive nerve transmission pathways often are overridden.[5] The reflexes most often stimulated are the stretch reflex, tendon reflex, flexor reflex, and crossed extensor reflex.

The stretch reflex. The stretch reflex is activated by the muscle spindles, which sense muscle stretching. In response to massage methods that stretch muscles, a muscle spindle produces nerve impulses that stimulate a somatic sensory neuron in the posterior root of the spinal nerve. When the motor nerve impulse reaches the stretched muscle, a muscle action potential is generated, which causes the muscle to contract. Muscle contraction stops spindle cell discharge. The muscle stretch stimulates the stretch reflex, resulting in shortening of the muscle. The sensitivity of the muscle spindle in response to stretching influences the level of muscle tone throughout the body.

Therapeutic massage methods can make use of this reflex to stimulate weak muscle patterns by stretching the muscles and initiating the stretch reflex. An awareness of this reflex response is important in all stretches that are intended to lengthen and relax the muscles. In these instances the reflex must be avoided. Often this system of reflexes becomes hyperactive, which results in an increase in muscle tension. Massage techniques that use isometric and isotonic muscle contraction to relax and lengthen muscles are helpful in normalizing excess muscle tension.

The tendon reflex. The stretch reflex operates as a feedback mechanism to control muscle length by causing muscle contraction. The tendon reflex, on the other hand, operates as a feedback mechanism to control muscle tension by causing muscle relaxation. This reflex is mediated by the tendon organs, which detect and respond to changes in muscle tension caused by the pull of muscular contraction.

The most common massage technique used to stimulate the tendon reflex is postisometric relaxation (see Chapter 9). This technique increases tension at the tendon. The tendon organ is stimulated, which sends a signal along

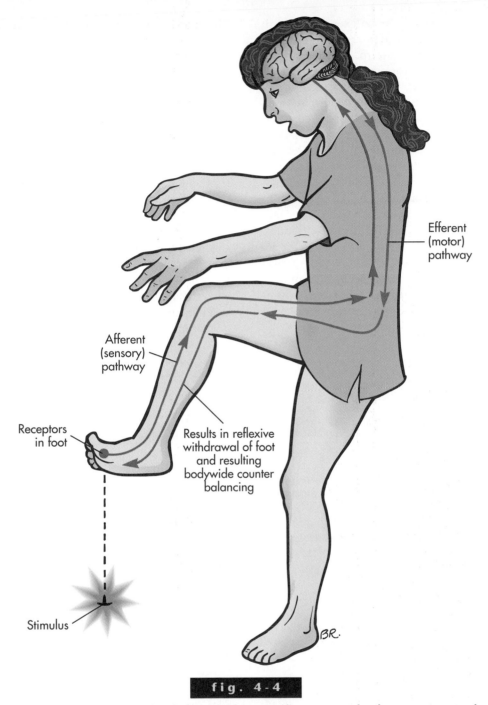

Efferent
(motor)
pathway

Afferent
(sensory)
pathway

Receptors
in foot

Results in reflexive
withdrawal of foot
and resulting
bodywide counter
balancing

Stimulus

fig. 4-4

Reflex response. Localized stimulation of a few specific receptors leads to many outgoing impulses, which affect a large number of muscles.

a sensory neuron. In the spinal cord the sensory neuron synapses with an inhibitory association neuron, which inhibits motor neurons that innervate the muscle associated with the tendon organ. This inhibition causes the muscle to relax. The sensory neuron from the tendon organ also stimulates an association neuron in the spinal cord. This association neuron synapses with a motor neuron, controlling antagonistic muscles and causing them to contract. To sim-

plify, when one muscle contracts, its antagonist, or opposing muscle group, must relax; this is called *reciprocal innervation.* Massage practitioners often use reciprocal innervation to avoid the stretch reflex response and prepare a muscle for lengthening and stretching.

The flexor and crossed extensor reflexes. The flexor (withdrawal) and crossed extensor reflexes are polysynaptic reflex arcs. Stimulation of these reflexes affects both sides of the body through a series of intersegmental reflex arcs that usually are linked in a pattern. A single sensory neuron can activate several motor neurons. The flexor reflex is involved in moving away from a stimuli, and the crossed extensor reflex is involved in maintaining balance. Synchronized control over the muscles that are contracting and those that are inhibited (allowing for relaxation) is achieved through contralateral reflex arcs, or reflex arcs on both sides of the body.

By creating a noxious signal (i.e., pain or an unpleasant sensation), therapeutic massage can stimulate a withdrawal response to stimulate opposite-side patterns of tension or weakness. This is a powerful response because withdrawal reflexes take priority over all other reflex activity occurring at the moment. These reflex patterns also explain why tension patterns seldom occur only on one side of the body. The linked patterns of the reflex influence explain why dysfunctional patterns of groups of muscles often are identified.

The influence of massage on neuromuscular mechanisms. When working with the neuromuscular mechanism in massage, the basic premises are (1) to substitute a different neurologic signal stimulation to support a normal muscle resting length through lengthening and stretching of muscles and connective tissue and (2) to reeducate the muscles involved (e.g., take the joint through its increased range of motion).

Movement, stretch, and pressure methods of massage focus on the activities of the muscles, tendons, joints, and ligaments to stimulate the proprioceptors. Massage methods can stimulate the resetting of unproductive reflex actions.

The effects of therapeutic massage depend heavily on the reflex mechanism. The effectiveness of the techniques depends on how efficiently the receptors for these reflexes are stimulated. The targeted receptor must be accessed with the appropriate technique and intensity so that the stimulated reflex can function appropriately.

Various neurologic laws come into play when explor-

NEUROLOGIC LAWS AND THEIR IMPLICATIONS FOR MASSAGE

All-or-none (Bowditch's) Law
The weakest stimulus capable of producing a response produces the maximal response contraction in cardiac and skeletal muscle and nerves.[2]

Implication for massage: Techniques need not be extremely intense to produce a response; all that is needed is enough sensory stimulation to begin the process.

Arndt-Schulz Law
Weak stimuli activate physiologic processes; very strong stimuli inhibit them.[21]

Implication for massage: To encourage a specific response, use gentler methods. To shut off a response, use deeper methods.

Bell's Law
Anterior spinal nerve roots are motor roots and posterior spinal nerve roots are sensory roots.[22]

Implication for massage: Massage along the spine is a strong sensory stimulation.

Cannon's Law of Denervation
When autonomic effectors are partly or completely separated from their normal nerve connections, they become more sensitive to the action of chemical substances.[6]

This denervation supersensitivity involves injured nerves, which respond to all sensory stimulation regardless of whether the stimulation is specific to that nerve. Denervation supersensitivity is a universal phenomenon that affects muscles, nerves, salivary glands, sudorific glands, autonomic ganglion cells, spinal neurons, and even neurons in the cor-

tex. Changes in muscle structure and biochemistry, as well as progressive destruction of the contractile elements of fibers, also occur. Furthermore, unlike normal muscle fibers, which resist innervation from foreign nerves, degenerated muscle fibers accept contacts from other motor nerves, preganglionic autonomic fibers, and even sensory nerves.

Implication for massage: An injured area may hyperreact even after healing to all sensory stimulation. If a person has a cold or is stressed at work or cannot sleep, previously injured areas may flare up.

Hilton's Law
A nerve trunk that supplies a joint also supplies the muscles of the joint and the skin over the insertions of such muscles.[22]

Implication for massage: It is difficult to figure out if a pain originates from the joint itself, the muscles around a joint, or the skin over a joint; stimulation of each area affects all parts.

Hooke's Law
The stress used to stretch or compress a body is proportional to the strain experienced, as long as the elastic limits of the body have not been exceeded.[22]

Implication for massage: Methods that lengthen the tissue must be intense enough to match the existing shortening but must not exceed it.

Law of Facilitation
When an impulse has passed through a certain set of neurons to the exclusion of others one time, it will tend to

ing the effects of therapeutic massage on the somatic nervous system (Box 4-2). A **law** is a scientific statement that is uniformly true for a whole class of natural occurrences.

Some controversy exists about the validity of some of these laws, primarily Pflüger's laws; however, it is valid to consider these neurologic laws in attempting to understand the physiologic effects of massage.

The Vestibular Apparatus and Cerebellum

The vestibular apparatus (inner ear balance mechanism) and the cerebellum are interrelated. The output from the cerebellum goes to the motor cortex and brainstem. Stimulating the cerebellum by altering muscle tone, position, and vestibular balance stimulates the hypothalamus to adjust ANS functions to restore homeostasis.

The influence of massage on the vestibular apparatus and cerebellum. The techniques that most strongly affect the vestibular apparatus and therefore the cerebellum are those that produce rhythmic rocking during the application of massage. Rocking produces movement at the neck and head that influences the sense of equilibrium. Rocking stimulates the inner ear balance mechanisms, including the vestibular nuclear complex and the labyrinthine righting reflexes, to keep the head level. Pressure on the sides of the body may stimulate the body-righting reflex. Stimulation of these reflexes produces a bodywide effect involving stimulation of muscle contraction patterns, which pass throughout the body.

Massage alters body positional sense and initiates specific movement patterns that change sensory input from muscles, tendons, joints, and the skin. This feedback information, which adjusts and coordinates movement, is relayed directly to the motor cortex and the cerebellum.

Hyperstimulation Analgesia

In 1965 Melzack and Wall proposed the **gate control theory.** Although some aspects of the original theory have been modified over the past 30 years, the basic premise remains viable. According to this theory, a gating mecha-

---

box 4-2

NEUROLOGIC LAWS AND THEIR IMPLICATIONS FOR MASSAGE—CONT'D

take the same course on a future occasion, and each time it traverses this path the resistance will be smaller.[21]

Implication for massage: The body likes sameness, which produces habitual patterns. After a pattern has been established, less stimulation is required to activate the response.

Law of Specificity of Nervous Energy

Excitation of a receptor always gives rise to the same sensation regardless of the nature of the stimulus.[22]

Implication for massage: Whatever the method used, if a sensory receptor is activated, it will respond in a specific way.

Pflüger's Laws

Law of generalization

When the irritation becomes very intense, it is propagated in the medulla oblongata, which becomes a focus from which stimuli radiate to all parts of the cord, causing a general contraction of all muscles in the body.[21]

Implication for massage: This response must be avoided if possible. It is important to keep invasive massage measures (e.g., frictioning) below the intensity level that causes a general body response.

Law of intensity

Reflex movements usually are more intense on the side of irritation; at times the movements of the opposite side equal the movements in intensity, but they usually are less pronounced.[21]

Implication for massage: See Law of symmetry.

Law of radiation

If the excitation continues to increase, it is propagated upward, and reactions take place through centrifugal nerves coming from the higher cord segments.[21]

Implication for massage: See Law of Symmetry.

Law of symmetry

If the stimulation is increased sufficiently, motor reaction is manifested not only on the irritated side but also in similar muscles on the opposite side of the body.[21]

Implication for massage: By using increasing levels of massage intensity, a bilateral effect can be created, even if only one side of the body is massaged. This is especially useful for massage applications to painful areas. By massaging the unaffected side, the painful areas can be addressed without receiving direct massage work.

Law of unilaterality

If a mild irritation is applied to one or more sensory nerves, the movement will take place usually on one side only and on the side that has been irritated.[21]

Implication for massage: Light stimulation remains fairly localized in response to massage.

Weber's Law

The increase in stimulus necessary to produce the smallest perceptible increase in sensation bears a constant ratio to the strength of the stimulus already acting.[22]

Implication for massage: For a massage method to change a sensory perception, the intensity of the method must match and then just exceed the existing sensation.

nism functions at the level of the spinal cord; that is, pain impulses pass through a "gate" to reach the lateral spinothalamic system. Painful impulses are transmitted by large-diameter and small-diameter nerve fibers. Stimulation of large-diameter fibers prevents the small-diameter fibers from transmitting signals. Stimulation (e.g., rubbing, massaging) of large-diameter fibers helps suppress the sensation of pain, especially sharp pain.

The skin over the entire body is supplied by spinal nerves that carry somatic sensory nerve impulses to the spinal cord. Each spinal nerve serves a specific segment of the skin, called a *dermatome*. Dermatomes, which can be affected by massage techniques that stimulate the skin, may account for **hyperstimulation analgesia.** The reduction of pain through stimulation (hyperstimulation analgesia) produced by massage and acupuncture has been used for many years.[10] In recent years transcutaneous electrical nerve stimulation (TENS) has become a popular method of producing hyperstimulation analgesia.

Massage and the production of hyperstimulation analgesia. Stimulation of the peripheral nervous system may produce analgesia by inducing neurophysiologic and neurohumoral inhibitory effects at the spinal gating mechanism (gate control theory). Evidence suggests that the development of analgesia depends on the stimulation of specific points in the muscle that correspond to certain types of muscle receptors. These same points correspond with many traditional acupuncture points (see Fig. 4-2). If massage stimulates these points at a sufficient intensity, the large-diameter fibers can be stimulated and the gating mechanism and hyperstimulation analgesia may be activated.

Tactile stimulation produced by massage travels through the large-diameter fibers. These fibers also carry a faster signal. In essence, massage sensations win the race to the brain, and the pain sensations are blocked because the gate is closed. Many parents and small children seem to know this instinctively. They rub the injured spot, thus activating large-diameter fibers. Stimulating techniques such as percussion or vibration of painful areas to activate "stimulation-produced analgesia," or hyperstimulation analgesia, also are effective.

Counterirritation

Taber's Cyclopedic Medical Dictionary defines **counterirritation** as superficial irritation that relieves some irritation of deeper structures.[22] Counterirritation may be explained by the gate control theory. Inhibition in central sensory pathways, produced by rubbing or shaking an area, may explain counterirritation. Noxious stimuli suppress nociceptive (pain) impulses. Changing the perception of pain by introducing a different pain signal is akin to stepping on a person's foot to relieve the pain in the thumb just hit by a hammer.

Inhibition in central sensory pathways may explain the effect of counterirritants. Stimulation of the skin over an area of pain or dysfunction produces some relief from the pain. The old-fashioned mustard plaster works on this principle, and various rubs and creams on the market also work in this manner.

Massage and the production of counterirritation. All methods of massage can be used to produce counterirritation. Many people have learned from practical experience that touching or shaking an injured area diminishes the pain of the injury.

Any massage method that introduces a controlled sensory stimulation intense enough to be interpreted by the client as a "good pain" signal will work to create counterirritation.

Massage therapy in many forms stimulates the skin over an area of discomfort. Techniques that friction the skin and underlying tissue to cause reddening are effective.

Compression and movement methods require the body to attend to a different signal and temporarily ignore the original discomfort (Proficiency Exercise 4-4).

Trigger Points

A **trigger point** is an area of local nerve facilitation in the muscle or associate connective tissue that creates small areas of tension or microspasm. These points are sensitive to pressure and when stimulated become the site of painful neuralgia. Dr. Janet Travell spent much of her professional career researching and developing treatment for myofascial trigger points. A plethora of terms, including *myalgia, myositis, fibrositis, fibromyalgia, myofibrositis, fibromyositis, fasciitis, myofascitis, rheumatism, fibrositic nodule,* and *myogelosis* all seem to describe the myofascial trigger point.[5]

Opinions differ as to whether trigger points are more a neuromuscular or a connective tissue phenomenon, but the acknowledged effects of massage indicate a strong neuromuscular interphase as well as a neuroendocrine response.

The effect of massage on trigger points. Travell, Simons, and others suggest that the effects of massage on

---

4 - 4

PROFICIENCY EXERCISE

Can you think of two more forms of counterirritation?

myofascial trigger points are a result of the stimulation of proprioceptive nerve endings, the release of enkephalin, the stretch of musculotendinous structures that initiate reflex muscle relaxation through the Golgi tendon organ and spindle receptors, and increased circulation.[3,5,24] Various massage methods, including pressure, positioning, and lengthening, provide this stimulation. Trigger points are discussed in detail in Chapter 11.

Nerve Impingement (Entrapment, Compression)

Soft tissue often impinges on a nerve, a condition commonly called *pinched nerve.* Tissues that can bind are skin, fascia, muscles, ligaments, joint structures, and bones. Spastic muscles and shortened connective tissue (fascia) often impinge on major and minor nerves, causing discomfort.

Entrapment and compression are technically different dysfunctions. **Entrapment** results when soft tissue (e.g., muscles and ligaments) exerts inappropriate pressure on nerves. **Compression** occurs when hard tissue (e.g., bone) exerts inappropriate pressure on nerves.

Regardless of the source of impingement, the symptoms are similar; however, the therapeutic intervention is different. Soft tissue approaches are beneficial for entrapment but less so for compression.

The effect of massage on nerve impingement. Because of the structural arrangement of the body, impingement often occurs at major nerve plexuses (Fig. 4-5). The specific nerve root, trunk, or division affected determines the condition, such as thoracic outlet syndrome, sciatica, or carpal tunnel syndrome. Therapeutic massage techniques work in many ways to reduce pressure on nerves. The main ways are to (1) reflexively change the tension pattern and lengthen the muscles, (2) mechanically stretch and soften connective tissue, and (3) interrupt the pain-spasm-pain cycle caused by protective muscle spasm that occurs in response to pain.

THINK IT OVER Why might a combination of manipulations, such as chiropractic and massage, be a valid way to deal with nerve impingement?

The Effect of Massage on the Somatic Nervous System

Massage methods directly stimulate the reflex mechanisms of the somatic functions. In fact, the bulk of the influence of massage is exerted through the somatic stimulation. Often the ANS and the endocrine system are influenced by secondary reflex activity in response to homeostatic changes caused by somatic stimulation during massage. All massage methods are effective. The specific result depends on precise communication with the somatic sensory receptor. It is a language of pressure, pull, and movement.

Connective Tissue

Connective tissue, the structural component of the body, is the most abundant body tissue. Its functions include support, structure, space, stabilization, and scar formation. It assumes many forms and shapes, from fluid blood to dense bone. The pliability of connective tissue, which is based on its water-binding components, is significant in effective connective tissue support and function. Connective tissue is adaptive and responsive to a variety of influences, such as injury, immobilization, overuse (increased demand), and underuse (decreased demand).

Connective tissue is made up of various fibers and cells in a gelatinous ground substance. In bone this ground substance is impregnated with minerals that harden the bone. The combination of the fibers and the cells that produce the fibers and the ground substance is called the *connective tissue matrix.*

Healing of damage to body tissues requires the formation of connective tissue. The inflammatory response is one trigger that generates the healing process. Occasionally more tissue than is needed forms, and adhesions develop. An adhesion is a binding of connective tissue to structures not directly involved with the area of injury.

In areas of *acute* (active) dysfunction, connective tissue initially may not play a role in the dysfunctional pattern. Connective tissue dysfunction usually is suspected as a factor in disorders older than 12 weeks.[4]

With overuse, additional connective tissue is formed to provide stabilization to the musculoskeletal areas involved. When the soft tissue problem is chronic, the connective tissue becomes fibrotic and involves areas surrounding the dysfunctional area.[4] After this has occurred, either of the following conditions may exist:

- The connective tissue may have thickened or thinned, or it may have dried out or become water-logged.
- Ligaments and tendons may fail to support joint stabilization, or the connective tissue may bind, restricting movement and function.

Piezoelectricity is an electrical current produced by applying pressure to certain crystals such as mica, quartz, or Rochelle salt. Collagen seems to have a piezoelectric property. The piezoelectric phenomenon in some way affects the connective tissue properties. With its piezoelectric properties, the collagen portion of connective tissue may be the link to energy-related forms of bodywork.

The Effect of Connective Tissue Methods

Connective tissue massage was formalized in 1929 by Elizabeth Dicke, a German physiotherapist. Dr. James Cyriax also contributed extensively through his research on deep

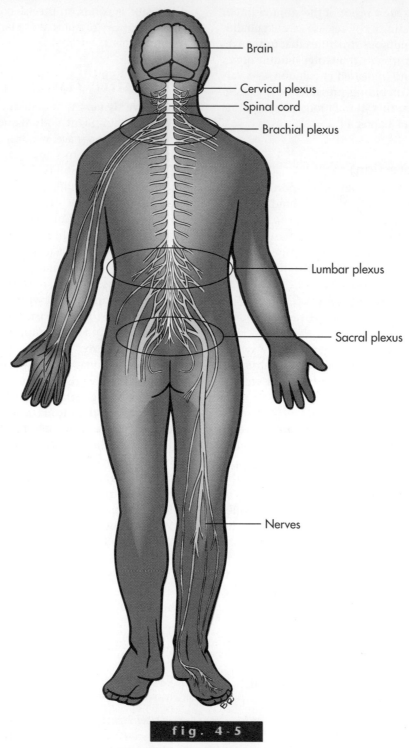

Brain

Cervical plexus

Spinal cord

Brachial plexus

Lumbar plexus

Sacral plexus

Nerves

fig. 4-5

Major nerve plexuses.

transverse friction massage. Fibrotic tissue responds well to the specific approaches of connective tissue massage (see Chapter 11). Studies indicate that massage may reduce the formation of adhesions and the scarring that often result from soft tissue injury. Similar approaches for the fascial or connective tissue component of muscles are called *myofascial techniques.* Connective tissue methods are primarily mechanical.

Connective tissue methods primarily affect the body structure. Methods that directly address the connective tissue do so by mechanically changing the consistency and pliability of the connective tissue, usually by softening it, and by creating physical space in the body. Mechanical dysfunctions call for more direct methods and depend on an actual physiologic change in the area. Cross-fiber frictioning (see Chapters 9 and 11) and inhibitory (direct) pressure approaches (see Chapter 9) are examples of mechanical massage methods.

Bodywork methods most often affect the superficial and deep fascial sheaths, the ligaments, and the tendons. Two basic approaches are used:

- Some methods address the *ground substance,* which is thixotropic, meaning that the substance liquefies on agitation and reverts to gel when standing. Ground substance is also a colloid. A colloid is a system of solids in a liquid medium that resists abrupt pressure but yields to slow, sustained pressure.
- Other methods address the *fibers* contained within the ground substance. The fibers are collagenous (ropelike), elastic (rubber band–like), or reticular (meshlike).

Methods that primarily affect the ground substance have a quality of slow, sustained pressure and agitation. Most massage methods can soften the ground substance as long as the application is not abrupt. Abrupt tapotement and compression (see Chapter 9) are less effective than slow effleurage or gliding methods that have a drag quality. Kneading, pétrissage, and skin rolling (see Chapter 9) that incorporate a slow pulling action are effective as well.

The fiber component is affected by methods that elongate the fibers past the elastic range (i.e., past the normal give) into the plastic range (i.e., past the bind or point of restriction). This creates either a freeing and unraveling of fibers or a small therapeutic (beneficial and controlled) inflammatory response that signals for change in the fibers. Transverse friction (see Chapter 11) also creates *therapeutic inflammation.*

Massage that provides for a gentle, sustained pull on the fascial component stimulates cutaneovisceral (skin to organ) reflex, and together with autonomic reflex pathways and endocrine responses produces the body-wide reactions to connective tissue massage. Connective tissue massage helps to harmonize the relationship between the sympathetic and parasympathetic divisions of the ANS. It helps to normalize the circulation between organs and organ systems and other tissues. Locally it improves the blood supply of the surface tissues in the area treated, especially in the particular connective tissue element. Connective tissue applications using massage methods are specifically addressed in Chapter 11.

Circulation

Three to five basic types of **circulation** have been recognized. All anatomy texts recognize arterial, venous, and lymphatic circulation. The other two types discussed here are respiratory and cerebrospinal fluid (CSF) circulation. These five systems depend on the pumping action of the skeletal muscles as they contract and relax. Arterial flow has the additional pumping action provided by the heart and muscle tissue in the arteries. Recent research indicates that the lymphatic system has it own rhythmic pumping action. The implication is that some of the benefits of massage may be a result of its influence on this rhythm.[17] These circulatory functions are both directly linked and interdependent. For example, the carbon dioxide level of CSF affects the respiratory center in the medulla, helping to control breathing.

Increases in the blood and lymph circulations are the most widely recognized physiologic effects of massage therapy. According to Dr. Yates' information, many studies validate the increase in lymphatic movement caused by massage. Application of a mechanical device that produced a rhythmic massage in a proximal direction reduced edema, increased lymphatic movement from the tissues to the blood, and improved blood circulation.[25]

The Effect of Massage on Circulation

Increased blood flow on a local level is achieved by compression of tissues, which empties venous beds, lowers venous pressure, and increases capillary blood flow, which is quickly counteracted by autoregulation. Massage stimulates the release of vasodilators, especially histamine. Blood flow changes also may be induced through the autonomic vascular reflexes. This particular increase in blood flow has a body-wide effect. Compression against arteries mechanically influences the internal pressure receptors in the arteries. It seems that there is no way to avoid affecting the blood and lymph circulations by giving a massage. Massage and other forms of bodywork mimic and assist the pumping action of the muscle and respiratory pump.

Arterial flow. The massage practitioner must know the anatomy and physiology of the blood and lymph circulations to understand the effect of massage on these systems. Circulation enhancement is fairly straightforward. Although it is true that more body fluids are moved by a 5-minute walk than by a 50-minute massage, for those unable to walk or even get out of bed, manual facilitation of the movement of body fluids can be a viable and significant therapeutic option.

Arteries carry blood under pressure from the heart as a result of the pumping action of the heart muscle. The arteries themselves also have a muscular component that contracts rhythmically, facilitating arterial flow. Direct compression into the area of an artery effectively crimps the artery, much like crimping a hose, and allows some back pressure to build up. When the pressure is released, the blood rushes through like a waterfall. Arteries basically are accessible to compressive pressure on the soft medial areas of the arms and legs. Compressions should begin proximal to the heart and move in a distal direction. Heavy pressure or sustained compression is not necessary; rather, moderate pressure is used in the right location to pump rhythmically at the client's current heart rate as the practitioner moves distally toward the fingers or toes. In style, it resembles shiatsu or sports massage.

An increase in arterial flow is beneficial in any situation in which an increase in oxygenated blood is desirable. Such situations include sluggish circulation in a sedentary person or the increased demand of an athlete (see Chapter 11).

Venous return flow. Venous return flow depends on contraction of the muscles against the veins. Back flow of blood is prevented by valves. Veins usually run more superficially than arteries. Because of the valve system in the veins and the fact that the blood is intended to flow back toward the heart, strokes to encourage venous flow move toward the heart. Short pumping, gliding, effleurage strokes are most effective in enhancing this flow.

Passive and active joint movement also encourages the muscles to contract against the deeper vessels, assisting venous blood flow. If this is not possible for the client, slow, meticulous mechanical work is required to drain the area. Placing the limb above the heart, allowing gravity to assist, is beneficial (see Chapter 11).

Lymphatic drainage. The massage procedures for lymphatic drainage are similar to those for venous return. Because lymph vessels open into tissue space, the surface work is performed over the entire body instead of being focused only over the major veins. Pumping of jointed areas with passive joint movement seems to assist the movement of lymph through the areas of lymph node filtration. Deep breathing assists lymph movement in the thorax. Unless the massage therapist is using manual lymph drainage as a specific therapeutic intervention in cases of a pathologic condition of the lymphatic system, it does not seem to be necessary to be precise about specific flow patterns. It is important to note that the lower abdomen (from the umbilicus down) drains into the inguinal area and that the right side (right arm and head) drains into the right lymphatic duct. Both major vessels dump into the vena cava (see Chapter 11).

Respiration

The muscular mechanism for the inhalation and exhalation of air is designed like a simple bellows system and depends on unrestricted movement of the musculoskeletal components of the thorax. The muscles of respiration include the scalenes, intercostals, serratus anterior diaphragm, abdominals, pelvic floor muscles, and lower leg muscles (which surprises many people). This can be demonstrated by contracting any of these muscle groups

and attempting to take a deep breath; you will note that the ability to breathe is restricted. Disruption of function in any of these groups inhibits complete and easy breathing. Often subclinical overbreathing, called **hyperventilation syndrome,** occurs, which causes many physical symptoms (Box 4-3).

Physiologists define *hyperventilation* as abnormally deep or rapid breathing in excess of physical demands. *Dyspneic fear* (no air) is a core factor in the etiology of panic attacks, which result in rapid breathing.

The effect of massage on respiration. All massage approaches that restore mobility to the thorax and the muscles of respiration affect the ability to breathe. Particularly with hyperventilation syndrome, breathing retraining often is ineffective because the mobility of the respiratory mechanism is disrupted. Often massage can restore the normal function of the soft tissue involved with breathing, allowing breathing retraining to become effective.

Cerebrospinal Fluid Circulation

CSF cools, nourishes, and protects the brain and nerves and influences breathing through carbon dioxide levels. The movement of this fluid has a pumping rhythm that can be palpated. This rhythm seems to affect the phenomenon of fascial movement and is independent of the other body rhythms. Entrainment is implicated as a factor in fascial movement.[17] More research must be done before the anatomic and physiologic mechanisms of the fascial movement phenomenon can be understood scientifically. Techniques of craniosacral therapy specifically affect CSF circulation (Fig. 4-6).[8] General massage also may influence this mechanism indirectly.

Energy Systems (Biofield)

Both styles of massage, mechanical and reflexive, influence the energy component of the body by stimulating both electrical-chemical and electrical-magnetic effects.

Scientific technology is just now enabling researchers to measure this subtle component of the body. Consequently, the validity of the effectiveness of any method based on the reaction of the electrical-chemical or electrical-magnetic component of the body is controversial. The term *subtle energies* or *biofield therapies* covers a wide range of techniques that affect the subtle electrical fields of the body. These electrical fields exist. Animal behavior studies have shown that the platypus detects a living food source by sensing the weak electrical field around its prey.[1]

Some methods of massage, especially the more subtle approaches, have not yet been researched enough to be scientifically validated. However, research is underway in these areas. These methods, based on the subtle electrical energy of the body, have been around for eons. Most ancient healing practices are based on the interaction with

box 4-3

HYPERVENTILATION SYNDROME

Hyperventilation syndrome is a complex set of behaviors that leads to overbreathing despite the absence of a pathologic condition. It is considered a functional syndrome because all the parts are working effectively, therefore a specific pathologic condition does not exist. Instead the breathing pattern is inappropriate for the situation, resulting in confused signals to the CNS, which sets up a whole chain of events.

Increased ventilation is a common component of fight-or-flight responses. However, when our breathing rate increases but our actions and movements are restricted or do not increase accordingly, we are breathing in excess of our metabolic need. Blood levels of carbon dioxide (CO_2) fall, and symptoms may occur. Because we exhale too much CO_2 too quickly, our blood becomes more acidic. These biochemical changes can cause many of the following signs and symptoms:

- *Cardiovascular:* Palpitations, missed beats, tachycardia, sharp or dull atypical chest pain, "angina," vasomotor instability, cold extremities, Raynaud's phenomenon, blotchy flushing of blush area, capillary vasoconstriction (face, arms, hands)
- *Neurologic:* Dizziness; unsteadiness or instability; sensation of faintness or giddiness (rarely actual fainting); visual disturbance (blurred or tunnel vision); headache (often migraine); paresthesia (numbness, uselessness, heaviness, pins and needles, burning, limbs feeling out of proportion or as if they "don't belong") commonly of the hands, feet, or face but sometimes of the scalp or whole body; intolerance of light or noise; enlarged pupils (wearing dark glasses on a dull day)
- *Respiratory:* Shortness of breath, typically after exertion; irritable cough; tightness or oppression of chest; difficulty breathing; "asthma"; air hunger; inability to take a satisfying breath; excessive sighing, yawning, and sniffing
- *Gastrointestinal:* Difficulty swallowing, dry mouth and throat, acid regurgitation, heartburn, hiatal hernia, nausea, flatulence, belching, air swallowing, abdominal discomfort, bloating
- *Muscular:* Cramps, muscle pain (particularly occipital, neck, shoulders, and between scapulae; less commonly the lower back and limbs), tremors, twitching, weakness, stiffness, or tetany (seizing up)
- *Psychologic:* Tension, anxiety, "unreal" feelings, depersonalization, feeling "out of body," hallucinations, fear of insanity, panic, phobias, agoraphobia
- *General:* Feelings of weakness; exhaustion; impaired concentration, memory, and performance; disturbed sleep, including nightmares; emotional sweating (axillae, palms, and sometimes the whole body); woolly or thick head

Cerebral vascular constriction, a primary response to hyperventilation syndrome, can reduce the oxygen available to the brain by about one half. Among the resulting symptoms are dizziness, blurring of consciousness, and possibly, because of a decrease in cortical inhibition, tearfulness and emotional instability.

Other effects of hyperventilation syndrome that therapists should watch for are generalized body tension and chronic inability to relax. In addition, individuals prone to hyperventilation syndrome are particularly prone to spasm (tetany) in muscles involved in the "attack posture"; they hunch their shoulders, thrust the head and neck forward, scowl, and clench their teeth.[23]

---

these subtle energy fields. The massage profession, as well as the health care and scientific professions, would be wise not to discount these methods just because current technology is not advanced enough to verify what the human being can perceive.

In time many of the methods probably will show validity, or their use would not have stood the test of time. It is possible that the effectiveness of the energy approaches is reflexive: touch here, and it causes something to happen there.

Entrainment is now being considered as a mechanism to explain the benefits of the more subtle approaches.[17] Currently the electrical energy generated by the body can be measured by electroencephalograms, electrocardiograms, magnetic resonance images, and other sophisticated scientific equipment. However, the lack of sufficient Western scientific validation of the ancient energetic flows of chi, prana, meridians, chakras, auras, or whatever else they may be called causes us to represent this area of bodywork to the public carefully.

Until our technology can prove the validity of energy techniques, it is important to remember the wisdom of Hippocrates, "Do no harm," and also Bernie Siegal's belief, "There is no false hope." It is important to represent subtle techniques simply, professionally, and free of false expectations and mysticism. Additional training is required to learn to use the subtle energy approaches purposefully. It is also important not to discount the stimulation of the powerful placebo effect. If touch can activate it, why not use it?

It will be exciting to watch science "discover" the validity of more and more of the ancient energy concepts.

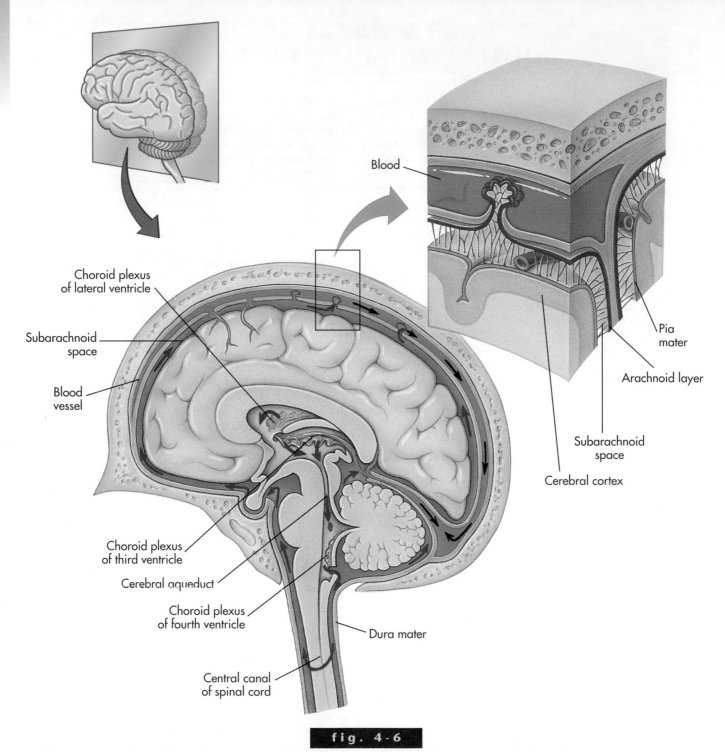

Blood

Choroid plexus of lateral ventricle

Subarachnoid space

Blood vessel

Choroid plexus of third ventricle

Cerebral aqueduct

Choroid plexus of fourth ventricle

Central canal of spinal cord

Dura mater

Pia mater

Arachnoid layer

Subarachnoid space

Cerebral cortex

fig. 4-6

Flow of CSF. Filtration of the blood by the choroid plexus of each ventricle produces the CSF, which flows inferiorly through the lateral ventricles, the interventricular foramen, the third ventricle, the cerebral aqueduct, the fourth ventricle, and the subarachnoid space into the blood. (From Thibodeau GA, Patton KT: *The human body in health and disease,* ed 2, St Louis, 1997, Mosby.)

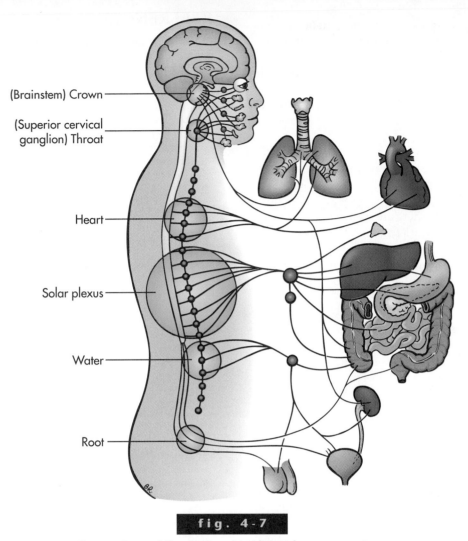

(Brainstem) Crown

(Superior cervical ganglion) Throat

Heart

Solar plexus

Water

Root

fig. 4-7

Comparison of the ANS and traditional energy centers.

The Effect of Massage on Body Energy

Physiologically, sufficient research exists to demonstrate that methods using "energy" have an effect through ANS activity and endocrine responses in regard to entrainment, motor nerve points, and the piezoelectric properties of connective tissue fibers. Acupuncture points and meridians can be correlated directly to the nerve tracts and motor nerve points; chakras are located over nerve plexuses and biologic oscillators (Fig. 4-7).

The interrelationship among all the body's systems is sufficient to cause the body to respond to the stimulation of the innate electrical-chemical energy with massage approaches. Therapeutic massage stimulates the nervous system and applies pressure on the connective tissues to produce a measurable electrical current via the piezoelectric properties of the connective tissue. The generalized therapeutic approach of massage seems to have a normalizing effect on the body's energetic processes.

SUMMARY

Therapeutic massage methods are simple and effective in producing responses mediated through the nervous system, the interaction with the endocrine system, the connective tissue, and the circulatory systems. Massage techniques can replace pharmaceuticals in cases of mild manifestations of symptoms in some illnesses and as a supporting adjunct to medication therapy can reduce dosages and duration of treatment, thereby reducing the risk of side effects. The use of massage for anxiety, depression, and chronic pain is beneficial in conjunction with an overall treatment protocol. Most forms of musculoskeletal pain and discomfort respond, at least temporarily, to massage. General daily stress responds well to massage.

With an understanding of the physiologic effects of massage, it is hoped that professionals, in consultation with medical personnel, will consider the use of these very old and effective methods. When provided by trained professionals, therapeutic massage can be beneficial in conservative treatment plans for chronic pain and stress-induced disease processes before a resort is made to more invasive measures. Therapeutic massage can play an important role in prevention programs by providing a natural mechanism for stimulating the body to adjust to the stress of daily life and restore the natural homeostatic balance.

Professional experience shows that most clients get a massage because it feels good and helps them feel better. It is difficult to research "good" and "better" scientifically. The massage professional can provide the services of this art and be confident that there are scientific reasons to explain why massage works and feels good. Let us not forget, as professionals, the importance of the "feel-good" aspect of massage. Clients do care about how much you know, but they care more about how much you care and about how good they feel after a massage.

The massage profession needs more research. Therefore the massage profession needs to cooperate with researchers and appreciate that research is tedious, painstaking work. The medical profession and the public need the research to strengthen their belief in massage so that they can justify receiving or recommending massage. The massage profession needs the public and the medical profession to support massage. We all need touch because it is so beneficial and, most of all, because it feels good. Whatever the massage or bodywork system used, the beneficial effects of therapeutic massage are elicited from the client's physiology as it adjusts to the external sensory information supplied by massage and responds to the compressive forces of massage.

As indicated at the beginning of this chapter, it is easy to validate massage. Additional information can be obtained by locating and studying the resources listed as references in this chapter and in Appendix D. Applying the techniques that bring about the physiologic effects is discussed in more depth in Chapters 9, 10, and 11.

THINK IT OVER

Can the various effects of massage really be separated from one another? Can you *only* massage connective tissue, or *only* affect circulation, or *only* affect the ANS?

REFERENCES

1. Alcock J: *Animal behavior: an evaluatory approach,* Sunderland, Mass., 1989, Sinawer.
2. Anderson K, Anderson LE, Glanze WD, editors: *Mosby's medical, nursing, and allied health dictionary,* ed 4, St Louis, 1990, Mosby.
3. Baldry PE: *Acupuncture, trigger points and musculoskeletal pain,* New York, 1989, Churchill Livingstone.
4. Cailliet R: *Soft tissue pain and disability,* Philadelphia, 1977, FA Davis.
5. Chaitow LND: *Soft tissue manipulation,* Rochester, Vt., 1988, Healing Arts Press.
6. deGroot J, Chusid JG: *Correlative neuroanatomy,* ed 20, San Mateo, Calif., 1985, Appleton & Lange.
7. Ernest M, Lee MHM: Sympathetic effects of manual and electrical acupuncture of the tsusanli knee point: comparison with the huko hand point sympathetic effects, *Exp Neurol* 1986.
8. Gewirtz D: Touchpoints 1(1): 1993.
9. Greenman PE: *Principles of manual medicine,* ed 2, Baltimore, 1996, Williams & Wilkins.
10. Gunn CC: *Reprints on pain, acupuncture and related subjects,* Seattle, 1992, University of Washington.
11. Hooper J, Teresi D: *The three pound universe,* New York, 1986, Dell.
12. Horacek J Jr: *Brainstorms,* Northvale, New Jersey, 1998, Jason Aronson.
13. Knaster M: Tiffany Field provides proof positive scientifically, *Massage Therapy Journal* 37(1):84, 1998.
14. Levin SR: *Acute effects of massage on the stress response,* Greensboro, N.C., 1990, University of North Carolina (master's thesis).
15. Longworth JCD: Psychophysiological effects of slow-stroke back massage in normotensive females, *Nurs Sci* 4:44, 1982.
16. McCraty R, Tiller WA, Atkinson M: *Head-heart entrainment: a preliminary survey,* 1995, Institute of HeartMath, PO Box 1463, 14700 West Park Ave, Boulder Creek, Calif. 95006. Hrtmath@netcom.com http://www.heartmath.org/researchpapers/Head/Heart/Headheart.html
17. Oschman JL: What is healing energy? III. Silent pulses, *Journal of Bodywork and Movement Therapies* 1(3):179, 1997.
18. Research at TRI: *Touch Therapy Times* 5(5): 1994.
19. Selye H: *The healing brain: understanding stress, stress without distress,* Institute for the Study of Human Knowledge, Los Altos, Calif., ISHK Paperbacks.
20. Shealy NC: *The neurochemical substrate of behavior: the psychology of health, immunity and disease,* vol B, Mainsfield Center, Calif., 1992, National Institute for the Clinical Application of Behavioral Medicine.
21. St John P: *Workshop notes: seminar I,* St John neuromuscular therapy seminars, Largo, Fla., 1990, Self.
22. Thomas CL, editor: *Taber's cyclopedic medical dictionary,* ed 16, Philadelphia, 1985, FA Davis.
23. Timmons BH, Ley R: *Behavioral and psychological approaches to breathing disorders,* New York, 1994, Plenum Press.
24. Travell JG, Simons DG: *Myofascial pain and dysfunction: the trigger point manual,* Baltimore, 1984, Williams & Wilkins.
25. Yates J: *Physiological effects of therapeutic massage and their application to treatment,* Vancouver, British Columbia, 1990, Massage Therapists Association.

WORKBOOK SECTION

Short Answer

1. What are the five basic physiologic effects of massage?

   _____

   _____

   _____

   _____

2. In what way do chronic problems affect the connective tissue?

   _____

   _____

   _____

   _____

3. What are the five types of circulation?

   _____

   _____

   _____

   _____

4. What three words describe the sympathetic ANS functions?

   _____

   _____

   _____

   _____

5. What words describe the parasympathetic functions?

   _____

   _____

   _____

   _____

6. What is the importance of state-dependent memory to the massage therapist?

   _____

   _____

   _____

   _____

7. What is hyperstimulation analgesia?

   _____

   _____

   _____

   _____

8. How does massage promote the body's ability to maintain self-regulation and structural and functional balance?

   _____

   _____

   _____

   _____

9. Why is it easy to validate massage?

   _____

   _____

   _____

   _____

10. Why are research and its replication to verify the positive biochemical and behavioral responses to touch important?

    _____

    _____

    _____

    _____

11. Is it possible to separate the somatic, emotional, and cognitive elements in the response to massage? Is it possible to separate the mechanical, neural, chemical, and psychologic effects?

    _____

    _____

    _____

    _____

WORKBOOK SECTION

12. How does the gate control theory explain hyperstimulation analgesia and counterirritation?

_____

_____

_____

_____

13. What role does massage play in relieving nerve impingement?

_____

_____

_____

_____

14. Why are reflexes important to the understanding of why massage works?

_____

_____

_____

_____

15. How does massage interact with the powerful body/mind phenomenon?

_____

_____

_____

_____

16. How does massage stimulate the release of neurotransmitters, endorphins, and enkephalins?

_____

_____

_____

_____

17. What seem to be the effects of massage on myofascial trigger points?

_____

_____

_____

_____

18. In what ways does massage encourage circulation?

_____

_____

_____

_____

19. What are the possible physiologic mechanisms that support energy methods?

_____

_____

_____

_____

WORKBOOK SECTION

Matching

I. Match the term with the best definition.

1. Autoregulation _____

2. Body/mind _____

3. Centering _____

4. Cognitive _____

5. Counterirritation _____

6. Endogenous _____

7. Endorphins _____

8. Feedback _____

9. Gate control theory _____

10. Toughening/hardening _____

11. Hyperstimulation analgesia _____

12. Intuition _____

13. Law _____

14. Nerve impingement _____

15. Noxious stimulation _____

16. Placebo _____

17. Reflex _____

18. Science _____

19. Somatic _____

20. Subtle energies _____

a. the ability to focus on a specific circumstance by screening sensation

b. superficial stimulation that relieves deeper sensation by stimulating different sensory signals

c. weak electrical fields that are said to surround and run through the body

d. an involuntary response to a stimulus; the response is specific, predictable, adaptive, and purposeful

e. the interaction between thought and physiology connected to the limbic system, the hypothalamic influence of the ANS, and the endocrine system

f. a controlled pain sensation; "good pain"

g. a scientific statement found to be true for a whole class of natural occurrences

h. a method of teaching the body to deal with stress

i. a method of autoregulation to maintain internal homeostasis that interlinks body functions

j. made in the body

k. one of the endogenous opioid peptides that have morphinelike analgesic properties, behavioral effects, and neurotransmitter and neuromodulator functions

l. reduction of perception of a sensation by stimulation of large-diameter nerve fibers

m. awareness with perception, reasoning, judgment, intuition, and memory

n. knowing something by using subconscious information

o. the hypothesis that painful stimuli can be prevented from reaching higher levels of the CNS by stimulating larger sensory nerves

p. pressure against a nerve by skin, fascia, muscles, ligaments, and joints

q. a treatment for an illness that influences the course of the disease even if it is not specifically validated

r. pertaining to the body

s. the intellectual process of understanding through observation, measurement, accumulation of data, and analysis of the findings

t. control of homeostasis by alteration of tissue or function

WORKBOOK SECTION

II. Match the scientific laws affecting massage with their descriptions.

a. Hilton's law

b. law of unilaterality

c. law of facilitation

d. Hooke's law

e. law of generalization

f. Arndt-Schulz law

g. all-or-none (Bowditch's) law

h. Bell's law

i. law of specificity of nervous energy

j. Weber's law

k. law of symmetry

l. law of intensity

m. law of radiation

n. Cannon's law of denervation

1. _____ The weakest stimulus capable of producing a response produces the maximal response contraction in cardiac and skeletal muscle and nerves.

2. _____ Anterior spinal nerve roots are motor roots, and posterior spinal nerve roots are sensory roots.

3. _____ When an impulse has passed once through a certain set of neurons to the exclusion of others, it tends to take the same course on a future occasion, and each time it transverses this path, the resistance is smaller.

4. _____ The stress used to stretch or compress a body is proportional to the strain experienced, as long as the elastic limits of the body have not been exceeded.

5. _____ Excitation of a receptor always gives rise to the same sensation regardless of the nature of the stimulus.

6. _____ The increase in stimulus necessary to produce the smallest perceptible increase in sensation bears a constant ratio to the strength of the stimulus already acting.

7. _____ A nerve trunk that supplies a joint also supplies the muscles of the joint and the skin over the insertions of such muscles.

8. _____ If a mild irritation is applied to one or more sensory nerves, the movement usually occurs on only one side, the side that is irritated.

9. _____ If the stimulation is increased sufficiently, motor reaction is manifested not only on the irritated side but also in similar muscles on the opposite side of the body.

10. _____ Reflex movements usually are more intense on the side of irritation; at times the movements of the opposite side equal them in intensity, but they usually are less pronounced.

11. _____ If the excitation continues to increase, it is propagated upward, and reactions take place through centrifugal nerves coming from the higher cord segments.

12. _____ When the irritation becomes very intense, it is propagated in the medulla oblongata, which becomes a focus from which stimuli radiate to all parts of the cord, causing a general contraction of all muscles in the body.

13. _____ Weak stimuli activate physiologic processes; very strong stimuli inhibit them.

14. _____ When autonomic effectors are partly or completely separated from their normal nerve connections, they become more sensitive to the action of chemical substances.

WORKBOOK SECTION

III. Match the visceral functions with their sympathetic or parasympathetic controls. Column 1 lists visceral functions. Choose the best response from the Control List below and place the corresponding letter in column 2. In column 3, write either "S" for sympathetic or "P" for parasympathetic, depending on the control response.

Column 1	*Column 2*	*Column 3*
1. Heart muscle	_____	_____
2. Digestive tract	_____	_____
3. Skeletal muscle blood vessels	_____	_____
4. Smooth muscle blood vessels	_____	_____
5. Urinary bladder	_____	_____
6. Iris	_____	_____
7. Pilomotor muscles	_____	_____
8. Adrenal medulla	_____	_____
9. Sweat glands	_____	_____
10. Digestive glands	_____	_____

Control List

a. increases secretion of digestive juices

b. increases secretion of sweat

c. slows heartbeat

d. constricts blood vessels

e. relaxes bladder

f. increases peristalsis

g. dilates blood vessels

h. increases secretion of epinephrine

i. stimulates goose pimples

j. constricts pupil

WORKBOOK SECTION

Labeling

Label the major nerve plexuses for fig. 4-8.

> **Brachial plexus**
> **Brain**
> **Cervical plexus**
> **Lumbar plexus**
> **Nerves**
> **Sacral plexus**
> **Spinal cord**

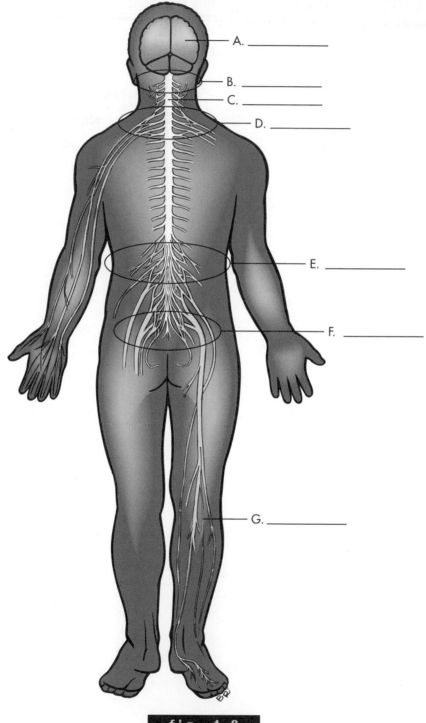

A. _____

B. _____

C. _____

D. _____

E. _____

F. _____

G. _____

f i g .   4 - 8

WORKBOOK SECTION

Problem-Solving Exercises

1. A physician refers a client to you for basic relaxation massage to ease chronic pain of undetermined cause. Using the information presented in this chapter, list at least four principal reasons why the massage could benefit the client.

   _____

   _____

   _____

   _____

2. After a series of massages, a client finds that her anxiety and impatience have diminished. How would you explain this?

   _____

   _____

   _____

   _____

3. A client brings in a research article about the use of massage for a specific condition, but he doesn't understand what this means. What steps would you take to explain it to him?

   _____

   _____

   _____

   _____

Professional Applications

1. Make a list of your daily experiences with ANS functions. Make a second list of ANS functions you encounter while performing massage.

   _____

   _____

   _____

   _____

2. Read through the various therapeutic massage journals. Find one or two articles on bodywork, and classify the information presented according to the following effects:
   a. Mechanical or reflexive
   b. Nervous system primarily affected; benefits primarily somatic, visceral, peripheral, central or autonomic connective tissue, or circulatory
   c. Chemical (i.e., hormone) and neurotransmitters stimulated
   d. Sensory receptor responsible for responding to the stimulation

Research for Further Study

Design a possible research study. Develop an idea (a hypothesis), narrow the topic, then decide what measurements will be used. Identify possible outcomes. Identify other factors that may influence the outcome. Look at other research studies for examples of research design. Locate resources on ways to develop a research study.

_____

_____

_____

_____

_____

WORKBOOK SECTION

ANSWER KEY

Short Answer

1. Neuromuscular, connective tissue, circulation, ANS, and electrical-chemical or electrical-magnetic effects.
2. The connective tissue becomes fibrotic, and the fibrosis extends to areas surrounding the dysfunctional area.
3. Arterial flow, venous return flow, lymphatic drainage, respiration, and CSF circulation.
4. Fight, flight, and fear.
5. Relaxation response.
6. Massage may recreate state-dependent memory patterns for the client.
7. It is a protective mechanism of sensory overload caused by sustained stimulation.
8. Because of the effect on the ANS and associated functions, massage produces feelings of general well-being and comfort, allowing clients to control their own emotional state.
9. Massage has an extensive base of historical literature and current research, and it works by stimulating simple physiologic mechanisms.
10. This type of information gives the effects of the massage back to the client. Instead of a force from outside that in some mystical way exerts power over the body, this type of research shows that the effects of massage come from within the client and that massage is a great form of sensory simulation to "get the ball rolling." Many claims are made about alternative health measures; some are valid, and some are not. The effects of massage are simple and basic and require validation in order to separate fact from mere speculation.
11. In actual practice it is impossible to divide up the wholeness of massage; this is one of the things that makes massage special. In research it is possible to study one aspect, and in the education process it is possible to study one method, but in application the elements mingle. For example, individual ingredients make up a cookie, but they do not become the cookie until all ingredients are mixed together and a chemical reaction takes place. After the cookie is a cookie, it is almost impossible to separate the individual components.
12. Stimulation that activates the large-diameter nerve fibers wins the race to the brain and closes the "gate," so that the pain sensations are not processed. Hyperstimulation is stimulation that uses extensive or sustained sensation; counterirritation is stimulation of a different sensory fiber.
13. Tissues that can bind nerves through shortening or a shift in position are skin, fascia, muscles, ligaments, and joints. Massage can stretch the connective tissues and change the tension of muscle to relieve the pressure on a nerve.
14. Reflexes are fast, predictable, autonomic responses to a change in the environment that help maintain homeostasis. Many of the beneficial responses of massage depend on the specific stimulation of a reflex. Reflexes are important movement and protective mechanisms. Because they take priority in a sensory signal, stimulation of reflexes can result in a shift in homeostasis and nonproductive nerve transmission pathways can be overridden.
15. Massage stimulates the secretion of certain neurotransmitters, hormones, and other endogenous chemicals, such as endorphins, and also stimulates ANS functions. The combination of endocrine and ANS functions plays a part in the body/mind phenomenon.
16. Massage can create a controlled but slightly more intense stimulus than the existing pain or stress. The increase in intensity is sufficient to trigger the release of these substances. The stimulus must last long enough to allow blood levels to rise in order for the client to feel the effects, which have a fairly long-lasting response in the body.
17. Research seems to suggest that massage stimulates proprioceptive nerve endings, releases enkephalins, stretches the musculotendinous structures to stimulate reflex mechanisms, Golgi tendon organs, and spindle receptors, and increases circulation.
18. Massage encourages circulation on a local level through compression of vessels, which changes the internal pressure and releases vasodilators, which opens the capillaries. On a systemic level, massage shifts the autonomic vascular reflexes.
19. Entrainment, piezoelectric properties of connective tissue, nervous system stimulation, and neuroendocrine responses.

WORKBOOK SECTION

Matching

I.

1. t	11. l
2. e	12. n
3. a	13. g
4. m	14. p
5. b	15. f
6. j	16. q
7. k	17. d
8. I	18. s
9. o	19. r
10. h	20. c

II.

1. g	8. b
2. h	9. k
3. c	10. l
4. d	11. m
5. I	12. e
6. j	13. f
7. a	14. n

III.

1. c, p	6. j, p
2. f, p	7. I, s
3. g, s	8. h, s
4. d, s	9. b, s
5. e, s	10. a, p

Labeling

A. Brain
B. Cervical plexus
C. Spinal cord
D. Brachial plexus
E. Lumbar plexus
F. Sacral plexus
G. Nerves

Problem-Solving Exercise

1. Counterirritation, hyperstimulation analgesia, release of endorphins and serotonin, toughening/hardening, placebo effect
2. Reduction of sympathetic arousal responses, increased ability to restore homeostasis, increased energy as a result of reduced generalized muscle tension, increased circulation, which produces a generalized increase in efficient functioning, restoration of effective parasympathetic restorative function
3. No specific answer—the validity of the response to the question is based on the student's ability to justify the response.

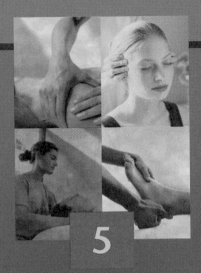

5

INDICATIONS AND CONTRAINDICATIONS FOR THERAPEUTIC MASSAGE

o b j e c t i v e s

After completing this chapter, the student will be able to perform the following:

■ Define *indication* and *contraindication*

■ Define *therapeutic change, condition management,* and *palliative care*

■ Use a clinical reasoning model to determine the appropriate intervention process

■ Develop a basic understanding of pathology and its connection to contraindications to massage

■ Explain the stress response, inflammatory response, and pain response

■ Identify indications for massage therapy and justify those indications

■ Understand when to refer clients to licensed medical professionals

THE massage professional must be able to identify indications and contraindications for therapeutic massage. An **indication** is when an approach is beneficial for health enhancement, treatment of a particular condition, or support of a treatment modality other than massage. A **contraindication** is when an approach could be harmful. The following types of contraindications occur:

1. General avoidance of application—Do not perform any massage techniques.
2. Regional avoidance of application—Do massage but avoid a particular area.
3. Application with *caution,* usually requiring supervision from appropriate medical or supervising personnel—Do perform massage but carefully select the type of methods to be used, duration of the massage, and frequency of application.

INDICATIONS FOR MASSAGE

section objectives

Using the information presented in this section, the student will be able to perform the following:

- Identify and chart the benefits of massage
- Explain the difference between objective and subjective massage benefits
- Explain the benefits of massage to others

Indications for massage are based on its objective and subjective health-enhancing benefits. That is, some results of massage can be measured (objective), whereas others are assumed effective based on experience (subjective). The effects of massage are both physical (objective, physically measured observation) and mental (subjective perception reporting) (Box 5-1) (Proficiency Exercise 5-1).

---

5 - 1

PROFICIENCY EXERCISE

1. *In the spaces provided, write two dialogues that explain the benefits of massage. Direct one discussion to a group of health care professionals such as physicians, chiropractors, nurses, physical therapists, and psychologists and the other to a group of business professionals, factory workers, construction workers, food service workers, and athletes.*

Choose one: physicians, chiropractors, nurses, physical therapists, psychologists

Type of health professional: _____

Choose one: business professionals, factory workers, construction workers, food service workers, athletes

Type of group: _____

box 5-1
THE GENERAL BENEFITS OF MASSAGE THERAPY

Massage manipulations can be applied in a systematic approach or plan to influence conditions that affect physical function.

Skeletal muscles respond with direct biomechanical effects. Within this response, biomechanical effects encourage or produce reflex reactions that involve the nervous system and chemical responses. A variety of responses are reached at many levels. The nervous system can respond through the reflex arc, secretion of endorphins and other neural chemicals, and the release of histamine and other cellular secretions. The release of chemical substances affects a structure or system of the body directly or indirectly.

The foundation for the benefits of massage therapy is understanding the nature of the effects on circulation, elimination, and nervous system control. Circulation is primarily improved by direct biomechanical responses to manipulations. A secondary benefit is obtained through reflex responses encouraging chemical secretion, which affects nervous system control.

Circulation improvement occurs as nutrients, oxygen, and arterial blood components are delivered to the local area being manipulated or distributed to the general circulation. The benefit of circulatory improvement is the secondary effect of improved filtration and elimination of carbon dioxide, metabolites, and biochemical byproducts that are transported in the venous blood. Improved circulation, with its ability to affect elimination, generally enhances the abilities of the structures to benefit and support normal function. When nutrition is improved and elimination enhanced, the structures of localized areas, tissues, and systems are given the opportunity to maximize the potential for normal function.

Massage manipulations directly benefit restrictions to muscle tissue function. Mechanical benefits and reflex responses combine to help the muscular soft tissues respond through circulation improvement and elimination of byproducts. Mechanical effects on muscular tissues include influence on the stretch receptors, tendon apparatus, and direct manual stretching of the muscle fibers. The reflex effects encourage relaxation of the tissues through change in the motor nerve output and chemical secretions.

Clients receiving massage therapy report a variety of sensations, emotions, feelings, and mental perceptions that are subjective, difficult to measure, and unique to the individual.

Massage therapy benefits conditions by encouraging the body through the phases involved in rehabilitation, restoration, and normalization of anatomic and physiologic function and ability. Psychologic benefits occur subjectively according to the individual in response to therapy with secondary effects that influence sensation and pain perception. Objective and subjective results of therapy combine to create individual responses that affect the desired health outcome.

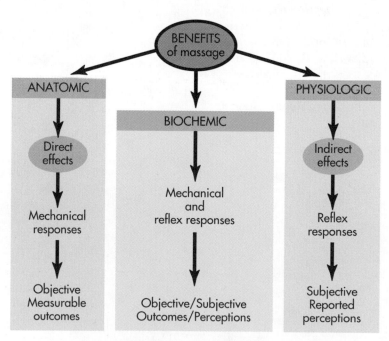

The benefits, effects, responses, and outcomes
can occur separately, combined, or as a
result of one another

(Courtesy Emily E.S. Cowall, Reg. MT.)

APPROACHES TO CARE

section objectives

Using the information presented in this section, the student will be able to perform the following:

- Define *therapeutic change*
- Explain the concepts of condition management and palliative care
- Implement a clinical reasoning process to make appropriate decisions as to the type of care most beneficial for the client

The benefits of massage occur as a result of therapeutic change, condition management, and palliative care. This section explains each of these approaches to care.

Therapeutic Change

Therapeutic change is defined as "beneficial alteration produced by a bodywork process that results in a modification of physical form or function that can affect the physical, mental and/or spiritual state of a client."

Any change process, including beneficial change, requires energy and resource expenditure on the part of the client. Important decisions include the ability of the client to expend the energy required for active change and the availability of the support and resources often necessary during a change process. The practitioner requires appropriate knowledge and skills (current or acquired) and often a network of support from other professionals to facilitate a change process. The client requires motivation and resources (information, finances, time, social support, and coping mechanisms) to complete a change process.

Careful assessment helps to identify if a change process program holds a likely chance for success. If these components are not sufficient or in place, or the existing situation supports some sort of coping mechanism or has secondary gain for the client, the client will not be able to commit the necessary motivation to the change process.

If the conditions are not suitable for active change, other intervention processes can be developed. The wise professional understands and considers the complex dynamics involved in the lives of the people they serve. Although change is often indicated, it may not be realistically possible at a particular time or under a current set of circumstances.

When the likelihood of a successful change outcome is not good, condition management and palliative care can be offered. These allow clients to be more effective within their current set of circumstances and suffer less.

Condition Management

Condition management involves the use of massage methods to support clients who are not able to undergo a therapeutic change process but wish to be as effective as possible within an existing set of circumstances. When a client is dealing with a chronic health condition or set of life circumstances that creates chronic stress (e.g., caring for an ailing parent or child, stressful work environment, strain within a relationship, ongoing financial strain), condition management is beneficial. Condition management is beneficial when the likelihood of the situation changing is not a viable possibility (e.g., amputation, diabetes, job-related repetitive strain) or the timeframe for changing a situation needs to be postponed for a period of time (e.g., pregnancy, chemotherapy, graduation from school).

On a physical level, massage can offer benefits by managing the existing physical compensation patterns and sometimes slowing the progress of chronic conditions or preventing a situation from becoming worse. On an emotional level, massage can assist in the management of physical stress symptoms to allow the person to cope better with life stresses that cannot be altered.

Condition management accounts for the largest client base for therapeutic massage. Many people find themselves in undesirable circumstances and search for ways to cope with—not change—the existing conditions. Most of us can relate to the importance of being able to remain resourceful and responsive to life events. Although it may be ideal to bring about a change when life is not as we would like it to be, we all know that sometimes this is not possible for many reasons. Therapeutic massage offers support, acceptance, compassion, and a short-term respite.

Palliative Care

To *palliate* is to soothe or relieve. Massage is soothing and provides comfort regardless of whether one is seeking relaxation to meet pleasure needs or to cope with chronic pain of some type.

In a health care context, the term **palliative care** means to relieve or reduce the intensity of uncomfortable symptoms but not to produce a cure. Palliative care is provided when the condition is most likely going to become worse and degenerative processes will continue (e.g., terminal illness, dementia). It often relates to approaches that reduce suffering.

Because the term *suffering* is inherently subjective and multi-faceted, it is often difficult to totally understand this experience in the client. **Suffering** can be defined as an overall impairment in quality of life. Some say that we may not have a choice about whether or not we experience pain (physical, emotional, or spiritual), but we can choose to suffer or not. Often managing pain does not alleviate suffering. Dealing with only the physical aspects of pain may not address the mind and spirit of the client because suffering is often a mental and spiritual issue. Many times suffering overshadows the client's ability to create or participate in meaningful experiences or experience pleasure.

Palliative care is also appropriate when the condition should not be changed or the person does not desire a specific outcome other than pleasure and relaxation. Providing massage to a woman during labor, receiving a massage while on vacation, supporting an athlete during training for an event, providing massage at a public event such as a health fair, giving a massage to someone just before surgery, and providing massage to a wedding party the day before the event are all examples of the appropriate use of palliative care.

Massage approaches have great efficacy in palliative care. When presented through massage, the pleasurable experiences of touch and human connection may be one of the greatest therapeutic gifts our profession offers.

Based on the aforementioned information, questions then arise:

- When is change appropriate?
- When is change not desirable and condition management and palliative support more appropriate?
- How does the professional determine what type of care is appropriate: therapeutic change, condition management, or palliative care?
- How does the professional know when these transi-

tions in care types (therapeutic change, condition management, and palliative care) occur?

Palliative care can progress to condition management, and, with the gradual restoration of energy, the client may even progress to a change process. Eventually a change process will end or transform, and management, such as stress management, becomes the professional focus once again (Proficiency Exercise 5-2).

Chapter 3 detailed intake procedures, including a client history, physical assessment, and methods to develop this information into care/treatment plans. The clinical reasoning model provides a decision-making process to analyze whether therapeutic change or approaches to maintain or support an existing state is the best approach. The ability to analyze data collected during assessment procedures is crucial in making decisions about what massage therapy intervention to use and whether the outcome is a therapeutic change process, condition management, or palliative care. These factors are considered when developing a plan that best serves the client (Proficiency Exercise 5-3).

Text continued on p. 196.

5-2
PROFICIENCY EXERCISE

Metaphor

Clean house—offer palliative and management care, decrease suffering, and encourage better coping in the existing situation

or

Remodel the house—an active change process

For both the professional and the client, list the differences between "cleaning house" and "remodeling the house" in terms of skill levels, cost, time, materials, difficulties, disruption in daily living, and other factors.

Example:

Cleaning house:
Professional—ongoing service
Client—ongoing appointments
Remodeling:
Professional—defined number of appointment with specific outcome
Client—commitment to specific set of appointments

Your Turn
List three differences in each area.

Cleaning house:
Professional:

1.

2.

3.

Client:

1.

2.

3.

Remodeling:
Professional:

1.

2.

3.

Client:

1.

2.

3.

PROFICIENCY EXERCISE

After reading the following client case situations, decide whether you would introduce therapeutic change, condition management, or palliative care. Explain your reasons for the decision using the clinical reasoning model. An example is provided.

Example:

A male client, age 47, is experiencing fatigue and neck and shoulder pain. He is a cross-country truck driver. He is married with three children and has the normal financial obligations of a house payment, car payment, and other responsibilities. One child just started college, and the client is somewhat concerned about the tuition expenses. He likes his job and is content with his family and social life. He can't seem to understand why he is tired or why his shoulder hurts. He can think of no reason for the pain other than the strain of the driving position and the long hours. This pain never bothered him before. He went to the doctor for a physical examination, and nothing out of the ordinary was identified. The physician thinks that an old football injury coupled with some age-related changes are responsible. The doctor also thinks that the pain in the shoulder might be interfering with sleep and be a cause of fatigue. The doctor recommends an over-the-counter antiinflammatory agent and painkiller such as aspirin, and suggests massage might help. The doctor also recommends that he cut back on his work hours and relax more. Aspirin helps the shoulder pain but upsets his stomach. He does not want to cut back on work hours. He is seeking help for shoulder pain and would like more physical energy.

Identify the Facts

Questions that help with this process are the following:

What is considered normal or balanced function?
The ability to work pain free with reasonable stamina at a job that one enjoys.

What has happened? (Spell out events)
Nothing substantial has occurred to account for the changes other than age-related influences and a prior football injury.

What caused the imbalance? (Can it be identified?)
A prior injury, long work hours, static seated position with arms evaluated on the steering wheel. Repetitive looking to the left during driving.

What was done or is being done?
Aspirin

What has worked or not worked?
Aspirin works but upsets stomach. He has chosen to maintain his current work schedule.

Brainstorm the Possibilities

Questions that help with this process are the following:

What are the possibilities? (What could it all mean?)
The fatigue and pain could be a result of age-related changes and prior injury coupled with repetitive use and pain interfering with sleep as suggested by the doctor.
The situation could be more related to emotional stress resulting from financial concerns.
There could be an undiagnosed health condition that is not sufficiently evident for a definitive diagnosis to be made.

What is my intuition suggesting?
I think that we are likely dealing with a combination of the doctor's diagnosis and unexpressed emotional stress over financial concerns, particularly the tuition costs for the child in college.

What are the possible patterns of dysfunction?
It is possible the static driving position is aggravating the old football injury.

What are the possible contributing factors?
Worry, postural distortion for the static position, and age-related tissue changes because we become somewhat less flexible with age and lack of exercise.

What are possible interventions?
Job change
Stretching program
Massage therapy
Short-term mental health support
Different medication that does not upset stomach

What might work?
Massage and a stretching program

What are other ways to look at the situation?
The client does not seem to want to use medications, does not want to change his job, and does not seem to think that there is anything wrong with his emotional or social life. Maybe if the financial situation were different, the stress load would be low enough so that the energy levels would increase and he could ignore the pain. Maybe a financial advisor would be helpful, or maybe his wife could get a job.

What do the data suggest?
Data seem to suggest that an age-related process affects a prior injury aggravated by repetitive job strain and static seated position.

Consider Logical Outcomes of Each Possibility

Questions that help determine outcomes are the following:

What is the logical progression of the symptom pattern, contributing factors, and current behaviors?
If the pain remains or worsens and sleep continues to be interrupted so that fatigue worsens, the immune system can

Continued.

be compromised and other disease processes might occur. He could become unable to work. His mood would be altered, affecting family and social relationships.

What is the logical cause and effect of each intervention identified? What are the pros and cons of each intervention suggested?

Job change—*Remove repetitive strain on the shoulder and eliminate static position: drastic change in lifestyle, finances, and work environment.*

Stretching program—*Increase flexibility and counterbalance static position: could make the situation worse if the stretching is too aggressive, not progressive, and intermittent instead of used daily; is self-initiated and once learned would not incur any ongoing costs; does not need regular appointment schedule because he is on the road; requires discipline to do the stretches*

Massage therapy—*Help pain symptoms and support better sleep: does not require extensive self-discipline other than making regular appointments; would incur a financial obligation; would support a daily stretching program; would reduce the use of medication*

Short-term mental health support—*Does not require extensive self-discipline other than making regular appointments: would incur a financial obligation; does not address physical condition but does address emotional strain*

Different medication that does not upset stomach—*Help pain symptoms and support better sleep: does not require extensive self-discipline; would incur a small financial obligation; does not need regular appointment schedule because he is on the road; possible side effects and development of dependency on the medication*

Financial advisor—*Better control of finances, eliminate basis for worry and emotional stress: does not address physical conditions, long work hours, or job stress*

Wife get a job—*Would eliminate financial burden: could create stress in relationship, requires action on part of person other than self; does not address physical conditions, long work hours or job stress*

What are the consequences of not acting?

Situation could stabilize and resolve itself. Situation could become more problematic, requiring more drastic intervention measures in the future.

What are the consequences of acting?

Problem remains stable or improves. Client is better able to cope with current situation.

Identify the Effect of Each Possibility on People Involved

Questions that help identify possible effects are the following:

In terms of each intervention being considered, what would be the impact on the people involved: client, practitioner, and other professionals working with the client?

Job change—*Client not supportive, wife may or may not like idea*

Stretching program—*Client does not like to fuss with himself and avoids activities having to do with self-care*

Massage therapy—*Client open to idea but nervous; wife supportive, doctor supportive, massage practitioner supportive*

Short-term mental health support—*Both client and wife not open to this possibility at this time; they do not think this is an emotional problem; massage practitioner is hesitant about the client being unwilling to seek mental health services and does think emotion is involved (worry over finances) and would like client to remain open to this possibility*

Different medication that does not upset stomach—*Client does not like to take medication, and the doctor is unwilling to prescribe at this time until other measures are explored*

Financial advisor—*Both client and wife thought this was a good idea and would pursue this possibility*

Wife get a job—*Not an option at this time*

How does each person involved feel about the possible interventions?

Job change—*Not supportive*

Stretching program—*Client ambivalent, massage practitioner and wife supportive*

Massage therapy—*All supportive*

Short-term mental health support—*Massage therapist supportive; client and wife not supportive*

Different medication that does not upset stomach—*Doctor and/client not supportive*

Financial advisor—*Client and wife supportive*

Wife get a job—*Not an option*

Is the practitioner within his/her scope of practice to work with such situations?

Yes

Is the practitioner qualified to work with such situations?

Yes

5 - 3
PROFICIENCY EXERCISE—CONT'D

Does the practitioner feel qualified to work with such situations?

Practitioner is concerned about the ambivalence to a stretching program and nonsupport about a mental health referral. These concerns raise questions concerning the ability to work effectively with the physical problems when other causal factors may exist.

Is there a feeling of cooperation and agreement between all parties involved?

There is a degree of cooperation as well as some resistance. There is agreement for the use of massage therapy.

Based on this analysis of the information provided, the massage practitioner would recommend a condition management program instead of a therapeutic change process. Causal factors are involved that the client may not be able to address during a change process. He is also resistant to the idea of an exercise or stretching program that would interfere with his driving schedule.

Case 1

A 17-year-old volleyball player is in training for a playoff tournament in 4 weeks. She has been somewhat sore after practice and anxious about the playoffs. Her game is a bit "off," which is adding to the anxiety. Both her coach and parents thought massage would be helpful. She is in good health, taking no medications, but she does have an erratic eating pattern and has been recently drinking soda with caffeine in it. She has also been working with visualization and progressive relaxation before sleeping. She thinks these methods help her sleep better.

Identify the Facts
Questions that help with this process are the following:

What is considered normal or balanced function?

What has happened? (Spell out events?)

What caused the imbalance? (Can it be identified?)

What was done or is being done?

What has worked or not worked?

Brainstorm the Possibilities
Questions that help with this process are the following:

What are the possibilities? (What could it all mean?)

What is my intuition suggesting?

What are the possible patterns of dysfunction?

Continued.

5 - 3
PROFICIENCY EXERCISE—CONT'D

What are the possible contributing factors?

What are possible interventions?

What might work?

What are other ways to look at the situation?

What do the data suggest?

Consider Logical Outcomes of Each Possibility
Questions that help determine outcomes are the following:

What is the logical progression of the symptom pattern, contributing factors, and current behaviors?

What are the pros and cons of each intervention suggested?

What is the logical cause and effect of each intervention identified?

What are the consequences of not acting?

What are the consequences of acting?

---

5 - 3

PROFICIENCY EXERCISE—CONT'D

Identify the Effect of Each Possibility on People Involved

Questions that help identify effects are the following:

In terms of each intervention being considered, what would be the impact on the people involved: client, practitioner, and other professionals working with the client?

How does each person involved feel about the possible interventions?

Is the practitioner within his/her scope of practice to work with such situations?

Is the practitioner qualified to work with such situations?

Does the practitioner feel qualified to work with such situations?

Is there a feeling of cooperation and agreement between all parties involved?

Based on this analysis of the information provided, the massage practitioner would recommend _____ for the following reasons:

Case 2

A 39-year-old female is experiencing mood swings and headaches. She had a car accident 3 years ago, resulting in whiplash that was treated successfully with physical therapy; she still has some residual stiffness in her neck. She visited her doctor and is premenopausal. No treatment other than stress management and moderate exercise was recommended at this time. Her only child just graduated from high school has entered the military. She was divorced 2 years ago. She has a supportive circle of friends and is financially stable and secure in her job. She expresses that she wants to feel more in control of her body and wants to be able to self-manage the mood swings and headaches. She is not opposed to hormone therapy for the menopause but would like to see if she can manage without it. She is seeking massage as part of her lifestyle self-care program and is motivated.

Identify the Facts

Questions that help with this process are the following:

What is considered normal or balanced function?

What has happened? (Spell out events?)

Continued.

PROFICIENCY EXERCISE—CONT'D

What caused the imbalance? (Can it be identified?)

What are the possible contributing factors?

What was done or is being done?

What are possible interventions?

What has worked or not worked?

Brainstorm the Possibilities
Questions that help with this process are the following:

What are the possibilities? (What could it all mean?)

What might work?

What are other ways to look at the situation?

What is my intuition suggesting?

What do the data suggest?

What are the possible patterns of dysfunction?

Consider Logical Outcomes of Each Possibility
Questions that help determine outcomes are the following:

What is the logical progression of the symptom pattern, contributing factors, and current behaviors?

5-3

PROFICIENCY EXERCISE—CONT'D

What are the pros and cons of each intervention suggested?

How does each person involved feel about the possible interventions?

What is the logical cause and effect of each intervention identified?

What are the consequences of not acting?

Is the practitioner within his/her scope of practice to work with such situations?

Is the practitioner qualified to work with such situations?

What are the consequences of acting?

Does the practitioner feel qualified to work with such situations?

Identify the Effect of Each Possibility on People Involved

Questions that help identify effects are the following:

In terms of each intervention being considered, what would be the impact on the people involved: client, practitioner, and other professionals working with the client?

Is there a feeling of cooperation and agreement between all parties involved?

Based on this analysis of the information provided, the massage practitioner would recommend _____ for the following reasons:

Case 3

A 26-year-old male with asthma is experiencing an increase in symptoms. He is recently married and just moved to a new city because of a job transfer. His wife is 3 months pregnant. He takes good care of himself and is careful with

Continued.

PROFICIENCY EXERCISE—CONT'D

his diet. His exercise program has been disrupted by the move and he has not reestablished a regular exercise program. Medication is effective in treating the asthma. His respiratory therapist recommended massage because she feels that the increased stress is a possible cause for the more severe asthma.

Identify the Facts

Questions that help with this process are the following:

What is considered normal or balanced function?

What has happened? (Spell out events?)

What caused the imbalance? (Can it be identified?)

What was done or is being done?

What has worked or not worked?

Brainstorm the Possibilities

Questions that help with this process are the following:

What are the possibilities? (What could it all mean?)

What is my intuition suggesting?

What are the possible patterns of dysfunction?

What are the possible contributing factors?

What are possible interventions?

What might work?

What are other ways to look at the situation?

What do the data suggest?

PROFICIENCY EXERCISE—CONT'D

Consider Logical Outcomes of Each Possibility
Questions that help determine outcomes are the following:

What is the logical progression of the symptom pattern, contributing factors, and current behaviors?

What are the pros and cons of each intervention suggested?

What is the logical cause and effect of each intervention identified?

What are the consequences of acting?

Identify the Effect of Each Possibility on People Involved
Questions that help identify effects are the following:

In terms of each intervention being considered, what would be the impact on the people involved: client, practitioner, and other professionals working with the client?

How does each person involved feel about the possible interventions?

Is the practitioner within his/her scope of practice to work with such situations?

Is the practitioner qualified to work with such situations?

Continued.

---

5 - 3

PROFICIENCY EXERCISE—CONT'D

Does the practitioner feel qualified to work with such situations?

Is there a feeling of cooperation and agreement between all parties involved?

Based on this analysis of the information provided, the massage practitioner would recommend _____ for the following reasons:

PATHOLOGY, HEALTH, AND THERAPEUTIC MASSAGE

section objectives

Using the information presented in this section, the student will be able to perform the following:

- **Define** *health, dysfunction,* **and** *pathology*
- **Recognize when a client's condition should be evaluated by a primary health care provider**
- **List the mechanisms and risk factors that predispose people to disease processes**
- **Recognize the warning signs of cancer**
- **Explain the general inflammatory response**
- **Explain the mechanisms of pain and evaluate pain for referral purposes**
- **List the endangerment sites for massage**

Pathology is the study of disease. To practice safely, massage therapists need a basic understanding of pathologic processes. Although the diagnosis of disorders is not a function of a massage professional, to refer appropriately the massage therapist must be able to recognize when the client's condition represents an irregularity that should be evaluated by his or her primary health care provider. When working with a referral and under proper supervision, the massage professional also must be able to alter the application of massage in terms of any present disease process so that the client receives the benefits of massage without harm. Massage students should have both a general awareness of the types of disorders that occur in each major body system and more specific knowledge of the

signs and symptoms of selected disorders that could endanger the health of either the client or the practitioner. See Appendix A for specific contraindications to massage. The massage professional also needs a basic understanding of pharmacology and the possible interactions between medications and massage. See Appendix C for specific information.

It is also important to understand the way in which a disease process develops. The body is designed for health, and it requires a sequence of events for disease to occur. Trauma also requires the body to use healing energy. Trauma is an abrupt shock or injury to the body or psyche.

To understand disease we need first to understand the definition of health. **Health** is optimal functioning with freedom from disease or abnormal processes. Health is influenced by many factors, including inherited (genetic) and constitutional conditions. Lifestyle, activity level, rest, loving relationships, exercise, a balanced diet, empowering beliefs and attitudes, self-esteem, authentic personality, and freedom from self-hindering patterns all support health. When a state of health no longer exists or is interrupted, dysfunction begins.

Dysfunction is the in-between state of "not healthy" but also "not sick" (experiencing disease). Unfortunately, many people experience dysfunctional states. Western medicine has a difficult time identifying and dealing with dysfunctions because these are prepathologic states and are often not apparent within current diagnostic methods. Actual pathology usually needs to exist before medical tests and diagnostic methods can determine an actual disease state.

Recent prevention methods, many modeled after more "Eastern" or "holistic" approaches, are beginning to address this area called *dysfunction*. Many ancient healing methods are more focused on the process of dysfunction, introducing restorative methods before a system breaks down into a disease process. When used in the prepathology state of dysfunction, these methods of mind/body medicine, stress management, and prevention are very effective. When applied to an active pathologic process, these methods are less effective, although they remain an important part of the total healing program. Often more aggressive approaches are required to reverse the pathologic condition and allow healing to begin.

Disease or pathology occurs when homeostatic and restorative body mechanisms break down and can no longer adapt. It is seldom one thing that contributes to pathology, but instead a series of events occurs.

For example, influenza, or the flu, is caused by a virus, but not everyone exposed to the virus gets the flu. Consider one person who gets the flu and another who does not. The person who has the flu smokes, had a minor car accident 2 weeks ago, is experiencing a short-term financial setback, and got in an argument with a co-worker 3 days before the onset of the flu. The person who does not have the flu did not experience anything out of the ordinary for the last 3 months, exercises moderately, and follows a fairly supportive dietary plan with lots of fruits and vegetables.

Functioning Limits

The body has anatomic and physiologic functioning limits. The heart can only beat so fast, the endocrine glands secrete a maximal amount of hormones, the skeletal muscles can only lift so much weight or jump so high. Extraordinary events push the body's limits of functioning. Athletes often function at the end of their body limits.

Under normal conditions the body functions within a margin of safety. Normal physiologic mechanisms inhibit the tendency to function at the body limits. We usually do not run as fast as we can, work as long as we could, or exert all of our energy to complete a task. Instead the body signals fatigue, pain, or strain before the anatomic or physiologic limits are reached and we back off. This very important protective mechanism allows us to live within a healthy range of energy expenditure while keeping functioning energy reserves in place in case of an emergency or extraordinary demand. Each time we tap into this reserve the body tends to work to restore what was used and if possible add a little more to the reserve.

Dysfunction occurs when the reserve runs low because restorative mechanisms are not able to function effectively or when the body begins to limit function in an attempt to maintain higher energy reserves.

Dysfunction Related to Low Reserves

For example, a new mother with a fussy baby is unable to get restorative sleep. This continues for 6 months. The mother gets a cold that lingers. The infant is prone to recurring ear infections over the next 3 years, which continues to disturb the sleep pattern of the mother. In addition, the mother's diet becomes limited and begins to consist of mostly snack foods. The mother begins first to have headaches, then neck and shoulder pain. Finally, 5 years after the birth, just as the child begins school, the mother develops chronic fatigue syndrome with fibromyalgia.

Massage intervention early in the process may help support restorative sleep, especially if help with the baby is provided. Massage and other similar stress-management systems could at least slow the progression of dysfunction. After the headaches appear, massage could be used to manage the pain and reduce the muscle tension patterns in an attempt to support innate body healing and restorative mechanisms. After chronic fatigue symptoms begin with fibromyalgia pain, a multidisciplinary team and lifestyle approach are necessary to reverse pathology.

Dysfunction Related to Attempts to Maintain Higher Energy Reserve

For example, if a person plays tennis and overstretches the shoulder reaching for the serve, the body senses a danger of harm to the joint. Neurologic sensors may reset muscle patterns, limiting range of motion slightly to prevent this from happening again. Physiologically, protective space has been deposited in the body reserves even though range of motion has been sacrificed. If this continues, eventually the limited of range of motion interferes with the ability to play tennis. Dysfunction occurs. If perpetuated and compensated for over a period of time, pathology usually develops. The person could end up with a frozen shoulder.

Massage intervention just after the first event, coupled with a more conservative playing style, might reverse the process and dysfunction would not develop. Intervention applied at the point that range of motion limits were first observed would mostly still be effective in reversing the dysfunctional process. However, the intervention plan would be more complex and time consuming. Interventions introduced after pathology has begun are complex, sometimes aggressive, and occasionally too late to support repair and restoration of function.

Massage professionals serve many people at the beginning of dysfunctional patterns—when the client does not feel his or her best but is not sick yet. It is important to monitor the client to make sure they do not continue to progress further into dysfunctional patterns. Early intervention and referral to appropriate health care professionals are important to the identification of potential problems before they actually develop. The benefits of massage are most effectively focused in assisting people to stay within the healthy range of functioning.

Development of Pathology

Because therapeutic massage has widespread effects on the physiologic functions of the body, it is the massage professional's responsibility, when applying bodywork techniques, to have a knowledge of pathology, contraindications, and endangerment sites. It is difficult to obtain a consensus on such information, however, because all sources do not agree.

Because many diseases have similar symptoms, it is difficult to determine the specific underlying causes of pathology. The massage professional must refer clients to qualified, licensed health care providers for specific diagnosis.

Disease conditions are usually diagnosed or identified by signs and symptoms. **Signs** are objective abnormalities that can be seen or measured by someone other than the patient. **Symptoms** are the subjective abnormalities felt only by the patient. A **syndrome** is a group of different signs and symptoms, usually from a common cause. A disease is classified as **acute** when signs and symptoms develop quickly, last a short time, then disappear. Diseases that develop slowly and last for a long time (sometimes for life) are called **chronic** diseases.

Communicable diseases can be transmitted from one person to another. The study of communicable diseases is an important process for the massage therapist and is discussed in further detail in Chapter 6.

Homeostasis is the relative constancy of the body's internal environment. If homeostasis is disturbed, as occurs in a disease process, a variety of feedback mechanisms usually attempt to return the body to normal. A disease condition exists when homeostasis cannot be restored easily. In acute conditions, the body recovers its homeostatic balance quickly. In chronic diseases a normal state of balance may never be restored and compensation develops. **Compensation** is the process of counterbalancing a defect in body structure or function.

Risk Factors

Certain predisposing conditions may make the development of a disease more likely. Usually called *risk factors,* these conditions may put an individual at risk for developing a disease but do not actually cause the disease. Several major types of risk factors exist.

Genetic factors. Several types of genetic risk factors exist. An inherited trait may sometimes put a person at a greater-than-normal risk for developing a specific disease. Family history of disease processes and causes of death usually can reveal the possible genetic traits. Steps can be taken to support the body against the genetic tendency toward a disease process. Changes in diet and lifestyle may also be beneficial.

Age. Biologic and behavioral factors increase the risk for developing certain diseases at certain ages in life. For example, musculoskeletal problems are common between the ages of 30 and 50 years.

Lifestyle. The way we live and work can put us at risk for some diseases. Some researchers believe that the high-fat, low-fiber diet common among people in developed nations increases their risk of developing certain types of cancer and cardiovascular diseases.

Environment. Some environmental situations put us at greater risk for contracting certain diseases. For example, living in an area with high concentrations of air pollution may increase the risk for development of respiratory problems.

Preexisting conditions. A primary (preexisting) condition can put a person at risk of developing a secondary condition. For example, a viral infection can compromise the immune system, rendering the individual more susceptible to bacterial infection.

Stress. *Stress* may be defined as any substantial change in routine or any activity that forces the body to adapt. Stress places demands on physical, mental, and emotional resources. Research has shown that as stresses accumulate, especially if the stress is long term, the individual becomes increasingly susceptible to physical illness, mental and emotional problems, and accidental injuries.

General adaptation syndrome. Selye labeled the body's response to stress as the **general adaptation syndrome** (GAS), which involves three stages. The first stage is alarm, or the "fight-or-flight" response, which is the body's initial reaction to the perceived stressor. The second stage is known as the *resistance reaction.* This stage, through the secretion of regulating hormones, allows the body to continue fighting a stressor long after the effects of the alarm reaction have dissipated. The third stage is exhaustion, which occurs if the stress response continues without relief. General adaptation is a uniform, consistent, general response to the perceived stimuli.

The GAS describes the way the body mobilizes different defense mechanisms when threatened by harmful (actual or perceived) stimuli. In generalized stress conditions the hypothalamus acts on the anterior pituitary gland to cause the release of adrenocorticotropic hormone, which stimulates the adrenal cortex to secrete glucocorticoid. In addition, the sympathetic subdivision of the autonomic nervous system (ANS) is stimulated by the adrenal medulla, so the release of epinephrine and norepinephrine occurs to assist the body in responding to the stressful stimulus. Unfortunately, during periods of prolonged stress, glucocorticosteroids may have harmful side effects, including a decreased immune response, decreased blood glucose levels, altered protein and fat metabolism, and decreased resistance to stress.

Considering the variety and number of organs and glands innervated by the ANS, it is no wonder that autonomic disorders have varied and broad consequences. This is especially true of stress-induced diseases. A prolonged or excessive physiologic response to stress, the fight-or-flight response, can disrupt normal functioning throughout the body. Stress has been cited as an indirect cause or an important risk factor in many conditions.

Pathologic Conditions and Indications for Massage

Inflammatory Response

Inflammation may occur as a response to any tissue injury. The **inflammatory response** is a combination of processes that attempts to minimize injury to tissues, thus maintaining homeostasis. Inflammation may also accompany specific immune system reactions. The inflammatory response is an active and important part of a healing process. The inflammatory response has four primary signs—heat, redness, swelling, and pain.

Heat and redness. As tissue cells are damaged, they release inflammation mediators such as histamine, prostaglandins, and compounds called *kinins*. Some inflammation mediators cause blood vessels to dilate, increasing blood volume in the tissue. Increased blood volume produces the redness and heat of inflammation. This response is important because it allows immune system cells (white blood cells) in the blood to travel quickly and easily to the site of injury.

Swelling and pain. Some inflammation mediators increase the permeability of blood vessel walls. When water leaks out of the vessel, tissue swelling or edema results. The pressure caused by edema triggers pain receptors. The fluid that accumulates in inflamed tissue is called *inflammatory exudate* and has the beneficial effect of diluting the irritant. Inflammatory exudate is removed slowly by lymphatic vessels. Bacteria and damaged cells are held in the lymph nodes and are destroyed by white blood cells. Occasionally, lymph nodes enlarge when they process a large amount of infectious material.

Sometimes the inflammatory response is more intense or prolonged than desirable. Inflammation can be suppressed by antihistamines, which block the action of histamine, and aspirin, which disrupts the body's synthesis of prostaglandins.

Inflammatory Disease

Local inflammation occurs in a limited area: for example, a small cut that becomes infected. Systemic inflammation occurs when the irritant spreads through the body or when inflammation mediators cause changes throughout the body. Conditions involving chronic inflammation are classified as *inflammatory diseases*. Inflammatory conditions such as arthritis, asthma, eczema, and chronic bronchitis are among the most common.

indications for massage

Therapeutic massage seems to be beneficial in cases of prolonged inflammation. Possible theories regarding this include the following:

1. The stimulation from massage activates a release of the body's own antiinflammatory agents.

2. Certain types of massage increase the inflammatory process to a small degree, triggering the body to complete the process.
3. Massage may facilitate the dilution and removal of the irritant by increasing lymphatic flow.

Tissue repair. The processes of inflammation trigger tissue repair. Tissue repair is the replacement of dead cells with living cells. In a type of tissue repair called *regeneration*, the new cells are similar to those they replace. Another type of tissue repair is *replacement*. In replacement the new cells are formed from connective tissue and are different from those they replace, resulting in a scar. Often, fibrous connective tissue replaces the damaged tissue, resulting in a condition called *fibrosis*. Most tissue repairs are a combination of regeneration and replacement. A goal in the healing process is to promote regeneration and keep replacement to a minimum. Massage has been shown to slow the formation of scar tissue and keep scar tissue pliable when it does form.

Therapeutic inflammation. Because the inflammatory response is part of a healing process, the deliberate creation of inflammation can generate or "jump start" healing mechanisms. Certain methods of massage can be used to create a controlled, localized area of therapeutic inflammation. Deep frictioning techniques and connective tissue stretching methods are the most common approaches. In some healing practices the skin is burned to create inflammation. Acupuncture may also create very small localized areas of inflammation to generate healing mechanisms. These methods are most beneficial in resolving connective tissue dysfunction, particularly fibrotic changes of muscle tissue and areas of scar tissue adhesion.

The benefit derived from the use of therapeutic inflammation depends on the body's ability to generate healing processes. If healing mechanisms are suppressed, do not use methods that create therapeutic inflammation. Therapeutic inflammation is not used in situations in which sleep disturbance, compromised immune function, a high degree of stress load, or systemic or localized inflammation is already present, or if any condition such as fibromyalgia that consists of impaired repair and restorative functions exists, unless carefully supervised as part of a total treatment program.

Consideration needs to be given to the use of antiinflammatory medications. If a person is taking such medication, either steroidal or nonsteroidal, the effectiveness of therapeutic inflammation is negated or reduced, and restoration mechanisms are inhibited. When these medications are present, any methods that create inflammation are to be avoided.

Pain

The massage therapist especially needs to understand the mechanisms of pain. Chapter 4 provides reasons why massage is beneficial for the symptomatic reduction of pain perception. Here we will consider the types of pain and the ways massage can be indicated or contraindicated for pain. Understanding the various types of pain helps the massage practitioner know when to refer the client to a physician.

Pain is a complex, private, abstract experience that is difficult to explain or describe. It is the main symptom or complaint that causes people to seek health care. Its effective management is a major challenge. Defining pain in descriptive and measurable terms is not easy because pain has physiologic, psychologic, and social aspects. The massage professional needs to recognize that pain is what the client says it is and exists when the client says it does. The fourth edition of *Mosby's Medical, Nursing, & Allied Health Dictionary* defines *pain* as "an unpleasant sensation caused by noxious stimulation of the sensory nerve endings. It is a subjective feeling and an individual response to the cause."[1]

Pain sensations. Pain provides information about tissue-damaging stimuli, and thus often enables us to protect ourselves from greater damage. Pain initiates our search for medical assistance. The subjective description and indication of the location of the pain helps pinpoint the underlying cause of disease.

The receptors for pain, called *nociceptors,* are simply the branching ends of the dendrites of certain sensory neurons. Pain receptors are found in almost every tissue of the body and may respond to any type of stimulus. When stimuli for other sensations, such as touch, pressure, heat, and cold, reach a certain intensity, they stimulate the sensation of pain as well. Injured tissue may release prostaglandins, making peripheral nociceptors more sensitive to the normal pain response (hyperalgesia). Aspirin and other nonsteroidal antiinflammatory drugs inhibit the action of prostaglandins and reduce pain.

Excessive stimulation of a sensory organ causes pain. Additional stimuli for pain receptors include excessive distention or dilation of a structure, prolonged muscular contractions, muscle spasms, inadequate blood flow to tissues, or the presence of certain chemical substances. Because of their sensitivity to all stimuli, pain receptors perform a protective function by identifying changes that may endanger the body.

Pain receptors adapt only slightly or not at all. *Adaptation* is the decrease or disappearance of the perception of a sensation, even though the stimulus is still present. (An example is the way we get used to our clothes soon after dressing.) If adaptation to pain occurred, pain would cease to be sensed and irreparable damage could result.

Sensory impulses for pain are conducted by the central nervous system along spinal and cranial nerves to the thalamus. From here the impulses may be relayed to the parietal lobe. Some awareness of pain occurs at subcortical levels. Recognition of the type and intensity of most pain is ultimately localized in the cerebral cortex. Pain is usually classified as acute, chronic, intractable, or phantom.

Acute pain. Acute pain is either a symptom of a disease condition or a temporary aspect of medical treatment. It acts as a warning signal because it can activate the sympathetic nervous system. Acute pain is usually temporary, of sudden onset, and easily localized. The client frequently can describe the pain, which often subsides with or without treatment.

Chronic pain. *Chronic pain* is a major health problem for approximately 25% of the population. Chronic pain is pain that persists or recurs for indefinite periods, usually for longer than 6 months. It frequently has an obscure onset, and the character and quality of the pain changes over time. Chronic pain is usually diffuse, poorly localized, and often requires the efforts of a multidisciplinary health care team, which may include a massage therapist, for its effective management.

Intractable pain. When chronic pain persists even when treatment is provided, or when it exists without demonstrable disease, it is called *intractable pain*. Intractable pain represents the greatest challenge to all health care providers. Short, temporary, symptomatic relief for this type of pain may be provided by massage. This is accomplished by flooding the sensory receptors with sensation, distracting the client temporarily from the perception of pain.

Phantom pain. A type of pain frequently experienced by clients who have had a limb amputated is called *phantom pain*. These clients still experience pain or other sensations in the area of the amputated extremity as if the limb were still there. This pain probably occurs because the remaining proximal portions of the sensory nerves that previously received impulses from the limb are being stimulated by the trauma of the amputation. Stimuli from these nerves are interpreted by the brain as coming from the nonexistent (phantom) limb.

Evaluation of pain. Because pain is a primary indicator in many disease processes, the massage practitioner must have a basic evaluation protocol for pain to refer his or her clients to the appropriate health care provider. The following guidelines for evaluating pain will help in this process.

Pain has many characteristics. *Location* can be divided into four categories:

1. Localized pain is pain confined to the site of origin.
2. Projected pain is typically a result of proximal nerve compression. This pain is perceived in the tissue supplied by the nerve.
3. Radiating pain is diffuse pain, which is not well localized, around the site of origin.
4. Referred pain is felt in an area distant from the site of the painful stimulus.

Pain may be divided into five types:

1. *Pricking or bright pain*—This type of pain is experienced when the skin is cut or jabbed with a sharp object. It is short-lived but intense and easily localized.
2. *Burning pain*—This type is slower to develop, lasts longer, and is less accurately localized. It is experienced when the skin is burned. It often stimulates cardiac and respiratory activity.
3. *Aching pain*—Aching pain occurs when the visceral organs are stimulated. It is constant, not well localized, and is often referred to areas of the body far from where the damage is occurring. This type of pain is important because it may be a sign of a life-threatening disorder of a vital organ.
4. *Deep pain*—The main difference between superficial and deep sensibility is the different nature of the pain evoked by noxious stimuli. Unlike superficial pain, deep pain is poorly localized, nauseating, and frequently associated with sweating and changes in blood pressure. Deep pain can be elicited experimentally from the periosteum and ligaments by injecting them with hypertonic saline. Pain produced in this fashion initiates reflex contraction of nearby skeletal muscles. This reflex contraction is similar to the muscle spasm associated with injuries to bones, tendons, and joints. The steadily contracting muscles become ischemic, and ischemia stimulates the pain receptors in the muscles. The pain, in turn, initiates more spasms,

creating a vicious circle called the **pain-spasm-pain cycle** (Fig. 5-1).

5. *Muscle pain*—If a muscle contracts rhythmically in the presence of an adequate blood supply, pain does not usually result. However, if the blood supply to a muscle is occluded (closed off), contraction soon causes pain. The pain persists after the contraction until blood flow is reestablished. If a muscle with a normal blood supply is made to contract continuously without periods of relaxation, it also begins to ache because the maintained contraction compresses the blood vessels supplying the muscle.

The origins of pain can be divided into two types, somatic and visceral. *Somatic pain* arises from stimulation of receptors in the skin (called *superficial somatic pain*), or from stimulation of receptors in skeletal muscles, joints, tendons, and fascia (called *deep somatic pain*). *Visceral pain* results from stimulation of receptors in the viscera (internal organs).

The ability of the cerebral cortex to locate the origin of pain is related to past experience. In most instances of somatic pain and in some instances of visceral pain, the cortex accurately projects the pain back to the stimulated area.

Referred pain. The pain may also be felt in a surface area far from the stimulated organ. This phenomenon is called **referred pain.** In general, the area to which the pain is referred and the visceral organ involved receive their inner-

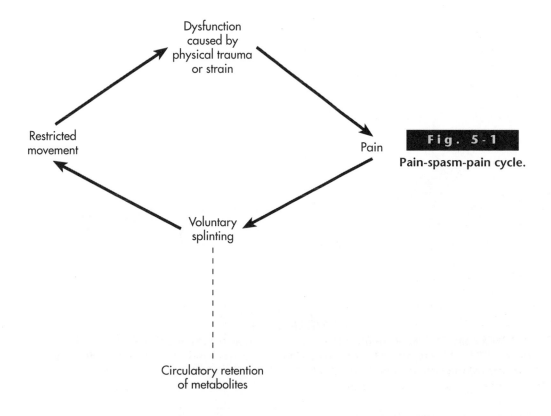

Fig. 5-1

Pain-spasm-pain cycle.

vation from the same segment of the spinal cord. Fig. 5-2 illustrates cutaneous regions to which visceral pain may be referred. If the client has a recurring pain pattern that resembles patterns on the chart, he or she should be referred to a physician for a more specific diagnosis.

As already stated, irritation of the viscera frequently produces pain that is felt not in the viscera but in some somatic structure that may be located at a considerable distance. Such pain is said to be referred to the somatic structure. Deep somatic pain may also be referred, but superficial pain is not. When visceral pain is both local and referred, it sometimes seems to spread (radiate) from the local to the distant site. Visceral pain, like deep somatic pain, initiates reflex contraction of nearby skeletal muscle. Because somatic pain is much more common than visceral pain, the brain has "learned" to project the pain to the somatic area.

Obviously, knowledge of referred pain and the common sites of pain referral from each of the viscera is very important to massage therapists and other health care professionals. However, sites of reference are not stereotyped, and unusual reference sites occur with considerable

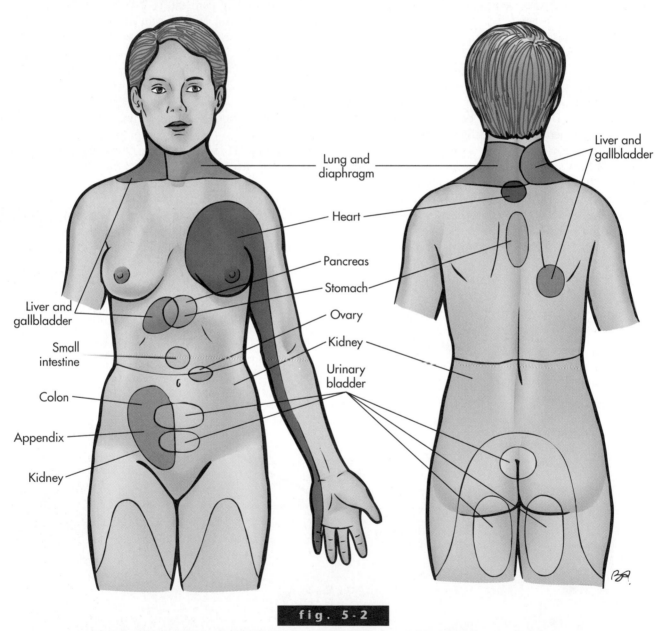

fig. 5-2

Referred pain. The diagram indicates cutaneous areas to which visceral pains may be referred. The professional encountering pain in these areas needs to refer the client for diagnosis to rule out visceral dysfunction.

frequency. Heart pain, for instance, may be experienced as purely abdominal, may be referred to the right arm, and may even be referred to the neck. Any client with a referred or unexplained pain pattern should be referred to a physician, especially if the pattern is similar to visceral referred pain patterns (see Fig. 5-2). When pain is referred, it is usually to a structure that developed from the same embryonic segment or dermatome as the structure in which the pain originates (Fig. 5-3).

Pain may be caused by mechanical, electrical, thermal, or chemical stimuli. We do not appear to adapt to pain or accommodate it. We may be distracted from it or ignore it, but it recurs unchanged if we pay attention to it. Subjective measurements of pain intensity are more reliable than observable ones. Only the client in pain can determine the amount of severity experienced. Pain is rarely the same at all times. It is felt (perceived) differently over time and differs with various precipitating and aggravating factors. Pain can range from excruciating to mild and may be difficult for the client to verbalize.

indications for massage

Pain is a complex problem with physical, psychologic, social, and financial components. Many ways exist to alleviate pain. The massage professional, as part of a health care team, can contribute valuable manual therapy in various pain conditions using direct tissue manipulation and reflex stimulation of the nervous system and the circulation. As a therapeutic intervention, massage may help reduce the need for pain medication, thus reducing the side effects of medication. All medications, including over-the-

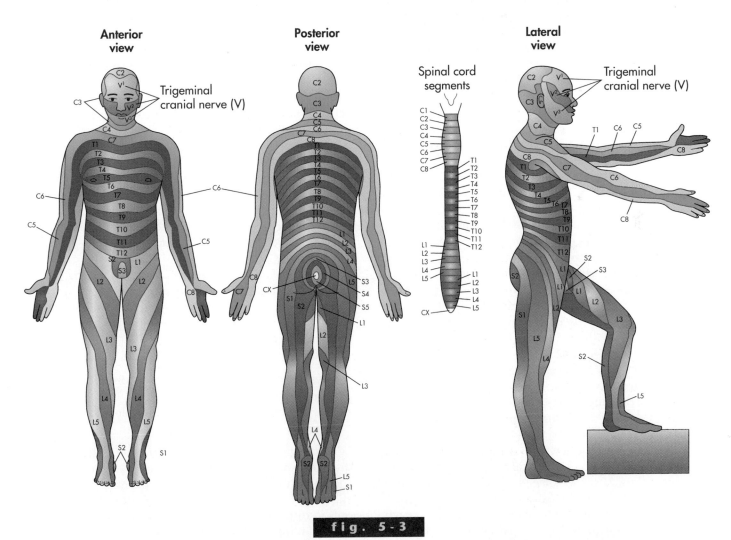

fig. 5-3

Dermatomes. Segmental dermatome distribution of spinal nerves to the front, back, and side of the body. *C,* Cervical segments; *T,* thoracic segments; *L,* lumbar segments; *S,* sacral segments; *CX,* coccygeal segment. (From Thibodeau GA, Patton KT: *The human body in health and disease,* ed 2, St Louis, 1997, Mosby.)

counter medication available without a prescription, have some side effects. Obviously, clients in extreme pain must have their massage therapy monitored by a doctor or other appropriate health care professional. Most people experience pain in less severe forms occasionally throughout life. Massage may provide temporary symptomatic relief for moderate pain brought on by daily stress, replacing over-the-counter pain medications or reducing their use.

Acute pain and chronic pain are managed somewhat differently; therefore it is important to make the distinction between the two. Intervention for acute pain is less invasive and focused to support a current healing process. Chronic pain is managed with either symptom relief or a more aggressive rehabilitation approach incorporating a therapeutic change process.

Impingement Syndromes

The two types of nerve **impingement syndromes** are compression and entrapment. As explained in Chapter 4, compression is pressure on a nerve by a bony structure, and entrapment is pressure on a nerve from soft tissue. Massage is beneficial for entrapment and can manage some symptoms of nerve compression, even though the direct causal factor is not addressed.

Cervical plexus. If the cervical plexus is being impinged, the person experiences headaches, neck pain, and breathing difficulties. The muscles most responsible for pressure on the cervical plexus are the suboccipital and sternocleidomastoid muscles. Shortened connective tissues at the cranial base will also press on these nerves.

The cervical plexus is formed by the ventral rami of the upper four cervical nerves. The phrenic nerve is part of this plexus. It innervates the diaphragm. Any disruption to this nerve affects breathing. Many cutaneous (skin) branches of the cervical plexus transmit sensory impulses from the skin of the neck, ear, and shoulder. The motor branches innervate muscles of the anterior neck.

Brachial plexus. The brachial plexus is situated partly in the neck and partly in the axilla and provides virtually all the nerves that innervate the upper limb. Any imbalance that brings pressure on this complex of nerves results in shoulder pain, chest pain, arm pain, wrist pain, and hand pain.

The muscles most often responsible for impingement of the brachial plexus are the scalenes, pectoralis minor, and subclavius. Muscles of the arm occasionally impinge branches of the brachial plexus. Brachial plexus impingement is responsible for thoracic outlet symptoms, which are often misdiagnosed as carpal tunnel syndrome. Whiplash injury involves the brachial plexus.

Lumbar plexus. Lumbar plexus nerve impingement may give rise to low-back discomfort with a belt distribution of pain, as well as pain in the lower abdomen, genitals, thigh, and medial lower leg. The main muscles that impinge the lumbar plexus are the quadratus lumborum and the psoas. Shortening of the lumbar dorsal fascia exaggerates a lordosis and causes vertebral impingement of the lumbar plexus.

Sacral plexus. The sacral plexus has approximately a dozen named branches. Almost half of these serve the buttock and lower limb; the others innervate pelvic structures. The main branch is the sciatic nerve. Impingement of this nerve by the piriformis muscle gives rise to sciatica.

Ligaments that stabilize the sacroiliac joint can affect the sacral plexus. Pressure on the sacral plexus can cause gluteal pain, leg pain, genital pain, and foot pain.

indications for massage

Massage methods can soften and stretch connective tissues that may impinge nerves as well as normalize muscle tension patterns, restoring a more normal resting length to shorten muscles to reduce pressure on nerves.

Psychologic Dysfunctions

Science has validated the body/mind link in terms of health and disease. Many risk factors for the development of physical (body) pathology are mental (mind) influenced, such as stress level and lifestyle choices. The same is true for mental health and pathology. The physical state of an individual has a strong influence on mental functioning. Usually when people feel well physically, they also feel well mentally, and again the reverse is often the case—feeling bad mentally results in physical dysfunctions.

The major mental heath dysfunctions affecting Western society are the following: trauma and posttraumatic stress disorder, pain and fatigue syndromes coupled with anxiety and depression, anxiety and depression, and stress-related illness.

Trauma is defined as follows:

- Physical injury caused by violent or disruptive action or toxic substance
- Psychic injury resulting from a severe emotional shock, either short term or long term

Posttraumatic stress disorder as defined by the *DSM IV,* the effects of which may be long term, includes experiencing flashback memory, state dependent memory, somatization, anxiety, irritability, sleep disturbance, concentration difficulties, times of melancholy or depression, grief, fear, worry, anger, and avoidance behavior.

Pain and fatigue syndromes are defined as multicausal and often chronic nonproductive patterns that interfere with well-being, activities of daily living, and productivity. Some current conditions in this area include fibromyalgia, chronic fatigue syndrome, Epstein-Barr virus, sympathetic reflex dystrophy, headache, arthritis, chronic cancer pain, neuropathy, low back syndrome, idiopathic pain, somatization disorder, and intractable pain syndrome. Acute pain can be a factor as well as acute "episodes" of chronic conditions.

Anxiety and depressive disorders are characterized by anxiety and depression. Anxiety is an uneasy feeling usually connected with increased sympathetic arousal responses. Depression is characterized by a decrease of vital functional activity and mood disturbances of exaggerated emptiness, hopelessness, and melancholy, or unbridled periods of high energy with no purpose or outcome.

It is common to see anxiety and depressive disorders in conjunction with fatigue and pain syndromes. Panic behavior, phobias, and a sense of impending doom, along with the sense of being overwhelmed and hopeless are common with these disorders. Mood swings, hyperventilation, sleep disturbance, concentration difficulties, memory disturbances, outbursts of anger, fatigue, changes in habits of daily living, appetite, and activity levels are symptoms of these disorders.

Stress-related illness is defined as an increased stress load or reduced ability to adapt that depletes the reserve capacity of individuals, increasing their vulnerability to health problems. Stress-related illness can encompass the previously mentioned conditions as the primary cause of dysfunction or as the result of the stress of the dysfunction. Excessive stress sometimes manifests as cardiovascular problems, including hypertension; digestive difficulties, including heartburn, ulcer, and bowel syndromes; respiratory illness and susceptibility to bacterial and viral illness; endocrine dysfunction, particularly adrenal or thyroid dysfunction and delayed or reduced cellular repair; sleep disorders; and hyperventilation syndrome, just to mention a few (Proficiency Exercises 5-4 and 5-5).

Text continued on p. 210.

5-4

PROFICIENCY EXERCISE

After reading the following case study, use the clinical reasoning model to develop a statement validating the indication for the use of therapeutic massage. An example is provided as a model.

Example:
Client is a 45-year-old female. She works 6 to 8 hours per day on the computer. She is experiencing mind fatigue and mid-back tension with pain. Her left arm is tingling during sleep and waking her up. She has a chronic compressed disk at L-4. Currently she is involved with a large writing project with a deadline to meet. Her exercise and stretching program has become sporadic. She also finds herself regularly driving for 3 and 4 hours at a time, which aggravates the nerve impingement in her low back. What are the indications for massage?

Identify the Facts
Questions that help with this process are the following:

What is considered normal or balanced function?
Regular movement without prolonged static positions
What has happened? (Spell out events?)
Workload and a deadline are requiring more time at the computer. Long periods of time are required in the car. The exercise and stretching program has been interrupted.
What caused the imbalance? (Can it be identified?)
Static seated position with the arm held in fixed position
What was done or is being done?
Exercise and stretching, but this pattern has been interrupted.

What has worked or not worked?
Exercise and stretching, but this pattern has been interrupted.

Brainstorm the Possibilities
Questions that help with this process are the following:

What are the possibilities? (What could it all mean?)
Muscles could be shortening in the front, changing the posture and straining the back muscles. Something may be interfering with circulation. Nerves could be impinged. Pain and increased tension could be contributing to mind fatigue.

What is my intuition suggesting?
She is tired, overworked, and sitting in one position too long.

What are the possible patterns of dysfunction?
The existing back disk dysfunction could be causing compensation, which is being aggravated by the ongoing static seated position. Fixed position of the shoulder while driving or at the computer may cause muscle tension that is impinging a nerve. Stress from the deadline for the project is interfering with sleep.
What are the possible contributing factors?
Preexisting injury to back, age, wrong position at the computer, or an ergonomically incorrect chair
What are possible interventions?
Massage, stretching, exercise, progressive relaxation, changing position of equipment

Continued.

What might work?

A combination of the possible interventions might be beneficial.

What are other ways to look at the situation?

Excessive workload with equipment that is positioned to aggravate the problem

What do the data suggest?

Multicausal factors

Logical Outcomes of Each Possibility

Questions that help determine outcomes are the following:

What is the logical progression of the symptom pattern, contributing factors, and current behaviors?

If the condition remains unchanged, the symptoms are likely to worsen. After the deadline is reached, the main causal factor will be eliminated and the condition could reverse itself.

What are the pros and cons of each intervention suggested? What is the logical cause and effect of each intervention identified?

Massage: Pros—reduces muscle tension, supports sleep

Cons—time away from work, effects may be short term

Logical outcome—massage may provide temporary relief until the condition changes

Stretching: Pros—able to be done throughout the day, would not require time away from job

Cons—effects short lived

Logical outcome—stretching would temporarily relieve tension pattern and provide a counterbalancing activity to the static seated position

Exercise: Pros—reduces muscle tension, supports sleep, clears mind fatigue

Cons—time away from work, effects may be short term

Logical outcome—exercise may provide temporary relief until the condition changes while supporting ongoing health maintenance

Progressive relaxation: Pros—supports sleep and helps relieve muscle tension; able to be done throughout the day, would not require time away from job

Cons—effects short lived

Logical outcome—progressive relaxation would provide some symptomatic relief

Changing position of equipment: Pros—would address a possible causal factor, would not require any other energy expenditure

Cons—would not address emotional stress or physical symptoms

Logical outcome—if equipment position is a causal factor, a change here could eliminate a source of the problem

What are the consequences of not acting?

Situation may worsen or resolve itself after project is completed.

What are the consequences of acting?

Symptoms and further compensation patterns may be managed.

Identify the Effect of Each Possibility on People Involved

Questions that help identify effects are the following:

In terms of each intervention being considered, what would be the impact on the people involved: client, practitioner, and other professionals working with the client? How does each person involved feel about the possible interventions?

Massage: Client supportive, massage therapist supportive

Stretching: Client supportive

Exercise: Client supportive

Progressive relaxation: Client does not feel benefits enough to justify time spent

Changing position of equipment: Client supportive

Is the practitioner within his/her scope of practice to work with such situations?

Yes

Is the practitioner qualified to work with such situations?

Yes, with cautions for disk compression

Does the practitioner feel qualified to work with such situations?

Yes

Is there a feeling of cooperation and agreement between all parties involved?

Yes

Based on this analysis of the information provided, the massage practitioner would recommend MASSAGE, STRETCHING, EXERCISE, and EQUIPMENT CHANGE for the following reasons:

The condition is short term until the project is completed. The client previously used stretching and exercise and needs encouragement to begin to use the methods again. Minor changes in the position of the computer may offer benefits. Massage is indicated to support sleep and address the general stress, the possible minor nerve impingement, the muscle tension from the static position, and management of muscle pain.

PROFICIENCY EXERCISE—CONT'D

Case

Client is an 81-year-old male in good health for his age. He took a fall 6 months ago but recovered nicely. He is active with his church and works in his garden. His wife died 18 months ago after a long illness. Lately his age-related aches and pains are bothering him more, especially his knees. This is interfering with his activities. He has mild hypertension and is taking medication for the condition. Currently it is controlled. He takes aspirin for the arthritis as needed. During his last physical, no problems were detected. What are the indications for massage?

Identify the Facts

Questions that help with this process are the following:

What is considered normal or balanced function?

What has happened? (Spell out events?)

What caused the imbalance? (Can it be identified?)

What was done or is being done?

What has worked or has not worked?

Brainstorm the Possibilities

Questions that help with this process are the following:

What are the possibilities? (What could it all mean?)

What is my intuition suggesting?

What are the possible patterns of dysfunction?

What are the possible contributing factors?

Continued.

5 - 4

PROFICIENCY EXERCISE—CONT'D

What are possible interventions?

What are the pros and cons of each intervention suggested? What is the logical cause and effect of each intervention identified?

What might work?

What are other ways to look at the situation?

What do the data suggest?

What are the consequences of not acting?

Consider Logical Outcomes of Each Possibility

Questions that help determine outcomes are the following:

What is the logical progression of the symptom pattern, contributing factors, and current behaviors?

What are the consequences of acting?

5 - 4

PROFICIENCY EXERCISE—CONT'D

Identify the Effect of Each Possibility on People Involved

Questions that help identify effects are the following:

In terms of each intervention being considered, what would be the impact on the people involved: client, practitioner, and other professionals working with the client? How does each person involved feel about the possible interventions?

Is the practitioner within his/her scope of practice to work with such situations?

Is the practitioner qualified to work with such situations?

Does the practitioner feel qualified to work with such situations?

Is there a feeling of cooperation and agreement between all parties involved?

Based on this analysis of the information provided, the massage practitioner would recommend _____

_____

for the following reasons:

5 - 5

PROFICIENCY EXERCISE

Do a self-evaluation listing all your predisposing risk factors for disease in the space provided.

Now, pick one risk factor and research a wellness plan to provide support for your body to prevent or lessen the possibility of the development of the pathologic condition.

indications for massage

Massage intervention has a strong physiologic effect from the comfort of compassionate touch as well as a physical influence on mental state through the effect on the ANS and neurochemicals. Therefore benefits may be derived from massage for those experiencing mental health problems. Management of pain is a strong factor. Because therapeutic massage can often offer symptomatic relief from chronic pain, the helplessness that accompanies these difficulties may dissipate as the person realizes that management methods exist. Soothing of any ANS hyperactivity or hypoactivity provides a sense of inner balance. Normalization of the breathing mechanism allows the client to breathe without restriction and can reduce the tendency toward hyperventilation syndrome, which feeds anxiety and panic.

Therapeutic massage can provide intervention on a physical level to restore a more normal function to the body, which supports appropriate interventions by qualified mental health professionals. Certainly strong and appropriate indications exist for the use of massage therapy in restoration of mental health, but caution is indicated in terms of the establishment of dual roles and boundary difficulties. It is very important to work in conjunction with mental health providers in these situations.

CONTRAINDICATIONS TO MASSAGE THERAPY

section objectives

Using the information presented in this section, the student will be able to perform the following:

- ■ **Evaluate a client's status to determine whether massage is contraindicated**
- ■ **Effectively refer a client to a primary health care provider**
- ■ **Interpret the reference list of indications and contraindications provided in Appendix A**

As mentioned earlier in this chapter, a *contraindication* is any condition that renders a particular treatment improper or undesirable or when cautions concerning treatment exist and supervision is required. Contraindications to massage are the responsibility of both responsible physicians and massage practitioners. The massage professional is not expected to diagnose any condition but should learn the client's particular condition by taking a thorough history and completing a physical assessment. The massage professional must be able to recognize indications and contraindications based on this information.

The massage practitioner also should have a current medical dictionary available to research unfamiliar terms and names of pathologic conditions. A massage practitioner is not a physician nor a mental health professional and is not expected to know the symptoms of all diseases, but resources must be available to locate specific information as needed.

Massage practitioners should not rely on lists of specific contraindications but rather on a set of medical and therapeutic guidelines pertinent to clinical applications and recent research developments. The present difficulty is that such guidelines are not consistent in current literature. Contraindications are unique to each client, as well as to each region of the body. The ability to reason clinically is essential to make appropriate decisions about the advisability of, modifications to, or avoidance of massage interventions. It is important to understand when to refer a client for diagnosis and when to obtain assistance in modifying the approach to the massage session so that it will best serve the client. A medical (including mental health) professional must always be consulted if any doubt exists concerning the advisability of therapy. *When in doubt, refer!*

Contraindications can be separated into regional and general types:

- *Regional contraindications* are those that relate to a specific area of the body. For our purposes, regional contraindication means that massage may be provided, but not to the problematic area. However, the client should be referred to a physician to obtain a diagnosis of the condition and rule out any underlying conditions.
- *General contraindications* are those that require a physician's evaluation to rule out serious underlying conditions before any massage is indicated. If massage is recommended by the physician, the physician will need to help the therapist develop a comprehensive treatment plan. Mental health dysfunctions fall into the general contraindication category.

Therapeutic massage is often beneficial for clients who are receiving treatment for a specific medical or mental health condition, but *caution is indicated*. In general, massage is indicated for musculoskeletal discomfort, circulation enhancement, relaxation, stress reduction, and pain control, as well as in situations in which analgesics, antiinflammatories, muscle relaxants, antianxiety, and antidepressive medications may be prescribed. Massage therapy, appropriately provided, can support the use of these medications and in mild cases may be able to replace the medications.

The general effects of stress and pain reduction, increased circulation, and physical comfort of therapeutic massage complement most other medical and mental health treatment modalities. However, when other therapies, including medication, are being used, the physician must be able to evaluate accurately the effectiveness of each treatment the client is receiving. If the physician is not aware that the client is receiving massage, the effects of other therapies may be misinterpreted.

Immediately refer patients with any vague or unexplainable symptoms of fatigue, muscle weakness, and general aches and pains to a physician. Many disease processes share these symptoms. This recommendation may seem overly cautious, but in the early stages of some very serious illnesses, the symptoms are not well defined. If the physician is able to detect a disease process early in its development, there is often a more successful outcome. A specific diagnosis is essential for effective treatment. Massage should be avoided in all infectious diseases suggested by fever, nausea, and lethargy until a diagnosis is received and recommendations given by a physician can be followed.

Tumors and Cancer

Benign tumors remain localized within the tissue from which they arise and usually grow very slowly. **Malignant** tumors (cancer) tend to spread to other regions of the body. The cells migrate by way of lymphatic or blood vessels. This manner of spreading is called **metastasis**. Cells that do not metastasize can also spread by growing rapidly and extending the tumor into nearby tissues. Malignant tumors may replace part of a vital organ with abnormal tissues, which is a life-threatening situation.

Early detection of cancer is important because cancer is most treatable in the early stages of primary tumor development, before metastasis and the development of secondary tumors. Box 5-2 lists the warning signs of cancer, as summarized by oncologists, or cancer specialists.

It is possible that the massage practitioner may be the first to recognize the early warning signs of cancer.

Although it is important to refer the client for proper evaluation to find out if a cancer process is developing, the massage practitioner is cautioned never to suggest to the client that cancer is evident. Instead, the practitioner should simply point out the changes, and explain that it is important that the changes be evaluated by a qualified professional.

Massage is not necessarily contraindicated for those

---

box 5-2
THE WARNING SIGNS OF CANCER

- Sores that do not heal
- Unusual bleeding
- A change in appearance or size of a wart or mole
- A lump or thickening in any tissue
- Persistent hoarseness or cough
- Chronic indigestion
- A change in bowel or bladder function

---

with cancer. Current research indicates that massage can support the immune system battle with cancer cells. However, massage must be used as part of the entire treatment program and supervised by qualified medical personnel. As in any stressful condition, when working with those with cancer it is important to not overtax the system but instead use massage for a general support to the healing mechanisms of the body.

Medications

The massage professional needs to be aware of the client's **medications.** The massage therapist should have a current *Mosby's GenRx, Physician's Desk Reference, Medical Economics,* or similar drug reference book so that all medications the client lists on the client information form can be researched. The client may also be able to provide information about each medication being taken.

In general, a medication is prescribed to do one of the following:

- Stimulate a body process
- Inhibit a body process
- Replace a chemical in the body

Therapeutic massage can also stimulate, inhibit, and replace body functions. When the medication and massage both stimulate the same process, the effects are **synergistic** and the result can be too much stimulation. If the medication inhibits a process and massage inhibits the same process, the result is again synergistic but this time with too much inhibition. If the medication stimulates an effect and massage inhibits the same effect, massage can be **antagonistic** to the medication. Although massage seldom interacts substantially with a medication that replaces a body chemical, it is important to be aware of possible synergistic or inhibitory effects.

Massage can often be used to manage undesirable side effects of medications. In particular, medications that stimulate sympathetic ANS function can cause uncomfortable side effects such as digestive upset, anxiety or restlessness, and sleep disruption. The mild inhibitory effects of massage resulting from stimulation of parasympathetic activity can sometimes provide short-term relief of the undesirable effects of the medication without interfering with its desired action. Especially in these instances, caution is required and close monitoring by the primary care physician is necessary.

For example, a side effect of some medications is anxiety. The massage either may help the client by reducing anxiety or may be the cause of an adverse reaction. If the doctor is using the level of anxiety to monitor the correct medication dose and anxiety levels are lowered through massage, there is a possibility that the dosage would then appear to be too high.

The massage therapist should be able to assess the effects of medications and discover the way massage may interface with these effects. Massage practitioners need to be specifically aware of antiinflammatories, muscle relaxants, anticoagulants (blood thinners), analgesics (pain modulators), and other medications that alter sensation, muscle tone, standard reflex reactions, cardiovascular function, kidney or liver function, or personality. They should be aware of over-the-counter medications, herbs, and vitamins as well. If a client is taking medication, it is important to contact the physician for recommendations about the advisability of therapeutic massage. (See Appendix C for a list of medications and possible interactions with massage.)

Endangerment Sites

Endangerment sites are areas in which nerves and blood vessels surface close to the skin and are not well protected by muscle or connective tissue. Consequently, deep, sustained pressure into these areas could damage the vessels and nerves. Areas containing fragile bony projections that could be broken off are also considered endangerment sites. The kidney area is included as such a site because the kidneys are loosely suspended in fat and connective tissue. Heavy pounding is contraindicated in that area. Avoidance or light pressure is indicated if working over an engagement site to avoid any damage to the area.

The following areas are commonly considered endangerment sites for the massage therapist. Refer to Fig. 5-4 to locate the specific sites (Proficiency Exercise 5-6).

Other endangerment sites and activities include the following:

- Eyes
- Inferior to the ear—fascial nerve, styloid process, external carotid artery
- Posterior cervical area: spinous processes, cervical plexus
- Lymph nodes
- Medial brachium—between the biceps and triceps
- Musculocutaneous, median, and ulnar nerves
- Brachial artery
- Basilic vein
- Cubital (anterior) area of the median nerve, radial and ulnar arteries, and median cubital vein
- Deep stripping over a vein in a direction away from the heart is contraindicated because of possible damage to the valve system
- Application of lateral pressure to knees
- Some acupuncture authorities indicate the ankle area on pregnant women

---

5 - 6
PROFICIENCY EXERCISE

Locate all endangerment sites on a fellow student.

Referrals

Referral is a method by which a client is sent to a health care professional for diagnosis and treatment of a disease. When a client is ill, he or she is aware of it. If the client is very sick, it shows. Common sense should be the guide. Although massage cannot cure anything, it can assist in the client's healing process. Massage professionals may pick up subtle changes in the tissue before the client consciously recognizes that something is out of balance. When this happens, the client should be referred to a qualified professional for specific diagnosis.

Massage practitioners are advised to become familiar with the health professionals in their area, including medical doctors, osteopathic doctors, podiatrists, chiropractors, physical therapists, occupational therapists, psychologists, licensed counselors, and dentists. Some health care providers provide alternative therapy such as acupuncture and homeopathy. Because clients trust the massage practitioner, before referring a client to a specific health professional, the massage practitioner should take the time to get to know that professional. This can be done by calling that person's office and making an appointment for a short visit, during which the professional's feelings about massage could be discussed. Information about massage should be left for reference.

Clients must always be referred to their personal health care professionals. The massage therapist should make no attempt to direct them to different health care professionals. If the client does not have a doctor, chiropractor, or counselor, then a list of professionals who have been contacted and educated about therapeutic massage should be provided.

When referral is indicated, the massage practitioner simply explains to the client why a referral to a health care professional is being recommended: "The observed set of signs or symptoms should be evaluated by someone who has more specific training." No specific condition should be named. The client should be given the massage professional's business card or brochure to give to the health care professional to facilitate contact. The client must sign a release of information before information can be exchanged between professionals.

For example, a therapist named Sandy has been seeing Ms. Jones for massage every other week for about 1 year. Ms. Jones has a mole on her left shoulder. During the last two visits Sandy notices that the mole has started to change shape and looks different. Sandy feels that these signs should be evaluated by someone who has more specific training. She says to Ms. Jones, "The mole you have on your left shoulder looks a little different to me. Have you noticed any change? It is important to have your doctor look at any changes in a mole. Will you please make an appointment with your personal physician to have the mole examined? Have your doctor give you a written statement that you were seen and that massage may be continued, along with any special instructions. It is im-

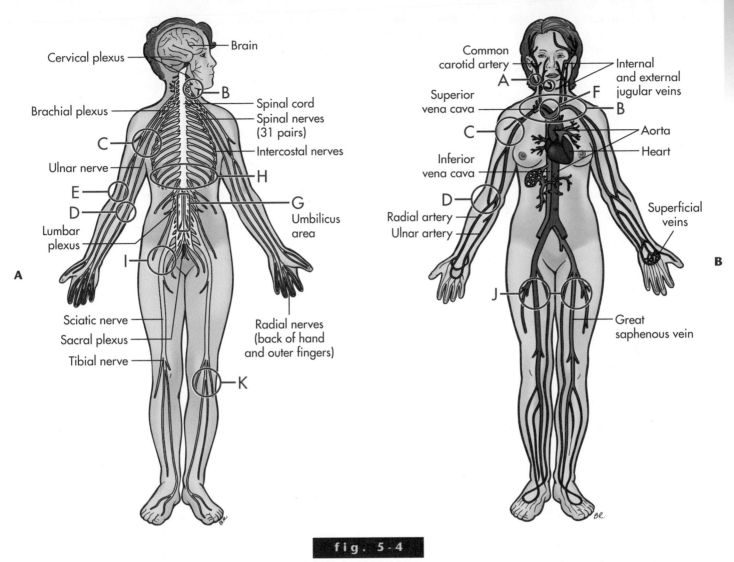

fig. 5-4

Endangerment sites of the nervous system **(A)** and cardiovascular system **(B).** *A,* Anterior triangle of the neck—carotid artery, jugular vein, and vagus nerve, which are located deep to the sternocleidomastoid. *B,* Posterior triangle of the neck—specifically the nerves of the brachial plexus, the brachiocephalic artery and vein superior to the clavicle, and the subclavian arteries and vein. *C,* Axillary area—the brachial artery, axillary vein and artery, cephalic vein, and nerves of the brachial plexus. *D,* Medial epicondyle of the humerus—the ulnar nerve. *E,* Lateral epicondyle—the radial nerve. *F,* Area of the sternal notch and anterior throat—nerves and vessels to the thyroid gland and the vagus nerve. *G,* Umbilicus area—to either side; descending aorta and abdominal aorta. *H,* Twelfth rib, dorsal body—location of the kidney. *I,* Sciatic notch—sciatic nerve (the sciatic nerve passes out of the pelvis through the greater sciatic foramen, under cover of the piriformis muscle). *J,* Inguinal triangle located lateral and inferior to the pubis—medial to the sartorius, external iliac artery, femoral artery, great saphenous vein, femoral vein, and femoral nerve. *K,* Popliteal fossa—popliteal artery and vein and tibial nerve.

portant for you to do this before we schedule the next massage. After I determine it is a good idea to refer a client, and I put that on your record, I need written verification from the doctor to see you again." If the client does not have a personal physician, Sandy could say, "I have talked with various health care professionals in our area and have developed a referral list. I am sure one of

the doctors listed will be able to help you, or you can ask a family member or friend for a recommendation." Ms. Jones may say, "What do you think the change in the mole is?" Sandy replies, "I am trained to notice changes in the body and when to refer a client, but I am not trained to be able to diagnose what any specific condition is. That is the role of a physician. It is best for you to go and have it checked by someone who has much more training in this area."

If the therapist feels it is necessary to refer a client for diagnosis, some sort of written permission from the doctor is needed to continue to see the client. The client should obtain the written documentation and bring it to the next massage session. This information is kept in the client's file. If the doctor or other health care professional has given any specific directions or recommendations, they must be followed exactly. The care plan of the physician must never be interfered with or contradicted, nor should the massage therapist assume the role of counselor. If it is necessary to contact the health care professional directly, the massage professional should always work through the receptionist. Leave whatever information is needed with the front desk, and if the doctor feels it is nec-

essary to speak with the massage therapist directly, he or she will call.

The referral and the date must be noted on the client's record, along with the signs and symptoms. If the client responds in any unusual way, such as by panicking or refusing to go to the doctor, this must be indicated on the client record as well. The written permission for continuation of the massage from the health professional must then be placed in the client's file.

Most disease processes present a few basic symptoms. See Appendix A for more comprehensive information. Always refer for diagnosis when the symptoms listed in Box 5-3 do not have a logical explanation (i.e., if the client has been up late or working long hours, naturally he or she will display the symptom of fatigue). Use common sense tempered with caution (Proficiency Exercises 5-7 and 5-8).

---

5 - 7

PROFICIENCY EXERCISE

1. *Using the reference section in Appendix A, list five regional contraindications to massage that you have encountered (or think you may encounter) with practice clients.*

   1.

   2.

   3.

   4.

   5.

2. *List five general contraindications that you think you will encounter most often.*

   1.

   2.

   3.

   4.

   5.

3. *Using the Oregon Model in Appendix A, list two specific disease conditions that correspond to the 12 basic symptoms listed in Box 5-3.*

   1.

   2.

   3.

4. *Choose a condition from each of the categories in the Oregon Model in Appendix A. Pretend that clients display symptoms of that condition or actually role play in the classroom, having a fellow student act out the signs and symptoms of the condition. Write down what things you would notice about each condition that would make you want to refer. Write down or act out a referral process with the pretend client.*

5. *Choose two medications from Appendix C and describe the possible interactions with massage.*

   1.

   2.

6. *On a separate piece of paper, write down the names of health care providers in your area whom you would like to place on a referral list. Because they need to support your work, set up a plan to meet and interview each one. Write down a list of questions to be asked and information that you must provide about your skills. Have at least three professionals from each category so that the client has a choice. If time permits, contact these people while you are still a student.*

box 5-3

INDICATIONS FOR REFERRAL

- Pain—local, sharp, dull, achy, deep surface
- Fatigue
- Inflammation
- Lumps and tissue changes
- Rashes and changes in the skin
- Edema
- Mood alterations—e.g., depression, anxiety

- Infection—local or general
- Changes in habits, such as in appetite, elimination, and sleep
- Bleeding and bruising
- Nausea, vomiting, and diarrhea
- Temperature—hot (fever) or cold

5-8

PROFICIENCY EXERCISE

After reading the following case study, use the clinical reasoning model to identify whether contraindications exist for the use of therapeutic massage and whether referral is necessary. If you determine that referral is necessary, list reasons for the referral.

A 32-year-old female client is seeking massage for stress management and pain management for headaches. A co-worker recommended massage therapy. Over the last 3 months she has been increasingly unable to maintain her work schedule, and work time missed is increasing to the point where her job is in jeopardy. She is a production line worker in a small plastic factory. The work environment has adequate ventilation but requires repetitive movement of the arms. She is getting afternoon headaches almost daily. She has been moody and temperamental, which is unusual for her. Her weight has increased by 15 pounds over the past year. She sporadically exercises and crash diets. She has close family ties in a nearby town and is single with no children. Her last physical examination was 5 years ago, and at that point no problems were identified. Her menstrual cycle is somewhat erratic, with periods of heavy bleeding during the last two periods. She is prone to hay fever and is currently self-medicating with an over-the-counter antihistamine as well as taking aspirin for the headaches. She is taking a multiple vitamin. She is taking no other medications. She thinks the cause is job stress but does not feel a job change is viable at this time.

Identify the Facts
Questions that help with this process are the following:

What is considered normal or balanced function?

What has happened? (Spell out events?)

What caused the imbalance? (Can it be identified?)

What was done or is being done?

What has worked or not worked?

Brainstorm the Possibilities
Questions that help with this process are the following:

What are the possibilities? (What could it all mean?)

Continued.

5 - 8

PROFICIENCY EXERCISE—CONT'D

What is my intuition suggesting?

What do the data suggest?

What are the possible patterns of dysfunction?

Consider Logical Outcomes of Each Possibility
Questions that help determine outcomes are the following:

What is the logical progression of the symptom pattern, contributing factors, and current behaviors?

What are the possible contributing factors?

What are the pros and cons of each intervention suggested?

What are possible interventions?

What is the logical cause and effect of each intervention identified?

What might work?

What are other ways to look at the situation?

PROFICIENCY EXERCISE—CONT'D

What are the consequences of not acting?

What are the consequences of acting?

Identify Effects on People Involved

Questions that help identify effects are the following:

In terms of each intervention being considered, what would be the impact on the people involved: client, practitioner, and other professionals working with the client?

How does each person involved feel about the possible interventions?

Is the practitioner within his/her scope of practice to work with such situations?

Is the practitioner qualified to work with such situations?

Does the practitioner feel qualified to work with such situations?

Is there a feeling of cooperation and agreement between all parties involved?

Based on this analysis of the information provided, the massage practitioner would identify the following contraindications _____

_____

for the following reasons:

Is referral indicated? What are the reasons for referral?

SUMMARY

Indications for massage are based on the physiologic effects that provide the benefits of massage. Massage is beneficial for most people, yet contraindications do exist. The responsible massage professional always refers a client for diagnosis and treatment by a qualified health professional, without delay, as soon as any condition is noticed that may suggest an underlying physical or mental health problem. After a condition has been diagnosed and appropriate treatment established, the massage professional may provide massage under the supervision of the medical professional. Massage may prove beneficial and supportive to the interventions of the health care professional and may enhance the healing process by temporarily reducing pain, relaxing the client, reducing stress responses, increasing circulation, and much more. In addition, the client's subjective experience with the one-on-one contact given by the massage professional may provide support and compassionate touch during a difficult time, thereby reducing feelings of frustration, isolation, anxiety, and depression that often accompany illness or periods of stress.

REFERENCE

1. Anderson K, Anderson LE, Glanze WD, editors: *Mosby's medical, nursing, and allied health dictionary,* ed 4, St Louis, 1990, Mosby.

WORKBOOK SECTION

Short Answer

1. What is an indication for massage?

2. What is a contraindication to massage?

3. What are the three approaches to care? Define them.

4. Define *health*.

5. What is dysfunction as defined in this text, and how does massage provide benefit in dysfunctional situations?

6. How do acute and chronic conditions affect homeostasis?

7. Why would a massage practitioner need to be aware of risk factors?

8. Why does the massage practitioner need to understand tumor pathology?

9. Why does the massage therapist need to understand the inflammatory response?

10. Define *therapeutic inflammation*.

11. Under what conditions should therapeutic inflammation not be used?

12. Why is describing pain difficult?

13. What would be the benefits of massage for acute pain, chronic pain, and intractable pain?

14. What is the difference between localized pain, radiating pain, referred pain, and projected pain?

WORKBOOK SECTION

15. What is the difference between somatic and visceral pain?

_____

_____

_____

16. Why is the knowledge of referred pain patterns important?

_____

_____

_____

17. What role do dermatomes play in the pain pattern?

_____

_____

_____

18. What is phantom pain?

_____

_____

_____

19. What is the difference between entrapment and compression impingement, and when is massage most indicated?

_____

_____

_____

20. What are endangerment sites?

_____

_____

_____

21. What are some important warning signs that indicate that the client should be referred to a medical doctor for specific diagnosis?

_____

_____

_____

22. What resource materials should the massage practitioner have available to help understand medications and terminology?

_____

_____

_____

23. Why should the massage therapist understand the action of medications?

_____

_____

_____

24. How do you refer a client to a health care professional?

_____

_____

_____

25. How can the student best make use of the appendix on massage interactions with medications?

_____

_____

_____

WORKBOOK SECTION

Matching

Match the term to the best definition.

1. Acute pain _____

2. Arterial circulation _____

3. Autonomic nervous system _____

4. Cerebral spinal fluid _____

5. Chronic diseases _____

6. Chronic pain _____

7. Connective tissue _____

8. Contraindication _____

9. Dermatome _____

10. Disease _____

11. Endangerment site _____

12. General contraindications _____

13. Health _____

14. Homeostasis _____

15. Indication _____

16. Inflammatory response _____

17. Intractable pain _____

18. Lymphatic drainage _____

19. Metastasis _____

20. Pain _____

21. Pain-spasm-pain cycle _____

22. Pathology _____

23. Phantom pain _____

24. Referral _____

25. Referred pain _____

26. Regeneration _____

27. Regional contraindications _____

28. Respiration _____

29. Risk factor _____

30. Signs _____

31. Somatic pain _____

a. cutaneous (skin) distribution of spinal nerve sensations

b. tumor cell migration by way of lymphatic or blood vessels

c. an unpleasant sensory and emotional experience associated with actual or perceived tissue damage or described in terms of such damage

d. the most abundant tissue of the body, its functions include support, structure, space, stabilization, and scar formation

e. a warning signal that activates the sympathetic nervous system, it can be a symptom of a disease condition or a temporary aspect of medical treatment; it is usually temporary, of sudden onset, and easily localized

f. dynamic equilibrium of the internal environment of the body through processes of feedback and regulation

g. diseases that develop slowly and last for a long time

h. pain arising from stimulation of receptors in the skin or skeletal muscles, joints, tendons, and fascia

i. encoding and storage of a memory based on the ANS and the resulting chemical balance of the body; only retrievable during a similar situation in the body

j. any substantial change in routine or any activity that causes the body to have to adapt, including changes for the better and for the worse

k. a diffuse, poorly localized discomfort that persists or recurs for indefinite periods, usually for more than 6 months

l. regulates energy using sympathetic fight-or-flight and fear responses and the restorative parasympathetic relaxation response; sympathetic and parasympathetic systems work together to maintain homeostasis through a feedback loop system

m. subjective abnormalities felt only by the patient

n. a collection of different signs and symptoms, usually with a common cause, that present a clear picture of a pathologic condition

o. the return of deoxygenated blood to the heart by way of the veins

WORKBOOK SECTION

32. State dependent memory _____

33. Stress _____

34. Symptoms _____

35. Syndrome _____

36. Venous circulation _____

37. Visceral pain _____

p. pain that results from stimulation of receptors in the internal organs

q. an abnormality in a body function that threatens well-being

r. a liquid that nourishes and protects the brain and nerves

s. movement of oxygenated blood under pressure from the heart to the body through the arteries

t. healing process where the new cells are similar to those they replace

u. method to send a client to a health care professional for specific diagnosis and treatment of a disease

v. a therapeutic application that promotes health or assists in a healing process

w. any condition that renders a particular treatment improper or undesirable

x. a normal mechanism that usually speeds recovery from an infection or injury characterized by pain, heat, redness, and swelling

y. physical, mental, and social well-being—not merely the absence of disease

z. the study of disease

aa. a kind of pain frequently experienced by patients who have had a limb amputated

bb. the steady contraction of muscles that causes them to become ischemic, which stimulates the pain receptors in the muscles; the pain, in turn, initiates more spasms, setting up a vicious circle

cc. a specific type of massage that enhances lymphatic flow

dd. chronic pain that persists even when treatment is provided or exists without demonstrable disease

ee. area of the body where nerves and blood vessels surface close to the skin and are not well protected by muscle or connective tissue; deep sustained pressure into these areas could damage these vessels and nerves

ff. findings that require a physician's evaluation to rule out serious underlying conditions before any massage is indicated

WORKBOOK SECTION

gg. contraindications that relate to a specific area of the body

hh. movement of oxygen in the body during breathing

ii. predisposing conditions that may make the development of disease more likely by the client than by some other person

jj. objective abnormalities that can be seen or measured by someone other than the client

kk. pain felt in an area different than the source of the pain

Match the correct words with the primary responses.

1. Heat and redness _____

2. Swelling and pain _____

a. histamine, prostaglandins, and kinins are released

b. increased permeability of vessel walls

c. enlargement of lymph nodes

d. dilation of blood vessels

e. edema pressure triggers pain receptors

f. irritant diluted through excess fluid

g. white blood cells destroy bacteria

h. increase in blood volume

WORKBOOK SECTION

Labeling

1. *Using the list of words below, label the areas of re-ferred pain in Fig. 5-5 using the corresponding letters. Words may be used more than once.*

A. Urinary bladder
B. Colon
C. Appendix
D. Heart
E. Lung and diaphragm
F. Liver and gallbladder
G. Ovary
H. Pancreas
I. Small intestine
J. Kidney
K. Stomach

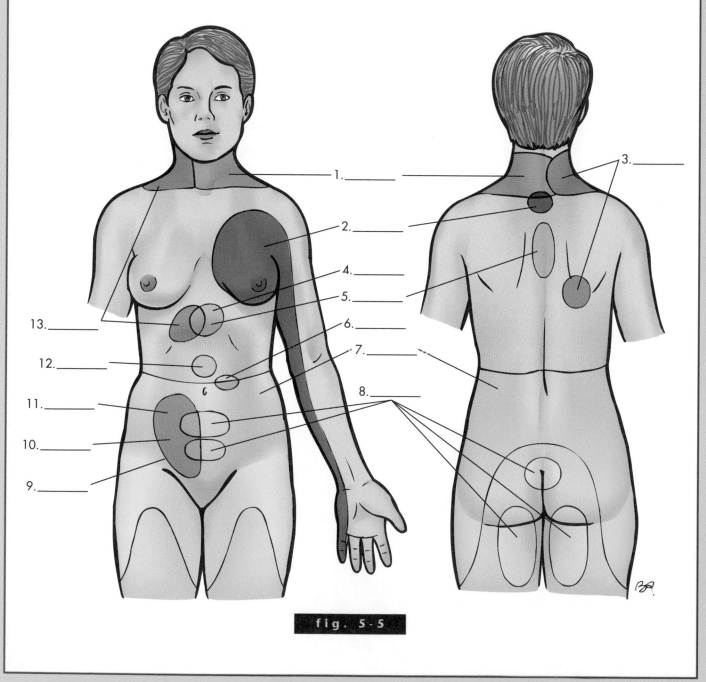

fig. 5-5

WORKBOOK SECTION

Using the list of words below, label the endangerment sites for Fig. 5-6 using the corresponding letters. Words may be used more than once.

A. Anterior triangle of neck
B. Posterior triangle of neck
C. Axillary area
D. Ulnar nerve
E. Radial nerve
F. Vagus nerve, nerves and vessels to thyroid gland
G. Abdominal and descending aorta
H. Kidney
I. Sciatic nerve
J. Inguinal triangle
K. Tibial nerve, popliteal artery and nerve

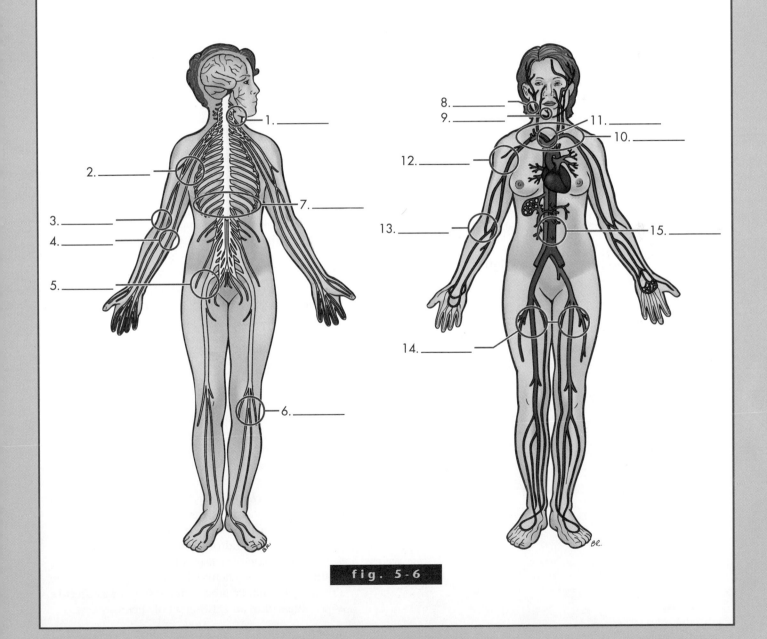

fig. 5-6

WORKBOOK SECTION

Risk Factors Exercise

1. List all the risk factors for developing disease, and write down separate columns for your personal risk factors and the risk factors of two friends.

_____

_____

_____

_____

_____

_____

2. When interviewing a client or doing a massage, how would you find out if that person has any possible warning signs for cancer? A list of the signs is found below; state how or when you would find out the information if the client did not reveal it.

The warning signs of cancer:

Sores that do not heal
Unusual bleeding
A change in a wart or mole
A lump or thickening in any tissue
Persistent hoarseness or cough
Chronic indigestion
A change in bowel or bladder function

Example:
Sores that do not heal:

Noticed during proper draping techniques—skin on body has open wounds

_____

_____

_____

_____

_____

Problem-Solving Exercise

You just ran into a friend you have not seen in 5 years. That friend is now a college professor, teaching anatomy and physiology. When you mention you are studying massage, the friend says, "It sounds interesting, but I don't think I'd ever need one." Take 5 minutes to list all the reasons you think your friend may need a massage.

_____

_____

_____

_____

_____

_____

_____

_____

_____

ANSWER KEY
Short Answer

1. An *indication* is when an approach would be beneficial for health enhancement, treatment of a particular condition, or support of a treatment modality other than massage.
2. A *contraindication* is when an approach could be harmful. The following types of contraindications occur:
   a. General avoidance of application—Do not do massage.
   b. Regional avoidance of application—Do massage but avoid a particular area.
   c. Application with *caution,* usually requiring supervision from appropriate medical or supervising personnel—Do massage but carefully select the type of methods to be used, duration of the massage, and frequency.
3. Therapeutic change, condition management, and palliative care

   Therapeutic change is a beneficial alteration produced by a bodywork process that results in a modification of physical form or function that can affect the physical, mental, and/or spiritual state of a client.

   Condition management involves the use of massage methods to support clients who are not able to undergo a therapeutic change process but wish to be as effective as possible within an existing set of circumstances.

WORKBOOK SECTION

Palliative care is provided when the condition is most likely going to become worse and degenerative processes will continue (e.g., terminal illness, dementia). It often relates to approaches that reduce suffering. Palliative care is also considered general relaxation massage for pleasure.

4. Besides being the absence of disease, health is the optimal functioning of the body and mind.

5. Dysfunction is the in-between state of "not healthy" but also "not sick" (experiencing disease). Massage professionals serve many people at the beginning of dysfunctional patterns—when the client does not feel his or her best but is also not yet sick. It is important to monitor the client to make sure he or she does not progress further into dysfunctional patterns. Early intervention and referral are important in the identification of potential problems before they develop. The benefits of massage are most effectively focused in assisting people to stay within the healthy range of functioning.

6. In acute conditions, homeostatic balance is recovered quickly. In chronic diseases, the body is stressed, and a fully normal state of balance may never be restored.

7. Risk factors may put a client at risk for developing a disease. Sometimes signs and symptoms may be contraindications or may show a need for referral to a physician.

8. A massage therapist may be the first to recognize the early warning signs.

9. To determine whether a massage will benefit or interfere in the process, and whether a client needs to be referred to another health care professional

10. The use of methods of massage to deliberately create a controlled localized area of inflammation to generate healing mechanisms

11. Therapeutic inflammation should not be used in situations in which sleep disturbance, compromised immune function, a high degree of stress load, or systemic or localized inflammation is already present. It also should not be used if any condition, such as fibromyalgia, that consists of impaired repair and restorative functions exists unless carefully supervised as part of a total treatment program. If a person is taking an antiinflammatory medication, either steroidal or nonsteroidal, the effectiveness of therapeutic inflammation is negated or reduced and restoration mechanisms are inhibited. When these medications are present, any methods that create inflammation are to be avoided.

12. Because it is a complex, private, abstract experience

13. For acute pain, massage can activate the parasympathetic nervous system, thereby relaxing the client. For chronic pain, a massage therapist needs to work as part of a multidisciplinary health care team to provide symptomatic relief for pain and initiate hardiness. With intractable pain, massage can provide short, temporary, symptomatic relief.

14. Localized pain is confined to a specific area at the site of origin. Projected pain is a nerve pain that is continued along the nerve tract. Radiating pain is diffused around the site of origin and is not well localized. Referred pain is felt in an area distant from the site of the painful stimulus.

15. *Somatic pain* arises from stimulation of receptors in the skin (called *superficial somatic pain*) or skeletal muscles, joints, tendons, and fascia (called *deep somatic pain*). *Visceral pain* results from stimulation of receptors in the viscera (internal organs).

16. If the client has a recurring pain pattern that resembles referred pain patterns, he or she should be referred to a physician for a more specific diagnosis.

17. When pain is referred, it is usually to a structure that developed from the same embryonic segment or dermatome as the structure in which the pain originates.

18. Phantom pain is a type of pain frequently experienced by clients who have had a limb amputated. These clients experience pain or other sensations in the area of the amputated extremity as though the limb were still there.

19. Entrapment is pressure on a nerve from soft tissue. Compression is pressure on a nerve from bony structures. Massage is most often indicated for entrapment.

20. Endangerment sites are areas in which nerves and blood vessels surface close to the skin and are not well protected by muscle or connective tissue. Areas with fragile bony projections that could be broken off are also considered endangerment sites.

21. Fatigue; inflammation; lumps and tissue changes; rashes and changes in skin; edema; mood alterations (e.g., depression and anxiety); infection (local or general); changes in appetite, elimination, or sleep; bleeding and bruising; nausea, vomiting, or diarrhea; and temperature (hot [fever] or cold)

22. Have a current *Mosby's GenRx, Physician's Desk Reference,* or similar reference book and a medical dictionary

23. The massage therapist should be able to assess the effects of the medications and discover the ways massage may interface with these effects.

WORKBOOK SECTION

24. Clients must always be referred to their personal health care professionals. The massage therapist should make no attempt to direct them to different health care professionals. If the client does not have a doctor, chiropractor, or counselor, then a list of the professionals who have been contacted and educated about therapeutic massage should be provided.

25. As a reference, this list can assist with the clinical reasoning necessary to determine the possible interactions between massage and medications and guide the development of appropriate referral and/or massage intervention.

Matching

1. e	14. f	26. t
2. s	15. v	27. gg
3. l	16. x	28. hh
4. r	17. dd	29. ii
5. g	18. cc	30. jj
6. k	19. b	31. h
7. d	20. c	32. I
8. w	21. bb	33. j
9. a	22. z	34. m
10. q	23. aa	35. n
11. ee	24. ll	36. o
12. ff	25. kk	37. p
13. y		

1. a, d, h
2. b, c, e, f, g

Labeling

Labels for Fig. 5-5:	Labels for Fig. 5-6:
1. E	1. B
2. D	2. C
3. F	3. E
4. H	4. D
5. K	5. I
6. G	6. K
7. J	7. H
8. A	8. A
9. J	9. A
10. C	10. B
11. B	11. F
12. I	12. C
13. F	13. D
	14. J
	15. G

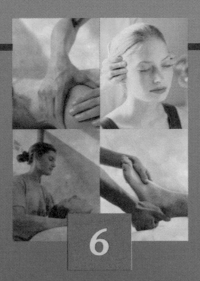

6

HYGIENE, SANITATION, AND SAFETY

o b j e c t i v e s

After completing this chapter, the student will be able to perform the following:

- Identify good health and personal hygiene practices
- Explain the major disease-causing agents
- Describe methods for preventing and controlling disease
- Give specific recommendations for sanitary practices for massage businesses
- Implement universal precautions
- Provide information about HIV, AIDS, and hepatitis
- Establish a hazard-free massage environment

THIS chapter discusses hygiene and sanitation practices in a professional setting. The information may seem to be mere common sense, but specific skills are needed to practice massage in a way that protects the safety of both the client and the massage professional. Many local and state laws governing massage deal extensively with sanitary procedures. The Oregon health code requirements, which have been used as a model for part of this chapter, are both typical and well defined.

The primary importance of **sanitation** is to prevent the spread of contagious disease. Diseases caused by "germs," or viruses, bacteria, fungi, and parasites, are considered contagious. Some contagious diseases are rare, and others are becoming more common. Until recently, tuberculosis, a bacterial disease, was considered to be under control; however, the incidence of the disease has begun to rise, and strains resistant to current medications have emerged. Various streptococci bacteria also are becoming resistant to the antibiotics currently available. The common cold and influenza (or "the flu") are caused by viruses that constantly mutate, thwarting scientific development of any sort of consistent vaccine. The key, then, is prevention: contagious diseases are best controlled before infection occurs, by the use of sanitary practices.

Considerable concern, misinformation, and misunderstanding has arisen about the spread of hepatitis, the human immunodeficiency virus (HIV), and acquired immunodeficiency syndrome (AIDS). Intense education of the public through the media about HIV and AIDS has dispelled some of the misunderstanding about these conditions. Better care and research developments are beginning to move the prognosis of HIV infection to that of a chronic disease. The rate of new infection is declining in the United States, but elsewhere in the world the spread of the virus is almost epidemic, with up to 26% of the population infected in some places. The infection rate for hepatitis is increasing alarmingly, which poses a significant health danger. In hopes of providing accurate information about hepatitis, HIV, and AIDS and to detail the massage practitioner's responsibilities, an extensive section of this chapter is devoted to these topics.

Because new information about the spread and control of contagious diseases becomes available almost daily, it is important to stay up to date. As information emerges, the federal Centers for Disease Control and Prevention (CDC) adjusts its standards and guidelines for communicable diseases. Massage practitioners are responsible for updating themselves semiannually on changes in the CDC's recommendations and following the most recent standards and guidelines.

Besides a sanitary environment, the massage professional must provide a safe environment. It is important to consider fire and accident prevention for both the client and the professional. The massage professional is well served by becoming certified in first aid and cardiopulmonary resuscitation (CPR) through the Red Cross or a similar organization.

Let's begin with the personal care of the massage practitioner. It is important to take care of ourselves not only so that we function at our best, but also because, as wellness and health professionals, we set an example for our clients. Clients notice the way we look and act, as well as our energy and vitality levels. Clients respect a professional who cares for herself as she teaches them to care for themselves. The ethical principle of respect, discussed in Chapter 2, is reflected in the way we care for ourselves and for our clients.

PERSONAL HEALTH, HYGIENE, AND APPEARANCE

section objectives

Using the information presented in this section, the student will be able to perform the following:

- Identify the basic hygienic procedures important to a professional environment

One of the best ways to control disease is to stay healthy. If our bodies are strong and our immune systems are functioning properly, we do not become sick easily. If injured, we heal better if we are healthy. Diet, sleep, rest, body mechanics (the way we use our bodies), exercise, and lifestyle must be considered in the overall health picture. It is important to keep to a schedule of regular physical checkups because early detection of disease leads to more successful treatment.

Smoking

Smoking is considered one of the leading causes of disease. It is directly linked to cardiovascular disease and is the leading cause of lung cancer.[3] Exposure to secondhand smoke has been found to cause cancer and other health problems in nonsmokers. Besides the dangerous health effects, smoking is offensive to many people. Smoke odors linger in the air and on hands, hair, and clothing. Many nonsmokers find this smell obnoxious. The smell of smoke can cause reactions in sensitive individuals. Because the massage professional works physically close to the client, any smoke odors from the professional are reason for concern.

The massage professional should never smoke in the massage therapy room, even when clients are not present, because the smell of smoke lingers in carpets, draperies, and other furniture. If the practitioner must smoke during business hours, it should be done outside, away from any access doors or windows. The practitioner who smokes should wash his hands carefully before touching a client and inform clients when they make appointments. If the client is bothered by smoke odors, referral to a different massage professional is appropriate.

Alcohol and Drugs

Alcohol and drugs interfere with the ability to function as a massage professional. Because they affect thinking, feeling, behavior, and functioning, the practitioner must never be under the influence of alcohol or illegal drugs when working with a client. Any prescription or over-the-counter medications that affect mental or physical abilities must be considered carefully because use of these substances by the massage professional can place the client at risk. A massage professional should wait at least 12 hours after the last alcoholic drink before working with a client because it takes this long for the direct effects of alcohol to wear off. The indirect effects will last for the next 24 hours. In this condition, often called a *hangover,* the body is exhausted and toxic; it is not a good condition to be in while giving a massage. Clients should be referred or rescheduled if the professional's ability to function is affected.

Hygiene

The massage professional must pay careful attention to personal hygiene. Preventing breath and body odor without using chemical cover-ups is essential. The massage professional should not wear perfume, aftershave, or perfumed hair products because many clients are sensitive to these odors.

The massage professional should bathe or shower at the start of each workday. Using soap or a similar cleaning agent, the armpits, genitals, and feet should be washed carefully. Women professionals must be especially mindful of odor during menstruation.

Because breath odor is offensive, careful brushing and flossing of the teeth after each meal is important. Any food that may cause breath odor should be avoided during work hours. Gum chewing is unprofessional and irritating to many people and is ineffective in combating breath odors. Breath mints, however, may help with breath odor.

Hair should be kept clean. Chemicals such as hair spray or gel must be avoided because they may cause an allergic reaction in sensitive people. The hair must not fall onto the professional's face or drag on the client. If it is long, it should be kept pulled back.

Proper care of the hands is especially important. Nails should be short and well manicured and should not extend past the tips of the fingers. Fingernails can harbor bacteria and other pathogens. Care must be taken to keep the space under the nails clean, which is best accomplished with a nailbrush. Any hangnails, breaks, or cracks in the skin of the hands must be kept clean and covered during a massage. An intact, strong skin is the professional's first line of defense against infection. Nail polish and synthetic nails promote the growth of bacteria, and hand jewelry can harbor pathogens; these should not be worn while giving a massage.

Massage uniforms should be loose and made of cotton or a cotton blend. Because body temperature increases while the professional is giving a massage, clothing must "breathe" and absorb and evaporate perspiration. Sleeves should be above the elbow, but the uniform should not be sleeveless. All clothing should be opaque and modest. T-shirts and shorts usually are inappropriate. If skirts or shorts are worn, they should be knee length or longer; loose pants are preferable.

White clothing is not necessary or even desirable because lubricant stains are less evident on colored clothing. Clothing should be laundered in a disinfectant, usually bleach, and the uniform chosen must be able to withstand this type of laundering. If perspiration is heavy or the clothing becomes stained, it may be necessary to change clothes. A spare uniform should be kept available. Underclothing must be changed daily, more often if perspiration is heavy. Many professionals use uniforms called *scrubs.* Scrubs meet all the criteria, are inexpensive, and are easy to obtain.

Clean, comfortable shoes should be worn while giving a massage. It is not sanitary or professional to go barefoot or wear only stockings. Changing socks daily helps prevent foot odor.

Makeup should be modest to avoid a painted, severe appearance; heavy makeup is never appropriate. Male practitioners must keep facial hair shaved or neatly trimmed.

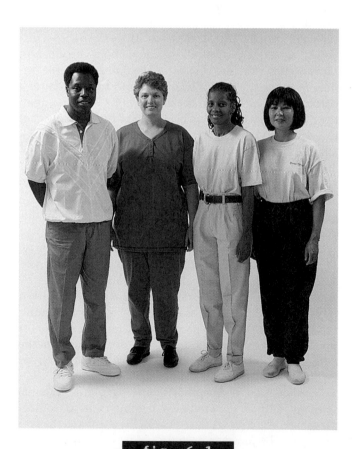

fig. 6-1

Properly groomed massage professionals.

Jewelry should not be worn while giving a massage. Necklaces and bracelets can become tangled or can drag on the client, and rings can scratch the client (Fig. 6-1).

If the client or professional is ill and if any concern exists that the condition might be contagious, the massage professional should refer or reschedule the client until the condition changes (Proficiency Exercise 6-1).

SANITATION

section objectives

Using the information presented in this section, the student will be able to perform the following:

- Identify the transmission routes for disease-causing pathogens
- Implement sanitation practices, including universal precautions, to prevent and control the spread of disease

Sanitary massage methods promote conditions that are conducive to health. This means that pathogenic organisms must be eliminated or controlled. Pathogens are spread by direct contact, through blood or other body fluids, or by airborne transmission.

Pathogenic Organisms

Pathogenic organisms cause many diseases. These organisms include viruses, bacteria, fungi, protozoa, and pathogenic animals.

Viruses

Viruses invade cells and insert their own genetic code into the host cell's genetic code. They use the host cell's nutrients and organelles to produce more virus particles. By bursting the cell membrane, the new virus particles may escape to infect other cells.

Bacteria

Bacteria are primitive cells that have no nuclei. They cause disease in one of three ways: (1) by secreting toxic substances that damage human tissues, (2) by becoming parasites inside human cells, or (3) by forming colonies in the body that disrupt normal function. Because bacteria can produce resistant forms, called *spores,* under adverse conditions, it is difficult for the human body to destroy pathogenic bacteria.

Fungi

Fungi are a group of simple parasitic organisms that are similar to plants but have no chlorophyll (green pigment). Most pathogenic fungi live on the skin or mucous membranes (e.g., athlete's foot, vaginal yeast infections). Yeasts are small, single-celled fungi, and molds are large, multicellular fungi. Because fungal, or mycotic, infections can be resistant to treatment, they can become quite serious.

Protozoa and Pathogenic Animals

Protozoa are one-celled organisms that are larger than bacteria. They can infest human fluids and cause disease by parasitizing (living off) or directly destroying cells.

Pathogenic animals, sometimes called *metazoa,* are large, multicellular organisms. Most are worms that feed off human tissue or cause other diseases.

Many of these pathogens cause skin diseases when the pathogen commonly is spread through direct contact. Because massage professionals spend much time working directly with skin, they would be wise to learn to recognize these various skin conditions. Most anatomy, physiology, and pathology textbooks have color plates showing different skin diseases.

An intact skin (skin integrity) prevents infection and various skin diseases, whereas abrasions and cuts breach the protective layer of the skin. Therefore it is important that the massage professional obtain additional information about pathologic skin conditions. (See Appendix D for the list of recommended texts for this chapter; also see Appendix B for color illustrations showing examples of skin disorders.)

Disease Prevention and Control

The key to preventing many diseases caused by pathogenic organisms is to prevent the organisms from entering the body. This sounds simple enough, but often it is difficult to accomplish. Following are three of the primary means by which pathogens can spread:

- **Environmental contact.** Many pathogens are found in the environment—in food, water, and soil and on various surfaces. Diseases caused by environmental pathogens often can be prevented by avoiding contact with certain materials and by following safe sanitation practices.
- **Opportunistic invasion.** Some potentially pathogenic organisms are found on the skin and mucous membranes of nearly everyone. These organisms do not

---

6 - 1

PROFICIENCY EXERCISE

1. Design your ideal uniform and ask three massage professionals their opinion of your idea.
2. Develop a class project in which fellow students' personal hygiene and professional appearance are evaluated anonymously.
3. Ask honest, trusted family members or friends if you have breath or body odor.

cause disease until they have the opportunity to do so. Preventing opportunistic infection involves avoiding conditions that promote infection. Changes in the pH (acidity), moisture, temperature, or other characteristics of skin and mucous membranes often promote these infections. Aseptic treatment and cleansing of wounds can prevent them.

- **Person-to-person contact.** Small pathogens often can be carried in the air from one person to another. Direct contact with an infected person or with materials handled by the infected person is a familiar mode of transmission. The rhinovirus that causes the common cold often is transmitted in these ways. Some viruses, such as the hepatitis B virus (HBV), are transmitted when infected blood, semen, or other body fluids enter the bloodstream.

Aseptic Technique

Aseptic technique kills or disables pathogens on surfaces before they can be transmitted (Table 6-1).

Most sanitation conditions for massage require disinfection. Occasionally protective apparel is necessary. In rare instances use of a mask, gown, and gloves may be appropriate to protect the massage professional or the client. These cases are discussed later in the chapter.

Hand washing. Proper hand washing is the single most effective deterrent to the spread of disease (Fig. 6-2). The hands must be washed before and after each massage, after blowing the nose or coughing into the hands, and after using the toilet. Hands and forearms must be washed in hot, running water to remove any infectious organisms. Soap or another antiseptic hand washing product must be used, and a clean towel is used to dry the hands and forearms. Faucets and door handles are contaminated and should not be touched after washing the hands. The towel should be used to turn off the water and open the door. Because frequent hand washing may dry and chap the skin, using a lotion after washing helps replace natural oils. Using the clean towel to hold the lotion bottle helps prevent contamination of the hands.

Suggested Sanitation Requirements

Box 6-1 provides a summary of sanitation procedures all massage professionals should observe. State and local laws may mandate additional procedures, and the professional should be aware of these (Proficiency Exercise 6-2).

Universal Precautions

Universal precautions, issued in 1987 by the CDC and in Canada in 1989 by the Bureau of Communicable Disease and Epidemiology, prevent the spread of both bacterial and viral infections. Developed initially to prevent the spread of blood-borne diseases, such as infection with HIV and HBV, the practice of universal precautions supports a safe and sanitary environment. HIV is not the only virus of concern. Other diseases, such as herpes and infection with the human papillomavirus (venereal warts), also are spread by body fluids or direct contact, including during sexual contact. Massage professionals must be concerned about the spread of all types of disease and should follow sanitation techniques and universal precautions.

The guidelines for universal precautions include specific recommendations for the use of gloves, a mask, and protective eye wear when contact with blood or body sections is possible. Universal precautions also include recommendations for clean-up procedures.

Indications for the Use of Universal Precautions

Under normal circumstances the massage professional does not come into contact with a client's blood, body fluids, or body substances (e.g., urine, feces, vomit). However, in rare cases an accident may occur in which such contact is possible. The best recommendation is always to make universal precautions part of the professional practice. Gloves are not necessary for most massage sessions unless the skin of the massage practitioner's hands or any skin area of the client has a rash, cut, abrasion, infection or any other condition that would allow the transmission of fluids. A mask may be appropriate if transmission of an airborne pathogen, such as the flu virus, is a concern. In most cases use of a mask protects the client from the massage professional's pathogens; therefore a mask is used with clients who have any form of immune suppression, including excessive stress, that makes the client more susceptible to infection.

Required Use of Universal Precautions

With additional training and under medical supervision, massage professionals may work with clients who have a contagious condition. In these cases knowledge of universal precautions is essential. However, it is wise to remember the importance of the massage professional's gentle, nurturing touch. The human connection becomes difficult through layers of protective coverings. We must remember that our normal germs can be very dangerous for

---

6 - 2

PROFICIENCY EXERCISE

1. *Contact your local health department and find out what information it has on disease control, health practices, and sanitation requirements.*
2. *Review your local and state laws concerning sanitation requirements.*

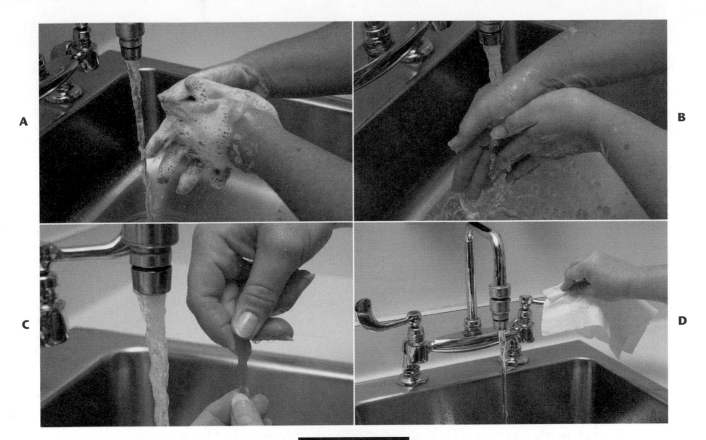

fig. 6-2

Hand washing technique. **A,** Create a lather with the soap. Interlace your fingers to wash between them, keeping your hands pointed down. **B,** Rinse the hands well, keeping your fingers pointed down. **C,** Use the blunt edge of an orangewood stick to clean under your fingernails. **D,** After drying your hands, use a dry paper towel to turn off the water. (From Zakus SM: *Clinical procedures for medical assistants,* ed 3, St Louis, 1995, Mosby.)

table 6-1

COMMON ASEPTIC TECHNIQUES FOR PREVENTING THE SPREAD OF PATHOGENS

Method	Action	Example
Sterilization	Destroys all organisms by means of heat	Pressurized steam bath, extreme temperature, irradiation
Disinfection	Destroys most or all pathogens (but not necessarily all microbes) on inanimate objects	Chemicals (e.g., iodine, chlorine, alcohol, soaps)
Isolation	Separates potentially infectious people or materials from uninfected individuals	Quarantine of infected patients; wearing of protective apparel while giving treatments; sanitary transport, storage, and disposal of body fluids, tissues, and other materials

box 6-1

SANITATION PRACTICES FOR MASSAGE PROFESSIONALS

The following sanitation requirements for practicing massage professionals have been developed from the State of Oregon Model:

- The massage professional must clean and wash the hands and forearms thoroughly with an antibacterial/antiviral agent before touching each client. Any professional known to be infected with any communicable disease or to be a carrier of such disease or who has an infected wound or open lesion on any exposed portions of the body is excluded from practicing massage until the communicable condition is alleviated.
- The professional must wear clean clothing. If at all possible, lockers or closets for personnel should be maintained apart from the massage room for the storage of personal clothing and effects.
- All doors and windows opening to the outside must be tight fitting and must ensure the exclusion of flies, insects, rodents, or other vermin. All floors, walks, and furniture must be kept clean, well maintained, and in good repair.
- All rooms in which massage is practiced must meet the following requirements: (1) heating must be adequate to maintain a room air temperature of 75° F; (2) ventilation must be sufficient to remove objectionable odors; and (3) lighting fixtures must be capable of producing a minimum of 5 footcandles of light at floor level; this level of lighting should be used during cleaning.
- All sewage and liquid waste must be disposed of in a municipal sewage system or approved septic system. All interior water distribution piping should be installed and maintained in conformity with the state plumbing code. The water supply must be adequate, deemed safe by the health department, and sanitary. Drinking fountains of an approved type or individual paper drinking cups should be provided for the convenience of employees and patrons.
- Every massage business must have a sanitary toilet facility with an adequate supply of hot and cold water under pressure, and it must be conveniently located for use by employees and patrons. Bathroom doors must be tight fitting, and the rooms must be kept clean, in good repair, and free of flies, insects, and vermin. A supply of soap in a covered dispenser and single-use sanitary towels in a dispenser must be provided at each lavatory installation, as well as a covered waste receptacle for proper disposal; a supply of toilet paper on a dispenser must be available for each toilet.

- Lavatory and toilet rooms must be equipped with fly-tight containers for garbage and refuse. These containers should be easily cleanable, well maintained, and in good repair. Any refuse must be disposed of in a sanitary manner.
- Massage lubricants, including but not limited to oil, alcohol, powders, and lotions, should be dispensed from suitable containers, to be used and stored in such a manner as to prevent contamination. The bulk lubricant must not come in contact with the massage professional. It should be poured, squeezed, or shaken into a separate container or the massage professional's hand. Any unused lubricant that comes into contact with the client or massage professional must be discarded.
- The use of unclean linen is prohibited. Only freshly laundered sheets and linens should be used for massage. All single-service materials and clean linens should be stored at least 4 inches off the floor in shelves, compartments, or cabinets used for that purpose only. All soiled linens must be placed in a covered receptacle immediately and kept there until washed in detergent and an antiviral cleaning agent (e.g., a 10% bleach solution, or nine parts water to one part bleach) in a washing machine that provides a hot water temperature of at least 140° F.
- Massage tables must be covered with impervious material that is cleanable and must be kept clean and in good repair. Equipment that comes into contact with the client must be cleaned thoroughly with soap or other suitable detergent and water, followed by adequate sanitation procedures before use with each individual client (a 10% bleach solution, made up daily, is recommended). All equipment must be clean, well maintained, and in good repair.
- When cleaning the massage area, observe the following rules:
  Do not shake linen, and dust with a damp cloth to minimize the movement of dust.
  Clean from the cleanest area to the dirtiest. This prevents soiling of a clean area.
  Clean away from your body and uniform. If you dust, brush, or wipe toward yourself, microorganisms will be transmitted to your skin, hair, and uniform.
  Used linens must be stored in a closed bag or container while in the massage room or during transport.
- Floors are dirty; any object that falls on the floor should not be used for a client.

Modified from Oregon Board of Massage Technicians: *Sanitation requirements for the state of Oregon,* Oregon Administrative Rules, July 1991.

any immune-suppressed client, and universal precautions must be used to protect the client from viruses and bacteria. Extra effort is required to follow universal precautions, but this extra effort should not hinder the safety of either client or practitioner.

Clients considered contagious may feel isolated and "unclean." We do not want to make such clients feel ashamed and guilty for having a contagious disease. Many of them desperately need to be touched in a supportive, nonjudgmental way. It is the pathogen that is undesirable, not the client, and all clients must be treated with respect, dignity, and kindness. The professional must remember to touch the person and not the disease, to see and listen to the person rather than the disease. These are *people* who are sick—not sick people.

The massage professional may need to wear gloves if a client is infected with a contagious, transmittable disease or if a client is in an immune-suppressed state, such as might occur with chemotherapy, and must be protected from germs. In these situations the massage therapist would be working under the supervision of a medical professional. It is important to follow all of his or her directions carefully.

If massage professionals work in the heath care setting (e.g., hospitals, extended care facilities, rehabilitation centers), it is essential that they follow universal precautions. Each setting has approved procedures posted. Most often special training is provided. If this is not the case and the massage professional is concerned in any way about the application of required sanitation procedures, she should speak directly to her supervisor.

Possible exposure to contaminants and body fluids.

Any person who touches a spill of blood or other body substances, such as vomit, urine, or feces, should wear single-use, disposable gloves (Fig. 6-3). Such contact conceivably could happen during a massage. The most common blood exposure is to menstrual blood, an incidence that can occur if the client's protective product is inadequate. In rare cases men who have a history of premature ejaculation could be stimulated indirectly by the general massage and ejaculate or leak fluid. An incontinent client could leak urine or feces, or a client could suddenly become sick and vomit. Universal precautions should be followed during any clean up.

Clean-Up Procedures Using Universal Precautions

A 10% bleach solution (one part bleach to nine parts water) should be used to clean up spills of body fluids. The spill should be surrounded with solution and then mopped or wiped up, with the professional working slowly and carefully inward to avoid splashes or aerosols (airborne particles). Stronger bleach solutions should be used if excessive amounts of blood or other substances are present. Afterward, the mop head or cloth should be soaked in the bleach solution. The mop head should be agitated carefully to ensure that all its surfaces are exposed to the cleaning fluid. All linens should be rolled away and double bagged in plastic, separately from other soiled linens. The outside bag should be marked "contaminated with body fluids." The table should be washed with a strong disinfectant solution and allowed to air dry. Latex gloves should be worn during the clean-up process.

If a contaminated substance comes into contact with a person's skin, the skin should be washed immediately with soap and water and an antiviral agent such as 10% bleach solution. If an open wound is exposed to a contaminated substance, it should be flushed immediately with large amounts of hydrogen peroxide or a 10% bleach solution. Hydrogen peroxide should *not* be used on mucous membranes or in any body orifice (e.g., mouth, vagina, anus, eyes, urethra).

Bleach is the preferred cleaning agent. A bleach and water solution should be prepared daily, and any leftover solution should be discarded at the end of the day. If blood or body fluid seepage is excessive, a stronger mixture of bleach should be used.

Although hot, soapy water kills HIV, dishes that are visibly soiled with blood or other body substances should be soaked in 10% bleach solution before they are washed in hot, soapy water.

Bathroom surfaces are hazardous only if they are visibly soiled with tainted bodily waste or substances. Any contaminated surface must encounter a mucous membrane surface or an open wound to transmit pathogens. Bathrooms should always be cleaned as if they were contaminated.

Approved cleaning solutions. The CDC has recognized the following three levels of solutions and products that destroy HIV, HBV, and other viral organisms. These recommendations should be followed in every practice.

- *High-level sanitation:* Products labeled "sterilant/disinfectant glutaraldehyde—air dry"; massage professionals do not need to practice high level sanitation techniques under normal conditions.
- *Medium level sanitation:* Bleach solution—1 part bleach to 9 parts water, made up daily (10% solution) or a hospital disinfectant labeled "tuberculocidal."
- *Low-level sanitation:* Hot, soapy water (with air drying) or a hospital disinfectant effective against viruses and bacteria. Hands are to be washed in hot, soapy water or with surgical soap.

Medium and low-level procedures are adequate for most therapeutic massage procedures. Cleaning up a body fluid spill might require high-level procedures. Massage professionals should update their information on recommended sanitary practices at least every 6 months (Proficiency Exercise 6-3). The CDC can provide current information. The telephone number for the CDC voice information system is (404) 332-4666 or (404) 639-3286. The Internet web site is http://www.cdc.gov.

---

6 - 3

PROFICIENCY EXERCISE

1. *Contact a local hospital, the police, the fire department, and an emergency rescue team, and investigate their procedures for universal precautions.*
2. *Practice putting on and taking off gloves.*

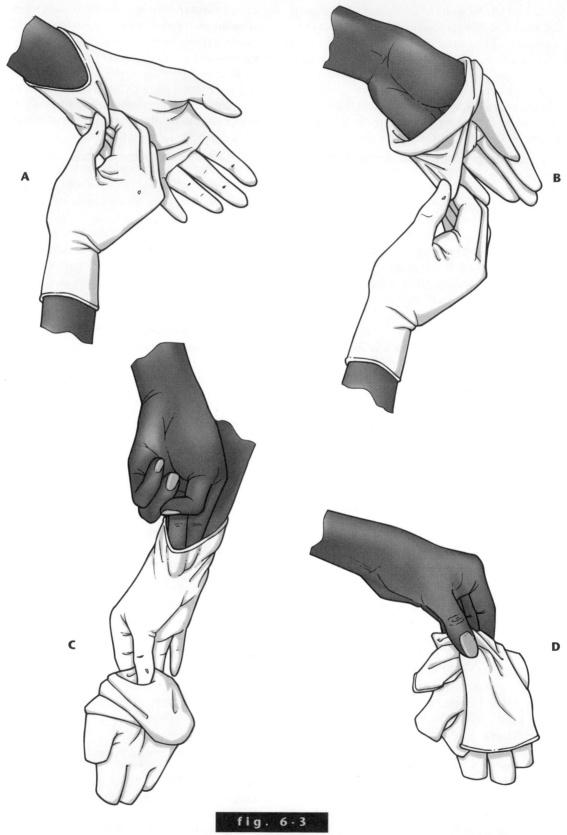

fig. 6-3

Procedure for removing gloves. A, Grasp the glove below the cuff. **B,** Pull the glove down over the hand, turning the glove inside out. **C,** Insert the fingers of the ungloved hand into the other glove. **D,** Pull the glove down and over the hand, turning the glove inside out. (Modified from Sorrentino SA: *Mosby's textbook for nursing assistants,* ed 4, St Louis, 1996, Mosby.)

PREVENTING THE TRANSMISSION OF HIV AND HEPATITIS

section objectives

Using the information presented in this section, the student will be able to perform the following:

- Define *AIDS* in detail
- Identify behavior that could result in transmission of HIV or HBV

A syndrome is a group of clinical symptoms that constitute a disease or abnormal condition. (*Clinical* means reported or observed symptoms not discovered by laboratory tests.) With syndromes, an individual need not have all the symptoms. Syndromes may be caused by many different things, but with **acquired immunodeficiency syndrome (AIDS)** the cause is a dysfunction in the body's immune system, one of the body's primary defenses against disease.

The diseases of AIDS are caused by germs we encounter every day. In fact, some of these germs live permanently in small numbers inside the human body. When the immune system weakens, these germs have the opportunity to multiply freely; therefore the diseases they cause are called *opportunistic diseases.*

The **human immunodeficiency virus (HIV)**, which seems to be responsible for AIDS, is a retrovirus. As a group, retroviruses can live in the host for a long time without causing any sign of illness. In most animals retrovirus infections last for life. These viruses die when exposed to heat, can be killed by many common disinfectants, and usually do not survive well if the tissue or blood they are in dries up. However, retroviruses have a high mutation rate and consequently tend to evolve very quickly into new strains. HIV shares this and other traits with other known retroviruses.

HIV replicates (lives) in the group of white blood cells called *lymphocytes,* or *T cells.* Among the T cells, HIV's favorite target is the T4 cell. The T4 cell, also called the *helper/inducer T cell,* performs a vital job in the immune system. HIV infection of the T4 cells creates a defect in the body's immune system, which may eventually result in AIDS. Long-term infection with HIV without the development of AIDS is becoming more common. Improved treatment, a better understanding of the disease on the part of health care professionals, increased public education, and less stress from public stigma support this process.

The Mechanics of Transmission

HIV must travel from the inside of one person to the inside of another person. Because viruses are unable to enter the body through intact skin, they must enter through an open wound or one of a number of possible body openings (most of which contain mucous membranes). *Mucous membranes* are thin tissues that protect most openings and passages in the human body. These membranes secrete mucus, which contains antigerm chemicals and keeps the surrounding tissues moist. Mucous membranes can be found in the mouth, inside the eyelids, in the nose and air passages leading to the lungs, in the stomach, along the digestive tract, in the vagina, in the anus, and inside the eye and the opening of the penis. From the surface of a mucous membrane, many viruses can travel through the membrane and enter the tiny blood vessels inside. The mucous membranes of the eyes and mouth often are doorways for highly infectious viruses such as the flu virus. The danger with HIV is very different. The major infection sites for this virus are the bloodstream and the central nervous system. HIV can be found in any body fluid or substance that contains lymphocytes.

The presence of HIV in a substance does not necessarily indicate that the substance is capable of transmitting the infection. In theory, all body fluids are capable of transmitting disease; in reality, however, the most dangerous substances seem to be blood, semen and preejaculate fluid, cervical and vaginal secretions, and perhaps feces. Despite much research, a clear-cut case of saliva causing transmission has not been found, although kissing theoretically could transmit the virus. The concentration of HIV (i.e., the number of viral particles per unit of volume) is very important in infectivity. If a substance has a high concentration of HIV, it is more likely to transmit the virus. A pregnant woman can transmit the virus to her unborn child. The concentration of HIV in mother's milk and in saliva, urine, and tears is low, but theoretically these are infectious substances that could transmit HIV infection. However, no cases have been reported to be caused by contact with these secretions. Sweat cannot transmit HIV.

HIV Survival Outside the Host

If HIV is present in a substance that leaves the body, the viral particles are capable of remaining infectious until the substance dries up. Depending on the circumstances, this could be a matter of minutes or hours. If the substance stays moist, the viral particles can survive much longer. For example, in water and blood solutions (10% blood, 90% saline), HIV can survive at room temperature for 2 weeks. In refrigerated blood, such as that used for transfusions, HIV can survive indefinitely.

The public has a widespread fear of contracting AIDS through casual contact, such as shaking hands, being in the same room with an individual infected with HIV, touching doorknobs, or sharing bathroom facilities. The fear is far, far greater than the risk. Diseases spread by casual contact invariably are spread via saliva or sputum, and they exist in the saliva or sputum in very high concentrations. The concentration of HIV in saliva and sputum is very low, if it exists in these substances at all. After 10 years of documentation of the AIDS epidemic, there are no known cases of AIDS or HIV infection being transmitted by casual social contact, not even among people living in the same household. In some cases household members have even shared toothbrushes with infected house-mates without contracting the virus.

To date no medical or health care workers have contracted HIV from casual contact. The contact between the massage professional and the client falls under this classification. We touch only the skin, which is not a transmission route.

Hepatitis

Hepatitis is an inflammatory process, an infection of the liver caused by a virus. Hepatitis A, a less serious form, usually is transmitted by fecal contamination of food and water. Hepatitis B is a potentially fatal disease caused by HBV, which is transmitted through routes similar to those for HIV. HBV is 100 times more contagious than HIV, and it is estimated that more than 1 million people in the United States are carriers of HBV. Two types of vaccine are available for preventing transmission of HBV. Hepatitis C accounts for 86% of new cases of hepatitis each year. The hepatitis D virus (HDV) infects only those who have hepatitis B, and its symptoms are more severe than other forms of hepatitis. Vaccines do not appear to be effective for HDV. Hepatitis E is transmitted through food and water contaminated by fecal material.

Universal precautions prevent the spread of hepatitis. It is important to be cautious of all behaviors where body fluids are contacted or unsanitary conditions may be present that may allow transmission of HIV and HBV (Proficiency Exercise 6-4).

PREMISE AND FIRE SAFETY

section objectives

Using the information presented in this section, the student will be able to perform the following:

■ **Recognize and avoid fire and safety hazards**

■ **Complete an accident report**

---

6 - 4

PROFICIENCY EXERCISE

1. *Call the National AIDS Hotline, which is open 24 hours, at (800) 342-AIDS (Spanish: [800] 344-7432 and TTY: [800] 243-7889) and ask a representative to send you information, or check the Internet web site at http://www.ashastd.org.*
2. *Contact the information center at the CDC in Atlanta, Georgia ([404] 639-3286). Request information about communicable diseases or check the Internet web site at http://www.cdc.gov.*

The massage professional's facility must be kept free of hazards. Some clients will need additional assistance to prevent falls or other injury. The following safety rules are guidelines for creating a hazard-free massage environment:

1. Infants and young children should not be left unattended. Parents or guardians should always be present during massage for minors.
2. Women in the last trimester of a pregnancy should not be left in the massage room alone and may need assistance getting on and off the massage table.
3. Elderly persons may be less steady on their feet and should not be left in the massage room unattended.
4. Any client whose mobility is impaired, including those with visual impairments, may need assistance getting on and off the massage table. Persons with disabilities should be asked what assistance they need, and their instructions should be followed carefully.

Preventing falls is very important. The massage professional should observe the following rules to prevent falls:

- Provide good lighting. Never perform a massage in a dark room.
- Do not use throw rugs, because they may slip or tangle in the feet.
- Avoid slippery tile floors.
- Keep floors and walkways uncluttered.
- Keep electrical and phone cords out of traffic areas.
- Regularly check all massage equipment to make sure that it is sturdy and in good repair.
- Make sure that all outside entrances are free of clutter and hazards caused by ice, snow, or rain.

If an accident occurs, all information about the accident must be written down. An insurance company will need the following information:

- Where and when the accident occurred
- Detailed information about the accident

---

6 - 5

PROFICIENCY EXERCISE

1. *Contact your local fire marshal and learn more about fire prevention.*
2. *Draw up a fire escape route and emergency plan for your massage business.*
3. *Contact the local building and safety inspector and find out more about accident prevention.*
4. *Contact a local insurance agent and find out about requirements for reporting accidents to the insurance company, as well as the insurance plan recommended for this type of protection.*
5. *Take basic and advanced first aid classes and learn CPR.*

- Names and addresses of the person or people involved in the accident
- Names of any witnesses to the accident
- Names of manufacturers, if equipment is involved

Most accidents can be prevented. Knowing the common safety hazards, recognizing which clients need extra assistance, and using common sense are all necessary to promote safety.

Fire prevention also is essential (Proficiency Exercise 6-5). The massage professional should observe the following rules to prevent fires:

- Provide a nonsmoking environment. In places where smoking is allowed, make sure proper ashtrays are used. Empty ashtrays only into a metal container that is partly filled with sand or water.
- Regularly check all electrical cords and equipment to make sure that they are in good condition. Do not plug more than two cords into an electrical outlet.
- Never use candles, incense, or any open flame.
- Make sure the massage area is equipped with a smoke detector and fire extinguisher. Check them regularly to make sure they are functional.

SUMMARY

The information in this chapter supports a safe professional practice. It is a good idea to review these procedures regularly to maintain the attention to detail needed to provide a safe, sanitary massage environment for our clients. It is our responsibility to act reliably in emergencies. As professionals, we must understand the use of universal precautions and fire and premise safety measures to serve our clients in a health-promoting and hazard-free manner.

REFERENCES

1. Board of Directors of Masseurs, Province of Ontario: *Ontario, Canada, therapeutic massage curriculum guidelines,* Toronto, 1992, Author.
2. Oregon Board of Massage Technicians: *Sanitation requirements for the state of Oregon, Oregon Administrative Rules,* July 1991, Author.
3. Thibodeau GA, Patton K: *Anatomy and physiology,* ed 3, St Louis, 1996, Mosby.

WORKBOOK SECTION

Short Answer

1. Why is the massage professional's hygiene so important?

_____

_____

_____

_____

2. What odors may be offensive or a health risk to clients?

_____

_____

_____

_____

3. Why does the use of alcohol and certain drugs interfere with the ability to function as an effective massage professional?

_____

_____

_____

_____

4. Why should the massage professional study pathogenic organisms?

_____

_____

_____

_____

5. Why is the integrity of the skin so important?

_____

_____

_____

_____

6. What are the main ways in which diseases caused by pathogenic organisms are spread?

_____

_____

_____

_____

7. What are the aseptic methods?

_____

_____

_____

_____

8. What are the main concepts presented in the section on sanitation requirements?

_____

_____

_____

_____

WORKBOOK SECTION

9. What is the main goal of universal precautions?

_____

_____

_____

_____

10. Why should the massage professional understand hepatitis, HIV, and AIDS?

_____

_____

_____

_____

11. What one sanitation method is most effective in controlling the spread of disease?

_____

_____

_____

_____

12. What are the main precautions necessary for preventing falls and accidents?

_____

_____

_____

_____

13. What are the main ways to prevent a fire?

_____

_____

_____

_____

14. Why should the massage professional study emergency care and CPR?

_____

_____

_____

_____

WORKBOOK SECTION

Matching

I. Match the term to the best definition. You may need to use your anatomy and physiology text or a medical dictionary to complete this exercise.

1. AIDS _____

2. Asepsis _____

3. Centers for Disease Control _____

4. Communicable disease _____

5. Contamination _____

6. Dermatosis _____

7. Dermatitis _____

8. Disinfection _____

9. First aid _____

10. Hazard _____

11. Hemorrhage _____

12. Host _____

13. Hygiene _____

14. HIV _____

15. Infection _____

16. Microorganism _____

17. Pathogen _____

18. Sanitation _____

19. Shock _____

20. Sterilization _____

21. Transmission _____

22. Universal precautions _____

a. the absence of pathogens

b. excessive loss of blood from a blood vessel

c. the human immunodeficiency virus

d. the formulation and application of measures to promote and establish conditions favorable to health, in particular public health

e. the process by which an object becomes unclean

f. procedures developed by the CDC to prevent the spread of contagious disease

g. a disease caused by pathogens that are easily spread, a contagious disease

h. skin inflammation

i. a condition that results from inadequate blood supply to body organs and tissues

j. the process by which all microorganisms are destroyed

k. a disease state that results from the invasion and growth of microorganisms in the body

l. the person, animal, or environment in which microorganisms live and grow

m. acquired immunodeficiency syndrome

n. a small living plant or animal that cannot be seen without the aid of a microscope

o. a microorganism that is harmful and capable of causing an infection; a virus, bacterium, fungus, protozoan, or pathogenic animal

p. emergency care given to an ill or injured person before medical help arrives

q. the spread or transfer of pathogens

r. the process by which pathogens are destroyed

s. a division of the U.S. Public Health Service that investigates and controls diseases with epidemic potential

t. any skin condition

u. anything that poses a safety threat

v. practices and conditions intended to promote health and prevent disease

WORKBOOK SECTION

II. Match the ways that pathogens can be spread or controlled with the proper description.

1. _____ Pressurized steam bath, extreme temperature, or irradiation

2. _____ Chemicals such as iodine, chlorine, alcohol, and soap

3. _____ Quarantine of affected individuals; protective apparel worn while giving treatments

4. _____ Pathogens found in the environment—in food, water, and soil and on assorted surfaces

5. _____ Disease that does not develop until the pathogens have the opportunity

6. _____ Transferal of pathogens from one person to another

7. _____ Killing or disabling of pathogens on surfaces before they can spread to other people

a. aseptic technique

b. person-to-person contact

c. opportunistic invasion

d. environmental contact

e. isolation

f. disinfection

g. sterilization

Professional Activity

List 20 suggested sanitation requirements developed from the state of Oregon model.

1. _____
2. _____
3. _____
4. _____
5. _____
6. _____
7. _____
8. _____
9. _____
10. _____
11. _____
12. _____
13. _____
14. _____
15. _____
16. _____
17. _____
18. _____
19. _____
20. _____

WORKBOOK SECTION

Professional Application

Completing an accident report

Most of us recognize that accidents happen daily. When they involve personal injury or property damage, information is needed so that the involved parties and any insurance companies can recognize and repair the damages. A massage practitioner, like any other business person, may be called on to fill out an insurance report.

Here is a practice story about an accident. After the story, some standard questions and the correct answers are supplied, so that you can see the way information is to be presented. (Please note that the following scenario is intended to be humorous.)

This afternoon you had a new client. He was the contortionist from the traveling circus, in town for the next week. He brought along his wife, who works with him, to observe your techniques so that she can help him as they travel. Unfortunately, some interesting things happened. You sit for a few minutes to recollect your thoughts, and this is what you remember:

You completed the massage with Mr. Gummy and had just asked him to roll over when you noticed that the table had started swaying. Ms. Gummy, who is an acrobat, was doing a handstand on Mr. Gummy's shoulders. Your table was sturdy enough, but because of the lubricant on your client's shoulders, his wife slid off and out the window. She was able to catch herself on the awning of the store below yours, but in doing so she bent the frame and tore the canvas. No one was injured, but the other tenant called emergency services, so reports had to be filed.

Because your immediate supervisor was not available, you had to complete the accident report yourself. Using your narrative, fill out the following information for the police and insurance companies.

1. State where and when the accident occurred.
2. Provide detailed information about the accident.
3. Give the names and addresses of the person or people involved in the accident.
4. Give the names of any witnesses to the accident.
5. Give the names of manufacturers, if equipment was involved.
6. Describe all property damage.
7. Detail any injuries to the people involved.

Answers to questions

1. The accident occurred at The Massage Center, 38 Falls Drive, Anytown, ML 48999, on Friday, June 12, 1997, at approximately 11:15 A.M.
2. The incident occurred during a massage therapy session at the above location, in room #4 on the second floor. As I was working with my client, Mr. Victor Gummy, his wife, Ms. Viola Gummy, began doing a handstand on Mr. Gummy's shoulders. Because of the lubrication on his shoulders, Ms. Gummy slid off of Mr. Gummy's shoulders and out the window. To prevent herself from hitting the sidewalk, Ms. Gummy caught the outer aluminum trim of the front door awning. The awning frame bent, and the canvas covering was torn.
3. The people involved in the accident included myself, Cathie Balevit, 38 Falls Drive, Anytown, ML 48999; my client, Victor Gummy; and his wife, Viola Gummy, of Fred's Traveling Funshows, 826 Cartwheel Drive, Caravan, FO 81234.
4. Mr. Victor Gummy and I both witnessed Viola Gummy fall out the window. Mr. William Bill of Bill's Locksmith Company, 41 Falls Drive, Anytown, ML, actually saw Viola catch herself on the awning as it gave way.
5. The awning was manufactured and installed by Art's Awning Company, 22 Tent Drive, Anytown, ML 48989.
6. The property damage was limited to the awning on the front of the building. An estimate of repair, provided by Art's Awning Company, is attached.
7. No one was injured.

Now that you have seen the way to prepare an accident report, read the following incident narration and provide the information requested.

Today's date is Monday, May 1, 0000. Your client, Mr. James Jackson, arrived for his weekly 4 P.M. massage appointment. Twenty minutes into the session, you asked him to roll over from his stomach to his side. As he did so, the table cracked and started to collapse. It did not collapse completely because the cable supports held it up. Other than being a little scared, Mr. Jackson was not injured, and you were able to help him off the table. Every Friday you check the tables for safety and perform any maintenance. This table had been checked the previous Friday, and no problems were found.

WORKBOOK SECTION

You immediately contacted the table distributor to tell him of the problem with the table. He works for Buy-Low Products, at 12 Buy-Low Drive in Badtown, VN 84848. He contacted the manufacturer, Fred's Cut Rate Tables, 480 W. Shady Lane, Market Town, MV 29341. The table is model #83, called "The Basic," and retails for $99.95.

1. State where and when the accident occurred.

_____

_____

_____

2. Provide detailed information about the accident.

_____

_____

_____

3. Give the names and addresses of the person or people involved in the accident.

_____

_____

_____

4. Give the names of any witnesses to the accident.

_____

_____

_____

5. Give the names of manufacturers, if equipment was involved.

_____

_____

_____

6. Describe all property damage.

_____

_____

_____

7. Detail any injuries to the people involved.

_____

_____

_____

ANSWER KEY
Short Answer

1. The massage professional represents all massage practitioners and therefore reflects the sanitary and safety practices of the massage business. If the professional's appearance does not reflect attention to hygiene and sanitation, concern may develop about the sanitation measures practiced by all massage professionals. Also, if massage professionals are not careful, they can become the agents of disease transmission between clients. Careful hygiene limits this possibility.

2. Tobacco smoke, breath odor, body odor, incense, and perfume are some of these odors.

3. Alcohol and drug abuse, along with use of some prescription medications, affects the ability to feel and reason. The sensitivity and perception of the massage professional are altered. This definitely interferes with the ability to give the very best massage possible and could even put the client in danger.

4. Pathogenic organisms can cause disease in a client who is stressed, fatigued, injured, or weakened. Bacteria usually can be controlled with various prescription antibiotics. Today there are many resistant strains of bacteria, which makes antibiotics less effective. Viruses are not easily controlled. The few antiviral agents available only slow the reproduction of the virus. The best resistance to a virus is the body's own immune system. Fungi, protozoa, and pathogenic animals can thrive only on or in a weakened host. The massage practitioner's main focus is wellness. If a disease is present, the body will be weak. Precautions must be taken to prevent the spread of disease and avoid putting a weakened body at further risk. The massage professional must understand the mechanisms of disease to practice massage safely.

5. The skin is the main defense against the invasion of pathogens and infection. The first signs of many serious diseases manifest as skin symptoms. Because the massage practitioner observes and touches so much of the client's skin, it is important to be able to recognize the major types of skin lesions. It also is important that the massage professional not massage over breaks in the skin, thereby preventing the spread of infection.

6. (1) Environmental contact (e.g., food, water, soil, contaminated surfaces); (2) opportunistic invasion (when a person is weakened and the conditions are right for invasion); and (3) person-to-person contact, either through droplet transmission from direct contact or airborne particles and body fluids.

WORKBOOK SECTION

7. Sterilization kills everything, disinfection kills almost everything, antisepsis slows or stops the growth of most pathogens, and isolation separates or puts up a barrier against pathogens. Disinfection procedures using hot, soapy water and a 10% bleach solution (freshly made each day) or a commercial disinfectant are adequate for most massage situations. Disinfection procedures are used for all laundry and cleaning, and the disinfectant is allowed to air dry on surfaces.

8. Keep things clean and disinfected. Keep areas or items that are contaminated separate from clean items. The massage environment must be constructed and maintained in such a way so as to prevent the spread of disease through insects and other vermin.

9. To prevent the spread of infection through person-to-person contact or through contact with body fluids. Methods of isolation, including the use of a mask, gloves, and gown, along with disinfection and sterilization procedures, prevent the spread of communicable disease.

10. There is much confusion, misinformation, and fear about these problems. It is the responsibility of the massage professional to stay current with new information, especially through the CDC. Massage professionals need to understand the contamination routes for hepatitis and HIV. They need to know when their own germs may pose a threat to those who are immune suppressed, including those with HIV infections or AIDS. Massage professionals need to understand that casual contact is not a transmission route for either hepatitis or HIV. If the skin is healthy, giving a massage poses no threat to the massage professional. Most of all, massage professionals who are educated enough continue to touch those who are immune suppressed, and we all need to be touched in a compassionate and healing way.

11. Careful hand washing.

12. Do not leave anyone who is at risk of falling alone in the massage therapy room. Keep all traffic areas hazard free. Provide good lighting. Regularly check all equipment for safety and make any repairs immediately.

13. Make sure all electrical equipment and wiring are in proper working order. Avoid any type of open flame. Do not allow any smoking in the facility.

14. Everyone should be skilled in first aid, CPR, and emergency care. The American Red Cross or similar organizations in other countries are best equipped to provide this training.

Matching

I.

1. m	7. h	13. v	18. d
2. a	8. r	14. c	19. i
3. s	9. p	15. k	20. j
4. g	10. u	16. n	21. q
5. e	11. b	17. o	22. f
6. t	12. l		

II.

1. g
2. f
3. e
4. d
5. c
6. b
7. a

Professional Activity

NOTE: Twenty-three suggested sanitation requirements have been listed; only 20 are required.

1. The massage therapist must clean and wash his or her hands thoroughly with an antibacterial/antiviral agent before touching each client.

2. The therapist must wear clean clothing.

3. Lockers or closets for personnel must be maintained apart from the massage room.

4. All doors and windows opening to the outside must be tight fitting and must keep out insects, rodents, or other vermin.

5. All floors must be kept clean, well maintained, and in good repair.

6. Walls and ceilings must be kept clean and well maintained.

7. Furniture must be kept clean and in good repair.

8. The room must be capable of maintaining a room air temperature of 75° F.

9. Ventilation must be adequate to remove objectionable odors.

10. Lighting fixtures must be capable of providing a minimum of 5 footcandles of light at floor level; this level of lighting must be used during cleaning.

11. All sewage and liquid waste must be disposed of in a municipal sewage system or an approved septic system.

12. The water supply must be adequate, deemed safe by the health department, and sanitary.

WORKBOOK SECTION

13. Drinking fountains of an approved type or individual paper drinking cups must be provided.
14. Every massage business must be provided with a sanitary toilet facility with an adequate supply of hot and cold running water under pressure; this facility must be conveniently located for use by employees and clients.
15. Restroom doors must be tight fitting, and restrooms must be kept clean, in good repair, and free of flies, insects, and vermin.
16. A supply of soap in a covered dispenser and single-use sanitary towels in a dispenser must be provided at each lavatory installation, along with a covered waste receptacle for proper disposal.
17. A supply of toilet paper on a dispenser must be available for each toilet installation.
18. Massage lubricants, including but not limited to oil, soap, alcohol, powders, and lotions, must be dispensed from suitable containers, which are to be used and stored so as to prevent contamination.
19. Any unused lubricant that comes into contact with the client or the massage therapist must be discarded.
20. Only freshly laundered sheets and linens are to be used.
21. All soiled (used) linens must be washed in a mechanical washing machine that provides a hot water temperature of at least 140° F, and antiviral agents must be used (e.g., 10% bleach solution [one part bleach to nine parts water]).
22. Massage tables must be covered with impervious material that is cleanable; they must be kept clean and in good repair.
23. Equipment that comes into contact with the client must be cleaned thoroughly with soap or some other suitable detergent and water, followed by adequate sanitation procedures, before use on each individual client.

Professional Application

1. The accident occurred on Monday, May 1, 0000, at approximately 4:20 P.M. (List your clinic name and address here.)
2. My client was receiving a massage during his weekly session. I asked that he turn from a prone position to a side-lying position. As he rolled to his side, we both heard a cracking sound. The massage table surface then partly collapsed downward. It was kept from fully giving way by the cable supports. The client was uninjured and able to climb off the table with some assistance.

   The massage table had been checked on Friday, April 28, 0000, as part of a weekly routine maintenance and safety check. No problems were found at that time.
3. I was working as the therapist. My name is (fill in your name and full address). The client was Mr. James Jackson (fill in his full name and address from your client information form). NOTE: It is always a good idea to provide phone numbers even if they are not requested.
4. The witnesses were myself and Mr. Jackson.
5. The table was model #83, "The Basic," with a retail price of $99.95. It is manufactured by Fred's Cut Rate Tables, 480 W. Shady Lane, in Market Town, MV 29341. It was sold to me by Buy-Low Products of 12 Buy-Low Drive, Badtown, VN 84848.
6. The property damage was limited to the table. The top surface is split, both the wood and the vinyl covering, the outer supports are cracked, and the hinge is bent. An estimate of repair costs will be forwarded when received.
7. No one was injured in the incident.
   NOTE: Because the client was involved, he will be asked to provide information. You must have his written permission to provide his name, address, and telephone number because you were providing a service to him and have guaranteed confidentiality.

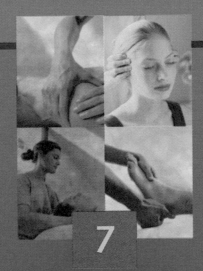

7

BODY MECHANICS

objectives

*After completing this chapter, the student
will be able to perform the following:*

- Use the body, especially the hands and forearms, in an efficient and biomechanically correct manner when giving a massage
- Alter position of both the client and the practitioner to maximize body mechanics

Student note: Most models in this chapter are pictured in leotards or sportswear to enhance and clarify the various body positions. The properly groomed massage professional would wear a uniform as shown in Fig. 6-1 on p. 232. Draping materials are not used in an effort to increase clarity.

BODY mechanics allows the massage practitioner's body to be used in a careful, efficient, and deliberate way. It involves good posture, balance, and the use of the strongest and largest muscles to perform the work. Fatigue, muscle strain, and injury, including overuse syndromes, can result from improper use and positioning of the massage practitioner's body while giving a massage. In this chapter the student will learn methods of working more efficiently so that providing 8 hours of massage in a day does not cause any dysfunction or pain. The ability to work for 8 full hours a day is important because to make a living doing bodywork full time, the practitioner must be able to give 15 to 30 sessions per week. Efficient use of the body helps prevent burnout.

The information in this chapter has been taken from standard recommendations for service professions, personal observation, and the author's professional and teaching experience. The principles of body mechanics presented in this text rely on leverage, balance, and biomechanics. Static and dynamic postures assumed at work and during recreational activities may have adverse effects on the body. These effects usually manifest in the musculoskeletal system. Safe professional practice must be considered.

The delivery of therapeutic massage has unique postural and physical demands. Body mechanics for most professionals are focused to lifting or exerting a force in an upward direction such as when a nurse lifts a patient from the bed to a chair. Other foci of body mechanics apply to dynamic movement such as for dancing and participating in athletics or the martial arts. By contrast, a majority of the effort exerted to give a massage is a sustained, restrained, and somewhat static movement with pressure focused down to deliver **compressive force.** The massage practitioner makes extensive use of the forearms, wrists, hands, fingers, and thumbs to deliver compressive force. Because of this difference, following standard recommendations provided to most professionals for the safe use of the body is of little use to the massage practitioner. In fact, attempting to modify these forms of body mechanics may actually result in injury to the massage professional.

Massage professionals need to consider their body types and musculoskeletal limitations. The suggestions in this chapter help most students develop the best personal body mechanics style for them as individuals.

DYSFUNCTIONS RESULTING FROM IMPROPER BODY MECHANICS

Areas of the body commonly affected in the massage professional who is not attentive to body mechanics include the neck and shoulder, wrist and thumb, lower back, knee, ankle, and foot. The following recommendations are methods to protect the practitioner's body.

Neck and Shoulder

Neck and shoulder problems result most commonly from the massage practitioner using upper body strength to push and exert the pressure for massage. These problems can be avoided if the student learns to use leverage and leans with the body weight to provide pressure. The arms and hands of the practitioner should be relaxed while giving a massage because tension in the arms and hands translates to the shoulder and neck.

Wrists and Hands

The massage professional needs to protect his or her wrists by avoiding excessive compressive forces developing from delivery of massage methods. Using a proper wrist angle and staying behind the massage stroke protects the wrist. Tense wrists and hands also contribute to shoulder problems. It is important to always maintain a relaxed hand and wrist while giving a massage.

Low Back

Some reasons for low back problems include inappropriate bending, bent static positions, twisting, improper knee position, improper foot position, and reaching for an area instead of moving to the area while giving a massage. The massage professional must learn to keep the lower back straight and avoid bending or curling at the waist while working. Maintaining a stable spinal line helps to avoid this problem. Frequent posture shifting of the massage practitioner's body also helps protect the lower back, as will learning to lift by leaning back during stretching. Use of an asymmetric stance, normal knee lock position in the weight-bearing leg, and variations using a short and tall stool provide protection for the back. The lower back is further supported by avoiding twisting and reaching while working and keeping the point of contact with the client below the practitioner's waist[1] (Fig. 7-1).

Knee

Knee problems can be avoided by respecting the basic stability design of the knee and frequently shifting the weight from foot to foot. The most efficient standing position involves the normal screw-home or knee-lock position in the last 15 degrees of extension. This position provides the least compressive force on the knee capsule and the least muscular action for stability. As the knee is flexed, compressive forces increase in the joint capsule, and muscular action for stability increases (Fig. 7-2). Full hyperextension is to be avoided.

Confusion and disagreement exist about the proper position of the knee while giving a massage. Some recommend a slightly flexed knee, opposing this text's recommendation of a "locked knee." Others express some concern with the locked knee position, opposing the blocking of body energy

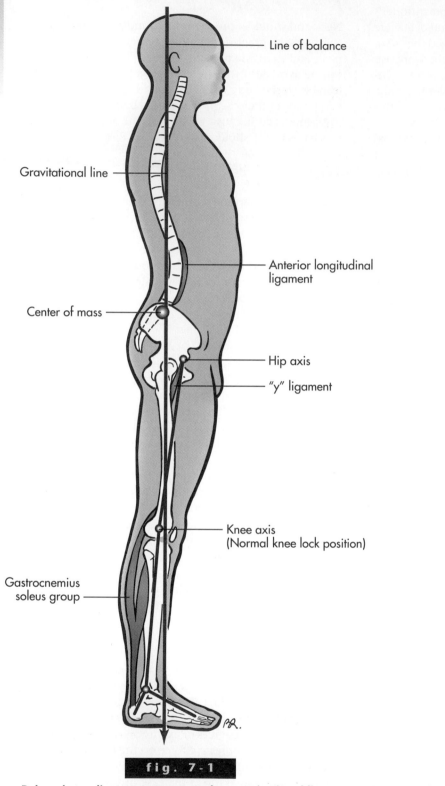

Line of balance

Gravitational line

Anterior longitudinal ligament

Center of mass

Hip axis

"y" ligament

Knee axis (Normal knee lock position)

Gastrocnemius soleus group

fig. 7-1

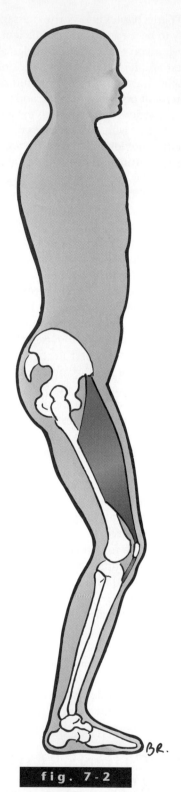

fig. 7-2

Relaxed standing posture supporting gravitational line with normal knee-locked position in the last 15 degrees of extension. The gravitational force line falls behind the hip joint, in front of the knee joint, and in front of the ankle joint. The only muscle group used for balance is the gastrocnemius-soleus muscles. The relaxed stance involves leaning on the y ligament or iliofemoral ligament, the anterior longitudinal ligament, and the posterior knee ligaments.

Improper leg position putting excessive strain on joints and requiring muscle activity to maintain balance. The gravitation line improperly falls behind the knees.

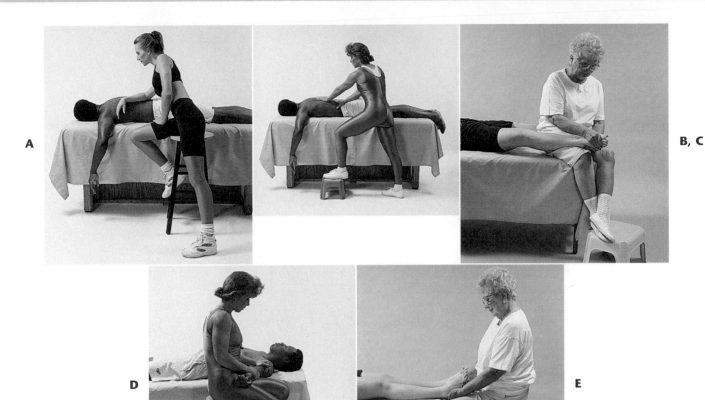

fig. 7-3

A, Use of high stool. **B,** Use of stool for massage practitioner's foot. **C,** Massage practitioner sits on table to protect the lower back with stability and grounding provided by the foot placement on the stool. (Note: appropriate sanitary draping is necessary whenever the practitioner's body comes in contact with the draping materials, such as when sitting on the table.) **D** and **E,** Massage practitioners using low stools to protect the lower back. Stability and grounding provided through the foot placement on the stool.

flow and interference with concepts of grounding and being centered. These concerns tend to arise from information founded on movement principles such as tai chi, forms of dance, and martial arts. Although a flexed knee is appropriate for these systems, massage requires the application of sustained pressure applied from a stable position with the least amount of effort, muscular activity, and compressive force to the joint.

The knee needs to be in a slightly flexed position as the massage practitioner changes position and moves around the table. However, when pressure is being applied, the anatomic design of the knee provides stability in the normal screw-home or knee-lock position in the last 15 degrees of extension. Practitioners must honor their own bodies in terms of the individualized approach to body position. The body mechanics presented in this chapter are developed to support the knee.[4,5]

Ankle and Foot

Asymmetric standing is the most efficient standing position. The weight is shifted from one foot to the other in an energy conservation mechanism. Symmetric standing with the weight equal on both feet is fatiguing, interferes with circulation, and should be avoided.[5] The ankle and foot are protected by the asymmetric stance, frequent position change, and sitting, when possible, to do massage. The body mechanics presented is based on the asymmetric stance to best use the massage professional's energy and avoid fatigue. Methods to support this stance, such as placing one foot on a stool, sitting on a high stool, or putting a knee on the table, protect the ankles, feet, and lower back and conserve energy (Fig. 7-3).

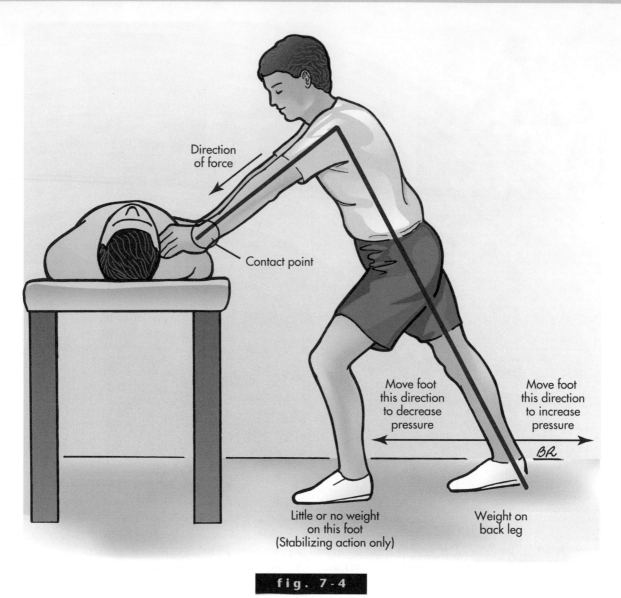

fig. 7-4

Correct body mechanics for compressive force required for massage.

APPLICATION OF COMPRESSIVE FORCES

The human body is designed for movement and range of motion and not the applied compressive forces required when giving a massage. Therefore it is vital to use body weight and not muscle strength to provide the pressure required during a massage.[3] This is accomplished by shifting the body weight so that the balance point is at the contact point between the massage professional's hand or forearm and the client's body. It is important to redistribute the body mass and change the location of the body's center of gravity. Increasing the amount of pressure to be applied is accomplished by widening the stance by moving the back leg further away from the point of contact (Fig. 7-4).

Massage uses primarily a force generated forward and downward. Therefore, it is necessary to redistribute the center of gravity and the weight force by keeping the weight on the back leg, the back straight, the leverage weight coming from the abdomen, and the balance point at the object-contact point. As the body's stance increases, it enlarges the base of support. The arm generating the pressure is opposite of the weight-bearing leg, which allows proper counterbalance and prevents twisting of the body.[3]

No one correct way exists to use the human body efficiently. The important thing is that the massage practitioner must learn to remain relaxed, to stay comfortable, and not to strain when doing massage. If a person feels and looks as though he or she is "working hard" while giving a massage, something is wrong with the body mechanics. If the proper body mechanics are used, the practitioner will look and feel relaxed and graceful while giving a massage. Shifts in balance are used to apply the various degrees of pressure, not

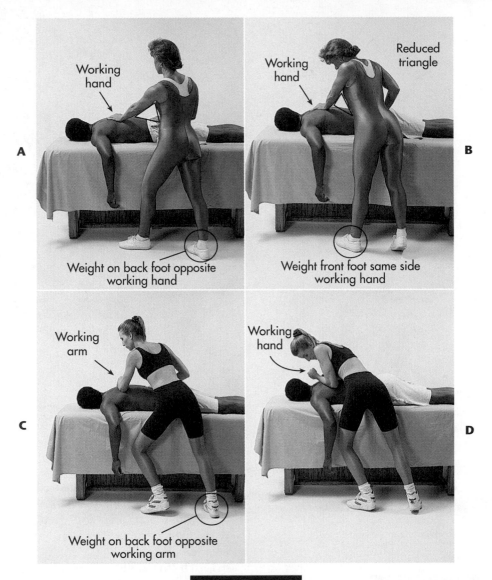

Working hand

Working hand

Reduced triangle

A

B

Weight on back foot opposite working hand

Weight front foot same side working hand

Working arm

Working hand

C

D

Weight on back foot opposite working arm

fig. 7-5

Comparison between correct and incorrect body mechanics in two positions. **A,** Correct position using hand. **B,** Incorrect position using hand. **C,** Correct position using forearm. **D,** Incorrect position using forearm. Note the equilateral triangle that is formed between hip, axilla, and client contact point in correct positions.

harder pushes. In fact, using body mechanics effectively eliminates the need for pushing to create compressive pressure when giving a massage (Fig. 7-5).

BASIC BODY MECHANICS PRINCIPLES
Leverage and Leaning

The basic concept of this style of body mechanics is the use of **leverage** by "leaning" on the client just as someone would comfortably lean against a wall or on a table. The practitioner seldom "pushes" against the client. Pushing

requires a tense body, using muscle contraction to exert pressure. By leaning, muscle tension in the practitioner's shoulders, neck, wrist, thumbs, elbows, and lower back is substantially reduced.

"Leaning" pressure can also be used to evaluate the client. Evaluation means gathering information but making no changes. If a change in soft tissue is desired, the signal to the tissues must be carefully overridden and intensified slightly to substitute a different pattern. For the client's body to accept this change, the new signal must be presented in a nonthreatening manner and applied slowly. As soon as clients feel trapped, pressed, or pushed on, they tense up to protect themselves. The old pattern is reinforced, and little or no change occurs.

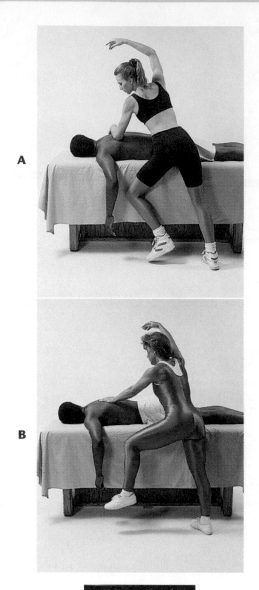

fig. 7-6

Comparison of correct leaning position to apply compressive force to exert pressure. Exaggerated leaning position for emphasis in two positions: **A,** forearm, and **B,** hand. When leaning correctly, the massage practitioner should be able to lift the front supportive leg from the floor and raise the opposite arm.

If the pressure levels are too intense or a sensitive area is touched, the client's body automatically responds with a protective movement by either pushing or moving away. These subtle evaluation cues are easily missed if the massage practitioner is pushing on the client and stabilizing the movement. The style of body mechanics presented in this text provides the essential component necessary to enable the practitioner to receive feedback through body signals. While leaning, the practitioner becomes extremely sensitive to subtle body changes in the client,

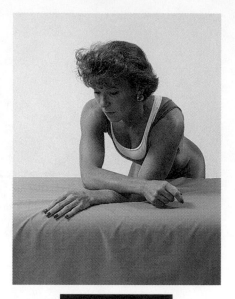

fig. 7-7

Self-massage.

which supports the ongoing assessment process during massage (see Chapter 10) (Fig. 7-6).

Balance Point

The practitioner's body is balanced and relaxed, which allows body weight to do the work. The point of contact between the practitioner and client is the **balance point.** With the balance point located at the point of contact with the client's body, the practitioner can be moved or swayed by the subtle movements of the client's body. This prevents the use of too much pressure and allows the client to direct the movement and pressure intensity of the massage without feeling pressed and pinned against the table. The client should never feel trapped or constrained by the massage practitioner.

Firm Pressure Distributed Over Wide Area

Clients appreciate a firm, even pressure that is distributed over a wide area. For example, firm pressure on the back using the forearm is pleasant. However, the same pressure using the point of the elbow or the thumb would be painful, because the pressure is concentrated in a small area instead of dispersed over a broad area. When the practitioner's weight is maintained on the back foot, the pressure levels are more even, but when the weight shifts to the front foot, the pressure becomes more concentrated and uneven and may be uncomfortable to the client.

ADDITIONAL BODY MECHANICS CONSIDERATIONS

Care of the Practitioner

Attention to body mechanics begins before the massage even takes place. The practitioner's body should be warmed up with general aerobic activity and stretching. The massage professional needs to be comfortable and dressed in loose, nonrestrictive clothing that does not interfere with movement. The massage professional should take breaks between each massage; all of the muscles used to give a massage should be stretched during these breaks. Besides getting a professional massage weekly, the practitioner should massage his or her own hands, arms, and shoulders during the day (Fig. 7-7).

Massage Table

The massage table must be at a comfortable height, which depends on the body size and style of the practitioner. Those with long torsos and long arms may need a shorter table than a person with short arms. A person with a short torso, short arms, and long legs needs a taller table.

A general rule is that the table height should reach the practitioner's fingertips or the first knuckle when the arms are hanging at the sides. For the purposes of leaning to provide the appropriate pressure, a table that is slightly short is better than one that is too tall. With a short table the stance can be opened a bit to accommodate, but appropriate accommodations are impossible for a table that is too tall. Practitioners will resort to upper body muscle strength to apply pressure if the table is too tall. These recommendations are only a place to begin, and each practitioner must experiment to find what table height is most comfortable.

A table that is 24 to 28 inches wide provides adequate space for the client to lie comfortably, but it is not so wide that the practitioner is reaching for the client in the middle of the table.

If the massage professional is carrying a portable table, attention should be paid to the body mechanics used to lift and move the table. Lifting the table is done with the knees and hips and not from the waist. A table that is 28 inches wide is easier to transport than a table that is 30 inches wide. The extra 2 inches of lift required to clear the ground requires additional effort, especially if the practitioner is short. Some manufacturers of tables have developed shoulder straps, wheel bases, and other aids to help with the transport of tables. These aids help to redistribute the weight load. If a table is carried into the location using the left arm, it should be carried out with the right arm. It could be harmful to carry the table on only one side of the body.

Floor Mats

If the massage professional chooses to work on a mat on the floor, the same body mechanics principles apply. The balance points will then be from the knees instead of the feet.

Stools and Chairs

It is helpful to have a short stool to put a foot on during the massage. A low stool or chair is helpful when working on the face, neck, and feet. It is appropriate for the practitioner to sit while doing massage as long as the practitioner is comfortable, relaxed, and can obtain the appropriate leverage for the pressure the client needs.

Sitting on the edge of the table to work on the client's feet is permissible, as is putting a knee on the edge of the table while working on the client's back. To do this effectively, the draping materials must be used to maintain sanitation. This is accomplished by using a bath towel or similar-sized piece of material to sit on. However, some professionals feel that sitting on the table is inappropriate. This decision is a personal choice. The various illustrations included in this chapter offer some ideas (Fig. 7-8).

BODY MECHANICS WHILE GIVING A MASSAGE

The following general rules apply to body mechanics:

1. The practitioner's body must be in good alignment, with the feet placed apart for support. The arm generating the downward pressure is opposite the back, weight-bearing leg (Fig. 7-9).
2. The body weight is kept on the back leg and foot and the client's body is in front of the practitioner. This position provides adequate leverage. Putting weight on the front leg and placing the client's body directly under the pressure results in no leverage; therefore all pressure results from pushing with the upper body muscles instead of using body weight. The front, non–weight-bearing leg is used to modulate pressure levels and provide some stability. The massage practitioner should be able to lift the front leg off the floor and still maintain a stable balance point at the client–practitioner contact point. It is important that the practitioner use body weight. Although muscle strength is not a big factor, leverage is essential.
3. It is important to stay behind the stroke. The practitioner should be able to look down the arm at a 45-degree to 60-degree angle and see the hand at the point of contact with the client. If the angle is 90 degrees, the practitioner is on top of the stroke, and muscle tension in the arm will result. If the student is pushing, a good practice technique is to lift the nonworking arm over

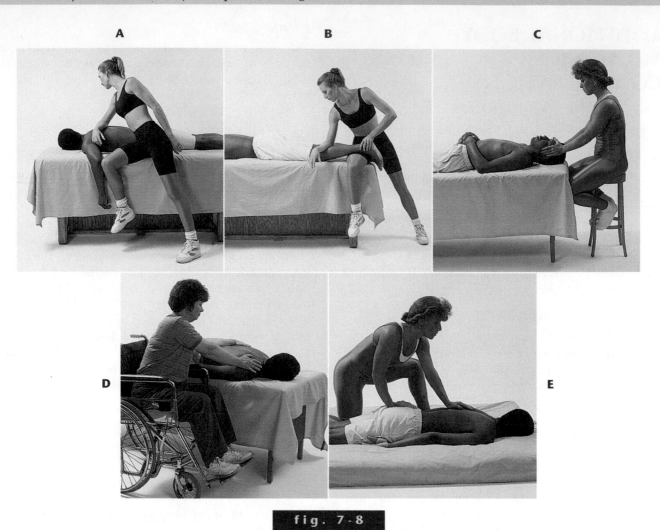

fig. 7-8

Various positions for use of tall tables, short tables, and massage mats. **A**, Tall table. **B**, Tall table with practitioner sitting on end of table. (Note: for **A** and **B**, appropriate use of draping material is required for sanitary purposes when sitting on the massage table.) **C**, Short table with stool. **D**, Short table with practitioner using a chair. **E**, Massage mat.

the head and keep the head up to prevent pushing and promote leaning (Figs. 7-10 and 7-11).

4. The wrists and hands must always be relaxed. Tension in this area transfers to the shoulder and may develop into shoulder and neck problems. When applying a manipulation, the practitioner should be sure the deltoid and shoulder muscles remain soft and the wrists and hands stay relaxed. When the practitioner is working with the hands, the elbow must remain straight. If the elbow is allowed to bend, pressure is unevenly distributed to the wrist (Fig. 7-12).

5. Avoid the use of the fingers and thumbs. These joints are not built for compressive forces. An eloquent description is provided by Emily Cowall, RMT, of Ontario, Canada[2]:

The thumb is a unique, versatile, and efficient aspect in relation to hand function. The ability of the thumb to perform the movement of opposition assists the massage practitioner in maximizing optimum performance during manipulations. Repetitive compressive force and incorrect use of the thumb and fingers, rigid positioning of the wrist, and excessive tension placed onto the hand can give rise to biomechanical dysfunctions . . . The combined activity of proper body mechanics is communicated down through the arms into the hands. Some massage manipulations and techniques can be accomplished by using leaning, lifting, and rocking. A variety of approaches can include use of the arm, specifically the forearm and elbow. Use of the arm reduces stress at the wrist and hand. However, the practitioner must accomplish biomechanical techniques to maximize the use of the hands during manipulation of the soft tissues. The hands deliver the resulting advantages of leverage and strength.

Most massage methods are performed using the whole hand or forearm. Creative use of the forearm and palm of the hand is important. Grasping manipulations, such as *pétrissage,* are stressful on the hands. Massage is not applied with the fingers. Instead, the fingers are used as a unit and

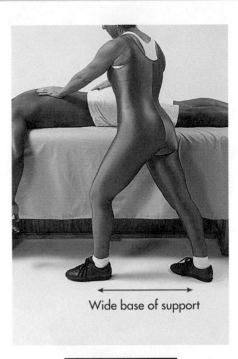

fig. 7-9

Practitioner's feet positioned to provide a wide base of support.

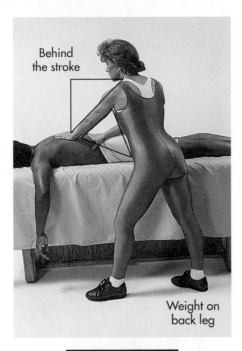

fig. 7-10

Correct position—weight on back leg. Wide base of support in asymmetric stance; equilateral triangles are maintained so the practitioner stays behind the stroke.

closed against the pad of the thumb. The position is similar to that of a lobster claw. Massage is provided with the palm of the hands. Direct pressure is best applied with the forearm and not the thumb, except in small areas when using the forearm is not feasible. The other hand is placed near the contact point to assess the tissue and the client's response when using the elbow or the forearm. The ulnar nerve can be damaged by the use of the triceps portion of the arm. The fleshy portion of the forearm most near the ulna below the elbow is best to use for massage (Fig. 7-13).

The practitioner follows the natural contours (hills and valleys) of the body and uses various methods of positioning the client's body. This allows the practitioner to lean "uphill" to provide pressure or conversely to slide "downhill" without pressure bearing to move to a new location while protecting the shoulders. Leaning keeps the lower back relaxed. Do not attempt to apply pressure on a downhill slide. Pressure is best applied while leaning uphill (Fig. 7-14).

The stroke should be kept at a 45- to 60-degree angle in front of the practitioner. An equilateral triangle is formed by the hip, shoulder, and client contact point. Reaching further may cause lower back strain and a shift of the weight to the front foot, requiring the use of upper body strength to apply pressure, which pins the client to the table. As soon as the angle increases beyond 60 degrees, the weight tends

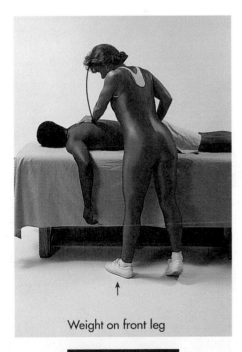

fig. 7-11

Incorrect position—weight is on front leg, moving the practitioner on top of the stroke and losing the triangles.

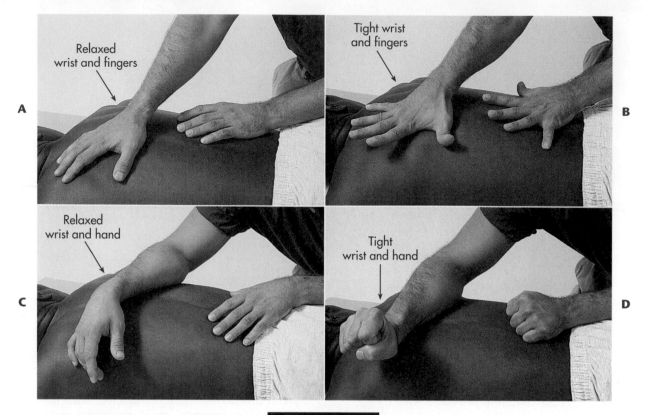

fig. 7-12

Comparison of correct and incorrect wrist and hand positions. **A,** Correct hand positions.
B, Incorrect hand positions. **C,** Correct forearm position. **D,** Incorrect forearm position.

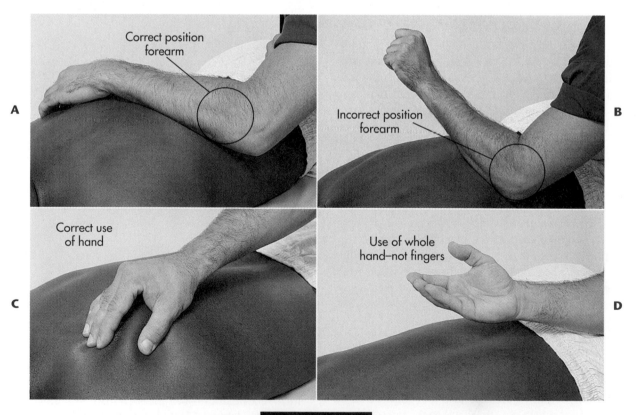

fig. 7-13

A and **B,** Comparison of correct and incorrect forearm positions. **C** and **D,** Demonstration
of effective use of the whole hand to apply massage.

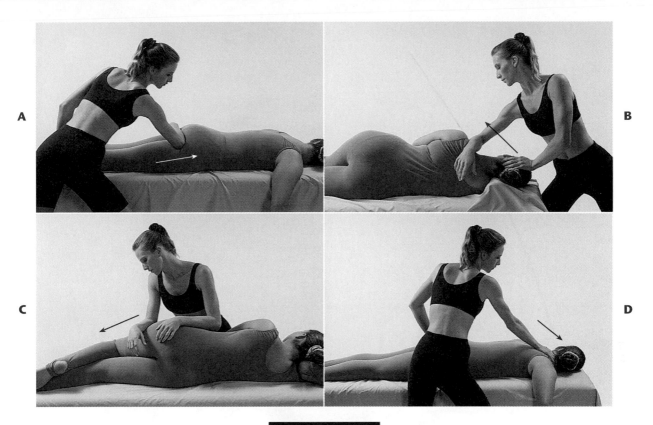

fig. 7-14

Examples of leaning uphill and sliding downhill. **A** and **B**, Correct leaning uphill to apply pressure. **C** and **D**, Correct sliding downhill without pressure as a focus to move to a different location on the body and maintain the flow of the massage.

to shift from the back foot to the front foot. If this happens, the practitioner should step forward without moving closer to the table and then redistribute weight bearing to the back leg (Fig. 7-15).

Hyperextension of the wrist or knees can cause damage. The weight-bearing knee moves into the normal knee-lock position; this is not hyperextension. The wrist angle must never be less than 110 degrees to avoid compression of the nerves in the wrist (Fig. 7-16).

The practitioner should face the area being worked on, with his or her navel and back weight-bearing foot pointed at the area being massaged. When the direction of movement is changed, the body must be turned, including both feet, and the weight shifted to the back foot (Fig. 7-17).

If using *pétrissage,* grasp and rock back to lift the tissue. A rhythm of rocking should be developed by moving forward as the tissue is grasped, and back as the tissue is kneaded and pulled (Fig. 7-18).

The practitioner should not push, even if intense pressure is required. Instead, the practitioner leans on the area of the client's body requiring the intense pressure and then, using the nonworking hand, lifts the body area into the practitioner's compressive force. By shifting the weight on the feet as the client's body is grasped, the client is automatically lifted into the practitioner. No set pattern or particular point to grasp is established. Anything available and

comfortable for the client can be used. The original contact arm pressure increases as the body area is pulled into it. As the pulling arm leans back, the contact arm moves forward into the client. This technique needs to be monitored by the client for pressure levels (Figs. 7-19 and 7-20).

Allowing the practitioner's body to rock and sway with the massage movements is important. Slow rocking keeps the massage manipulations slow. This is crucial for efficient adaptation or change in the client's muscle tissue or in the consistency of the connective tissue. The resulting rhythmic movement keeps the practitioner's body relaxed and is comforting to the client. Remember to work with smooth and even movements, shifting position often.

Body Mechanics Used During Range of Motion, Lengthening, and Stretching Methods

The same principles apply to stretching methods used during massage. Range of motion is most often restricted by faulty physiologic signals rather than an anatomic barrier (see Chapter 5). The protective proprioceptive mechanism sets up this physiologic barrier. Pushing or pulling the stretches or range-of-motion movements can bypass this physiologic barrier, which fully activates the protective

Text continued on p. 270.

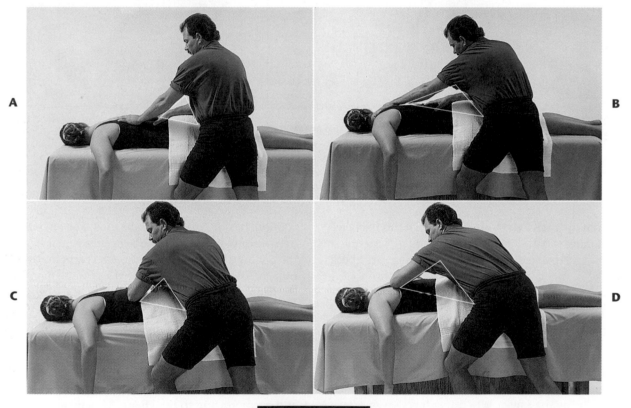

fig. 7-15

Comparison of correct position (45-degree to 60-degree angle of the stroke) and incorrect position (reaching for the stroke) in two positions—hand and forearm. **A,** Correct hand position. **B,** Incorrect hand position (reaching). **C,** Correct forearm position. **D,** Incorrect forearm position (reaching).

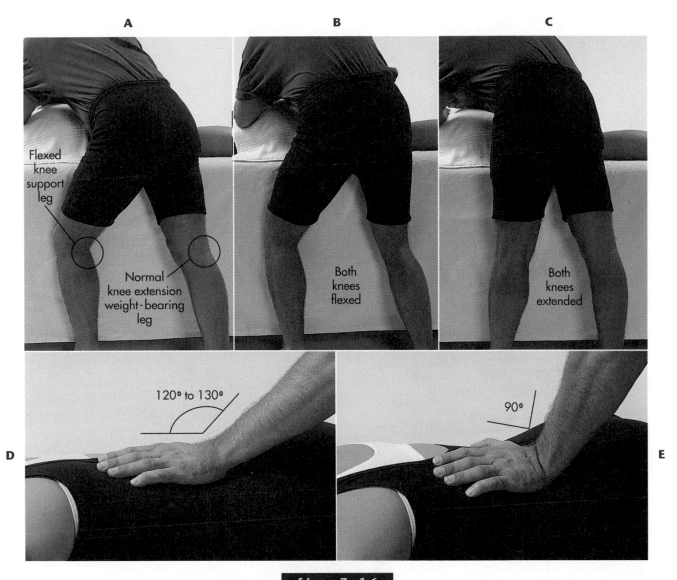

fig. 7-16

Comparison of correct and incorrect knee and wrist positions. **A,** Correct knee position.
B, Incorrect knee position, both knees flexed. **C,** Incorrect knee position, both knees
extended. **D,** Correct wrist position. **E,** Incorrect wrist position.

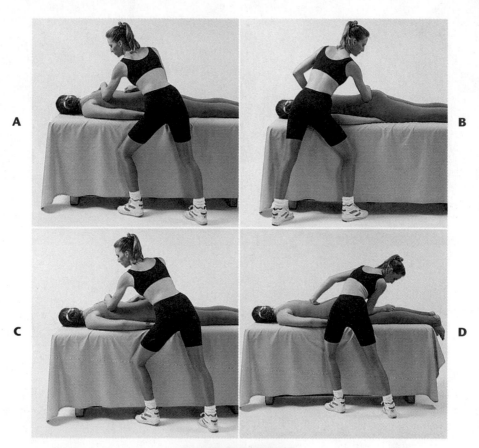

fig. 7-17

Comparison of facing the area to be massaged to avoid twisting and the incorrect twisted position. **A,** Correct starting position. **B,** Correct shifted position. Turn entire body; shift weight-bearing leg. **C,** Correct starting position. **D,** Incorrect (twisted) position. Feet did not move; torso becomes twisted.

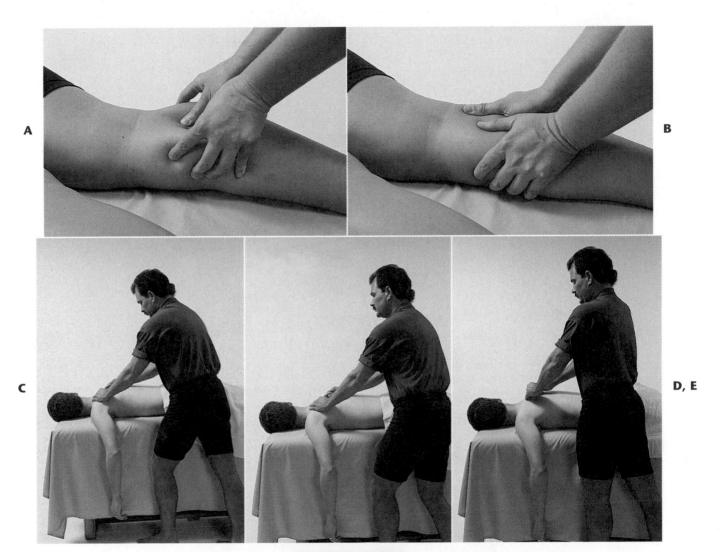

fig. 7-18

Comparison of correct grasp and rock back position for pétrissage and incorrect position of grasp and lift up. **A,** Correct finger position, pétrissage. **B,** Correct whole hand position, pétrissage. **C,** Correct position to begin pétrissage. **D,** Lean back and allow tissue to roll from grasp. **E,** Incorrect position. Instead of leaning back, massage practitioner is lifting up with his shoulders and pulling the tissue.

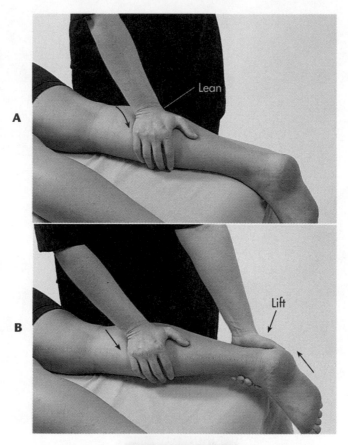

fig. 7-19

Lean and lift into the compression to increase pressure instead of pushing. **A,** Lean into area. **B,** Lift body area while maintaining compression to increase pressure.

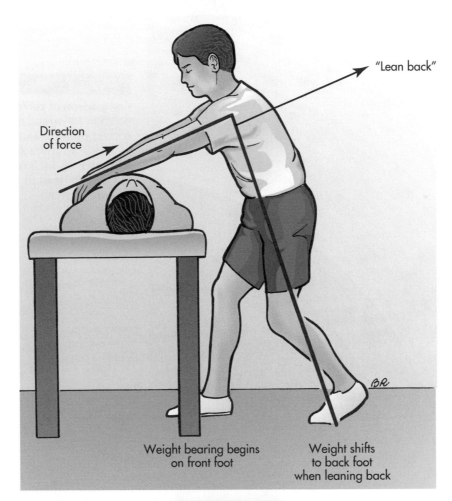

"Lean back"

Direction
of force

Weight bearing begins
on front foot

Weight shifts
to back foot
when leaning back

fig. 7-20

Proper position for lift and lean back for pétrissage and stretching.

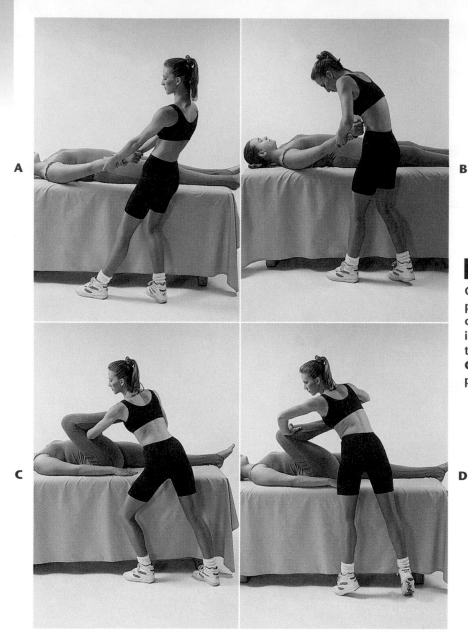

fig. 7-21

Comparison of correct and incorrect position for stretching using leaning for correct position and pushing or pulling in incorrect position. **A,** Correct—lean back to stretch. **B,** Incorrect—pull to stretch. **C,** Correct—lean to stretch. **D,** Incorrect—push to stretch.

neuromuscular mechanism. Spasms may result. Leaning and going slow with the lengthening and stretching movements automatically accesses the physiologic barrier. The practitioner can then feel the subtle push back as the stretch reflex response (Chapter 4) signals that the muscles have been stretched enough (Figs. 7-20 and 7-21).

Body Mechanics During General Transverse Friction

General transverse friction (Chapter 9) can be an energy-consuming and fatiguing massage manipulation. Adapting the frictioning process to use body mechanics prin-

ciples can reduce fatigue. Using compression on an area to be frictioned and simultaneously moving the joint or bone under the compression creates cross-fiber friction from the inside out, using the client's bone as the mechanism moving the tissue. The tissue can be felt moving. It is important that the compression does not slip so that tissue under the hand or forearm is effectively moved (Proficiency Exercise 7-1). The movement also acts as a distraction, which allows more pressure to be used. This is very important if the client is uncomfortable (Fig. 7-22).

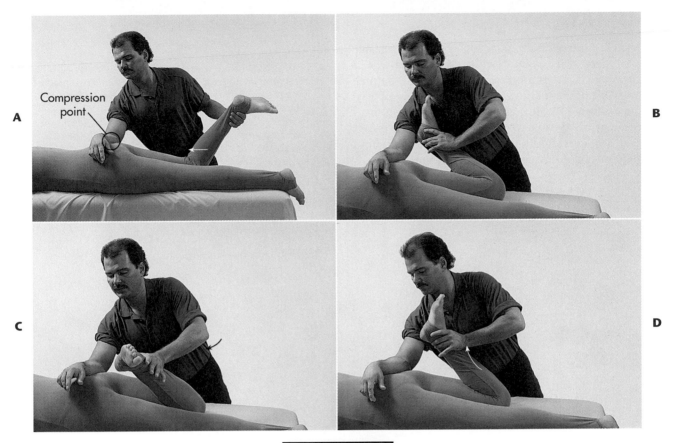

A

B

C

D

fig. 7-22

Friction using compression and movement. **A** through **D**, Move client's hip to various positions. Tissue moves under compression to create a friction movement.

7-1

PROFICIENCY EXERCISE

1. Practice leaning on a wall the correct way and the incorrect way. Feel the difference.
2. Videotape yourself giving a massage. Do you look graceful and relaxed, or are you working too hard?
3. Experiment with different positions with the client so that you can effectively "lean."
4. Tie one end of a short rope around your waist and the other end around your wrist. The length of the rope should allow you to reach out at a 45- to 60-degree angle, as in Fig. 7-15, C. Perform a massage. The rope will prevent you from reaching too far with the stroke and will tug at the waist when it is time to shift the body by taking a step forward.

5. Practice with a standing partner. Lean on your partner as you would lean on a wall. Pay attention to how you feel as your "wall" slightly changes position by moving forward, backward, or twisting. If your partner cannot easily move you with subtle body shifts, you are stabilizing your body and pushing.
6. Have your partner lie on the table and repeat Exercise 5.
7. Practice using the hand as a unit and grasping objects with the palm of the hand. Make sure not to pinch during the grasping movement.
8. Practice a massage using all of the positions illustrated and explained in this chapter.

SUMMARY

The massage professional's body is a vital, irreplaceable tool. It is crucial to use caution while giving a massage. If the professional is uncomfortable, the client will become uncomfortable. If the massage practitioner can give a massage in a relaxed, efficient, and energy-conserving manner, the client will be able to relax and more easily accept the touch. Students should practice again and again until their body mechanics are graceful and efficient.

REFERENCES

1. Birnbaum JS: *The musculoskeletal manual,* ed 2, Philadelphia, 1976, WB Saunders.
2. Cowall E: Personal communication, 1994.
3. Kreighbaum E, Barthels KM: *Biomechanics: a qualitative approach for studying human movement,* ed 2, New York, 1975, Macmillan.
4. Norkin CC, Levangie PK: *Joint structure and function: a comprehensive analysis,* ed 2, Philadelphia, 1992, FA Davis.
5. Smith LK, Weiss E, Lemkuhl LD: *Brunnstrom's clinical kinesiology,* ed 5, Philadelphia, 1996, FA Davis.

WORKBOOK SECTION

Short Answer

1. How do practitioners maintain good body mechanics?

_____

_____

_____

_____

2. How can massage professionals protect their necks and shoulders?

_____

_____

_____

_____

3. How can massage professionals protect their wrists?

_____

_____

_____

_____

4. How can massage professionals protect their thumbs and fingers?

_____

_____

_____

_____

5. How can massage professionals protect their lower backs?

_____

_____

_____

_____

6. How can massage professionals protect their knees?

_____

_____

_____

_____

7. How can massage professionals protect their ankles and feet while giving a massage?

_____

_____

_____

_____

8. What is asymmetric standing, and why should it be used instead of symmetric standing?

_____

_____

_____

_____

9. What are the basic principles of body mechanics?

_____

_____

_____

_____

10. Where is the balance point during a massage?

_____

_____

_____

_____

WORKBOOK SECTION

11. What premassage preparations are important to support good body mechanics?

_____

_____

_____

_____

12. What are the general rules for body mechanics?

_____

_____

_____

_____

13. How do the general principles of body mechanics apply to stretching?

_____

_____

_____

_____

14. How is general transverse friction adapted to this style of body mechanics?

_____

_____

_____

_____

Problem-Solving Activities

1. A female massage practitioner has been doing massage for 4 years. She tends to provide deep pressure with her forearms and the point of her elbow and works very hard to sustain the pressure throughout the massage. In the past 6 months she has developed shoulder pain with numbness and tingling. What might be problematic about her body mechanics, and what corrective action could be taken?

_____

_____

_____

_____

_____

_____

2. A male massage professional is experiencing tenderness in his wrist on the ulnar side. He has long arms and prefers a tall table. He tends to use the palm of his hands for a majority of his work because of concern about applying too much pressure with his forearm. What might be problematic about his body mechanics and what corrective action could be taken?

_____

_____

_____

_____

_____

_____

WORKBOOK SECTION

3. A female massage practitioner with 10 years of experience has been aware of right knee pain over the past 2 years. She learned to keep her knees flexed as part of her initial training. She tends to rotate her right leg externally, so she often does not line up her body so that her right foot is directed toward her application of pressure. What might be problematic about her body mechanics, and what corrective action could be taken?

_____

_____

_____

_____

_____

4. A female massage professional has recently developed low back pain. She tends to keep her weight on the front foot or evenly distributed between both feet in a symmetric stance. She has long legs, a short torso, and very short arms. She was told a year ago to work at a shorter table but never made this adjustment. What might be problematic about her body mechanics, and what corrective action could be taken?

_____

_____

_____

_____

5. A male massage practitioner with 2 years of experience is exhausted after giving five 1-hour massage sessions. He needs to be able to increase his client base by one massage per day but does not know whether his energy can hold out. He feels that he has good body mechanics. He usually stands and provides a variety of massage, but his specialty is a vigorous massage with lot of pétrissage and frictioning methods. He tends to adjust his position instead of altering the client position to his advantage. What might be problematic about his body mechanics, and what corrective action could be taken?

_____

_____

_____

_____

_____

_____

_____

_____

WORKBOOK SECTION

ANSWER KEY
Short Answer

1. To maintain good body mechanics, massage professionals need to be attentive to posture and balance, use the larger muscles to do the work, rely on leverage to apply the pressure, maintain a relaxed body, and avoid compressive forces on the joints.

2. Massage professionals must avoid using upper body strength to exert the pressure for massage. Tense wrists and hands also contribute to shoulder problems. These problems can be avoided if massage professionals learn to use leverage and leaning with the body weight to provide massage pressure. It is also important to avoid both pushing and the use of upper body strength, and to maintain relaxed hands and wrists while giving a massage.

3. Massage professionals can protect the wrists by avoiding excessive compressive forces. Using a proper wrist angle and staying behind the massage stroke (as presented in this chapter) will protect the wrist.

4. The thumb was not meant to endure compressive force. It is designed for grasping. Avoid using the thumbs and fingers for compression. Massage professionals must learn to use the olecranon process and ulnar side of the elbow instead. When the thumb must be used, a stabilized joint position protects the thumb. Massage professionals should use the hand as a unit and rely on the forearm for many massage strokes, including most effleurage and compression.

5. Massage professionals must learn to keep their lower backs straight and avoid bending or curling at the waist while giving a massage. Frequent posture shifting of the massage professional's body also helps protect the lower back, as does lifting by leaning back during stretching. The asymmetric stance presented in this chapter, along with variations using a short and tall stool, provides methods to protect the lower back. The lower back is further protected by avoiding twisting and reaching while working and keeping the point of contact with the client below the professional's waist.

6. Knee problems can be avoided by respecting the basic design of the knee and frequently shifting the weight from foot to foot. Avoid hyperextension of the knee. However, the most efficient standing position for the knee involves the normal screw-home or knee-lock position in the last 15 degrees of extension. This position

provides the least compressive force on the knee capsule and the least muscular action for stability.

7. The ankle and foot are protected by an asymmetric stance, frequent position change, and sitting when possible to do massage.

8. Asymmetric standing is the most efficient standing position. The weight is shifted from one foot to the other in an energy-conserving mechanism. Symmetric standing, with the weight equal on both feet, is fatiguing and interferes with circulation. Methods to support the asymmetric stance, such as using a stool to put one foot up on, using a high stool to sit on, or putting a knee on the table, further protect the lower back and conserve energy.

9. Leaning and using the body weight focused from the abdomen as leverage

10. At the client-practitioner contact point

11. The massage professional needs to be comfortable and dressed in loose, nonrestrictive clothing that does not interfere with movement. Before your massage day begins, warm up your body with some general aerobic activity and stretching. During the day, take stretch breaks between each massage and move all the muscles you do not use while giving a massage. Massage your own arms, hands, and shoulders after each massage. The massage professional should get a weekly massage. The massage table must be at a comfortable height. A stool to put a foot on is helpful. A high stool can be used to sit on while doing massage. A low stool or chair is helpful when working on the client's face, neck, and feet. If the massage professional carries a portable table, he or she must pay attention to the body mechanics used to lift and move the table. Lift the table with the knees and hip, not the waist. Do not reach for the table when moving it from the car. Avoid habitually carrying the table on only one side.

12. (a) Make sure your body is in good alignment and that your feet are in a wide base of support. The arm generating the downward pressure should be opposite the back weight-bearing leg. (b) The weight is kept on the back leg and foot and the client's body is in front of you. The front non–weight-bearing leg is used to modulate pressure levels and provide some stability. (c) It is important to stay behind your stroke. (d) If you find yourself pushing, lift the nonworking arm over your head and keep your head up. (e) Make sure that the wrists and hands are always relaxed. (f) Avoid using your fingers and thumbs. Keep pétrissage strokes to a

WORKBOOK SECTION

minimum. Grasping strokes such as pétrissage are stressful on the hands and forearms. Do not use the thumb for direct pressure. (g) Do not use the triceps portion of your arm. You can damage your ulnar nerve. Use the forearm just below the elbow. (h) Positioning the client's body to enable you to lean uphill, or conversely, to slide downhill, protects the shoulders. Leaning keeps the lower back relaxed. (i) Do not reach for the stroke. Keep the client close to you. (j) Never hyperextend the wrist or knees. The weight-bearing knee will move into the normal knee-lock position; this is not hyperextension, which damages the knee. Make sure the angle of the wrist is no more than 110 degrees to avoid compression of the nerves in the wrist and keep the elbows straight. (k) Change your position and method often. (l) Face the area you are working with to avoid twisting. (m) Turn your whole body when you change the direction of your movements, and shift the body weight to the back foot. (n) If using pétrissage, grasp the tissue and rock back to lift the tissue. Develop a rhythm of rocking forward as you grasp the tissue and rocking back as you knead and pull the tissue. (o) If intense pressure is required, do not push. Instead, lean and lift into you, shifting the weight on the feet as you lean back. (p) Work with smooth and even movements. (q) Allowing the therapist's body to rock and sway with the movements is important. Slow rocking keeps your strokes slow. The resulting rhythmic movement keeps your body relaxed and is comforting to the client.

13. Leaning and going slow on the stretches automatically accesses the physiologic barrier. The massage practitioner can then feel the subtle push back as the stretch reflex response signals that the muscles have stretched enough.

14. Use compression on an area and simultaneously move the joint or bone under the compression. This method creates cross-fiber friction from the inside out, using the client's bone as the mechanism moving the tissue.

Problem-Solving Activities

1. Most obvious would be the possibility that she is working with a tense hand and wrist, which is translating to the shoulder muscles. Also working with the point of the elbow puts pressure on the ulnar nerve as a possible contributing factor to the numbness and tingling. The table may be too high for her to lean with leverage to provide the pressure, so she finds herself pushing with her upper body muscles, which tenses the shoulder muscles.

   Corrective actions: Lower massage table; instruction in the proper use of forearm below the elbow

2. It is possible that he is bending his elbow to accommodate his long arms to a tall table, which is applying uneven pressure to the ulnar side of the wrist.

   Corrective actions: Keep arm straight when using the palm of the hand, use forearm more, and learn to adjust pressure with width of stance and lower table

3. The long-term increased compressive force in the knee capsule from the flexed knee position coupled with the extra strain of the external rotation may be causing the pain in the right knee.

   Corrective actions: Sitting more during the massage using both a high and low stool; becoming aware of the external rotation and minimizing it; learning to allow the knee of the weight-bearing leg to extend to the normal knee-lock position to reduce compressive forces in the knee joint

4. The table is likely to be too short, causing her to bend over while giving massage, and straining the low back. The symmetric stance often causes strain to the lower back.

   Corrective actions: Raise the table; use a short footstool for the front leg to provide extra stability, help keep the back straight, and support an asymmetric stance

5. He seems to be working hard while giving massage and would conserve and increase energy by working smarter.

   Corrective actions: Learn to sit more while giving massage; avoid the use of pétrissage and replace with methods that can be done with less energy using leaning methods such as effleurage and compression; limit frictioning to areas where it is essential and then use the compression with movements methods in this chapter; ensure that he is only providing pressure when leaning uphill and altering the position of the client to accomplish this; use the 'lean and lift' instead of the 'push harder' method to increase the pressure levels if necessary; make sure his body is relaxed and the pressure comes from body weight instead of muscle strength

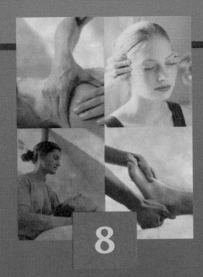

8

PREPARATION FOR MASSAGE

EQUIPMENT, SUPPLIES, PROFESSIONAL ENVIRONMENT, POSITIONING, AND DRAPING

THE massage practitioner must make certain preparations before beginning the massage. The room must be set up, and all necessary supplies must be gathered. The type of lubricant to be used must be considered, as well as the manner in which it will be dispensed properly, the temperature of the massage room, and the warmth of the practitioner's hands. Massage professionals must develop a method, referred to as *centering*, to help focus on the client and the session to come. Client positioning and modest, appropriate draping procedures also must be considered. The practitioner then uses history taking and assessment procedures to formulate the approach for the massage. The plan is discussed with the client, and informed consent is obtained. All this is done before the massage begins. This chapter helps the therapeutic massage professional develop these important premassage procedures that support the therapeutic relationship and professional environment first discussed in Chapter 2.

EQUIPMENT

section objectives

Using the information presented in this section, the student will be able to perform the following:

- Care for and protect his or her hands and general health
- Make informed decisions about the purchase of a massage table, chair, mat, body supports, draping materials, and lubricants
- Make the most effective use of massage equipment

Care of the Massage Practitioner's Hands and Body

For a massage professional, the most important pieces of equipment are the hands and body. Make sure to protect your hands from abrasion and damage by wearing gloves when doing outdoor chores or other work in which the hands may be injured. Using the forearms during a massage protects and limits use of the hands. In some circumstances the knees and feet are used for certain massage techniques. The massage practitioner has a professional responsibility always to be attentive to efficient and proper body mechanics (as presented in Chapter 7) and the maintenance of personal health.

The Massage Table

The next piece of equipment to consider is a surface on which the client may sit or lie while receiving the massage. The first choice of most practitioners for this purpose is a **massage table.** The table must be sturdy and properly assembled so that there is no chance of it collapsing while a client is lying on it. The two primary types of massage table are the portable table, which folds into a smaller unit and can be carried easily from place to place, and the stationary table, which remains in one location.

Most manufacturers offer a basic model, and many have more detailed tables with all sorts of features, such as automatic height and tilt adjustments, arm supports, and face cradles. The more features, the more expensive the table (Box 8-1).

Almost all portable tables are built with a hinge in the middle that allows them to fold in half for ease of carrying. This hinged area is a weak spot in the table; cable supports on the legs counterbalance this weakness. Most tables are strong and can hold about 300 pounds if the weight is distributed evenly over the entire surface of the table. Problems occur when the client sits in the middle of the table when lying down or sitting up, which focuses all the weight in one spot. With cumulative use the hinge weakens. It is important to check the cable tension consistently to ensure that no sag develops. Otherwise, the table may buckle, damaging the table and injuring the client (Fig. 8-1).

Stationary tables do not have the instability problem because the table is heavier; cross-bracing and leg supports make the table even safer. However, the lack of portability is a major drawback if the massage practice involves any on-site work (Fig. 8-2).

Adjustable legs allow the massage table to be lowered or raised to accommodate the various body builds of clients while allowing the practitioner to use proper body mechanics.

Ideally a massage professional would have both a stationary table and a portable one. A stationary table easily

---

box 8-1

FEATURES OF A PORTABLE MASSAGE TABLE

A portable massage table is the most versatile type of massage table. It should have the following features:

- Sturdy construction, including cable support on the legs
- Manual height adjustment
- A face cradle
- A washable covering (usually vinyl) that also can be cleaned with disinfectant
- Adequate padding to ensure comfort and firm support
- A width of 24 to 28 inches (most tables are about 6 feet long); tables narrower than 24 inches are too narrow for the client's comfort, and those wider than 28 inches are difficult to carry

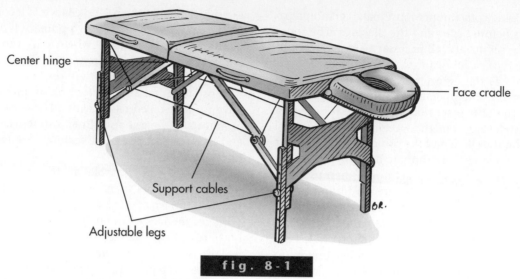

fig. 8-1

A generic portable massage table with center hinge, support cables, and face cradle.

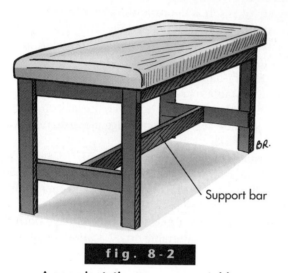

fig. 8-2

A generic stationary massage table.

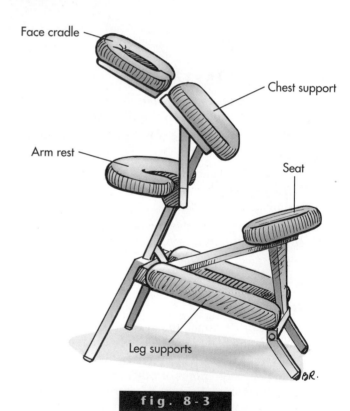

fig. 8-3

A generic massage chair.

can be built at home by an average carpenter for a reasonable cost. A portable table, however, should be purchased from an experienced manufacturer. It is worth the investment to buy a product that has been tested for safety. All massage tables must be checked daily for structural stability. It is important to perform a complete maintenance check on all connectors, bolts, cables, and hinges every week and to repair any defects immediately.

Many clients may be concerned about the sturdiness of the table. The lightweight portable tables may look weak, but a quality table is well built and strong. Before the massage, demonstrate the stability of the table or offer alternatives such as a chair or massage mat.

The Massage Chair

Instead of a massage table, equipment designed for seated massage can be used. A special **massage chair** can be pur-

chased for this purpose, and such chairs are a worthwhile investment (Fig. 8-3). The sit-down massage, often referred to as an *on-site* or *corporate massage,* usually takes place in a public setting (e.g., business location) and is done over clothing. Massage chairs also are excellent for working with clients who are more comfortable sitting upright, such as a woman in the last trimester of pregnancy or a person who has difficulty getting on and off a massage table (Box 8-2).

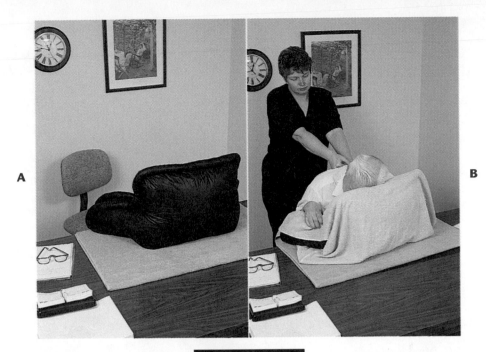

fig. 8-4

A, Use of a support pillow to provide massage in an office chair and at a desk. **B**, Positioning of the client for massage.

---

box 8-2

ADVANTAGES AND DISADVANTAGES OF A MASSAGE CHAIR

Advantages
1. Massage chairs, which are specially designed for that purpose, usually are very comfortable and easy to use.
2. Professionally manufactured equipment adds to the professional atmosphere of the massage setting and ensures safety through quality workmanship in construction and design.
3. Professionally manufactured massage chairs are lightweight and portable.

4. Clients with certain respiratory, vascular, and cardiac conditions are best given a massage in a seated position.

Disadvantages
1. Some people have difficulty getting into and out of the semi-kneeling position required to use the massage chair.
2. Access to certain body areas is limited.

A straight-backed chair with no arms also can be used. The client sits facing the back of the chair and leans on the chair back, supported by pillows. A stool or chair pushed up to a table or desk is another option. The client leans forward on a supporting pillow placed on the table. Special triangular or block-shaped foam forms can be purchased and used to provide support. A professionally manufactured desk-top support, which could replace the pillows, also is available (Fig. 8-4).

The Massage Mat

For some methods of massage, a mat on the floor is used (Box 8-3). The **massage mat** can be a futon or an exercise mat, but it must be protected by a sanitary covering (Fig. 8-5).

Body Supports

Body supports are used to bolster the body during the massage and give contour to the flat working surface (Fig. 8-6).

Commercial body support products are available that consist of various shapes and sizes of pillows and foam forms. As an alternative, the practitioner can buy assorted shapes and densities of hypoallergenic foam and make covers for them. A wedge, a round tube, and two or three square or oblong pieces will be needed, each with a differ-

KEY FEATURES, ADVANTAGES, AND DISADVANTAGES OF A MASSAGE MAT

Key Features

1. The mat should be soft enough and provide sufficient support to ensure the client's comfort.
2. It should be large enough to allow the massage practitioner to move around the client's body while staying on the cushioned surface, thereby protecting his or her own knees and body.
3. The mat should be made such that it can be covered with a sanitary covering.

Advantages

1. A mat often is less expensive than a massage table.
2. A mat may be lighter and thus easier to carry than a massage table.
3. Mats are particularly safe (i.e., there is little chance of a client falling off).
4. A mat is a popular choice when working with infants and children.
5. Mats are portable.
6. Because a mat is so safe and comfortable, it may be the best choice for working with clients who have certain physical disabilities; for example, a transfer from a wheelchair to a mat may be accomplished more easily.

Disadvantages

1. Proper training is needed to work effectively on the floor; many massage practitioners are not familiar with this kind of work.
2. The floor may be drafty or colder for the client.
3. Physically challenged or elderly clients may have difficulty getting down on or up from the floor.
4. Mats do not have face cradles to maintain alignment of the neck in the prone position

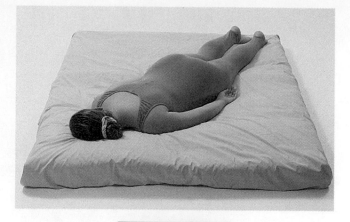

fig. 8-5

A generic massage mat covered with a sheet.

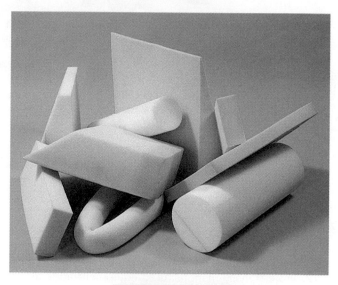

fig. 8-6

Various sizes and shapes of body supports.

ent depth and density. Additional supports are needed for working with pregnant women (Proficiency Exercise 8-1).

Draping Materials

Opaque **draping material** is used to provide the client with privacy and warmth. Standard bed linens are the coverings most commonly used because they are large enough to cover the entire body and are easily used for most draping procedures. Both full and twin-sized sheets fit nicely on most tables. The practitioner can either buy these linens and launder them in a sanitary fashion or use a linen service. Sheets made of cotton or cotton blends are the best choice because they do not slip on the client. Cotton flannel sheets are nice because they feel warm to the skin. Whatever linen is used, it must be able to withstand being washed in bleach or other disinfecting solution.

Large towels may be used for draping because they are both warm and opaque. They must be at least the size of a beach towel and have a soft texture. Be sensitive to the client's comfort, and provide a choice of towels or sheets. Because towels are smaller, a client may feel more exposed and may prefer the security offered by a sheet. As an alternative, both sheets and towels can be used, with a bath-size towel used as a chest covering.

Disposable linen also is available. Some higher quality disposable products may look and feel like a cotton fabric, but they do not provide the same warmth. Disposable linens are convenient, but they cannot be washed or recycled.

Draping Material Recommendations

Either a twin fitted sheet or a flat sheet should be put over the vinyl table top to protect the table; it is much less expensive to launder this additional sheet than to replace the covering on the table. A full or twin flat sheet then is placed over the protective covering. The top sheet can be either a full or a twin sheet. Twin sheets fit a bit better on the table but can be somewhat skimpy for draping. Full sheets provide more material, which facilitates draping, but can be cumbersome. Also, for sanitary purposes, care must be taken that sheets do not drag on the floor. Face cradles should be draped with a hand towel, a pillowcase, or an additional piece of fabric sewn just to fit the face cradle. All body supports and pillows are covered with pillowcases.

In addition to the sheets and pillowcases, a bath-size towel is used for various draping procedures. A large beach-size towel, a flannel sheet, or a light blanket should be available in case the client becomes chilled.

It is helpful to have different colors of sheets and towels. If all are the same color, it is difficult to distinguish between the top and bottom sheets.

A complete list of draping material for one client includes the following:

1 twin fitted sheet (table protector)
2 full or twin flat sheets (bottom and top drapes)
1 pillowcase or hand towel (face cradle)
Additional pillowcases (body supports)
1 bath-size towel
1 flannel sheet, light blanket, or beach-size towel (which is easiest to launder) for warmth

Some people are allergic to cotton blends, which may irritate their skin. If the client has sensitive skin, the practitioner should use white, pure cotton sheets to reduce the risk of a reaction. When possible, soft pastel colors should be chosen for draping materials because they withstand bleaching, are more opaque than white linens, and tend not to show lubricant stains.

At least 10 full sets of draping material are needed; this is sufficient for 2 standard business days, with laundry done every other day. If you use a laundry service, order enough linen for 10 days to make sure that you do not run out of linens should delivery be late. Whenever linens come into contact with the client, they must be laundered in an approved fashion before they are reused. Most linens must be replaced every 1 to 2 years if used often. Lubricants build up, and bleach wears out the fabric (Proficiency Exercise 8-2).

Lubricants

Lubricants serve only one purpose for the massage practitioner: they reduce friction on the skin during gliding-type massage strokes. Medicinal and cosmetic use of lubricants is out of the scope of practice for therapeutic massage.

Scented Lubricants

Because headaches and other allergic responses to lubricants often are caused by the volatile oils in scented products, scented lubricants should not be used. This recommendation does not discount the therapeutic benefit of aromatherapy; the sense of smell is a very powerful sensory mechanism, and many emotional and physiologic processes can be triggered by deliberate use of aroma. However, this textbook does not cover all these applications, and additional education is required to use aromas specifically, purposefully, and therapeutically. Until you receive this training, do not use them.

Lubricant Types

Oils and creams can be vegetable, mineral, or petroleum based, and powders can be talc or cornstarch based (Fig. 8-7). If possible, use the most natural products available and avoid using petrochemicals and talc, because many people are allergic to these substances. All lubricants must be dispensed from a contamination-free container.

The lubricant traditionally used for massage is oil. It is easy to dispense from a squeeze bottle and can be kept free of contamination. Natural vegetable oils can become rancid quickly. Some commercial products use additives that may cause allergic reactions in clients. Oils have some disadvantages: they are messy, they can spill and drip, and they stain linens. However, specialized laundry products are available for removing oil stains.

Massage creams must be dispensed in a contamination-proof way. Some creams are thin enough to be kept in a squeeze bottle. Others are thick, and the amount to be used must be removed in a sanitary fashion before the massage.

---

8 - 1

PROFICIENCY EXERCISE

1. Collect information from at least three manufacturers of massage tables and massage chairs. Compare the cost, quality, and construction of the equipment.
2. Research a variety of styles of body supports for clients with specific needs.
3. Locate a source for foam (an upholstery or a mattress company is a good start). See how many different body supports you can build from foam scraps.

---

8 - 2

PROFICIENCY EXERCISE

1. Obtain a set of sheets, some towels, and some disposable linen. Practice draping methods with them. Which type of material did you prefer to use?
2. Have another student or a massage practitioner give you a massage using the different draping materials. Which type did you prefer to have used on you?

New processing methods have produced many natural vegetable oil-based massage creams and lotions that do not feel greasy. Some products are water based, and these wash out of linens without leaving stains.

Powders are used when creams and oils are undesirable, usually because of skin conditions (e.g., acne) or excessive body hair. Do not inhale the dust from powders, because it could cause respiratory problems. Powders with a cornstarch base are preferable because they pose less of a risk of respiratory irritation. If the client and practitioner are in agreement, disposable masks can be used to reduce the risk of respiratory irritation even further.

Using Massage Lubricants

Only a small amount of lubricant needs to be used to give a massage. Remember that the reason for using lubricant is to reduce friction on the skin from the massage movements. More lubricant is required to work over body hair. In some cases powder may be a better choice. Sometimes the use of any type of lubricant is contraindicated, therefore it is important to be able to perform massage without a lubricant.

In Chapter 9 you will learn about different massage manipulations. The long, gliding methods are best for applying lubricant. Keep the application even and very thin. It is easy to apply more but difficult to remove excess. Keep a clean towel available in case removal is necessary.

Do not pour the lubricant directly onto the client. It first is warmed in the practitioner's palms by rubbing the hands together. Apply the lubricant to one area at a time rather than to the entire body. Do not use lubricant on the face or hair, because it disturbs makeup and hairstyles. The practitioner's hands must be cleaned before working in the area of the face. Some practitioners begin the massage with the face and head, before using any lubricant.

Some clients may appreciate having the lubricant removed after the massage. An alcohol-based product can do this, but alcohol is drying to the skin. Rubbing the skin with an absorbent towel removes most of the lubricant.

Additional Equipment

In addition to a massage table, draping material, supports, and lubricants, it is desirable to have disposable tissues, a clock, and music available.

Music

Music often is used to distract the client from or to block out surrounding noise. A less recognized use is to achieve interaction and modulation of the autonomic nervous system through entrainment. Simple, soft music with a base beat under 60 beats per minute tends to activate a parasympathetic response, which produces a soothing, relaxing effect. Music above 60 beats per minute encourages sympathetic responses, producing a stimulating, invigorating effect.

In using music, a practitioner must consider the effect to be created and whether both the client and the massage practitioner like the music being played. The best recommendation is that the massage practitioner keep on hand a variety of music from which the client is allowed to choose. An assortment of styles, rhythms, and instruments, as well as a cassette or CD player or other equipment, should be available. The volume should be kept low but loud enough so that the music can be heard without straining.

The music itself can be very helpful in pacing the massage. If the tunes are familiar, they can give the massage practitioner a sense of the passage of time without his having to look at the clock constantly (Proficiency Exercise 8-3).

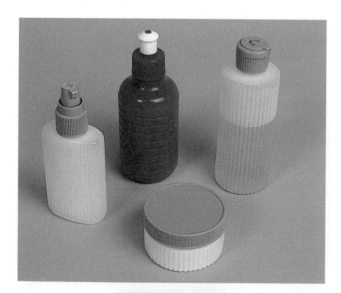

fig. 8-7

Massage lubricants.

8-3

PROFICIENCY EXERCISE

1. Obtain the three basic types of lubricant: oil, cream, and powder. Give a massage with each type. Which do you prefer to use?
2. Find a practice client with a hairy body, and again practice using the different types of lubricant. Which one was the easiest to use? Which one did the client prefer?
3. Have a fellow student give you a massage using all three types of lubricant on different parts of the body. While receiving the massage, compare and decide which type you preferred.
4. Practice giving a massage with as little lubricant as possible. See if you can give a massage with only 1 tablespoon of oil or cream.
5. Assemble a music library of four different types of tapes. Mark each 15-minute segment to assist with timing of the massage.

THE MASSAGE ENVIRONMENT

section objectives

Using the information presented in this section, the student will be able to perform the following:

- Design an efficient therapeutic massage environment
- Organize an office and massage room

Clients return for another massage because they appreciate the quality of the service and a professional personality and environment. Thoroughly plan the image that your massage environment is to convey to the public. To maintain the integrity of the professional relationship, the environment created for the massage setting, including decorations and the reading material provided for clients, should reflect the scope of practice of massage.

When most people think of massage, they picture a quiet, private room with low lighting and soft music. However, therapeutic massage can be done almost anywhere and under almost any conditions. Successful massage practices have been developed in noisy public locations, such as airports, in a client's home, in the workplace, and outdoors at sporting events or retreats. Whatever the physical location of the massage environment, the most important aspect is to present and deliver the highest standard of professional care to the public.

General Conditions

General conditions for massage areas that must be considered are the room temperature, the fresh air supply, privacy, and accessibility.

Room Temperature

The air temperature in the massage room should be kept at 72° to 75° F. Massage produces a vasodilation effect, which brings the blood closer to the surface and allows internal heat to escape, cooling the client. It is impossible for clients to relax if they are cold. The massage practitioner is active and fully dressed and can become warm while doing the massage. Some practitioners put an electric blanket on the table to keep clients warm. A piece of lamb's wool may be used because it traps and retains body heat. Placing a hot water bottle at the client's feet and another at the neck or wherever comfortable may increase body temperature.

The massage practitioner's uniform must be cotton or a cotton blend to wick away moisture and perspiration from the skin. It should have short sleeves and be loose fitting to help prevent the practitioner from becoming too warm.

Fresh Air and Ventilation

The room should have access to fresh air, but a window that opens to the outside is not always available. Ventilation of some sort is important. A small fan in the room pointed at the ceiling or the wall keeps the air moving without causing a draft on the client.

Privacy

Clients need privacy for removing their clothes in preparation for the massage treatment. If the massage room is separate from other public areas, the client can be left alone to get ready for the massage. Sometimes a screen or curtained area can be used to divide one large room into two distinct areas.

Accessibility

It is important to locate the massage practice so that it is easily accessible to clients with mobility impairments. Barrier-free access and restrooms are required.

Lighting

The massage area must be lit well enough to meet the standards for proper cleaning and safety (see Chapter 6). Bright overhead lighting often is too harsh and glaring for the client. Indirect or natural light from a window is much better. If the massage area has overhead lights, turn them off and use a lamp in the corner of the room instead. A dimmer switch is excellent because it allows adjustment of the lighting. Never work in a dark room, to prevent accidents caused by tripping, and never work by candlelight, because an open flame is a safety hazard.

Scents, Incense, Flowers, and Plants

Massage practitioners work with a variety of people during a day, each one with different ideas about what is pleasant and what is offensive. Many clients are also environmentally sensitive and react to scents, incense, and flowers. The best recommendation is to avoid using such items because the fragrance lingers and can cause problems for a client.

Nonflowering (foliage) plants usually are less of a problem. However, if the practitioner serves an allergic population, it may be best not to use them. If their use is not a problem, foliage plants are a wonderful natural air purifier that can supply oxygen to the massage areas.

Hygiene, Chemicals, Perfume, and Warm Hands

It is important for the massage professional to attend to personal hygiene and to prevent body odors because people are sensitive to these smells. Avoid heavy use of aftershave, perfume, scented cosmetics, or hair spray. Clients usually do not comment on offensive breath or body odors; they simply do not return for further sessions. Because it can be difficult to recognize odors on ourselves, ask a family member or friend who will answer truthfully if you have such a problem.

If the massage practitioner is a smoker, the smell of smoke can linger in fabric, carpeting, and furniture and on the practitioner. This can be very distasteful to a nonsmoking client. Because it is difficult to remove the odor, the massage environment should be located in a nonsmoking area. Refraining from smoking during professional hours may help prevent the smell from clinging to the hands, clothes, hair, and breath.

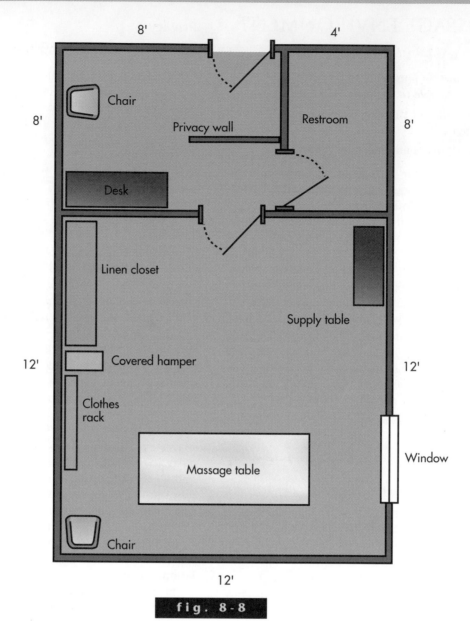

fig. 8-8

An example of the layout of a massage office with separate business office and massage area.

Cold hands are a real problem for many massage practitioners. The hands should be heated with warm water, on a hot water bottle, or by rubbing them together before touching the client.

A Typical Massage Room, Home Office, or Clinical Setting
Business and Massage Areas
The massage area must be kept separate from the business area. People associate behavior with locations and expect certain activities at those locations. It is important that these two activities remain separate in the client's mind. The interaction that takes place when appointments are made and money is taken is very different from the one that takes place during a massage.

The business or reception area should be near the entrance, but privacy must be provided for taking the client's history. If other clients are nearby, this area must be separate from the massage room. An appointment book, calendar, forms, receipts, pencils, and telephone, as well as a chair and a small table, should be set up in the business area. Reading material should be available for clients. The massage area should be located farther from the door or in an adjacent room (Fig. 8-8).

Make sure that the client has a place to sit and to hang his clothes. Use an enclosed cabinet to store linens and lubricants, and designate a place to keep the body supports. A covered hamper, located away from the massage table, is needed for used linens.

Hand washing and restroom facilities must be easily accessible. If the massage room has no sink, a liquid hand cleanser must be available. If there is no direct access be-

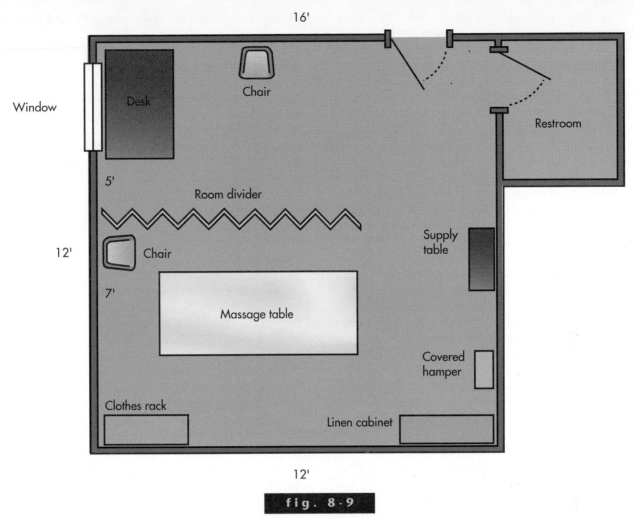

16'

Window

Desk

Chair

Restroom

5'

Room divider

12'

Chair

7'

Massage table

Supply table

Covered hamper

Clothes rack

Linen cabinet

12'

fig. 8-9

An example of the layout of a massage office with the business office and massage area in one room.

tween the massage room and the restroom, make sure the client uses the facilities before the massage session begins. It also is important to have a plan for getting the client to the restroom during the massage session if necessary. This can get tricky if the only way to the facilities is down a public hall, past offices that share the restroom facilities.

Room Size

The reception and business area can be small, about 8 feet by 8 feet (64 square feet). A room for massage should be at least 10 feet by 10 feet (100 square feet). If the two areas are in the same room, a space at least 12 feet by 12 feet (144 square feet) is needed to provide the necessary working area (Fig. 8-9).

The Office at the Practitioner's Home

Designating a professional area in your home is a business option if zoning regulations allow home office businesses (see Chapter 14). Establishing a professional office in the home involves special considerations. If at all possible, there should be a private entrance to the massage area

(zoning regulations usually require this). Barrier-free access and restrooms are a major consideration in planning a home office. Most homes are not designed with these accommodations.

If pets are in the home, potential clients must be informed in case of allergy or fear of animals. Pets should not be allowed in the business or massage areas. Family members must understand the privacy issue of the massage environment, and massage clients must understand the boundaries of the private home area. This more personal environment requires very careful attention to professional boundaries.

The Public Environment: Sports Massage, Demonstration Massage, On-Site or Corporate Massage

In the public setting, the massage practitioner goes to the location rather than having the client come to the practitioner's office. These public massage sessions normally last less than 30 minutes, and the client remains fully clothed. As the practitioner, you usually have little control over noise, lighting, and other conditions. Clear enough space to set up the massage table or chair. Try to locate this area in a corner, which gives two walls to provide some privacy.

Regardless of the massage location, it is always important to create both a business area and a massage area. Find a flat surface and use it to set up a portable office from a briefcase or similar carrying case that contains receipts, an appointment book, and handouts. Set up the massage area a few steps away.

Although the use of linen and lubricants usually is limited in these circumstances, it is still important to have them available. They should be carried in a closed bag to maintain sanitation. Make provision for hand washing or hand cleaning products to maintain hygiene and sanitation.

The Client's Residence (On-Site Massage)

On-site massage can be provided in the home for many reasons, including service and convenience for the client, especially if the person is housebound. A 60- or 90-minute massage usually is given in these situations. Because the massage takes place in the client's residence, this is the most difficult environment in which to maintain professionalism and professional boundaries. A professional uniform is especially important in this environment. A portable table most often is used, but a massage chair or mat also is acceptable.

Find a private location for the massage, but avoid the bedroom; opt for a family room or den. If the only room available is a bedroom, try to use the guest room or a child's room rather than the client's bedroom. Make sure it is near an area where hands can be washed. Set up a business area using a briefcase as the office and maintain the professional atmosphere. Don't sit at the kitchen table or in the living room because the professional role of the massage practitioner may be obscured in these traditional conversation locations.

Linens, body supports, and lubricants are needed. It also may be wise to carry a small fan to keep the air moving and drown out noise from other areas. Never lock the door because a locked door invites secrecy and creates an environment in which it is difficult to maintain professionalism. Under rare circumstances it could constitute entrapment, or the client could perceive it as a violation of the boundaries of the therapeutic relationship. Carry a sign to hang on the door that says, "Massage in session." If you are going to use music, bring a portable cassette or compact disc player.

Outdoors

Outdoor massage usually is provided at a sports massage event or promotional activity. Some massage professionals also work on boats, at family picnics, on the beach, and at poolside. Although these are very casual settings, the massage practitioner's behavior must reflect professional and ethical standards. Again, a professional uniform is especially important in these more casual and public environments.

Wind, sun, rain, and insects create special conditions. The wind blows the drapes, but picnic table clips can be used to prevent this. Instructing clients to wear a swimsuit or loose clothing for an over-the-clothing massage also helps. A firm, level location is needed for the table because tables that sink into the sand are dangerous. This can be avoided by putting sample carpet squares and coffee cans under the legs of the massage table. It is important to do massage in the shade to prevent sunburn.

A roof or canopy is helpful in case of rain. If the area is screened in, technically it is not outdoors. True outdoor massage has insects; just blend the brushing away of insects into the massage as best you can. If an area for wash-

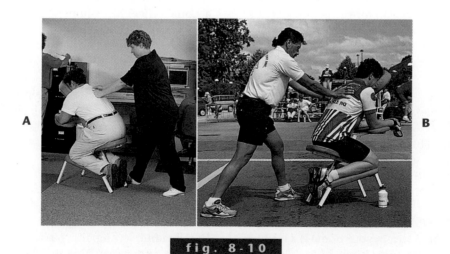

fig. 8-10

A, On-site massage in an office setting. **B**, Outdoor sports massage setting using a massage chair.

ing hands is not available, use a special disinfectant hand cleanser. Set up the portable office in an area away from the massage setting (Fig. 8-10) (Proficiency Exercise 8-4).

DETERMINING A NEW CLIENT'S EXPECTATIONS

section objective

Using the information presented in this section, the student will be able to perform the following:

- Interview a new client to better understand the client's expectations of massage in general and the outcome for a massage session in particular

It is important to explain the limitations of massage to the client carefully to put expectations into perspective and help define the outcome for the massage. It is important to do this in the beginning as part of the informed consent procedures before the massage begins (this information was first presented in Chapter 2).

The massage professional must be concerned with how the new client thinks a massage is to be given. If the client has never had a massage, his expectations will be determined by what he has heard, read, or observed. Because methods and applications of massage vary so much, the client may not expect the style of massage that is offered. The difference between what is expected and what is received may be confusing. The client's answer to a simple question such as, "What do you think a massage is like?" or "Describe for me how a massage is done" gives the massage practitioner an idea of the client's expectations for the session. The massage practitioner should explain the different approaches used so that the client is not on the table wondering why this massage is so different from what he expected.

If a new client has had a massage before from someone else, it is natural to compare the different styles. It is important for the massage practitioner to explain the procedures and methods used so that the client understands

that massage can be done in many ways. *Never* discount another massage professional's methods or approach and say that your way is better; this is unethical behavior. The only exception is if the previous massage violated professional ethics, scope of practice, and standards of practice. It is important to explain to the client that massage practitioners do not conduct themselves in a manner that violates professional codes of ethics. The code of ethics example in this textbook or one from a professional organization can be used as a framework for the discussion (see Chapter 2).

The outcome for massage is what the client can anticipate in response to the benefits of the proposed massage plan. Each massage manipulation has an anticipated response. A client can be made aware of these responses and any risks inherent in the proposed massage interventions.

Do not confuse expectations with outcome. Consider this example: A new client of yours has never had a massage, but a friend of hers in another city regularly receives therapeutic massage. The client explains that the massage her friend receives is for a chronic headache problem that seems to be related to daily stress and that the massage helps a lot (expectation). When you ask your client why she came for a massage (the outcome), she says that she has no real problems, although sometimes she has headaches just as her friend does. Your client thinks a massage would feel good. The outcome is a basic massage that feels good, not the more specific approach to address headaches.

The client's expectations were based on information from her friend. It is natural for a first-time client to consider this type of information, but the outcome may be very different. If the massage practitioner is not careful to differentiate the two, the massage provided for the client may not meet the client's expectations.

Some questions the practitioner can ask to help determine a new client's expectations are as follows:

- Why do you want a massage?
- How do you want to feel after the massage?
- What do you think massage will do for you?
- What results do you want from the massage?

After determining expectations, carefully go over all the client policies and procedures discussed in Chapter 2. Never assume that a client understands the complexities of massage practice. Explain everything in detail in terms the client can understand.

---

8 - 4

PROFICIENCY EXERCISE

1. Arrange to give a massage in each of the four basic environments. What was different about each experience?
2. Put together a briefcase office.
3. On separate pieces of paper, design three different set-ups for a clinical massage environment. Indicate the business and massage areas.

FEEDBACK

section objectives

Using the information presented in this section, the student will be able to perform the following:

- Elicit feedback from the client
- Provide the client with appropriate feedback

Feedback is a noninvasive, continual exchange of information between the client and the professional. Feedback is not social conversation. It is common for a client to talk during the massage and appropriate for a massage professional to listen to the client while remaining focused on the massage. *It is inappropriate for the professional to engage in social conversation with clients, particularly about their personal life.*

Client Feedback

Whether working with a new client or providing regular massage services to an existing client, it is important to encourage feedback from the client. Explain the importance of feedback concerning comfort levels (e.g., warmth, positioning, restroom needs) and the quality of any pain sensations (i.e., "good pain," such as is often experienced with deeper massage methods, and "undesirable pain," which the client may feel if the methods are too aggressive).

The practitioner benefits from feedback about the effectiveness or ineffectiveness of the various massage methods. Session-to-session reports of progress, postmassage sensations and experiences, and the duration of effects help the practitioner adjust the application of the massage. Feedback from the client about professionalism and the quality of the professional relationship also is valuable.

Some clients may find giving feedback difficult. They may not have enough body awareness to give an accurate report on sensations during the massage or the effectiveness of the methods used. With education from the practitioner, this communication can improve.

It is far more common for clients to have difficulty providing feedback about what they did not enjoy about the massage, methods that were uncomfortable or ineffective, and inappropriate behavior by the practitioner. People generally tend to avoid confrontational situations, or they try not to "hurt another's feelings." Both of these behaviors interfere with the client's ability to provide effective feedback to the practitioner. It is the massage professional's responsibility to develop a professional trust relationship that allows the client to feel safe in giving both positive and constructive feedback.

Clients should be told during premassage procedures about the importance of feedback. Explain to the client that all feedback is taken as constructive, that it is not personalized, and that it enhances the service of massage therapy. It is important to ease the client's concerns about the practitioner's possible reaction to "negative feedback." Gentle, open-ended questioning before, during, and after the massage encourages feedback. Reminder statements also are helpful.

Questions and reminder statements that could be used before the massage include the following:

- Is there a position in which you are most comfortable?

- Does the temperature of the room feel comfortable?
- Remember to tell me if a method is too deep or painful.
- I would appreciate it if you would indicate when a method seems particularly beneficial or enjoyable.

Questions and reminder statements that might be used during the massage include the following:

- I'll use three different pressure levels on your back; please tell me which you prefer.
- Might there be a more comfortable position for you?
- Are you comfortable with massage in this area?
- Remember that it's OK to tell me if you are uncomfortable.
- Remember to turn over slowly.

Questions and reminder statements to use after the massage include the following:

- What methods were most effective for you today?
- What might I improve on during the next session?
- Remember to evaluate the aftereffects of the massage, and we'll discuss them next session.

Instilling the idea of "client as a teacher" is one way to encourage feedback from the client. The client teaches the massage professional about himself and guides the practitioner in providing the best massage for them both. This knowledge and experience accumulate, adding depth to the knowledge base of the massage professional.

Practitioner Feedback

Massage practitioners also provide feedback to their clients. Practitioners must develop communication skills (see Chapter 2) to ensure that the feedback they give is not personalized by the client but rather taken as valuable information to be used.

Forms of feedback that the practitioner can give the client include the following:

- Do you notice that your breathing is beginning to slow a bit as you relax?
- Are you aware that you have a bruise on the back of your calf?
- The muscle tension in your shoulder seems higher today. Why do you think that's the case?
- You seem to tense up when I apply pressure to this area.
- I noticed that your skin color had improved after the massage.

Client Conversation

New clients often talk quite a bit during the first massage. This usually is the result of nervousness, and in future sessions, particularly those for relaxation and stress reduction outcomes, the talking diminishes.

Clients commonly talk more during the first 15 minutes of massage as they acclimate to the environment and begin to relax. Some talk during the entire massage; this is appropriate and should be accepted. Many people seek massage not only for the therapeutic physical benefit but also, unconsciously, for the social interaction. The professional respectfully listens to the client and limits conversation to appropriate feedback and necessary verbal exchanges to indicate understanding of what the client is saying.

The following is an example of an appropriate dialog:

Client: "My, it has been a very busy week. My son was in two band competitions. I was only able to attend one. It disturbs me when I miss these events. He placed second and third. I'm very proud of him. Do you remember that last week I told you he might get a scholarship to college for music?"

Practitioner: "Yes, I do remember you speaking of that possibility. If I remember correctly, it was to Mott College, right?"

Client: "Yes. You know, it's hard being a single parent. My work interferes with my ability to be with my son as much as I think is important."

Practitioner (replying with feedback): "Were you aware that your shoulders became more tense just now?"

Client: "Yes, it felt as if you were applying more pressure all of a sudden. Were you?"

Practitioner: "No, I didn't increase the pressure, but your muscles did tense while you were speaking about your time with your son."

Client: "What would you do about this if you were me?"

Practitioner: "I don't have the professional skills to help you with your feelings about your time availability with your son, but I can use some methods to relax your shoulders and teach you some methods to keep them relaxed throughout the week."

Here is the same dialog presented in an inappropriate way (Proficiency Exercise 8-5):

Client: "My, it has been a very busy week. My son was in two band competitions. I was only able to attend one. It disturbs me when I miss these events. He placed second and third. I am very proud of him. Do you remember that last week I told you he might get a scholarship to college for music?"

Practitioner: "Yes, I do remember you speaking of that possibility. If I remember correctly, it was to Mott College, right? My

daughter went to Mott College. She had difficulty with the registration procedure, and it took forever to work out the snag. Make sure your son doesn't work with Mrs. Jones. She was very rude."

Client: "Yes, Mott College is correct, but now I wonder if he'll be OK. You know, it's hard being a single parent. My work interferes with my ability to be with my son as much as I think is important."

Practitioner: "I sure do understand, because my sister is a single parent, and she just read a real good book about it. I told her she needs a day away once a month, and so do you. By the way, were you aware that your shoulders became more tense just now?"

Client: "Yes, it felt as if you were applying more pressure all of a sudden. Were you?"

Practitioner: "No, I didn't increase the pressure, but your muscles did tense while you were speaking about your time with your son."

Client: "What would you do about this if you were me?"

Practitioner: "Well, a social group or even a support group might help. I think I would talk with my son and see if the situation really bothers him, but you know teenage boys, he probably won't tell you anything. My daughter was so hard to get any information from when she was that age. I can use some methods to relax your shoulders and teach you some methods to keep them relaxed throughout the week, since you seem to get more upset when you think about these issues, and I am sure that this entire situation is a big reason for this muscle tension."

GENDER CONCERNS

section objective

Using the information presented in this section, the student will be able to perform the following:

- **Recognize differences based on gender in clients' expectations and interpretation of touch**

Male and female practitioners may experience some difference in a client's expectations and interpretation of touch. It is important to establish clear boundaries concerning the inappropriateness of sexual interaction and to create a safe, nonsexual professional environment with

---

8 - 5
PROFICIENCY EXERCISE

Compare the two dialogs and list three differences between them.

Example
In the first dialog, the client did most of the talking.

Your Turn
1.

2.

3.

first-time clients. These boundaries may need to be reinforced as the professional relationship evolves.

Without passing judgment on the correctness of the behavior, it often is observed that both men and women initially seem more comfortable with a woman practitioner. This appears to be based on several factors:

- Body image on the part of women clients—they are more comfortable having another woman see their bodies
- Women's male partners (e.g., husband) are not comfortable having a male massage professional interacting with them
- Women's concern about safe touch from men
- Men's discomfort over being touched in a pleasurable way by another man
- Men's social conditioning to accept comfort and touch in a caring manner from women
- Cultural influences

Male massage professionals must be aware of the possibility of encountering these preconceived ideas and present themselves in such a way as to alleviate concerns with education when possible and to respect the feelings of the individual client through referral to a female professional if necessary. As public awareness of massage increases, this gender difference probably will begin to dissipate.

PREMASSAGE PROCEDURES

section objectives

Using the information presented in this section, the student will be able to perform the following:

- Set up an orientation process for a new client
- Develop a personal method of focus and centering

Orientation Process

After the intake process, a new client is ready to enter the massage room. The orientation proceeds as follows:

1. Take the client to the massage area.
2. Show her where she may hang her clothes, and explain that she needs to remove only the amount of clothing necessary. Instruct her to leave her underclothing on. If you have any other special requirements about clothing, now is the time to explain them.
3. Demonstrate the massage table, how it is draped, and how the draping works. Explain the requested starting position on the table (prone, supine, or side-lying).
4. If you are using a massage chair or mat, show the client how to use the chair or mat for proper positioning.
5. Ask about the use of music and offer a few selections.

6. Show the client where the restroom is and how to get there if it is not next to the massage area.
7. Briefly explain any charts you may have on the walls.
8. Ask about a lubricant. Show the client what you have and offer a choice. It is important for clients to choose the type of lubricant or to have the option of no lubricant to avoid any misrepresentation by the massage practitioner of diagnosing or prescribing.
9. Explain that you will leave the room to allow the client privacy while she undresses. The exception to this is if a client is a very elderly person or a woman in an advanced stage of pregnancy who requests assistance, or any other special situation in which the client requires the practitioner's assistance. If you will be staying in the room, explain how you will help the client and maintain modesty. This usually is done by holding up a sheet in front of the client or by using a screen. If direct assistance is necessary for disrobing, present yourself in a professional and matter-of-fact way while providing the help needed.
10. Explain all sanitary precautions.
11. Show the client the sign on the door stating that a massage is in session, and explain why the door is not locked.
12. Give a general idea of the massage flow. For example, that the massage will start on the back and take about 10 minutes, and then the legs and feet will be done for 15 minutes. Explain the effect of any change in a basic pattern; for example, that spending more time on the neck means that less time will be available for the back.
13. Instruct the client to get on the table by sitting between the end of the table and the hinged area (if the table is a portable one) or in the middle of the table (if it is a free-standing table). Next, the client should lean on one side and roll to the supine or prone position. To get off the table, the client reverses the procedure: the person rolls to one side, pushes up to a seated position, and sits for a minute to prevent dizziness. She then gets off the table. If any chance exists that the client may fall or may need assistance getting on or off the table, stay in the room to help. Demonstrate the procedures if necessary, but do not use any draping materials on the table. It is unsanitary for anything or anyone to touch the drapes before the client uses them.
14. Ask the client if she has any questions.
15. Explain that you will be washing your hands and preparing for the massage while the client gets ready.
16. Tell the client how long you will be gone and that you will knock and announce yourself before entering the room.

Any modifications that need to be made because of the location and environment of the massage should be taken into consideration. People can become anxious if they do not know how to do what they are supposed to do. Do not assume that a client remembers the instructions or knows what is expected. Explain all steps in detail.

It is important to remind repeat clients of the previously mentioned procedures. Just as the information gathered during the intake procedure is updated each week and reassessment continues as the massage sessions progress, it is important to keep clients updated on any changes in procedures, new equipment, and so forth.

Focus/Centering

While waiting for the client to prepare for the massage, it is important for the practitioner to do the same through **focus/centering.** This can be done in many ways. Slow, deep breathing combined with stretching slows the mind and focuses the attention into the body. Looking at a nature scene or a painting is another way. Listening to music or performing some sort of repetitive behavior, such as washing your hands under warm water while visualizing the water carrying away all concerns for the next hour, can become a trigger for focus. The goal is to be present in the moment for the client and not focused on lists of things that need to be done. Developing a routine sequence for focusing enables the practitioner to become calm and centered much faster (Proficiency Exercise 8-6).

POSITIONING AND DRAPING THE CLIENT

section objectives

Using the information presented in this section, the student will be able to perform the following:

- **Position and drape a client and perform a massage using the four basic positions**
- **Drape effectively with two basic styles**

Positioning

Positioning is helping a client into the position that best enhances the benefits of the massage. The four basic massage positions are supine (face up), prone (face down), side-lying, and seated. This section explains the use of body supports and proper draping for these basic positions.

A client could use all four positions during a massage session, because staying in one position longer than 15 minutes may become uncomfortable. The exception is a painful situation that limits the client's ability to move with ease.

Pillows or other supports, such as folded towels, blankets, or specially designed pieces of foam, are used to make the client comfortable. The supports fill any gaps in contour when the client is positioned and provide soft areas against which the client can lean. Supports generally are used under the knees, ankles, and neck.

After the first trimester a pregnant woman probably will be most comfortable in a side-lying position. If a client has a large abdomen, supports should be used to lift the chest and support the abdomen. This can be done by using a foam form with an area cut out for the abdomen. Women with large breasts may need a chest pillow.

Side-lying positions require pillows or supports for the arms and a small support between the knees. Clients with lower back pain may be more comfortable with a support under the abdomen when lying prone.

Moving the client's position requires shifting of the body supports. All supports must be under the sanitary drape or protected with sanitary coverings that are changed after each client. If the supports are located under the sheets, simply fold the bottom sheet over the top to expose the supports and move them (Fig. 8-11).

Draping

Draping has two purposes:

1. *To maintain the client's privacy and sense of security.* The drape becomes the boundary between the practitioner and the client. It is a way to establish touch as professional. It is much more professional and less invasive

---

8 - 6

PROFICIENCY EXERCISE

1. Develop a checklist of everything the client needs to know before preparing for the massage.
2. Role play with three other students. One student is the first-time client, another is the massage practitioner, and the third evaluates the performance. Practice using the checklist and explaining procedures to the client. Switch roles so that each student plays all three parts.

3. Develop three different ways to focus your attention before beginning a massage. Make note of your ideas for future reference.
4. Work with three students and teach each other ways to focus. Discuss what works and what does not work in focusing.

fig. 8-11

Use of support in five positions

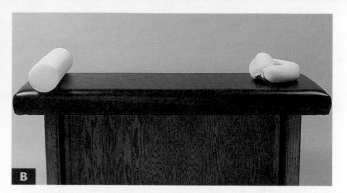

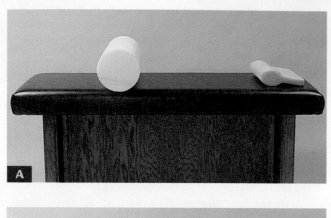

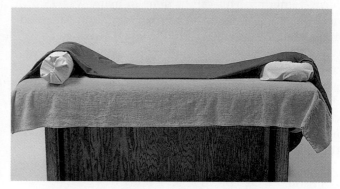

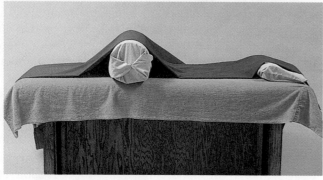

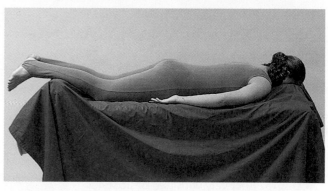

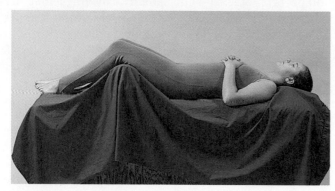

Supine

Prone

to skillfully undrape an area to be massaged and purposefully redrape the area than to slide the hands under the draping materials. Respect for the client's personal privacy and boundaries fosters an environment in which the client's welfare is safeguarded.

2. *To provide warmth.*

Draping Principles

Draping can be done in many ways. The main principles are as follows:

* All draping material must be freshly laundered us-

ing a bleach or other approved solution (see Chapter 6). Disposable linen must be fresh for each client.
* Only the area being massaged is undraped.
* The genital area is never undraped. The breast area of women is not undraped during routine wellness massage. Specific medical massage under the supervision of a licensed medical professional may require special draping procedures for the breast area in women. In Canada, breast massage for medical purposes has a specific methodology and a consent

fig. 8-11, cont'd

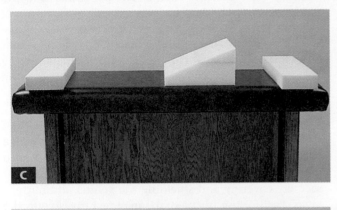

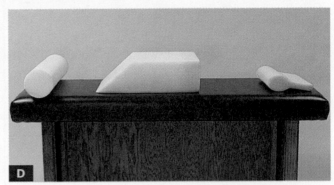

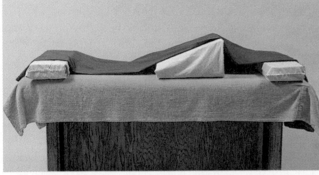

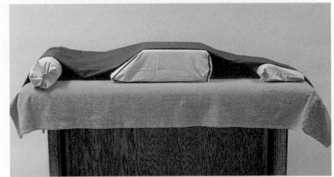

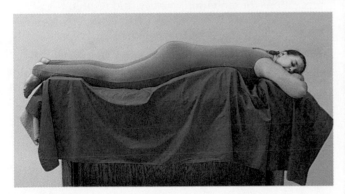

Large chest

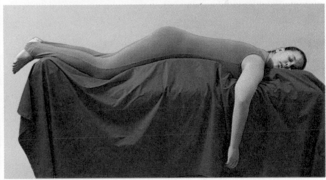

Low back support

Continued.

process. These methods are out of the scope of practice for the wellness massage practitioner. (Specific recommendations for therapeutic breast massage are provided in Chapter 12.)

• Draping methods should keep the client covered in all positions, including the seated position.

Draping materials can be a bit clumsy to use at first. To ensure the modesty of the first few practice clients, have them leave their clothing on.

If the client uses a dressing area away from the massage table, a robe, top sheet, or wrap large enough to cover the body will be needed for the walk to the massage area. If a wrap or top sheet is used, it can become the top drape once the client is on the table. The two basic types of draping are flat draping and contoured draping.

Flat Draping Methods

With flat draping, the top sheet is placed over the client in the same manner that a bed is made, with a bottom sheet and a top sheet. Instruct the client to lie supine, prone, or side-lying between the drapes on the massage table. The entire body is then covered. The top drape, and sometimes

fig. 8-11, cont'd

Use of support in five positions

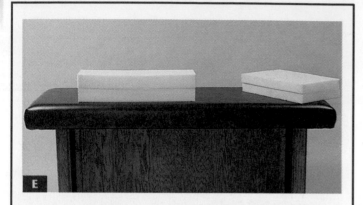

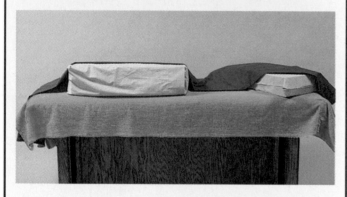

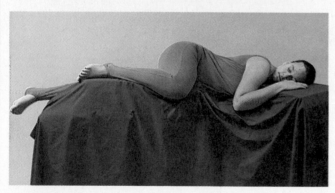

Side lying.

the bottom drape, is moved in various ways to cover and uncover the area to be massaged.

NOTE: To ensure the privacy of men, the massage practitioner should avoid smooth, flat draping over the genitals while the client is supine. The penis may become partly erect as a result of parasympathetic activation or a reflexive response to the massage. This response is purely physiologic and does not necessarily suggest sexual arousal. Loose draping that does not lie flat against the body provides for a visual shield and diminishes the client's embarrassment.

Contoured Draping

Contoured draping can be done with two towels or with a sheet and a towel. The drapes are wrapped and shaped around the client. This type of draping is very effective for securely covering and shielding the genital and buttock areas. Positioning of the drape may feel invasive to the client, but having the client assist in placement of the drapes preserves a sense of modesty. For women, a separate chest towel can be used to drape the breast area.

Alternative to Draping

As an alternative to draping, the client can wear a swimsuit or shorts and a loose shirt. The table or mat must have a sanitary covering, such as a bottom drape, and a top drape must be available because the client may become chilled even if partly clothed. When working with a client wearing clothing or a swimsuit, it still is necessary to observe all the precautions for sanitation, privacy, and respect.

Suggested Draping Procedures

The following photographs lead you step-by-step through several draping procedures. Practice them and then combine the methods to fit the particular needs of the client. (Fig. 8-12).

Notice how the draping material is placed so that the practitioner's clothing does not come into contact with the client. This maintains sanitation.

These draping procedures are a starting point for modest, secure use of towels and sheets for proper and appropriate draping. Many other methods are available and can be developed (Proficiency Exercise 8-7).

Text continued on p. 312.

8-7

PROFICIENCY EXERCISE

1. Receive three different professional massages and observe how the massage practitioner drapes and uses body supports.
2. With a fellow student or practice client, practice each draping method shown in Fig. 8-12.

fig. 8-12

Samples of draping sequences using sheets and towels

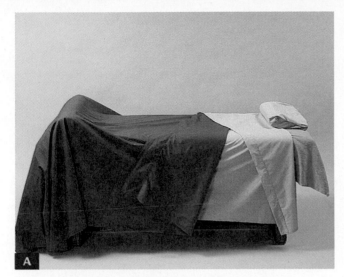

A

Basic table set up for draping.

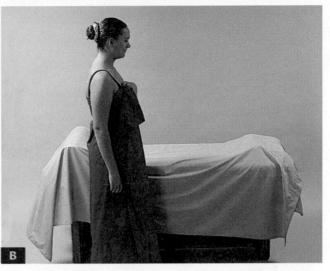

B

Client wrapped in top sheet. Top sheet is folded in half with fold at the top and end held in the front.

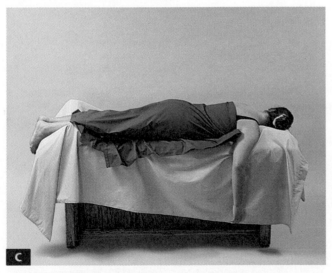

C

Client lies in prone position and sides of drape are moved to the side of the table.

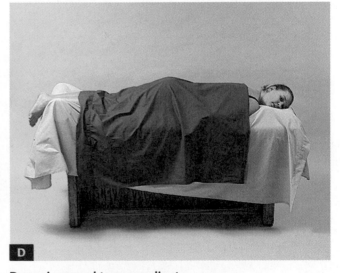

D

Drape is spread to cover client.

Continued.

Samples of draping sequences using sheets and towels

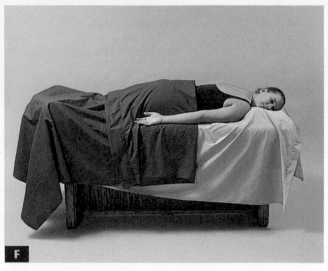

E

Client fully draped in prone position.

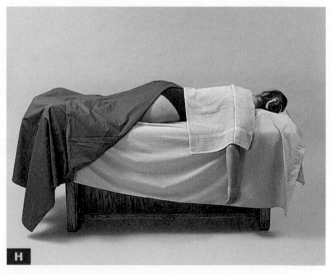

F

Drape is folded back to provide access to back.

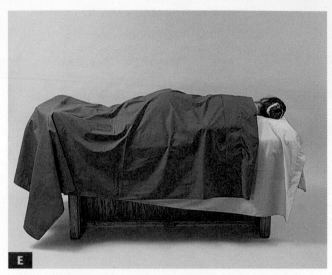

G

Drape is folded again on the diagonal to provide access to gluteal region.

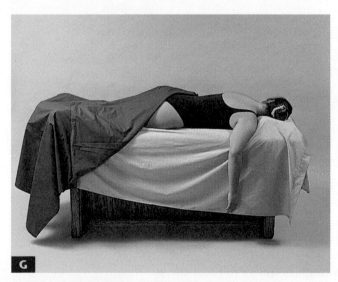

H

A towel is used to drape the back while the gluteal region is massaged.

fig. 8-12, cont'd

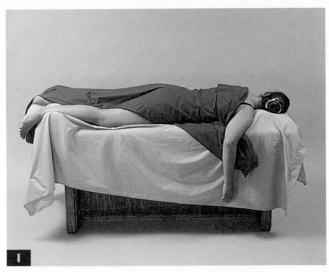

I

Drape is repositioned to cover client and towel is removed. The end of the drape is folded on the diagonal to provide access to the leg.

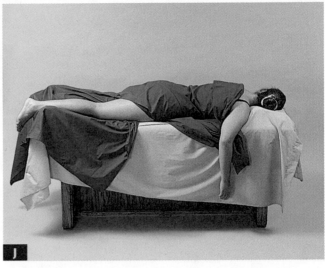

J

Drape is positioned under the leg to be massaged to secure it.

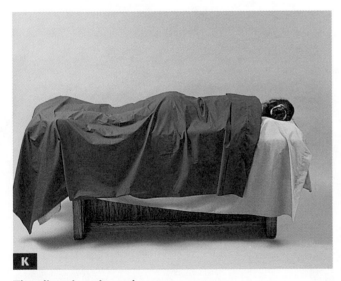

K

The client is redraped.

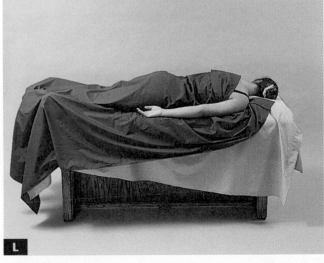

L

The arm is positioned over the drape, and the drape is held secure by the arm.

Continued.

Samples of draping sequences using sheets and towels

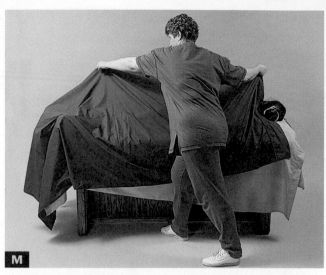

M

Position for holding the drape while the client turns to side. Drape is held in the middle in a tent fashion. The massage practitioner's knee secures the drape against the table.

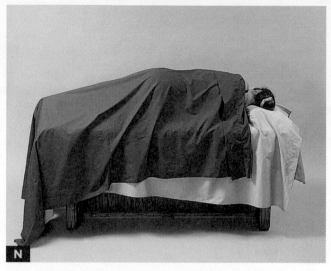

N

Client in side-lying position with full draping.

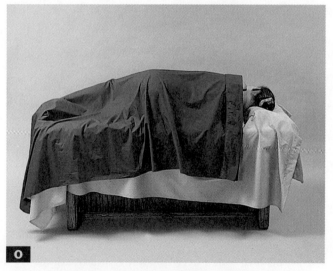

O

Client with top leg drawn up and supported with body support.

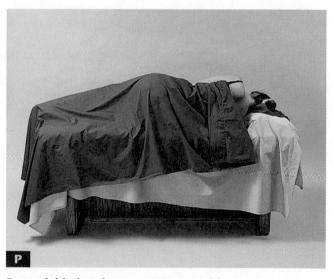

P

Drape folded under top arm to provide access to arm.

fig. 8-12, cont'd

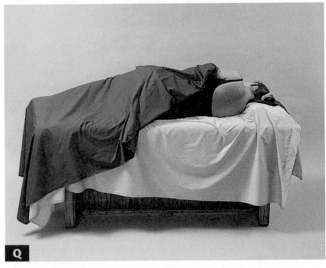

Q

Top corner of drape folded diagonally to provide access to back.

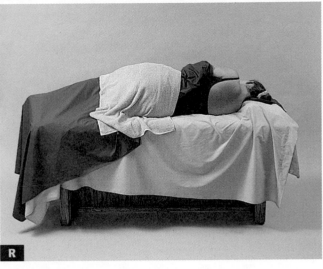

R

Towel positioned to drape the gluteal area.

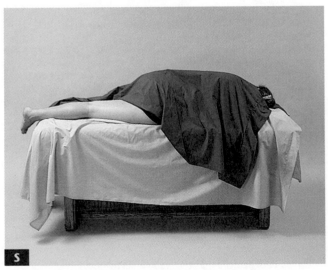

S

Client with back redraped and end corner of drape folded diagonally to provide access to leg.

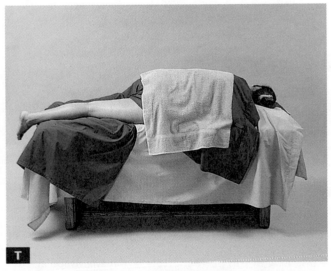

T

Drape moved under exposed lower leg and towel used to drape gluteal area. Drape is secured under lower leg.

Continued.

fig. 8-12, cont'd

Samples of draping sequences using sheets and towels

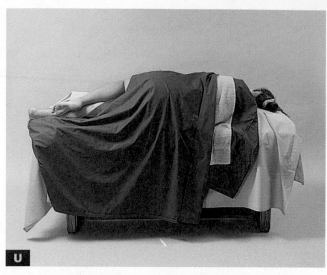

U

Lower leg is redraped and opposite end corner of drape is folded diagonally to provide access to upper leg.

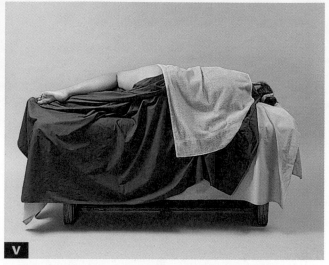

V

Folded corner of drape is brought through the legs and secured under upper leg. Towel is used to drape the gluteal and abdominal area.

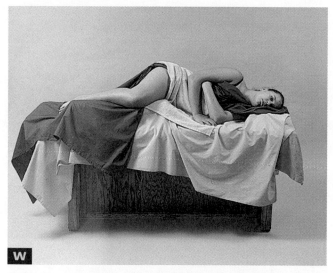

W

Front view of this position. Notice that the drape across the chest is secured under the client's head.

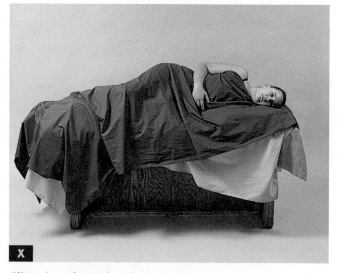

X

Client is redraped and towels are removed.

f i g .   8 - 1 2, cont'd

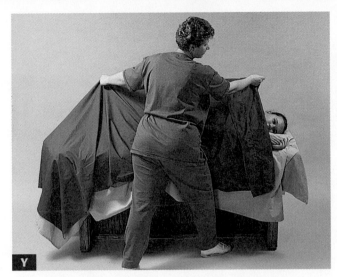

Y

Drape is held in tent fashion and secured against the table with the practitioner's knee as the client turns to supine position.

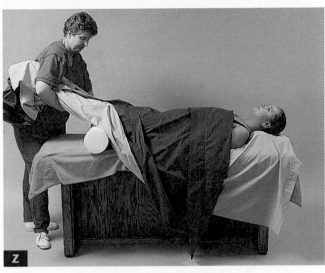

Z

Both top and bottom drape are folded over client's legs to provide access to body support; the body support is placed under the client's knees.

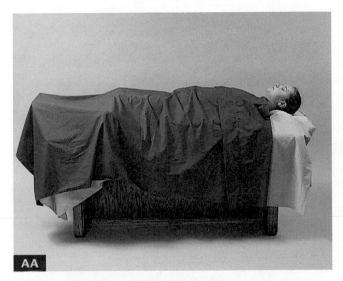

AA

Client is fully draped in supine position.

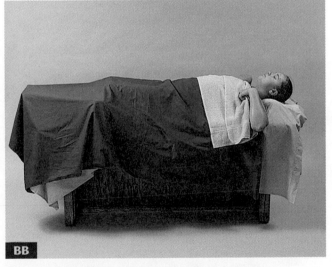

BB

Towel is placed on the client's chest over the top drape. Client holds the towel in place.

Continued.

fig. 8-12, cont'd

Samples of draping sequences using sheets and towels

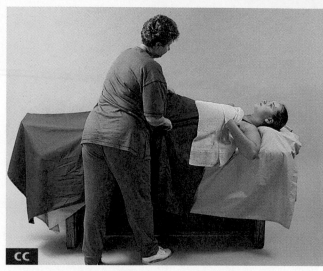

CC

The practitioner pulls the top of the drape from under the towel to provide access to the abdomen.

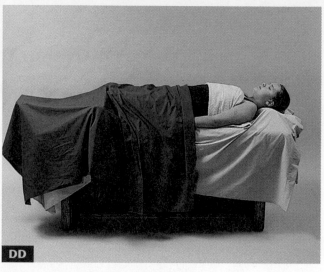

DD

Drape is repositioned over towel.

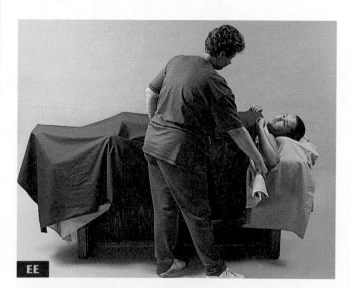

EE

Towel is removed from underneath the drape.

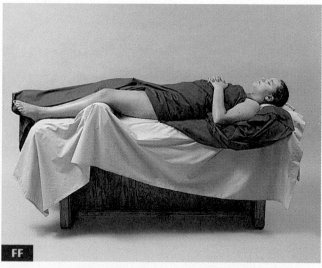

FF

The lower corner of the top drape is folded diagonally to provide access to client's leg.

fig. 8-12, cont'd

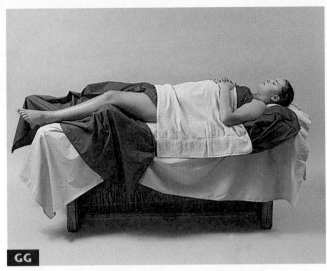

GG

Top drape is positioned under the client's leg and secured by the leg. Towel is placed over the client's abdomen and groin.

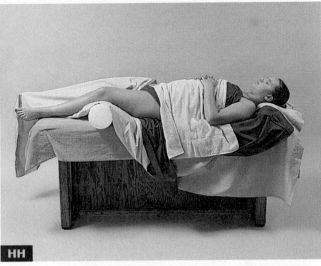

HH

Lower corner of bottom drape is brought under the leg diagonally and draped over the opposite leg. This exposes the secondary sanitary bottom drape. Notice that the client's leg does not touch the body support. This draping provides a secure groin covering during massaging, stretching, or providing range of motion to the leg.

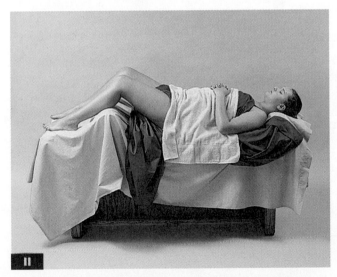

II

Alternate leg draping to provide access to both legs and to provide groin draping. Client bends knees and both end corners of the drape are folded diagonally and positioned between the knees. The corners are spread at either side of the table.

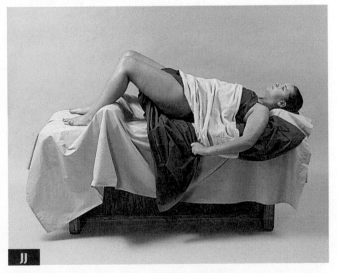

JJ

Client grasps each corner, lifts buttocks, and pulls drape under them.

Continued.

fig. 8-12, cont'd

Samples of draping sequences using sheets and towels

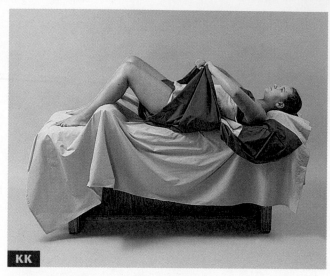

KK

Client or practitioner can then tie the ends together to secure the drape.

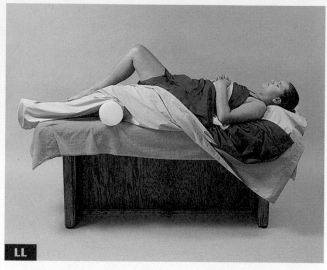

LL

One leg is lowered and the bottom drape is used to cover it, leaving only the area to be massaged exposed.

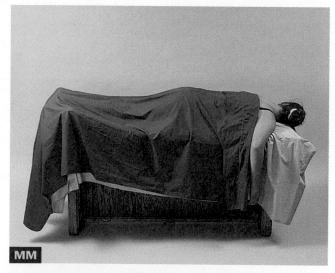

MM

Client prone and fully draped.

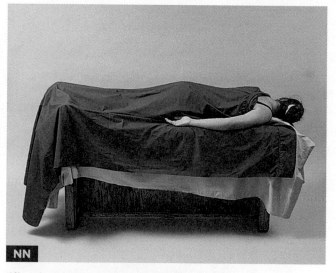

NN

Client's arm is positioned outside drape.

fig. 8-12, cont'd

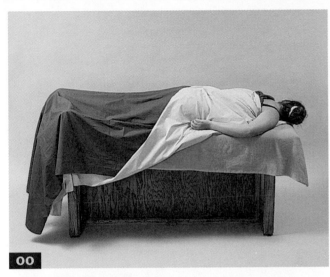

OO

The corners of both the top and bottom drapes are folded diagonally under the arm and over the back.

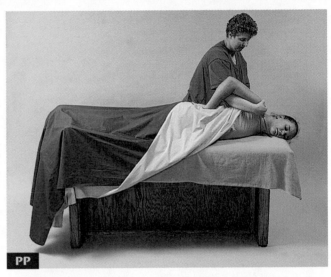

PP

Practitioner secures the bottom drape while moving the shoulder and arm.

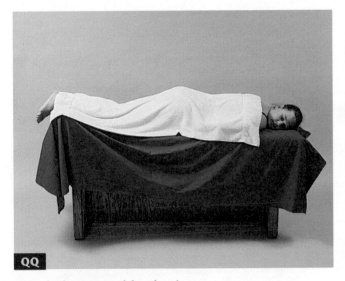

QQ

Use of a large towel for draping.

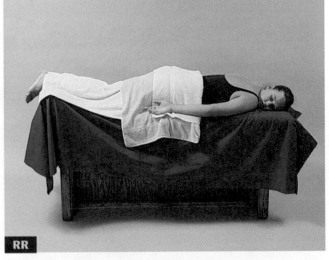

RR

Bath-size towel is placed over gluteal area for additional drape while top of towel is folded back to provide access to the client's back.

Continued.

f i g . 8 - 1 2, cont'd

Samples of draping sequences using sheets and towels

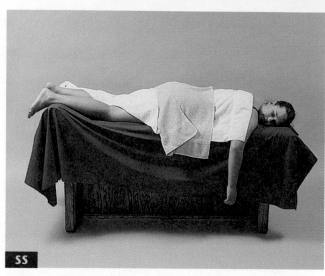

SS

Back is redraped and end corners of towel are folded diagonally to provide access to legs.

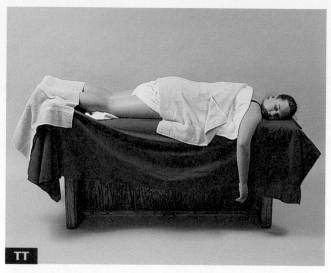

TT

Folded towel ends are placed between the client's knees, and additional towel is added to cover the feet.

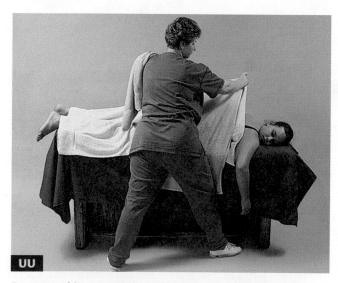

UU

Foot towel is removed, and large and small towel are secured against the table by the practitioner's knee and lifted to allow the client to turn to side position.

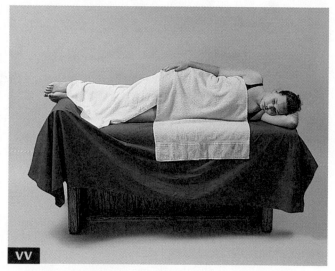

VV

Large towel and bath-size towel are repositioned over client.

fig. 8-12, cont'd

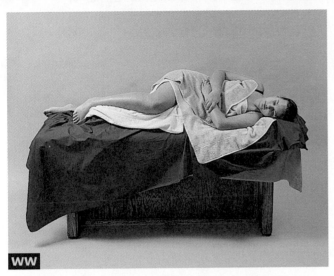

WW

Large towel end corner is folded diagonally to provide access to top leg and brought under top leg to be secured between leg and support under bent knee. Additional bath towel is placed over gluteal region.

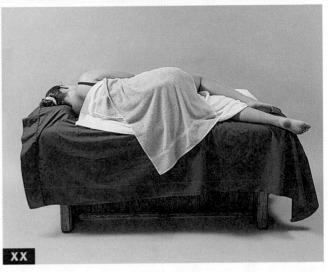

XX

Back view.

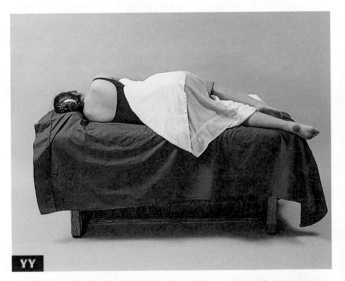

YY

Top end of drape folded diagonally to provide access to back.

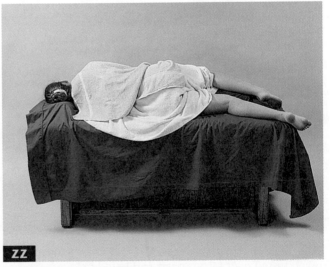

ZZ

Drape over gluteal area and bottom lower leg folded up to provide access to bottom leg.

Continued.

fig. 8-12, cont'd

Samples of draping sequences using sheets and towels

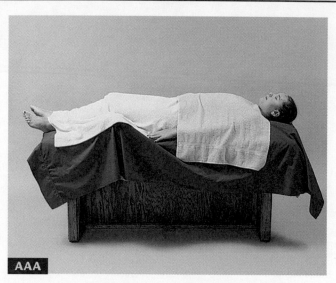

AAA

Client draped with towels in supine position.

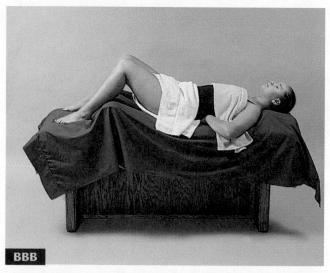

BBB

Client draped to provide access to abdomen and legs. Towel is used over large towel and held in place by the client as the practitioner pulls the large towel under and folds it back to expose the abdomen. Bottom ends of large towel are diagonally folded in and placed between the client's knees with the ends at the side of the table so the client is able to grasp the ends of the towel and pull it under her, providing secure draping of the groin.

AFTER THE MASSAGE

When the massage is finished, the client should be left alone for 5 to 10 minutes to rest. If necessary, reenter the massage area to help the client off the table.

Helping the Client Off the Massage Table

Use the following procedure when helping a client off the table (Fig. 8-13):

1. Reach under the client's neck and knees.
2. Support the sheet loosely around the client's neck, and hold it so that it does not slip when the client is lifted.
3. Lift the client's torso off the table while swinging the knees around to the edge of the table. Make sure the client's arm is over your shoulder and not around your neck.
4. In case of dizziness, stabilize the client for a moment after she is in the seated position.
5. Still holding the sheet, help the client to a standing position.
6. Shift the position of the sheet so that the client can hold it securely.

In rare instances the client may need help dressing. Let the client do as much as possible. Be matter-of-fact and deliberate with any assistance.

If a client is left to get off the table alone, remind him of the following:

1. Roll to one side.
2. Use your arms to push to a seated position.
3. Sit for a minute before getting up.
4. Leave the sheets on the table.
5. Get dressed and return to the business area.

Closing the Session, Collecting the Fee, and Making the Next Appointment

When the client is dressed and ready to leave, make the next appointment or provide a written reminder if it already has been made. If the fee has not been collected in advance, the client should pay at this time.

Saying Good-Bye

After the massage is finished, do not linger in conversation. The attitude in the business area is one of courteous completion. It often is difficult to get a client to leave. After spending time in a comfortable, caring environment, many people want to talk. It is difficult to break this pattern when business picks up, so it is best to establish a short, consistent departure routine in the beginning. Peo-

fig. 8-13

Assisting a client off the massage table

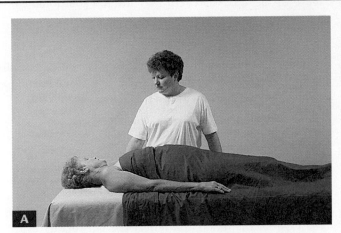

The procedure begins with the client prone.

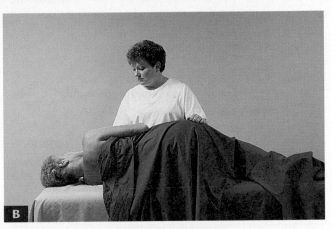

Client rolls to side and bends knees.

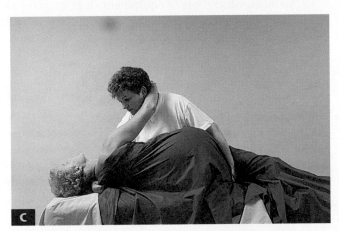

The client wraps her arm around the practitioner's shoulder (not the neck as shown in this illustration). The practitioner brings the sheet under the client's head and holds the front and back portions together while using the other hand behind the client's knees to provide support.

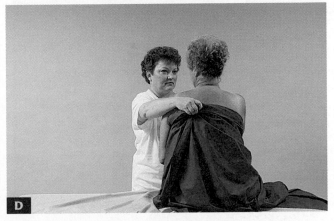

The practitioner lifts the client by standing up and leaning back while swinging the client's knees over the table to the seated position. The practitioner then adjusts the drape and assists the client from the table. The use of a foot stool for the client is helpful.

ple respond well to sameness. A client will get used to leaving and making the break from the massage practitioner in a reasonable period more easily if the sequence is always the same.

For example, the client approaches the desk, and the massage practitioner takes the money, writes a receipt, and confirms the next appointment. The massage practitioner gets up from the desk and says, "I really enjoyed working with you today. I am glad that you continue to feel that the massage is beneficial. It will be nice to see you again in 2 weeks. Remember to do the stretches we talked about, keep track of any changes, and we'll discuss them next time I see you."

The massage practitioner then extends a hand for a warm handshake. (In some situations, a quick, friendly hug is appropriate but *only* if initiated by the client and the practitioner is comfortable with the interaction. Pro-fessionally and respectfully accept hugs or physical contact initiated by the client.) Then say good-bye while gesturing or looking toward the door. At this point it is important for the massage practitioner to make a move to leave the area, or the client may initiate additional conversation.

After the Session

After the client has left, the practitioner should update all records, prepare the room for the next client, and attend to personal hygiene and self-care (Proficiency Exercise 8-8).

SUMMARY

The information discussed in this chapter is just as important as any other aspect of professional therapeutic massage. The different locations and environments for massage set the mood and reflect the personality of the massage practitioner.

Careful consideration of equipment (e.g., massage tables, body supports), supplies (e.g., oils, linens), music, and other amenities results in a professional yet personalized approach.

Taking time to explain massage procedures to a client, taking a basic history, and learning and understanding the expectations and outcome for each massage help create an approach that meets the client's needs. Providing safe, respectful touch by using careful, modest draping and positioning is very important.

This chapter has described professional skills that create the confidence, respect, and trust important to successful application of therapeutic massage. The professional massage practice requires attention to these details.

---

8 - 8

PROFICIENCY EXERCISE

1. Practice helping people off the massage table. Find 10 different body shapes and sizes to work with and note the difference in leverage needed for each client.
2. Write down your departure routine and practice it with other students. What will you do to end a massage session successfully with a client who does not want to leave? Have one of the students in your practice group role play this situation, and see how successful your procedure is.

WORKBOOK SECTION

Short Answer

1. What factors must be considered before the massage actually begins?

_____

_____

_____

_____

2. What is the most important piece of massage equipment?

_____

_____

_____

_____

3. How do massage practitioners protect their hands?

_____

_____

_____

_____

4. What types of massage equipment provide a surface that supports the client while the massage is given?

_____

_____

_____

_____

5. What features should be considered when looking for a massage table?

_____

_____

_____

6. What must be checked on the massage table to ensure the client's safety?

_____

_____

_____

_____

7. What are body supports?

_____

_____

_____

_____

8. What are drapes?

_____

_____

_____

_____

9. What types of draping materials are available?

_____

_____

_____

_____

10. What accommodation should be made for clients with sensitive skin?

_____

_____

_____

_____

WORKBOOK SECTION

11. What sanitary measures must be taken with draping materials?

_____

_____

_____

_____

12. What is the purpose of lubricants?

_____

_____

_____

_____

13. What types of lubricants are used?

_____

_____

_____

_____

14. What are some important things to remember about lubricants?

_____

_____

_____

_____

15. What are some general considerations for creating a professional massage environment?

_____

_____

_____

_____

16. What are the main types of massage environments?

_____

_____

_____

_____

17. What special considerations are needed with the use of music?

_____

_____

_____

_____

18. What considerations are needed with lighting in the massage room?

_____

_____

_____

_____

19. Why is a scentless environment so important?

_____

_____

_____

_____

20. What other considerations are necessary to ensure the client's comfort?

_____

_____

_____

_____

21. Why must the massage practitioner educate the client about appropriate expectations for the massage session?

_____

_____

_____

_____

22. Why should the massage practitioner carefully explain all procedures to the client before the massage?

_____

_____

_____

_____

WORKBOOK SECTION

23. What are the basic massage positions for a client, and how are body supports used in these positions?

_____

_____

_____

_____

24. What are the specific guidelines for draping?

_____

_____

_____

_____

25. In what way is the drape a type of boundary?

_____

_____

_____

_____

26. What are the two basic types of draping procedures?

_____

_____

_____

_____

27. How is a chest towel used?

_____

_____

_____

_____

28. How do you assist a client into a seated position?

_____

_____

_____

_____

29. What is the massage practitioner's attitude at the conclusion of the session?

_____

_____

_____

_____

30. After the client leaves, the massage practitioner should attend to what activities?

_____

_____

_____

_____

Problem-Solving Exercises

1. A client indicates on the client information form that he does not wish to have an oil-based lubricant used on his back, face, or chest. What are your options? List them on a separate piece of paper.
2. You are scheduled to travel to a client's home to do a massage. When you arrive you realize that there is no private location large enough to accommodate the massage table. What are some of your options? List them on a separate piece of paper.

Professional Application

You have been contracted to provide on-site massage in an office setting using a chair. Before you begin, you will have a chance to visit the location. On a separate piece of paper, list the specifics you will look for in locating the massage area, what supplies you need to include in the traveling office, and what materials you will need.

Research for Further Study

Check nursing texts and study the positioning and draping procedures; record any procedures that are applicable to massage.

WORKBOOK SECTION

ANSWER KEY
Short Answer

1. The set up of the massage area, supplies, client history and outcome, table supports for positioning, modest draping, types of lubricant, music, temperature of the massage area, and focus of the massage practitioner.
2. The massage practitioner's body, namely, the hands and forearms.
3. Always use proper body mechanics, warm up and stretch before beginning the massage, keep the hands and forearms clean and the nails carefully trimmed, and wear gloves when working outside or doing abrasive work.
4. Portable and free-standing massage tables, massage mats, massage chairs, and body supports for seated massage.
5. Simple, sturdy construction; portability if the table is to be moved often; a face cradle; adequate width and length; a washable covering; and adequate padding for comfort and firm support.
6. Structural stability, including all connectors, bolts, cables, and hinges.
7. Pillows, rolled towels, and specially cut pieces of foam are used to contour the flat surface of the massage table and provide stability and comfort.
8. Sheets, towels, or other large pieces of fabric used to cover the client during the massage to provide privacy, modesty, and warmth.
9. Cotton or cotton/polyester-blend sheets and towels and disposable linen.
10. Only white cotton sheets or towels are used to prevent possible allergic reactions.
11. All draping materials are laundered in bleach or other approved disinfecting solution. A fresh set of drapes always is used for each client.
12. Lubricants are used only to reduce friction on the skin from massage methods. Massage practitioners do not use lubricants for medicinal or cosmetic purposes.
13. Oils, creams, and powders.
14. Lubricants must be dispensed in a contamination-free manner, and they should be as natural as possible. Scents should be avoided, and powder should not be inhaled.
15. Temperature of 75° F, fresh air, designated areas for business operations and the massage session, and privacy if any clothing needs to be removed.
16. Private office or clinical setting, public setting, on-site at client's business or home, and outdoors.
17. Both the massage practitioner and the client must enjoy the music and want to listen to it. The rhythm and beat of the music must match the desired effect for the massage session.
18. The lighting must be indirect so that it does not cast a glare into the client's eyes. The practitioner also must be able to dim or reduce the intensity of the light, as well as increase it to provide visibility for cleaning the room. Practitioners never work in a dark or candlelit room.
19. Many people are sensitive to smells and chemical scents.
20. The massage practitioner must be attentive to cigarette or other smoke odors, cold hands, keeping pets out of the massage area, and other such considerations.
21. The client may have a specific medical focus for the massage that is outside the practitioner's scope of practice, or the client may have preconceived ideas that may interfere with the acceptance of the massage.
22. Clients respond better and are less anxious if they understand such procedural details as draping, where to hang their clothes, and what types of lubricant will be used. Conditions are safer for the practitioner and client if they both understand the use of the massage equipment, such as adjusting the face cradle on a table. The client then is better able to provide informed consent for the massage session.
23. Prone, with supports under the ankles and possibly around the chest. Supine, with supports under the knees and neck. Side-lying, with supports between the knees and under the arms and head.
24. Opaque materials must be used, and only the area being massaged is undraped. Neither the genital area nor a woman's breasts are ever undraped without a physician's supervision.
25. During a typical full-body massage, the client has removed most clothing. The drape is the separation from the massage practitioner and defines the personal space of the client.
26. Contour and flat draping.
27. A chest towel is used to drape women's breasts while the larger drape is pulled back to expose the abdomen. The towel is placed over the flat sheet and stabilized, and then the larger flat sheet is pulled out.

WORKBOOK SECTION

28. Place your arms under the client's neck and knees. Lift the torso and swing the knees to the side of the table. Be sure to secure the drapes so that they do not slip.

29. Polite and courteous completion. It is difficult for some clients to conclude the massage, and they may linger before leaving. Developing a sequence that is the same at the end of each massage helps the client break the contact that was created during the massage.

30. The practitioner washes his or her hands, updates the client's records, prepares the room for the next massage, and takes a small personal break. This takes about 15 minutes and should be considered in the scheduling of the massage sessions.

Problem-Solving Exercises

1. Powder or a water-based cream can be used during the massage. Compression-type massage over a clean sheet or towel can be done in these areas.

2. Switch to an over-the-clothing massage and ask the client to change into loose, nonrestrictive clothing. Turn the appointment into an educational session and teach others in the household some simple massage techniques. Do a seated massage in a private location.

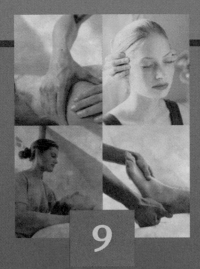

9

MASSAGE MANIPULATIONS AND TECHNIQUES

objectives

After completing this chapter, the student will be able to perform the following:

- Understand the basic theories for the physiologic effects of massage methods and techniques
- Organize massage methods and techniques into basic flow patterns
- Perform a full-body massage using the methods and techniques presented

Student note: Most models in this chapter are pictured in leotards or sportswear to enhance and clarify the various body positions. The properly groomed massage professional would, of course, wear a uniform as shown in Fig. 6-1 on p. 232. For draping procedures, see Chapter 8.

THIS core technical chapter includes definitions, descriptions, and directions for the application and use of the most common massage methods and techniques. The description of each massage approach incorporates background. As a therapeutic massage student, you must learn to problem solve, using clinical reasoning to generate variations of the application of the various massage methods. Massage routines offer limited benefits. Each session needs to be designed specifically for the individual client (see Chapter 10).

It is important to understand both why and where massage methods and techniques are used, and how to organize a process that uses the various therapeutic approaches efficiently. The next step is to examine each of the individual massage manipulations and techniques and learn to use them well. In the practice of therapeutic massage, practitioners use their fingers, thumbs, hands, forearms, and, for methods such as shiatsu, the knees and feet. This chapter focuses on methods that use the fingers, thumbs, hands, and forearms. You should always stay mindful of how to best use your body when applying massage manipulations and techniques (see Chapter 7).

The massage professional uses a structured, purposeful application of various forms of touch for specific reasons. Since the late 1800s these massage manipulations have used the French names of *effleurage, pétrissage, compression, vibration, tapotement,* and *friction.* The current trend is to use English descriptions; both are acceptable.

Mosby's Medical, Nursing, and Allied Health Dictionary[1] defines *manipulation* as "the skillful use of the hands in therapeutic or diagnostic procedures . . . see also massage." The same reference defines *massage* as "the manipulation of the soft tissue of the body through stroking, rubbing, kneading, or tapping." The word *manipulation* is used in this chapter to indicate each of these methods.

It is important to differentiate between the soft tissue manipulations of the massage professional and the joint manipulations of the chiropractor, osteopath, or physical therapist. The massage professional does not perform specific, direct joint manipulations. Massage techniques presented in this text incorporate passive and active joint movement within the comfortable limits of the joint, as well as lengthening and stretching methods. These may indirectly affect the range of motion of a joint through changes in the soft tissue. The particular focus of the massage professional is on the soft tissue and not the osseous structure of the joint.

Often a combination of soft tissue work and specific joint manipulation is required to achieve the functional goals of the client. In these instances the massage practitioner, with appropriate training, becomes part of the multidisciplinary team under the supervision of the health care professional. This team approach provides the skills and expertise of multiple professionals to best serve the client.

PHYSIOLOGIC EFFECTS

section objectives

Using the information presented in this section the student will be able to perform the following:

- Categorize the effects of massage methods and techniques into stimulating or inhibiting physiologic responses
- Classify massage manipulations and techniques into three categories based on reflexive, mechanical, and chemical effects

In general, massage manipulations and techniques either stimulate or inhibit a response. Simply stated, imbalances fall into two categories: "too much" or "not enough." Massage methods assist the body in restoration of balance by inhibition of "too much" conditions and by stimulation of "not enough" conditions. When thinking in terms of muscle responses, think of contraction or relaxation (reduction of the neural stimulation causing contraction) of the muscle with imbalance reflected as either a too tight or strong muscle or a too relaxed or weak muscle. Connective tissue methods deal with tissue that is too hard, too soft, too thick, or too thin. Circulation may have a rushing fluid flow or a sluggish fluid flow. With nervous system activity, think of overactivity or underactivity.

All massage methods use some form of external sensory information that can stimulate or inhibit body processes, depending on their use. Some methods are better at stimulation and others are better at inhibition. Some work better with mechanical effects, others with reflexive effects, and still others are better at initiating chemical responses. In general, fast, specific application of methods tends to stimulate, whereas slow general applications tend to inhibit.

It is not easy to generalize the mechanical, reflexive, or chemical effect of massage manipulations and techniques. It is often the combination of the effects of massage, coupled with the client's psychologic state and receptivity to the massage that causes the response.

Consider these general guidelines:

- Methods that move through the skin to the underlying tissue tend to be more mechanical and stimulate localized chemical responses.
- Massage manipulations and techniques that stay within the skin and superficial fascial layer tend to have a more direct reflexive effect on the nervous system because many sensory nerves are located in the skin. These methods also tend to stimulate the release of hormonal and other body chemicals that provide for a general systemic (whole-body) effect.
- Methods that move the body, cause muscles to contract and relax and joint positions to change, and deliver sensory input to the proprioceptors are more reflexive in nature.

- Methods that stretch (pull on) soft tissues are reflexive, mechanical, and chemical.

QUALITY OF TOUCH

section objectives

Using the information presented in this section, the student will be able to perform the following:

- ■ **Evaluate massage manipulations based on seven criteria**
- ■ **Effectively establish and adjust the physical contact with the client**

Gertrude Beard (1887-1971), one of the most respected educators in massage therapy as an integral part of physical therapy, described the components of massage as follows[4]:

The factors that must be considered as components in the application of massage techniques are: the direction of the movement, the amount of pressure, the rate and rhythm of the movements, the medium used, the frequency and duration of the treatment, the position of the patient and of the physical massage practitioner.

Beard's definition of *medium* was related to the application of lubricants or other instruments used. The definition of *frequency* reflected how often per day or week the massage was given. Individual massage methods vary in relation to the depth of pressure, drag, direction, speed, rhythm, frequency, and duration. From Beard's information and other sources, the following components for the quality of touch are considered in this textbook:

- **Depth of pressure** (compressive stress) can be light, moderate, deep, or variable.
- **Drag** is the amount of pull (stretch) on the tissue (tensile stress).
- **Direction** can move from the center of the body out (centrifugal) or in from the extremities toward the center of the body (centripetal). It can proceed from origin to insertion of the muscle following the muscle fibers, transverse to the tissue fibers, or in circular motions.
- **Speed** of manipulations can be fast, slow, or variable.
- **Rhythm** refers to the regularity of application of the technique. If the method is applied at regular intervals, it is considered even or rhythmic. If the method is disjointed or irregular, it is considered uneven or nonrhythmic.
- **Frequency** is the rate at which the method repeats itself in a given timeframe. In general, each method is repeated about three times before moving or switching to a different approach.
- **Duration** is the length of time that the method lasts or the manipulation stays in the same location.

Establishing and Adjusting Physical Contact

It is necessary to make contact with the client's body in a secure and confident way. Be sure the client is verbally informed that you are about to touch, that the approach of the touch is steady and not abrupt, and that your hands are warm.

After touch contact has been made with the client and the massage has begun, the *intention* of the contact should not be broken. *This means that the massage practitioner remains focused on the client for the entire session. Maintaining contact does not mean that the practitioner never removes his or her hands from the client.* It is nearly impossible to drape effectively or have the client change position or the practitioner change position to reapply lubricant without removing the practitioner's hands from the client's body. When the hands are removed, simply establish verbal contact by telling the client that you will be removing your hands for a moment, shifting the draping or altering position. Before reestablishing touch, again tell the client that you will be touching him and where so that he does not startle. Centering as presented in the preceding chapter facilitates this process of remaining focused on the client.

BASIC FLOW

section objectives

Using the information presented in this section, the student will be able to perform the following:

- ■ **Organize a massage sequence in four basic patterns**
- ■ **Use a specific massage pattern on the abdomen**

Organization of the various massage manipulations and techniques follows a cohesive pattern. During a full-body massage, all the soft tissues are addressed and the joints are moved within the limits of the client's comfortable range of motion. The following section provides some simple suggestion for organized flow patterns around the body. Some students will find these simple guidelines helpful, whereas others find it easy to develop a structure themselves. For purposes of learning, it is helpful to begin with four general patterns and then modify them as desired. Remember, these suggested flow patterns are only a place to begin to understand the organization of the application of massage.

The four patterns presented cover the client's beginning position as prone, supine, side-lying, and seated. The sequence used on the abdomen always remains the same.

The illustrations depict various ways to position and approach the body using massage. The different approaches can be combined in many different ways to create different massage patterns. It may be helpful to study the illustrations and incorporate the suggestions into your practice massage sessions. Use the illustrations while generating your own ideas and be open to experimentation, creation, and modification of massage applications based on individual clients according to body shape, style of massage, and equipment available.

Pattern 1: Prone Position (*Fig. 9-1*)

Beginning point BACK. Ending point FACE.
   Sequence:
   Left side back
   Left side gluteal region
   Move to head and contact both sides of back
   Neck
   Move to right side
   Right side back
   Right side gluteal region
   Right leg back
   Move to feet
   Contact both legs from back
   Move to left side
   Left leg back
   (Turn client to supine position)
   Right foot
   Right leg front
   Left foot
   Left leg front
   (Have client bend knees to prepare for abdominal massage)
   (Abdominal sequence)
   Left arm and hand
   Left shoulder and upper thorax (chest)
   Right arm and hand

---

fig. 9-1

Pattern 1: Prone position. Beginning point BACK. Ending point FACE

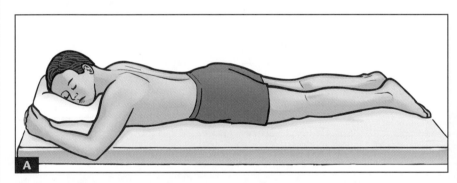

A Prone position.

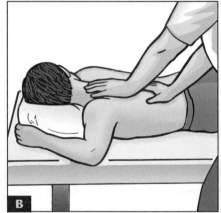

B Left side back.

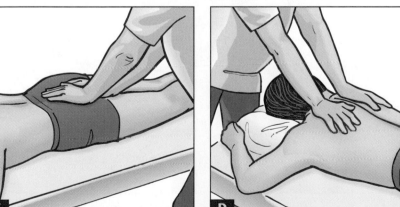

C Left side gluteal region.

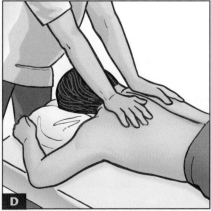

D Move to head and contact both sides of back.

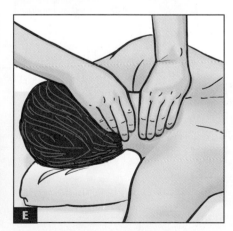

E Neck.

Continued.

fig. 9-1, cont'd

Pattern 1: Prone position. Beginning point BACK. Ending point FACE

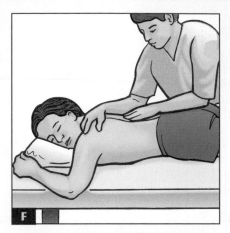

F Move to right side. Right side back.

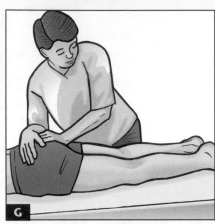

G Right side gluteal region.

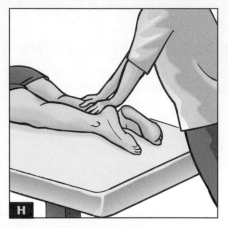

H Right leg back.

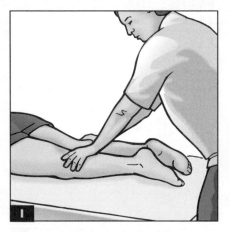

I Move to feet. Contact both legs.

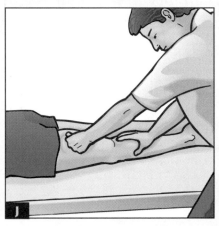

J Move to left side. Left leg back.

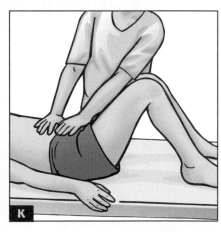

K Turn client to supine position.

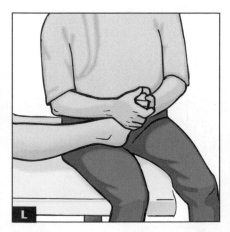

L Right foot.

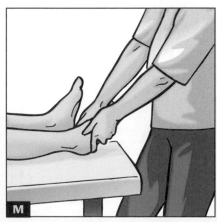

M Right foot continued.

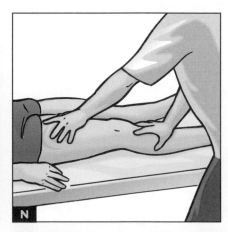

N Right leg front.

f i g . 9 - 1, cont'd

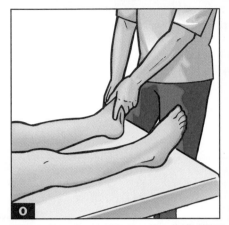

Left foot.

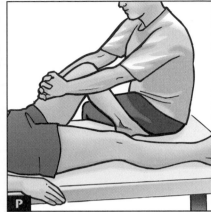

Left leg front.

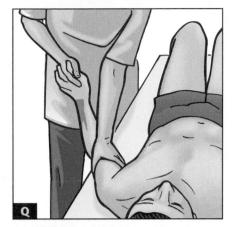

Left arm and hand.

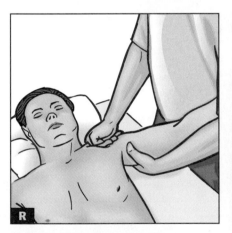

Left shoulder and upper thorax (chest).

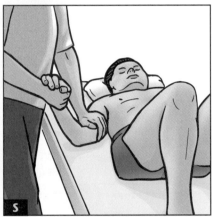

Right arm and hand.

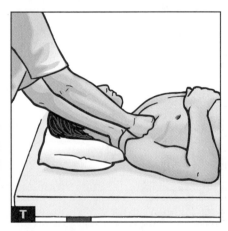

Right shoulder and upper thorax.

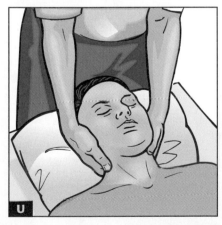

Neck.

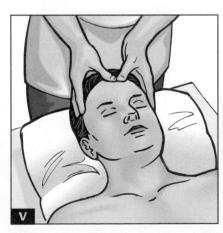

Head.

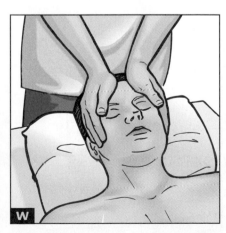

Face.

Right shoulder and upper thorax
Neck
Head
Face

Pattern 2: Supine Position *(Fig. 9-2)*

Beginning point FACE. Ending point BACK.
   Sequence:
   Face
   Head

Neck
Right shoulder and upper thorax
Right arm and hand
Left shoulder and upper thorax
Left arm and hand
(Have client bend knees to prepare for abdominal work)
(Left side for abdominal work [see special section for
    pattern for abdominal work])
Left leg in bent position
Front upper left leg
Medial upper left leg

---

fig. 9-2

Pattern 2: Supine position. Beginning point FACE. Ending point BACK

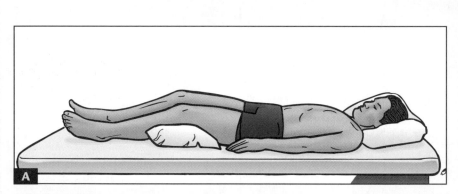

A Supine position.

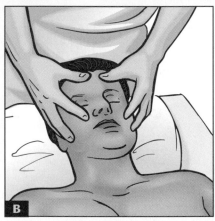

B Face.

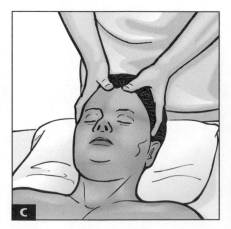

C Head.

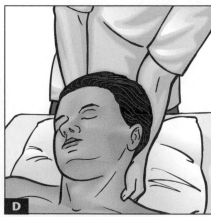

D Neck.

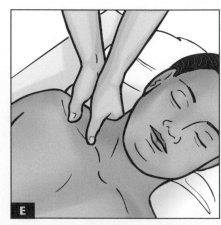

E Right shoulder and upper thorax.

Lateral upper left leg
Back upper left leg
Back lower left leg
Lateral lower left leg
Straighten left leg
Left foot
Right leg in bent position
Front upper right leg
Medial upper right leg
Lateral upper right leg
Back upper right leg

Back lower right leg
Lateral lower right leg
Straighten right leg
Right foot
(Turn client to prone position)
Right gluteal region
Right back
Left gluteal region
Left back
Neck
Head

f i g . 9 - 2, cont'd

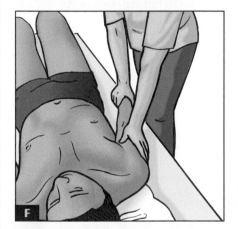

Right arm and hand.

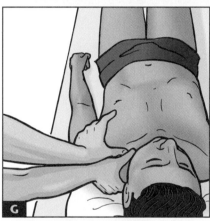

Left shoulder and upper thorax.

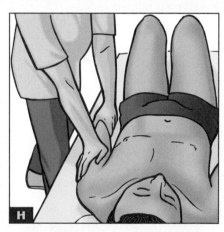

Left arm and hand. At this point, have client bend knees to prepare for abdominal work. From this position, begin abdominal work (see Fig. 9-5, abdominal sequence).

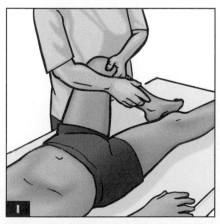

Left leg in bent position. Front upper left leg.

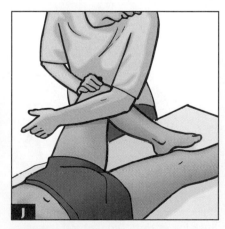

Medial upper left leg.

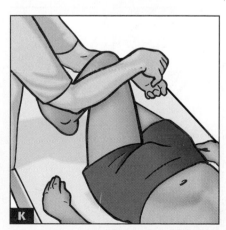

Lateral upper left leg.

Continued.

fig. 9-2, cont'd
Pattern 2: Supine position. Beginning point FACE. Ending point BACK

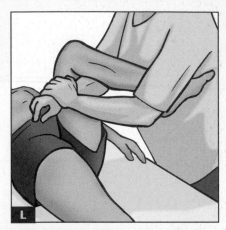

Back upper left leg.

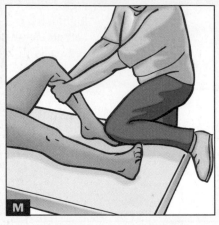

Back lower left leg. Lateral lower left leg.

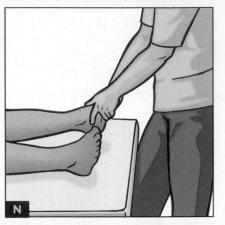

Straighten left leg. Left foot.

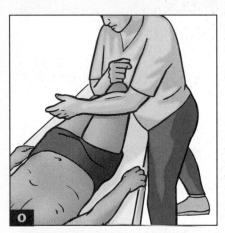

Right leg in bent position. Front upper right leg.

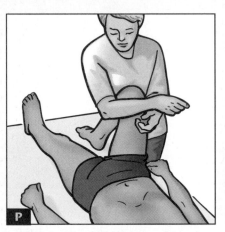

Medial upper right leg.

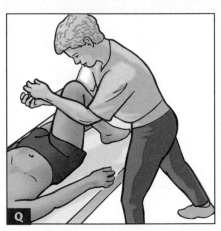

Lateral upper right leg.

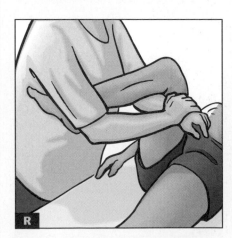

Back upper right leg.

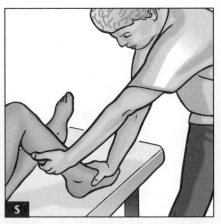

Back lower right leg. Lateral lower right leg.

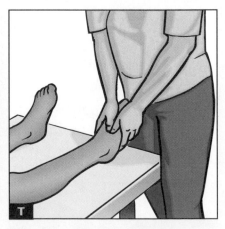

Straighten right leg. Right foot.

fig. 9-2, cont'd

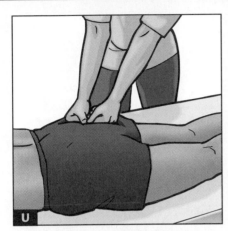

U Turn client to prone position. Right gluteal region.

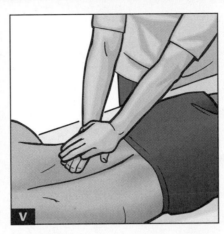

V Right back.

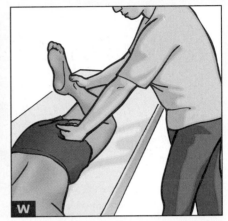

W Left gluteal region.

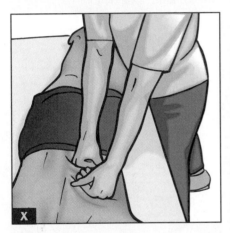

X Left back.

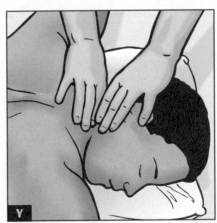

Y Neck.

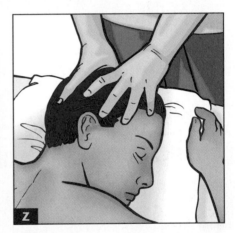

Z Head.

Pattern 3: Side-Lying Position (Fig. 9-3)

Beginning point HEAD. Ending point HEAD.
   Sequence:
   (Client lies on left side with right knee bent and supported)
Right side head
Right side face
Right side neck
Right side shoulder and upper thorax
Right arm and hand
Right side back
(Abdominal sequence)
Right side gluteal
Right back leg

Right lateral leg
Left medial leg
Left foot
(Turn client to right side with left leg bent and supported)
Right foot
Right medial leg
Left lateral leg
Left back leg
Left side gluteal
Left side back
Left side arm and hand
Left side shoulder and upper thorax
Left side neck
Left side head
Left side face

fig. 9-3

Pattern 3: Side-lying position. Beginning point HEAD. Ending point HEAD

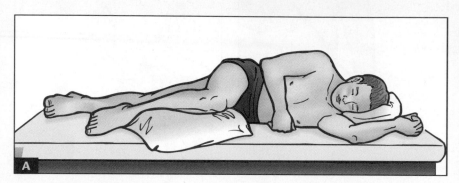

Side-lying position.

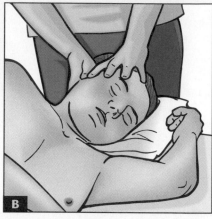

Client lies on left side with right knee bent and supported (legs not pictured). Right side head.

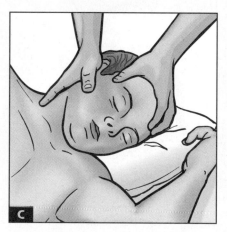

Right side face.

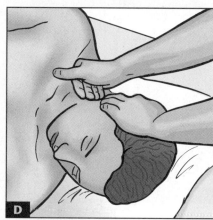

Right side neck.

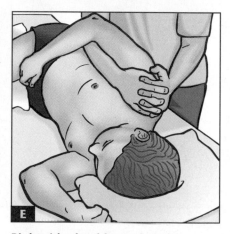

Right side shoulder and upper thorax.

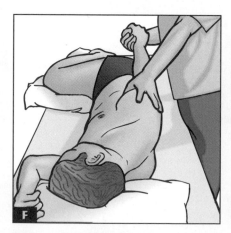

Right arm and hand.

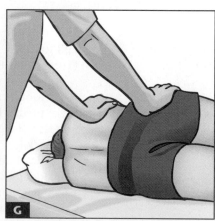

Right side back.

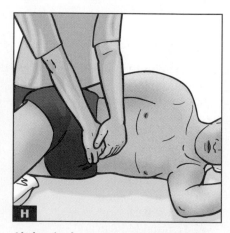

Abdominal sequence (see Fig. 9-5).

f i g . 9 - 3, cont'd

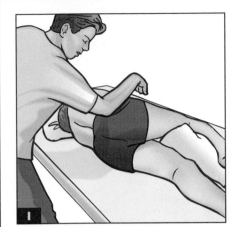

Right side gluteal.

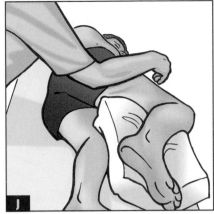

Right back leg.

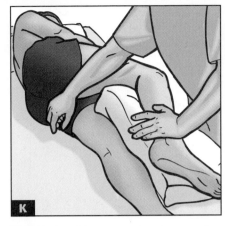

Right lateral leg.

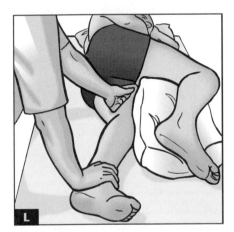

Left medial leg.

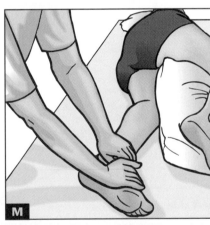

Left foot.

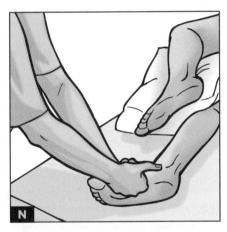

Turn client to right side with left leg bent and supported. Right foot.

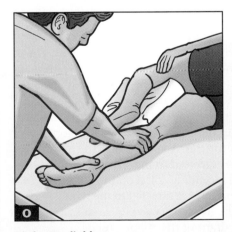

Right medial leg.

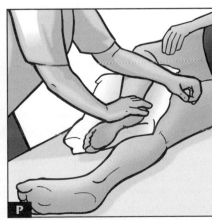

Left lateral leg.

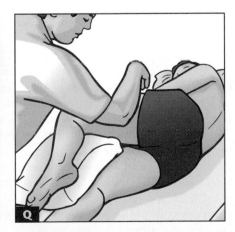

Left back leg.

Continued.

fig. 9-3, cont'd

Pattern 3: Side-lying position. Beginning point HEAD. Ending point HEAD

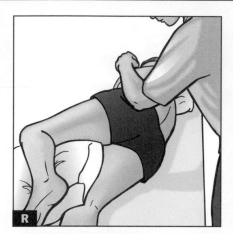

Left side gluteal.

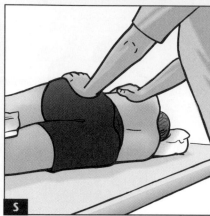

Left side back.

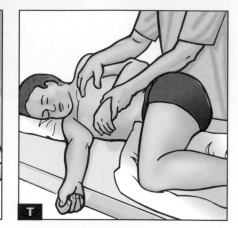

Left side arm and hand.

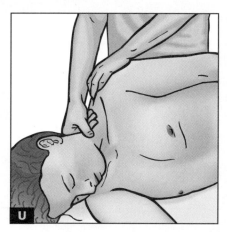

Left side shoulder and upper thorax.

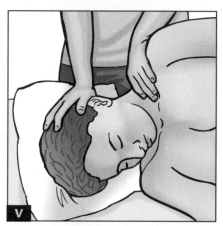

Left side neck.

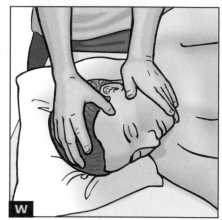

Left side head. Left side face.

Abdominal Sequence

Not all research agrees that massage has a substantial effect on peristalsis or even that the mechanical emptying of the colon is possible. Regardless of whether the researchers agree, it seems prudent with abdominal massage to approach the area as though massage does have an effect. Theoretically, to support peristalsis and mechanical emptying of the colon, all massage manipulations are directed in a clockwise fashion. To avoid any chance of impaction of fecal material, the manipulations begin in the lower right-hand quadrant at the sigmoid colon. The methods progressively contact the large intestine and eventually end up encompassing the entire colon area (Fig. 9-4).

Standing on the left side of the body when the client is in the supine position facilitates the body mechanics of the practitioner (Fig. 9-5). When the client is lying on his or her left side, body mechanics for the massage practitioner and elimination patterns are most efficient. The direction of flow for emptying of the large intestine and colon is as follows:

1. Massage down the left side of the descending colon, using short strokes directed to the sigmoid colon.
2. Massage across the transverse colon to the left side, using short strokes directed to the sigmoid colon.
3. Massage up the ascending colon on the right side of the body, using short strokes directed to the sigmoid colon.
4. End at the right ileocecal valve located in the lower right-hand quadrant of the abdomen.
5. Massage the entire flow pattern using long, light to moderate strokes from the ileocecal valve to the sigmoid colon. Repeat the sequence.

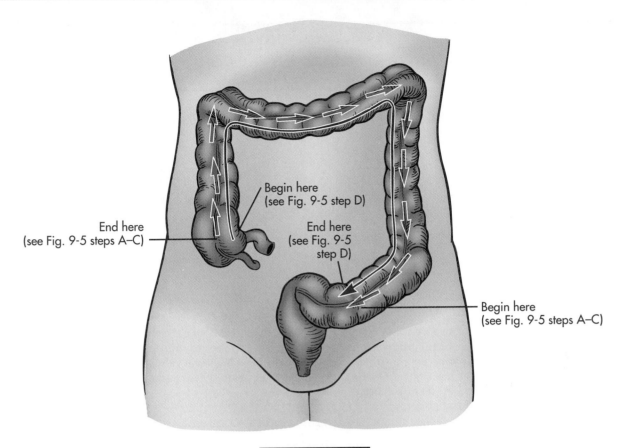

fig. 9-4

Colon with flow pattern arrows. All massage manipulations are to be directed in a clockwise fashion. The manipulations begin in the lower left-hand quadrant (on the right side as you view the illustration) at the sigmoid colon. The methods progressively contact all of the large intestine as they eventually end up encompassing the entire colon area.

fig. 9-5

Abdominal sequence. The direction of flow for emptying the large intestine and colon

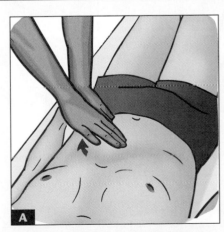

A

Massage down the left side of the descending colon using short strokes directed to the sigmoid colon.

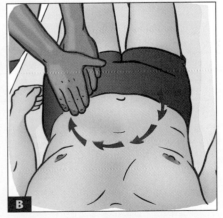

B

Massage across along the transverse colon to the left side using short strokes directed to the sigmoid colon.

Continued.

fig. 9-5, cont'd

Abdominal sequence. The direction of flow for emptying the large intestine and colon

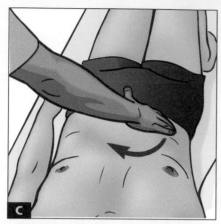

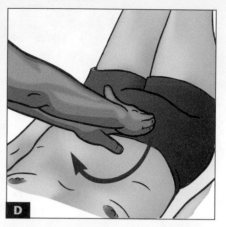

Massage up the ascending colon on the right side of the body using short strokes directed to the sigmoid colon. End at the right side ileocecal valve located in the lower right quadrant of the abdomen.

Massage entire flow pattern using long, light strokes to moderate strokes from ileocecal valve to sigmoid colon. Repeat sequence.

A   **B**   **C**

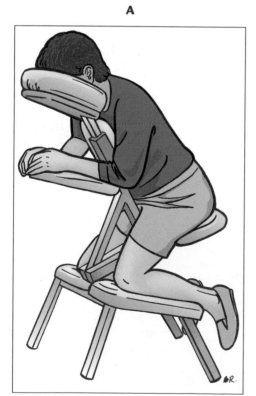

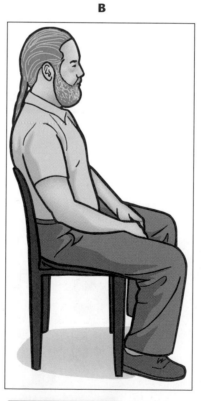

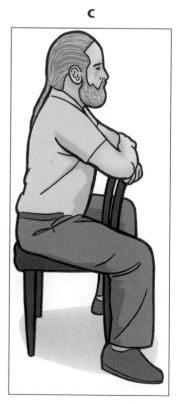

fig. 9-6

Seated massage may be performed in either a specially designed massage chair (**A**) or in straight-back chairs without arms (**B** and **C**).

Pattern 4: Seated Pattern
(Figs. 9-6 and 9-7)

It is important to be able to work efficiently when the client is seated. Specially designed massage chairs position the client comfortably and conveniently, but do not depend on such equipment. A regular straight-back chair can be used successfully; have the client sit facing the back of the chair. Use a pillow on the back of the chair so that he or she can lean comfortably.

In this position, which is not used for full-body massage, the clothing is left on. The focus is usually on the upper body only, but with practice the legs and feet can be addressed as well.

Beginning point HEAD. Ending point FEET.
Sequence:
Head
Face
Neck
Shoulders
Back—both sides simultaneously
Left arm
Right arm
Left lower leg and foot
Right lower leg and foot

Combination of Positions

It is appropriate to develop a combination of the prone, supine, side-lying, and seated positions during the massage session. As you will remember from Chapter 8, client comfort is important when using positioning and supports. Clients may appreciate a positional shift during the massage to maintain general comfort levels. Inquire about client comfort approximately every 15 minutes (Proficiency Exercise 9-1).

---

fig. 9-7

Pattern 4: Seated position. Seated in a regular chair. Begin at HEAD. End at FEET

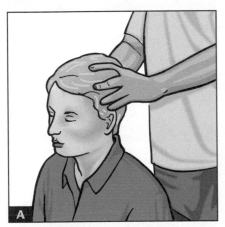
Head.

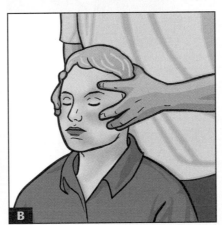
Face.

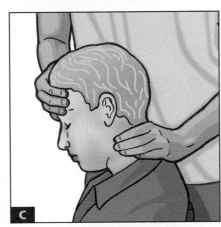
Neck.

Continued.

9-1

PROFICIENCY EXERCISE

Practice efficiency of movement and ease of positional shift by walking through the patterns. Do not do any massage at this point. Only touch the areas and position the body. Use each massage method illustrated with an entire-body focus for all four basic flow patterns.

For example, first move around the entire body using Pattern 1. The only technique used is the resting position (laying on of hands). Then use the resting position for the entire sequence of Patterns 2, 3, and 4. Repeat this exercise with effleurage, pétrissage, compression, and other manipulations.

f i g . 9 - 7, cont'd

Pattern 4: Seated position. Seated in a regular chair. Begin at HEAD. End at FEET

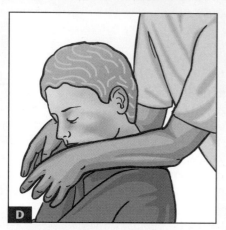

Shoulders (forearm position).

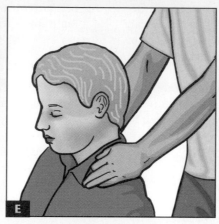

Shoulders (hand position).

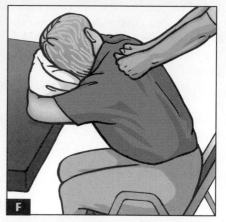

Back—both sides simultaneously.

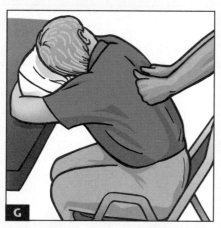

Back—both sides simultaneously, continued.

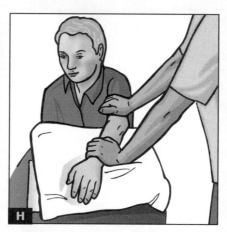

Left arm.

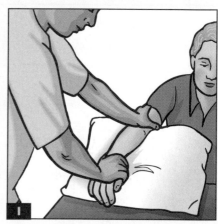

Right arm.

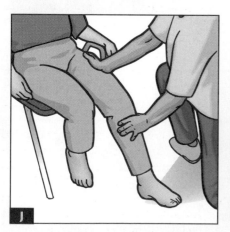

Lower left leg.

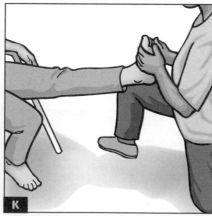

Left foot.

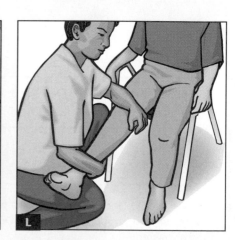

Right lower leg.

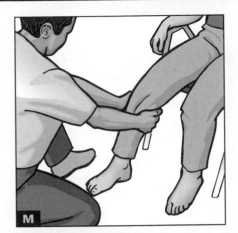

Right lower leg, continued.

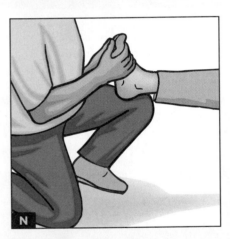

Right foot.

MASSAGE MANIPULATIONS

section objectives

Using the information presented in this section, the student will be able to perform the following:

- Perform eight basic massage manipulations
- Combine the eight massage manipulations into a basic full-body massage

Albert Baumgartner, in his 1947 book *Massage in Athletics*,[2] quotes Plato as saying "Massage must be simple." Baumgartner also says that "Many endeavor to introduce improvements into the science of massage but fail to gain adherents to their preventive methods. It would be well to advise these witty inventors of the new sub-methods to keep their improvements to themselves."

The massage manipulations and techniques in this textbook are explained and organized in a manner that consolidates, condenses, and simplifies therapeutic massage methods based on what seems to be the consensus from the historical material and currently accepted terminology and theory.

Massage Manipulation Terminology

In 1879, the terms *effleurage, pétrissage, friction,* and *tapotement* first appeared in the *VonMosegeil* (Proceedings of German Society for Surgery) to describe Mezger's methods. Since then, almost every textbook on massage has included these terms.[2] Kellogg described the resting position in terms of passive touch.[6] Most textbooks do not separate superficial stroking from effleurage, and many describe compression by classifying it as part of pétrissage or pressure. Current trends separate the methods of compression into a distinct description. The majority of references agree on "tapotement" or "percussion," yet resources seem evenly split between "vibration" or "shaking," being classified separately or together. "Friction" is classified many different ways but is usually defined with similar terms. This textbook refers to passive movements by the names developed through Ling and Mezger's work in combination with current usage; these are listed in the massage manipulations section. Active movements or gymnastics, as defined by Ling, Taylor, and others, are listed in the massage techniques section using current terminology.

Resting Position

The act of placing your hands on another person seems so simple, yet this initial contact must be made with respect and a client-centered focus. With the **resting position** technique, we enter the client's personal boundary space, as defined by sensitivity to changes in air movement and heat picked up by the sensory receptors in the skin. The root hair plexus is one of the most sensitive receptors to movement of air. Activation of the heat sensors indicates that something is close enough to cause physical harm. Because of these sensors, the fight-or-flight responses of the sympathetic autonomic nervous system are often activated with the initial contact.

Because of the instinctual survival and protective mechanisms designed to protect human beings from hand-to-hand combat, our physiologic safety zone is generally an arm's length. If another person is at this distance, the sensory mechanisms of sympathetic arousal are less sensitive than if the person is close enough to touch. This is why the first approach to touch by the massage professional is so important. The *resting position* provides time for the client to become acclimated to the proximity of another human being. It gives the client time to evaluate, on a subconscious level, whether this touch is safe. This first application of touch sets the stage for the first 15 to 30 minutes of the massage because it takes that long for the fight-or-flight response, which causes adrenaline to be released into the blood, to reverse itself.

The resting position also allows stillness when intermixed with the other movements of massage. The body needs time to process all the sensory information it receives during massage. Stopping the motions and simply resting the hands on the body provides for this moment of stillness.

The resting position is an excellent way to call attention to an area through stimulation of the cutaneous (skin) sensory receptors. Simple, sustained touch over an area of imbalance is often enough stimulation to cause a reflexive response. This position also adds body heat from the massage practitioner's hand to an area of the client's body. Additionally, it is an excellent way to reestablish contact with the client if the flow of the massage is interrupted or physical contact is broken.

How to Apply the Resting Position

An open, soft, relaxed, warm, and dry hand is best for application of the resting position. It is a signal to our survival mechanism that no weapon is nearby nor any intent to strike. A cool and clammy hand suggests sympathetic activation in the practitioner. Subconscious survival mechanisms in the client will recognize this and respond to perceived danger by tensing for protection.

Practice extending an open, relaxed hand. Rub your hands together to warm them, and then towel-dry them before touching the client.

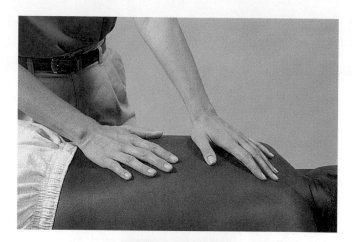

fig. 9-8

Open, relaxed hands.

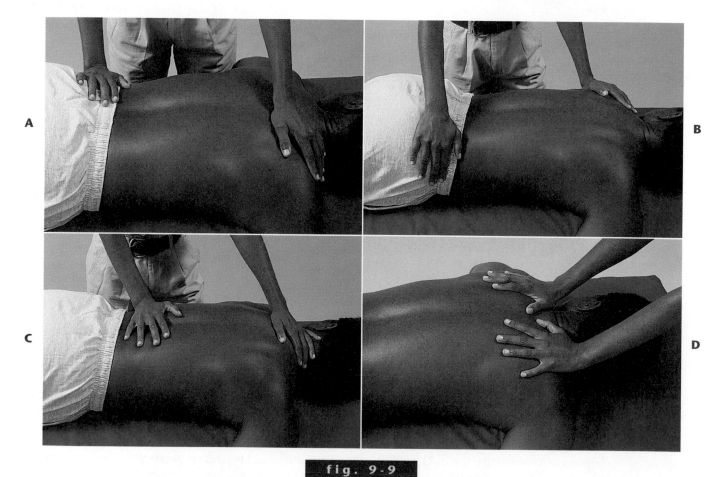

fig. 9-9

Four examples of the resting position on the back.

In most circumstances, a slow, steady approach by the practitioner with deliberate hesitation at the arm's-length boundary, coupled with a verbal announcement that you will begin touching, is the best way to avoid excessive sympathetic arousal. Most of the time the restorative parasympathetic state is what the massage practitioner seeks to activate for the client. Yet even in a situation in which the massage is designed to stimulate sympathetic activation, the first touch should be slow, gradual, and deliberate (Fig. 9-8).

Apply the resting position slowly and gradually, in a confident and secure manner. As part of the survival mechanism, the body will innately respond to a hesitant touch by withdrawing. An unsure touch is difficult to interpret and is unsettling to the client. When the application of the resting position is mastered, it is easy to flow into the other methods (Fig. 9-9) (Proficiency Exercise 9-2).

Effleurage, or Gliding Strokes

The current term for **effleurage** is "gliding stroke." Effleurage originates from the French verb meaning "to skim" and "to touch lightly on." The most superficial applications of this stroke do this, but the full spectrum of effleurage is determined by pressure, drag, speed, direction, and rhythm, making this manipulation one of the most versatile.

After the application of the initial touch or resting position, effleurage is often next in sequence, especially if a lubricant is used. The long, broad movement of this method is excellent for spreading the lubricant on the skin surface. The ease of the application makes this an effective manipulation to use repetitively while gradually increasing the depth of pressure. This is one of the preferred manipulations to warm or prepare the tissue for more specific bodywork. Because of the horizontal nature of the manipulation, the flow pattern of the massage can progress smoothly from one body area to another. It is a good method to use when evaluating for hard and soft tissue, hot and cold areas, or areas that seem stuck. Effleurage is also the preferred method for abdominal massage and massage to facilitate circulation.

The more superficial the stroke, the more reflexive the effect. Slow superficial strokes are very soothing, whereas fast superficial strokes are stimulating. If a deeper stroke pressure with a slower rate of application is used, the effect will be more mechanical.

How to Apply Effleurage, or Gliding Strokes

The distinguishing characteristic of effleurage, or gliding strokes, is that it is applied horizontally in relation to the tissues (Fig. 9-10).

During effleurage/gliding stroke, light pressure remains on the skin and moderate pressure extends through the subcutaneous layer of the skin to reach muscle tissue, but not so deep as to compress the tissue against the underlying bony structure. Moderate to heavy pressure that puts sufficient drag on the tissue mechanically affects the connective tissue and the proprioceptors (spindle cells and Golgi tendon organs) found in the muscle. Heavy pressure produces a distinctive compressive force of the soft tissue against the bone.

Depth of pressure is a result of leverage and leaning on the body. Pressure increases as the angle of the lean increases. Increases in pressure are NOT achieved by pushing with muscle strength.

Increasing pressure adds a compressive force and drag to the stroke. Light stroking is done with the fingertips or palm of the hand. Small body areas such as the fingers can be grasped and surrounded as effleurage is applied to the entire area. The surface contact increases with full hand and forearm application of the manipulations.

Effleurage that proceeds from the trunk of the body out, using superficial pressure, usually follows the dermatome distribution and is more reflexive in its effects (Proficiency Exercise 9-3). Strokes that use moderate pressure from the fingers and toes toward the heart following the muscle fiber direction are excellent for mechanical and reflexive stimulation of blood flow, particularly venous return and lymphatics. Light to moderate pressure, with short, repetitive effleurage stroking following the patterns for the lymph vessels is the basis for manual lymph drainage (see Chapter 11) (Fig. 9-11).

---

9 - 2
PROFICIENCY EXERCISE

1. Purposeful touch may be simple, but it is not easy. Diligent practice is required. If you enjoy animals, practice your approach with them. They do not hide responses as people do. Practice using the resting position to touch a dog, cat, or other animal while the animal is asleep, and see if you can do it without waking the animal.
2. Babies and young children are good for practice as well. Practice the resting position with a baby or child. Acceptance of the touch will be indicated by the child not startling or moving away.

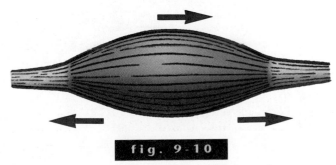

fig. 9-10
The focus of effleurage is horizontal.

fig.9-11

Examples of effleurage/gliding stroke applications

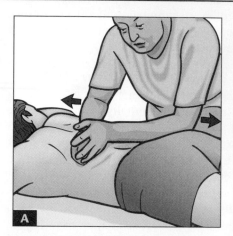

A

Double forearm effleurage.

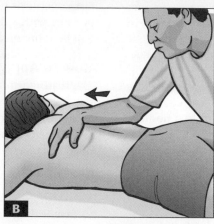

B

Single forearm effleurage to back.

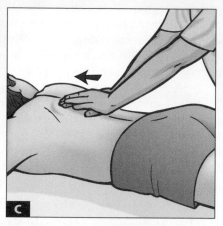

C

Supported hand effleurage.

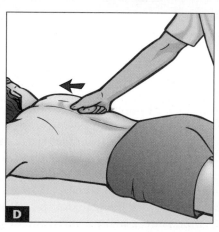

D

Loose fist effleurage.

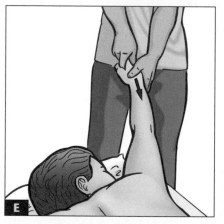

E

Surrounding grasp effleurage.

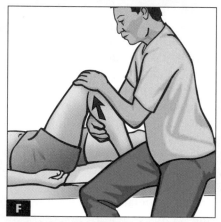

F

Single forearm effleurage to calf.

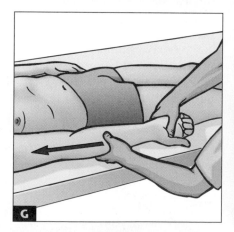

G

Single hand effleurage.

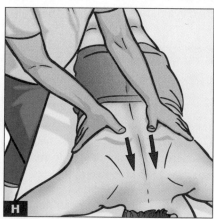

H

Double hand effleurage.

Pétrissage, or Kneading

Pétrissage, from the French verb *petrir* meaning "to knead," requires that the soft tissue be lifted, rolled, and squeezed by the massage technician (Fig. 9-12).

Just as effleurage is focused horizontally on the body, pétrissage focuses vertically. The main purpose of this manipulation is to lift tissue. After the tissues are lifted, the full hand is used to squeeze the tissue as it rolls out of the hand, while the other hand prepares to lift additional tissue and repeat the process (Fig. 9-13).

Because skin and the underlying muscles cannot be lifted without first pressing into them, compression is sometimes classified as pétrissage. This textbook separates compression into a distinct manipulation, but a compression element is part of the process of lifting tissue.

Pétrissage/kneading is very good for decreasing muscle tension. The lifting, rolling, and squeezing action affects the spindle cell proprioceptors in the muscle belly. As the belly of the muscle is squeezed (thus squeezing the spindle cells), the muscle feels less tense. When lifted, the tendons are stretched, thus increasing tension in both the tendons and the Golgi tendon receptors, which have a protective function. The result of this sensory input is to reflexively relax the muscle to keep it from harm. Pétrissage is a method of "tricking" the muscle into relaxation.

Pétrissage/kneading is very good for mechanically softening the superficial fascia. This type of connective tissue, located under the skin, is similar to gelatin. It is made up of a glycol (sugar) protein that binds with water. If gelatin is mixed with water and allowed to sit, it becomes thick and solidifies. If the gelatin is pressed into smaller pieces and stirred, it will soften. This is similar to the effect of pétrissage on connective tissue. The difference in feeling in the muscles after pétrissage is the same as comparing the stiffness of a brand new pair of shoes or jeans with the comfort of an old pair of jeans or a broken-in pair of shoes.

The fascia forms a major part of each muscle. Pétrissage has the mechanical effect of softening and creating space around the muscle fibers, making the tendons more pliable. The tension on the tendon as it is pulled during pétrissage deforms the connective tissue and mechanically warms it in a similar manner as a piece of metal bent back and forth becomes warm. Instead of metal fibers, collagen fibers are bent and warmed. When something is warm, its molecules are moving faster and are further apart. The space, which is created at a molecular level, translates into a softer and more pliable structure.

Pétrissage may incorporate a wringing or twisting component after the tissue is lifted. Changes in depth of pressure and drag determine whether the manipulation is per-

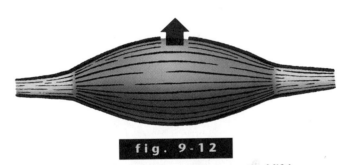

fig. 9-12

The focus of pétrissage/kneading is vertical lifting up.

9-3

PROFICIENCY EXERCISE

Do five massages and experiment with the following suggestions plus any other application of effleurage/gliding stroke you can create.

1. Use finger stroking of the face following the direction of the muscle fiber. Have a chart of the facial muscles available.
2. Using the forearm on the back, follow the muscle fiber directions from origin to insertion. Keep a muscle chart nearby.
3. Use the palm of the hand or pads of the fingers to lightly stroke the dermatome pattern from the spine to the fingers and toes. This method is sometimes called *nerve stroking*. Have a chart of dermatome distribution available.
4. Use the palm of the hand to glide from the toes and fingers toward the heart along the main pathways of the superficial vein. Use an anatomy chart as needed.
5. Grasp the fingers and toes and "milk" the tissue with effleurage.
6. Use the forearm to effleurage the quadriceps, hamstrings, abductors, fascia lata, and iliotibial band of the thigh. Use a muscle chart to follow the fiber direction.
7. Grasp the foot at the toes with both hands and glide to the ankle.
8. Use the knuckles to glide on the bottom of the foot from the toes to the base of the heel.
9. Use the thumbs to effleurage in a very specific pattern to gently separate the muscles in the hamstring and quadriceps groups.
10. Use the four basic flow patterns and design an entire massage with only effleurage/gliding strokes.

fig . 9 - 1 3

Examples of pétrissage/kneading applications

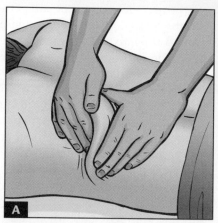

A

Two hands, with one hand pushing tissue into grasping.

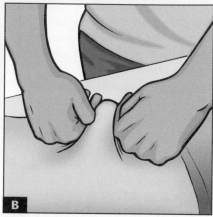

B

Two loose fists grasping and lifting tissue.

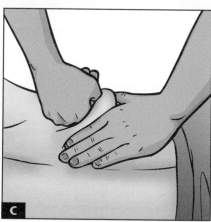

C

Two hands, with one hand pushing tissue into grasping.

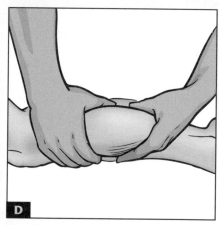

D

Two loose fists grasping and lifting tissue.

ceived by the client as superficial or deep. By the nature of the manipulation, the pressure and pull peak when the tissue is lifted to its maximum and decrease at the beginning and the end of the manipulation.

Skin Rolling

A variation of the lifting manipulation is **skin rolling**. Whereas deep pétrissage attempts to lift the muscular component away from the bone, skin rolling lifts only the skin from the underlying muscle layer. It has a warming and softening effect on the superficial fascia, causes reflexive stimulation to the spinal nerves, and is an excellent assessment method. Areas of "stuck" skin often suggest underlying problems. Skin rolling is one of the very few massage methods that is safe to use directly over the

spine. Because only the skin is accessed and the direction of pull to the skin is up and away from the underlying bones, the spine risks no injury, as is the case when any type of downward pressure is used.

Sometimes a client's tissue will not lift. This may be a result of excessive edema (swollen tissue), a heavy fat layer, scarring that extends into the deeper body layers, or thickened areas of connective tissue especially over aponeuroses (flat sheets of superficial connective tissue). If these conditions exist, applications of pétrissage or skin rolling will be uncomfortable to the client. Shifting to effleurage and compression may soften the tissue enough so that pétrissage can be used more effectively if applied later in the massage session.

Excessive body hair may interfere with the use of pétris-

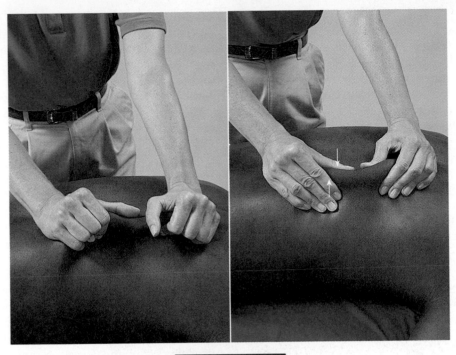

fig. 9-14

Skin roll.

sage. The massage practitioner must be careful not to pull the client's hair when using pétrissage or skin rolling.

How to Apply Pétrissage, or Kneading

Petrissage/kneading must be rhythmic to feel correct. The speed of the manipulation is limited. The speed and frequency of the application is determined by how much tissue can be lifted and how long it takes for that tissue to be rolled and squeezed through the hand. If the tissue is lifted quickly or squeezed too fast, it is uncomfortable to the client. Although the concept is hard to explain, much like milking a cow or goat, or kneading bread dough, the consistency of the material decides how it is to be kneaded.

Pétrissage/kneading begins with palmar compression on a 45-degree angle to push the tissue forward. The compression pressure results from leaning into the body—not pushing down using muscle strength. As the tissue bunches in front of the hand, the fingers, used as a unit combined with the palm of the hand, close over the mound of tissue. The tissue is then lifted, rolled, and squeezed through the hand as the practitioner rocks his or her entire body away from the initial direction used to produce the compressive force and initiates the lifting action. As the practitioner's body sways back, the tissues lift and roll through the grasping hands. The massage practitioner again rocks forward and leans into the body to apply a compression, and the movements are repeated to create a rhythmic pattern of pétrissage.

Except in very delicate areas such as the face, use of the fingers and thumbs to lift the tissue should be avoided because of a tendency to pinch and cause discomfort to the client (Fig. 9-14).

To get a feel for the method, practice with some clay. Keeping the fingers pressed together, use them as one unit against the thenar eminence (pad at the based of the thumb). Do not use the thumb itself. It is important to use as large a part of the palmar surface of the hand as possible. Extend the upward pull until you feel the end of the elastic give of the tissue. Kneading of this type works both on the skin and on the underlying muscular component, including the tendons. In most cases only one hand at a time is used to lift, squeeze, and twist the tissue. Pétrissage becomes continuous when a hand-over-hand rhythm is established. Two hands can also be used against each other on larger areas such as the hamstring muscle.

Skin rolling uses the entire hand to lift the skin; then the thumbs are used to feed the skin to the fingers in a rolling motion (Proficiency Exercise 9-4).

NOTE: Although pétrissage is very effective in softening and relaxing tissue, it is energy-consuming for the massage practitioner to use. The fingers should be used as a unit along with the thenar eminence of the thumb. Excessive use of this manipulation should be avoided. It is better to use pétrissage intermittently with effleurage and compression, which do not require such labor-intensive use of the hands. Constant attention must be paid to body mechanics.

Compression

Compression has developed as a distinct manipulation in recent years with the advent of sports massage and on-site corporate massage. It has always been the main method used in shiatsu and other Oriental approaches. This manipulation is a way of working over the clothing or without lubricant. Very specific pinpoint compression is called *direct pressure,* or *ischemic compression,* and is used on acupressure points and trigger points (Fig. 9-15).

Because compression uses a lift-press method, it is particularly suited for use when a lubricant is undesirable. It is also very good to use on hairy bodies because the manipulations do not glide on the skin, pull the tissue, or require lubricant. As with effleurage, the deeper the pressure, the more mechanical the effect will be. Likewise, the more superficial the pressure, the more reflexive the effect will be.

Compression moves down into the tissues with varying depths of pressure. The superficial application resembles the resting position but uses more pressure. The manipulations

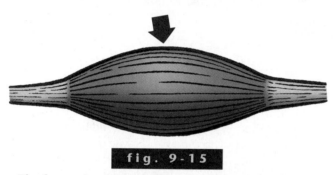

fig. 9-15

The focus of compression is a vertical pressing down.

9-4

PROFICIENCY EXERCISE

1. Knead a variety of sizes of bread dough. Small pieces can be used to practice the delicate applications used on the face and anterior neck, whereas larger pieces can mimic big muscles such as the gluteals. Bread dough is good for practice because it is resilient (like body tissue) and will not allow you to pétrissage too fast.
2. Pétrissage an inflated balloon. If it slips out of your grasp, it is a sign that you just pinched your "client." Using a balloon will help develop the use of the palm in place of the fingers.
3. For learning purposes only, practice using pétrissage or kneading for an entire body massage using all four basic flow patterns. Notice that some parts of the body are more easily kneaded. Because of the repetitive use of the hand for pétrissage, avoid extensive long-term use.

of compression usually penetrate the subcutaneous layer, whereas in the resting position they stay on the skin surface. Much of the effect of compression results from pressing tissue against the underlying bone, causing it to spread and be squeezed from two sides, similar to flattening out a tortilla or a ball of clay, or pressing pizza dough into a pan.

Compression disconnects from the body with each lift, and then reconnects with each press in a pistonlike fashion. Pressing rhythmically into connective tissue softens it mechanically. Pressing tissue against the underlying hard bone spreads the tissue mechanically, enhancing the softening effect of the connective tissue component of the muscle. Compression that takes all the slack out of the tissue then pushes or pulls in a 45-degree angle without slipping produces a drag on the tissue affecting the connective tissue.

Compression used in the belly of the muscle spreads the spindle cells, causing the muscle to sense it is stretching. To protect the muscle from overstretching, the spindle cell signals for the muscle to contract. The lift-press application stimulates the muscle and nerve tissue. These two effects combine to make compression a good method to stimulate muscles and the nervous system. Because of this stimulation, compression is a little less desirable for a relaxation or soothing massage. It is important to remember that not all people want to feel like a relaxed rag doll after a massage. If the client desires to be alert, then perform a stimulating massage.

A muscle needs to contract or at least have the nerve "fire" (as occurs in a contraction) before it can relax. This is due to the threshold stimulation pattern of the nerve and its effects on muscle tone. Nerves build up energy needed to spark the nerve impulse. The automatic response of muscle fibers to contraction is a period of relaxation called the *refractory period.* Sometimes the signals are enough to get everything ready to fire, but the signal is not strong enough to actually cause the contraction or discharge of the nerve. The result is that the muscle tenses but cannot quite contract and the tension remains. If stimulation to the nerves can be increased just enough for the nerve to discharge, then the muscle contracts and can reset to a normal resting length. Compression to the belly of the muscle and its effect on the spindle cell elicits this response. Any sustained and repetitive use of a stimulation method that causes muscle fibers to maintain a contraction or contract repeatedly eventually fatigues the muscle fibers. Compression used in this manner initiates a relaxation response in muscles.

How to Apply Compression

Compression can be done with the point of the thumb or stabilized finger, palm and heel of the hand, fist, knuckles, forearm, and in some systems, the knee and heel of the foot (Fig. 9-16).

When using the palm of the hand to do compression, avoid hyperextension or hyperflexion of the wrist by

fig.9-16

Examples of compression applications

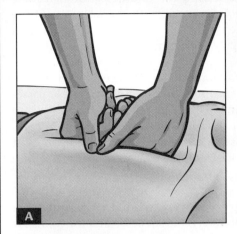

A Fist compression.

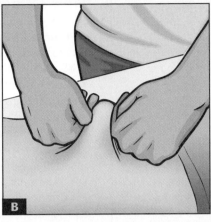

B Double loose fist compression.

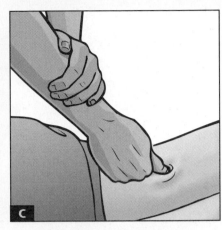

C Stabilized thumb compression.

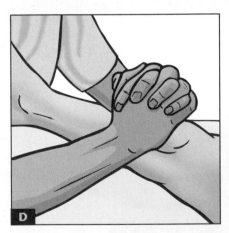

D Loose fist compression.

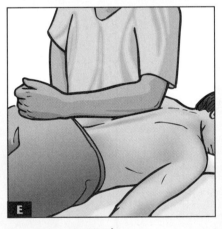

E Forearm compression.

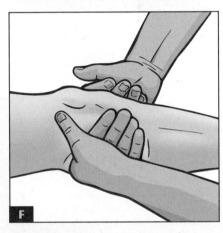

F Double hand compression.

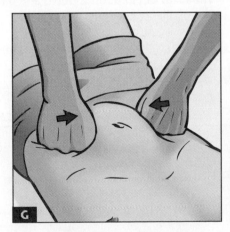

G Fists used in lateral compression.

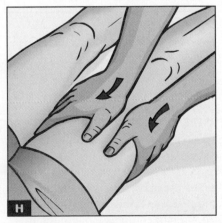

H Double palm compression.

Continued.

fig. 9-16, cont'd

Examples of compression applications

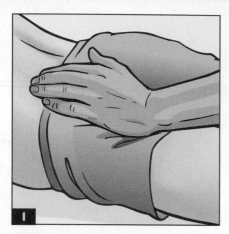

Single palm compression.

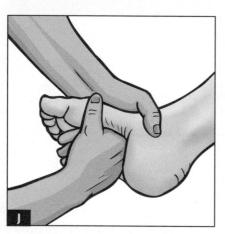

Fist application of compression to foot.

keeping the application hand in front instead of directly under the massage practitioner's shoulder. Even though the compressive pressure is perpendicular to the tissue, the position of the forearm in relation to the wrist is about 120 to 130 degrees. If using the knuckles or fist, make sure the forearm is in a direct line with the wrist. Use of the thumb should be avoided if possible. Extensive use of the thumb, especially on large muscle masses, could result in damage to it.

The tip or the radioulnar side of the elbow should not be used for compression. Because the ulnar nerve passes just under the skin and damage can result from extensive compression, use the forearm near the elbow for compression. The massage professional's arm and hand must be relaxed, or neck and shoulder tension will occur. Leverage applied through appropriate body mechanics does the work, not muscle strength.

Compression proceeds downward into the tissues; the depth is determined by what is to be accomplished, where compression is to be applied, and how broad or specific is the contact with the client's body.

Deep compression presses tissue against the underlying bone. Because of the diagonal pattern of the muscles, the massage practitioner should stay perpendicular or at a 90-

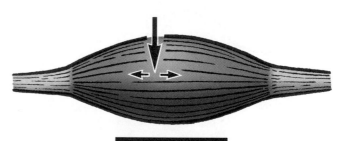

fig. 9-17

The focus of vibration is down and back and forth in a fast oscillating manner.

9-5

PROFICIENCY EXERCISE

1. Inflate a series of balloons with different internal pressures. Fill some with water and others with gelatin, and use these to represent the thickness or thinness of different tissue types. The use of balloons is great for practicing the angle and pressure of the manipulation. The best angle allows good firm compression into the balloon without it slipping out from under you.
2. Using pieces of foam with various densities, place them over objects of different sizes and shapes. Determine how much pressure it takes to feel each object. Pay attention to the difference with the low-density foam compared with the high-density foam.
3. Design a complete massage for each of the basic flow patterns using only compression. Pay very close attention to ways in which you can use compression manipulations in all of the variations to access the client's body successfully.

degree angle to the bone, with actual compression somewhere between a 45- and 90-degree angle to the body. Beyond those angles, the stroke may slip and turn into a glide.

Compression can be used to replace effleurage if for any reason gliding strokes cannot or should not be used. Examples include working on areas where there is excessive body hair, areas where people are ticklish, and areas where the skin is sensitive to lubricant. Compression bypasses the tickle response by activating deep touch receptors. Also, compression does not slip or roll on the tissue (Proficiency Exercise 9-5).

Vibration

Edgar Cyriax, one of the foremost authorities on massage and manual techniques, describes **vibration** as follows[4]:

almost every author who attempts to describe the modus operandi for generating these vibrations prefaces his remarks by stating that they are extremely tiring to produce. Vibration is generated by means of the operator tensing all the muscles of his or her arm (some even include the muscles of the shoulder) into a state of powerful complete tetanus. This method is very fatiguing: no one can sustain such a contraction evenly for more than a minute or so. The correct technique for production of manual vibrations is to set up a small amount of alternating contraction and relaxation in some of the muscles of the forearm, those of the upper arm and the shoulder being kept quite passive (unless required for fixation purposes).

Vibration is a very powerful stroke, if it can be done long enough and at an intensity sufficient to produce reflexive physiologic effects. Manual vibration can be used successfully by the massage practitioner to stimulate muscles by applying the technique at the muscle tendons for up to 30 seconds. When this is complete, the antagonist muscle pattern relaxes through neurologic reciprocal inhibition.

Another use for vibration is to break up the monotony of the massage. If the same methods are used repeatedly, the body adapts and does not respond as well to the sensation or stimulation. Because vibration is used to "wake up" nerves, it is a good method to stimulate nerve activity. The nerves of the muscles around a joint also innervate the joint itself. Muscle pain is often interpreted by the client as joint pain and vice versa. Used specifically and purposefully, vibration is a great massage manipulation to confuse and shift the muscle/joint pain perception (Fig. 9-17).

How to Apply Vibration

All vibration begins with compression. After the depth of pressure is achieved, the hand needs to tremble and transmit the action to the surrounding tissues. As described by Cyriax,[4] the muscles above the elbow should be relaxed. The action comes only from the alternating contrac-

tion/relaxation of the forearm muscles. Of all the massage methods, vibration may be the hardest to master.

To start with coarse vibration, place one hand on the client and compress lightly. Begin moving the hand back and forth using only the forearm muscles and limiting the motion to about 2 inches of space. Gradually quicken the back-and-forth movement, checking to make sure your upper arm stays relaxed. Next make the back-and-forth movement smaller until the hand does not move at all on the tissue but is trembling at a high intensity. This is vibration.

Because of the energy needed to perform this manipulation, it should be used sparingly and for short periods. It is suggested that a forearm effleurage follow vibration because the action of the effleurage essentially massages and relaxes the practitioner's arm, protecting it from repetitive use problems (Fig. 9-18).

Some professionals use mechanical vibrators to replace manual vibration. This is acceptable so long as the practice is allowed by any licensing regulations that may exist, the equipment is safe, and the client approves of its use (Proficiency Exercise 9-6).

Shaking

Shaking is a massage method that is effective in relaxing muscle groups or an entire limb. Shaking manipulations confuse the positional proprioceptors because the sensory input is too unorganized for the integrating systems of the brain to interpret; muscle relaxation is the natural response in such situations.

Shaking warms and prepares the body for deeper bodywork and addresses the joints in a nonspecific manner. Shaking is effective when the muscles seem extremely tight. This technique is reflexive in its effect, but there may be a small mechanical influence on the connective tissue as well because of the lifting and pulling component of the methods.

Shaking is sometimes classified as a vibration. However, the application is very different because vibration begins with compression and shaking begins by lifting.

How to Apply Shaking

Shaking begins with a lift-and-pull component. Either a muscle group or limb is grasped, lifted, and shaken. To begin to understand shaking, think of a dog shaking when it is wet, shaking out a rug or blanket, a dog or cat tugging on a toy, or the swish of a horse's tail.

The focus of the massage practitioner's shaking is more specific and less intense than shaking a rug, but the idea is still the same. There is a lift and then a fairly abrupt downward or side-to-side movement that ends suddenly as if throwing something off. Even the most subtle shaking movements deliberately move the joint or muscle tissue with the intention of a "snap" at the end of the movement.

Shaking is not a manipulation to be used on the skin or

Examples of vibration applications

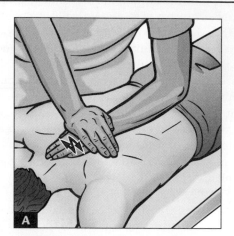

Stabilized hand.

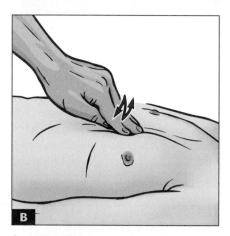

Stabilized fingers.

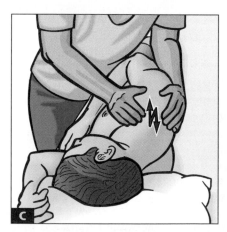

Double hand.

superficial fascia, nor is it effective to use on the entire body. Rather, it is best applied to any large muscle groups that can be grasped and to the synovial joints of the limbs. Good areas for shaking are the upper trapezius and shoulder area, biceps and triceps groups, hamstrings, quadriceps, gastrocnemius, and in some instances the abdominals and the pectoralis muscles close to the axilla. The joints of the shoulders, hips, and extremities also respond well to shaking.

The larger the muscle or joint, the more intense the method. If the movements are performed with all the slack out of the tissue, the focus point of the shake is very small and is extremely effective. The more purposeful the approach, the smaller the focus of the shaking. You should always stay within the limits of both range of motion of a joint and "elastic give" of the tissue. The goal is to see how small the shaking action can be and still achieve the desired physiologic effect. This can be accomplished by first lifting the tissue or limb, grasping it, then leaning back gently until the tissue becomes taut. Begin the shaking movement from this position (Fig. 9-20).

Rocking

Rocking is a soothing and rhythmic method that is used to calm people. Rocking is both reflexive and chemical in its effects (Fig. 9-21).

Rocking also works though the vestibular system of the inner ear and feeds sensory input directly into the cerebellum. It is probable that other reflex mechanisms are affected as well. Because of this, rocking is one of the most productive massage methods used to produce entrainment. For rocking to be most effective the body must move so that the fluid in the semicircular canals of the inner ear are affected, initiating parasympathetic mechanisms.

How to Apply Rocking

Rocking is rhythmic and should be applied with a deliberate full-body movement. Rocking involves the up-and-down and side-to-side movement of shaking, but no flick or throw-off snap occurs at the end of the movement. The action moves the body as far as it will go, then allows it to return to the original position. After two or three rocks, the client's rhythm can be sensed.

This attunement to the client's rhythms is a powerful interface point to synchronize entrainment. The massage practitioner works within the rhythm to maintain and amplify it by attempting to gently extend the limits of movement or by slowing the rhythm. Incorporation of a rocking movement that supports this entrainment process into all massage applications effectively individualizes the application and speed of the method. The client seems to relax more easily when a subtle rocking movement, matching his or her innate rhythm pattern, is incorporated as part of the generalized massage approach, along with such techniques as effleurage, pétrissage, compression, joint movement, and especially passive movements.

With a tense and anxious client who may initially resist rocking, begin the process with slightly bigger and more abrupt shaking manipulations. As the muscles begin to relax, switch to rocking methods.

Nothing is abrupt: there is an even ebb and flow to the methods. All movement is flowing, like a wind chime in a gentle breeze or a porch swing on a hot summer night. Rocking is one of the most effective relaxation techniques used by the massage practitioner. Many parasympathetic responses are elicited by the rocking of the body during effleurage, pétrissage, and compression (Proficiency Exercise 9-7).

Tapotement, or Percussion

The term *tapotement* comes from the French verb *tapoter*, which means "to rap, drum, or pat." Tapotement techniques require that the hands or parts of the hand administer springy blows to the body at a fast rate. The

---

9 - 6

PROFICIENCY EXERCISE

The first two exercises to teach vibration were developed by a professional magician who is also a massage practitioner and instructor. Many sleight-of-hand movements required for his illusions use the same movements as vibration. Perfecting these two balloon exercises will enhance your vibration skills.

1. Using a clear 5-inch balloon, put a penny inside, then inflate and tie the balloon. Grasp the tied end of the balloon, cupping it in the palm of the hand (Fig. 9-19, *A*). Using wrist action only, circle the balloon until the penny begins to roll inside. Once you can do this, make the wrist circles smaller and smaller while continuing to roll the penny in the balloon. Eventually the action will be the movement required for vibration.

2. Use the same balloon and put the fattest part in the palm of your hand. Place your other hand on top of the balloon. Using just the bottom hand, use a coarse vibration to get the penny to jump and dance in the balloon. Once you can do this, make the movements smaller and smaller until you can make the penny dance with fine vibration movements (Fig. 9-19, *B*).

3. Combine all the methods presented so far into a massage. Incorporate vibration at each tendon, paying attention to the results as the muscles contract or tense slightly in response to the stimulation.

---

fig. 9-19

Balloon exercises for vibration

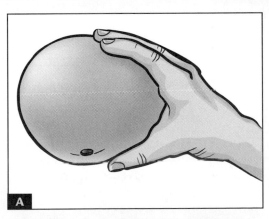

A

Hold balloon in the palm of the hand as shown.

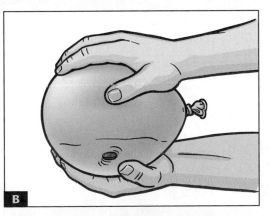

B

Hand placement for balloon exercise.

fig.9-20

Examples of applications of shaking

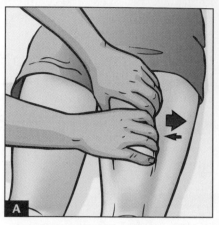
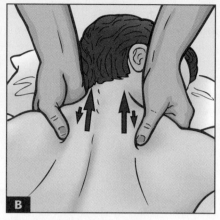

Lift tissue. Take out the slack. Apply abrupt shaking movement as directed by large arrow. Allow tissue to return in the direction of small arrow.

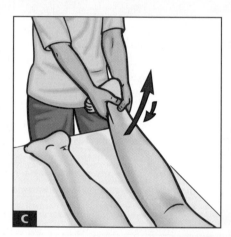
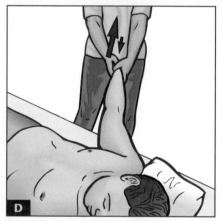

Grasp area and pull out slack in tissues. Apply abrupt shaking movement in direction of large arrows, and allow tissue to return in direction of small arrows.

fig.9-21

Rocking

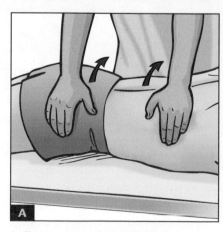
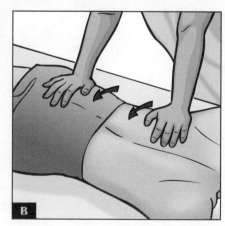

Pull area toward practitioner.

Rock area away from practitioner.

blows are directed downward to create a rhythmic compression of the tissue (Fig. 9-22).

Tapotement/percussion is divided into two classifications: light and heavy. The difference between light and heavy tapotement is determined by whether the force of the blows penetrates only to the superficial tissue of the skin and subcutaneous layers (light) or penetrates deeper into the muscles, tendons, and visceral (organ) structures, such as the pleura in the chest cavity (heavy).

Tapotement is a stimulating manipulation that operates through the response of the nerves. Because of its intense stimulating effect on the nervous system, tapotement initiates or enhances sympathetic activity of the autonomic nervous system. The effects of the manipulations are reflexive except for the mechanical results of tapotement in loosening and moving mucus in the chest. Children with cystic fibrosis are treated with tapotement, but massage therapy of this type is beyond the beginning skill levels of the massage technician.

The most noticeable effect of tapotement results from the response of the tendon reflexes. A quick blow to the tendon stretches it. In response, protective muscle contraction occurs. To obtain the best result, stretch the ten-

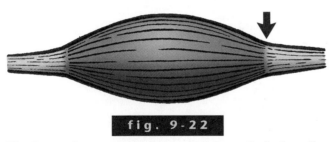

fig. 9-22

The focus of tapotement/percussion is vertical, abruptly snapped down.

don first. The most common example of this reflexive mechanism is the knee-jerk or patellar reflex, but this response happens in all tendons to some degree. Knowing this is very helpful when preparing the muscles for lengthening, for example, if a client indicates that his or her hamstrings are tight and need to be relaxed. With the client supine, the hip flexed to 90 degrees, and the knee flexed to 90 degrees, tapotement on the stretched quadriceps tendon will cause the quadriceps to contract. As a result, the hamstrings relax and it is easier to lengthen them to a more normal resting length.

When applied to the joints, tapotement affects the joint kinesthetic receptors responsible for determining the position and movement of the body. The quick blows confuse the system, similar to the effect of joint-focused rocking and shaking, but the body muscles tense instead of relax. This method is useful for stimulating weak muscles. The force used must move the joint but should not be strong enough to damage the joint. For example, one finger may be used over the carpal joints, whereas the fist may be used over the sacroiliac joint.

Tapotement/percussion is very effective when used at motor points that are usually located in the same area as the traditional acupuncture points. The repetitive stimulation causes the nerve to fire repeatedly, stimulating the nerve tract.

Tapotement/percussion focused primarily on the skin affects the superficial blood vessels of the skin, initially causing them to contract. Heavy tapotement or prolonged lighter application dilates the vessels as a result of the release of histamine, a vasodilator. Although prolonged tapotement seems to increase blood flow, surface tapotement enhances the effect of cold application used in hydrotherapy.

9-7

PROFICIENCY EXERCISE

1. Lay a sheet on your massage table or other flat surface. Lift one end and practice shaking the sheet to achieve a wavelike motion in the sheet from one end to the other. Practice directing the ripple to various locations on the table.
2. Swing in a playground swing, using your legs to pump yourself. This exercise will give the full-body effect of the shake. Pay close attention to the feeling as you reach the top of the swing and begin to head back.
3. Using your own body for practice, systematically shake each joint, lying down to do the legs. See how small you can make the movement and still feel the effects. Grab the muscles of your arm and leg. Lift and shake the tissue, paying attention to the sensations.

4. Sit in an old-fashioned rocking chair and let the chair rock you. See what happens when you rock the chair. Vary the speed to go faster and slower than the chair's movement. Put the chair on different surfaces, such as carpet, hard floor, sand, and grass. Again, let the chair rock you and notice the difference. Remember, each person has an individual rhythm that needs to be identified, supported, and respected.
5. Put on music with a 4/4 beat at less than 60 beats per minute. Pick up the sway of the music and rock with it. Repeat the exercise with different beats of music.
6. Design an entire massage for all four basic flow patterns using a combination of shaking and rocking.

fig. 9-23

Examples of tapotement

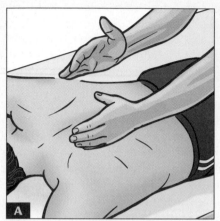

Hacking.

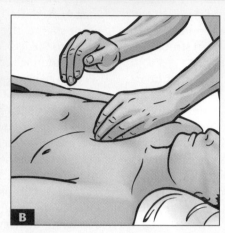

Cupping.

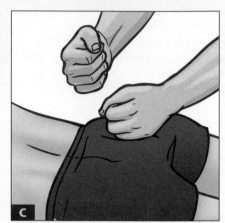

Fist beating.

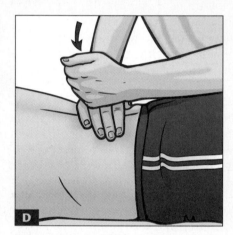

Beating over palm.

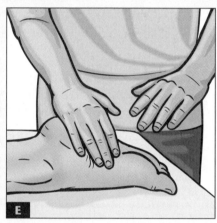

Slapping.

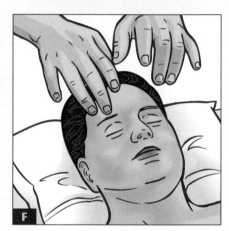

Finger tapping.

9-8

PROFICIENCY EXERCISE

1. Play a drum or watch a drummer, paying attention to the action of the arms and wrist and the grasp of the drumsticks. Notice that the drummer holds the drumstick loosely.
2. Get a paddleball or yo-yo and see what actions it takes to make these toys work. Play with a rattle or tambourine.
3. Use the foam from the compression exercises and practice the different methods and pressures of tapotement.
4. While shaking your hands very quickly, use hacking to strike the foam or a practice client. Without stopping, change hand positions so that all the methods are used.
5. Design a stimulating massage using all the basic flow patterns with various applications of tapotement.

How to Apply Tapotement/Percussion

In tapotement, two hands are usually used alternately. When tapping a motor point, one or two fingers can be used. The forearm muscles contract and relax in rapid succession to move the elbow joint into flexion and then allow it to quickly release. This action travels down to the relaxed wrist, extending it; the wrist then moves back and forth to provide the action of the tapotement. Tapotement/percussion is a controlled flailing of the arms as the wrists snap back and forth. Remember the wrist must always stay relaxed. Beginning students usually want to use the wrists to provide the snap action. This is especially tempting when using small movements of the fingers; however, it *should not be done* because it will damage the wrist.

Heavy tapotement should not be done over the kidney area, or anywhere there is pain or discomfort (Proficiency Exercise 9-8). Proper methods are classified as follows (Fig. 9-23):

- *Hacking*—Applied with both wrists relaxed and the fingers spread, only the little finger or the ulnar side of the hand strikes the surface. The other fingers hit each other with a springy touch. Point hacking can be done by using the fingertips in the same way. Hacking is used with the whole hand on the larger soft tissue areas such as the upper back and shoulders. Point hacking is used on smaller areas such as the individual tendons of the toes or over motor points.
- *Cupping*—Fingers and thumbs are placed as if making a cup. The hands are turned over and the same action as hacking is done. Used on the anterior and posterior thorax, cupping is good for stimulation of the respiratory system and for loosening mucus. If the client exhales and makes a monotone noise while cupping is being done, enough pressure is used so that the tone begins to break up from "AAAAAAAAAAAAHHHHHH" to "AH AH AH AH AH AH."
- *Beating and pounding*—These moves are performed using a soft fist with knuckles down, or vertically with the ulnar side of the palm (pictured). Beating and pounding is done over large muscles such as the buttocks and heavy leg muscles.
- *Slapping (splatting)*—The whole palm of a flattened hand makes contact with the body. This is a good method for release of histamine to increase vasodilation and its effects to the skin. It is also a good method to use on the bottom of the feet. The broad contact of the whole hand disperses the force laterally instead of down, and the effects remain in the superficial tissue. Kellogg[6] named this movement "splatting."
- *Tapping*—The palmar surface of the fingers alternately taps the body area with light to medium pressure. This is a good method to use around the joints, on the tendons, on the face and head, and along the spine.

Friction

One method of **friction** consists of small, deep movements performed on a local area. This method was formalized by James Cyriax and uses deep transverse friction massage while applying no lubricant. The skin moves with the fingers. Friction burns may result if the fingers are allowed to slide back and forth over the skin (Fig. 9-24). Friction creates therapeutic inflammation.

Friction manipulation prevents and breaks up local adhesions in connective tissue, especially over tendons, ligaments, and scars by creating therapeutic inflammation. This method is not used over acute injury or fresh scars. Modified use of friction, after the scar has stabilized or the acute phase has passed, may prevent adhesions and can promote a more normal healing process.

The Cyriax application also provides for pain reduction through the mechanisms of counterirritation and hyperstimulation analgesia. In many older textbooks, friction is explained as a back-and-forth, brisk movement focused on the skin and subcutaneous tissue for dilation of the vessels of the skin. Excessive use causes a friction burn on the skin similar to a rug burn. Historical literature on massage indicates that friction burns were done on purpose to produce long-term stimulation of the nerve. This is a method of counterirritation and is seldom used today.

Connective tissue has a high water content. For the connective tissue to remain pliable, it must remain hydrated. Friction increases the water-binding capacity of the connective tissue ground substance.

The movement in friction is usually transverse to the fiber direction. It is generally performed for 30 seconds to 10 minutes, with some authorities suggesting a duration of 20 minutes. The result of this type of friction is the initiation of a small, controlled inflammatory response. The chemicals released during inflammation result in the activation of tissue repair mechanisms with reorganization of connective tissue. This type of work, coupled with proper rehabilitation, is very valuable. Because of its specific nature and direct focus on rehabilitation, the use of deep transverse friction is not suitable for the beginning-level massage technician. Deep transverse friction is discussed in more depth in Chapter 11.

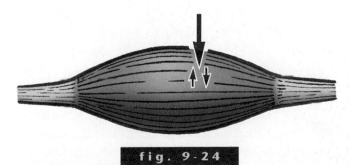

fig. 9-24

The focus of friction is a vertical pressing down, applying movement to underlying tissues.

fig.9-25

Examples of friction

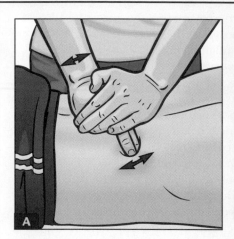

Stabilized finger friction.

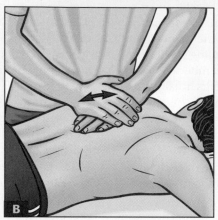

Stabilized hand friction.

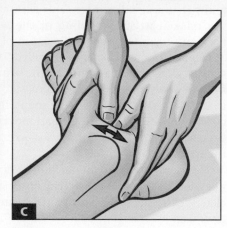

Double thumb friction.

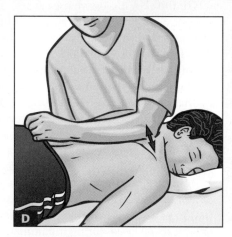

Forearm friction.

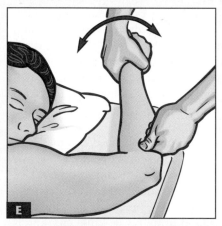

Thumb compression and movement of underlying tissue.

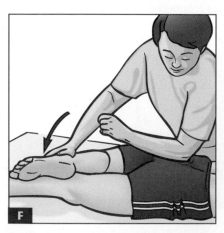

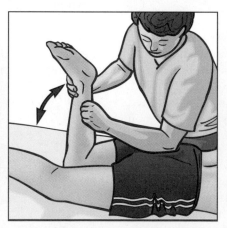

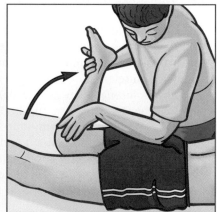

Forearm compression and movement of underlying tissue.

A modified application of friction, used to keep high-concentration areas of connective tissue soft and pliable, is appropriate for the beginner. The modified application is essentially the same as deep transverse friction in that the focus is transverse to the muscle fiber direction and moves the tissue beneath the skin, but the duration and specificity are reduced. The direction can be transverse or circular, pinpointed or more generalized, but the tissue under the skin is still affected.

Friction is a mechanical approach best applied to areas of high connective tissue concentration such as the musculotendinous junction. Microtrauma from repetitive movement and overstretching are common in this area. Microtrauma predisposes the musculotendinous junction to inflammatory problems, connective tissue changes, and adhesion. Friction is a good way to keep this tissue healthy. Experts disagree on whether an area that is to receive friction should be stretched or relaxed. Because both ways have merit, both positions should be included when frictioning.

Another use for friction is to combine it with compression. The combination adds a small stretch component. The movement includes no slide. This application has a mechanical, chemical, and reflexive effect, and is the most common approach today for the use of friction.

How to Apply Friction

The main focus when using friction is to move tissue under the skin. No lubricant is used because the tissues must not slide. The area to be frictioned should be placed in a soft or slack position. The movement is produced by beginning with a specific and moderate to deep compression using the fingers, palm, or flat part of the forearm near the elbow. After the pressure required to contact the tissue is reached, the upper tissue is moved back and forth across the grain or fiber of the undertissue for transverse or cross-fiber friction, or around in a circle for circular friction.

As the tissue responds to the friction, gradually begin to stretch the area and increase the pressure. The feeling for the client may be intense, but if it is painful, the application should be modified to a tolerable level so that the client reports the sensation as a "good hurt." The recommended way to work within the client's comfort zone is to use pressure sufficient for him or her to feel the specific area but not complain of pain. Friction should be continued until the sensation reduces. Gradually increase the pressure until the client again feels the specific area. Begin friction again and repeat the sequence for up to 10 minutes.

The area being frictioned may be tender to the touch for 48 hours after the technique is used. The sensation should be similar to a mild after-exercise soreness. Because the focus of friction is the controlled application of a small inflammatory response, this causes heat and redness from the release of histamine. Also, increased circulation results in a small amount of puffiness as more water binds with the connective tissue. The area should not bruise.

Another effective way to produce friction is a combination of compression and passive joint movement with the bone under the compression used to perform the friction. The process begins with a compression as just described, but instead of the massage practitioner moving the tissue back and forth (or in a circle), the massage practitioner moves the client's body under the compression. This automatically adds the slack and stretch positions for the friction methods. The result is the same. This method is much easier for the massage professional to perform and may be more comfortable for the client as well. The movement of the joint provides a distraction from the specific application of the pressure and generalizes the sensation. Broad general methods can be used with a higher degree of intensity than a pinpointed specific focus (Fig. 9-25) (Proficiency Exercise 9-9).

MASSAGE TECHNIQUES

section objectives

Using the information presented in this section, the student will be able to perform the following:

- **Use movement in a purposeful way to create a specific physiologic response**

- **Explain the proprioceptive mechanisms and their importance in the physiologic effects of massage techniques**

- **Move the synovial joints through the client's physiologic range of motion using both active and passive joint movement**

- **Incorporate muscle energy techniques to enhance lengthening and stretching procedures**

---

9 - 9

PROFICIENCY EXERCISE

1. Put toothpicks laid in a haphazard fashion under a towel. Use fingertip friction to line up all the toothpicks.
2. Use a piece of rope ½ inch in diameter. Use friction to separate the fibers of the rope.
3. Access as many surface areas of the musculotendinous junction as possible. Gently friction across the grain of the fibers using the fingers, palm, and ulnar side of elbow.
4. Using palmar or forearm compression on larger muscle groups, combine passive and active joint movement (see following section) to design a massage session.

In *An Illustrated Sketch of the Movement Cure*,[10] George H. Taylor said the following:

The purpose of an active movement, is to convey to, and concentrate upon a selected point, the nutrition and energies of the system. Such a movement may accomplish a twofold purpose, that of supplying a part, and of relieving another part more or less distant.

The mode of effecting this purpose is as follows: the person to receive the application, is placed in an easy unconstrained position, sitting, lying, half lying, kneeling, or in a convenient position that will suitably adjust all parts of the body to the purpose. The body is fixed either by the hands of an assistant, or by means of an apparatus so as to prevent as much as possible any motion of all parts of the body, except the acting part. The patient is in some cases directed to move the free part in a particular direction, the effort to do so is resisted by the operator, with a force proportionate to the exertion made very nicely graduated to the particular condition of the part and of the system at large. The resistance is not uniform, but varies according to the varying action of muscles, as perceived by the operator. In other cases the operator acts while the patient resists. The action is the same, but in one case the patient's acting muscles are shortened; and in the other lengthened. The operator is a wrestle, in which a very limited portion of the organism is engaged. The motion must be much slower than the natural movement of the part engaged, which fact strongly fixes the attention and concentrates the will. The act is repeated two or three times with all the care and precision the operator can command, being cautious not to induce fatigue.

The use of movement as described in this next section follows the guidelines and recommendations described by Taylor. The principles of massage today are built on the same principles as those shown in the historical literature. The names may be different and the physiologic explanations more precise, but the methods are the same.

The efficient use of massage techniques will reduce the need for repetitive massage manipulations. If used well, the neuromuscular mechanism can be activated and influenced quickly with less physical effort by the massage professional (Box 9-1).

Physiologic Influences of Massage Techniques

The techniques of passive and active joint movement and muscle energy presented in this chapter work with the neuromuscular reflex system to relax and *lengthen* muscles. In contrast, *stretching* has both a reflexive and mechanical aspect. The reflexive component of stretching is an initial neuromuscular lengthening phase used to prepare the area for the more mechanical stretching effect of elongating connective tissue. Stretching is discussed more completely on p. 383.

A working knowledge of the proprioceptive interaction between the prime mover and the antagonist, as well as bodywide reflex patterns, is necessary to understand and implement massage techniques. Methods are then chosen that provide specific information to the neuromuscular mechanism about current function to encourage a reset to the more normal neutral state, allowing the most optimal range of functioning. The neuromuscular mechanism

makes adjustments based on the information it receives. If the information is clear and accurate, the muscles operate as designed; however, if the information is unclear, incorrect, or inconsistent, imbalances can occur.

For example, if a client spends the day talking on the phone, holding the phone with the shoulder, the lateral neck flexors and shoulder elevators are in constant contraction, whereas the other side of the neck is in constant extension. An adaptation takes place so that when the neck muscles are used, painful resistance occurs to any use of the neck other than what is allowed by the new reset position. This type of interaction is responsible for most muscle tension.

The muscle imbalances result because the body adapts to a different muscle spindle set point and a new muscle resting length (usually shortened). Massage techniques can provide more clear neurologic information so that the body can restore optimal or as close to optimal function as possible. This allows the homeostatic mechanism of the body to restore a neutral mode.

All of the massage manipulations described previously affect proprioception reflexively but usually have a general nonspecific effect. The focus of this section is to learn ways to deliver accurate and specific information to the neuromuscular system supporting normal functioning. The difference is similar to that between providing a general announcement to a group of people (massage manip-

---

box 9-1

PRINCIPLES FOR THE APPLICATION OF MASSAGE TECHNIQUE BASED ON TAYLOR'S RECOMMENDATIONS

1. Be specific.
2. Be mindful of patterns of "too much" and "not enough."
3. Position the client purposefully.
4. Stabilize the body so that only the focused target area is affected.
5. You may move the area or may cooperate in the effort with the client.
6. Be sure that the force and exertion are gradual and vary with the demand.
7. Remember that the purpose is to lengthen shortened tissue and stimulate weakened muscles.
8. You are a facilitator in the process.
9. Make sure the application is slow and purposeful.
10. Repeat the movement two or three times but not to fatigue.

ulations) and calling out individuals' names and delivering a message (massage techniques).

Joint Movement

To understand **joint movement,** you must first understand the joint. A simplified review is included here. You are encouraged to consult anatomy and physiology resources for further clarification and understanding of individual joints (Fig. 9-26).

How Joints Work

Joints allow us to move. Joint position and velocity receptors inform the central nervous system regarding where and how the body is positioned in gravity and how fast it is moving. This sensory data is the major determining factor for muscle tone patterns.

Joint movement techniques focus on the synovial or freely movable joints in the body (see Chapter 3, p. 101). To a lesser extent, the joints of the vertebral column, hand, and foot are also considered, as are other joints such as the facet joints of the ribs, the sacroiliac joint, and the sternoclavicular joint. These joints are not directly influenced by muscles but move through indirect muscle action.

We can control some joint movements voluntarily: we can move our limbs through various motions such as flexion, extension, abduction, adduction, and rotation. These are referred to as *physiologic* or **osteokinematic movements.** For normal physiologic movement, other types of movements (*accessory* or **arthrokinematic movements**) must occur as a result of the inherent laxity or **joint play** that exists in each joint. This laxity allows the ends of the bones to slide, roll, or spin smoothly on each other inside the joint capsule. These essential movements occur pas-

Text continued on p. 364.

A

Finger adduction

B

Finger abduction

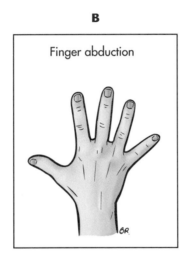

Finger extension

Finger flexion

C

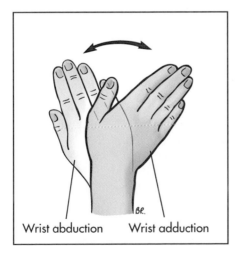

Wrist abduction   Wrist adduction

D

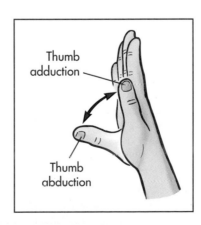

Thumb adduction

Thumb abduction

E

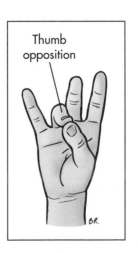

Thumb opposition

F

Continued.

fig. 9-26

Joint movements.

G

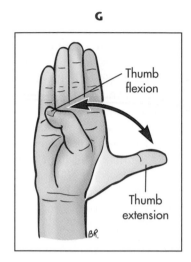

Thumb flexion

Thumb extension

H

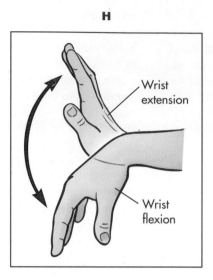

Wrist extension

Wrist flexion

I

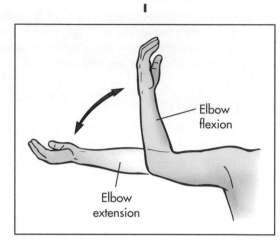

Elbow flexion

Elbow extension

J

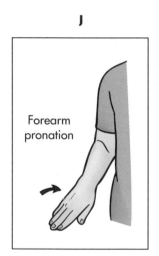

Forearm pronation

K

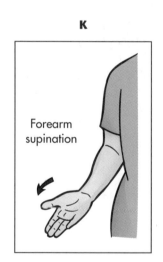

Forearm supination

L

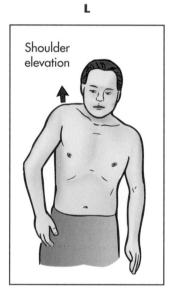

Shoulder elevation

M

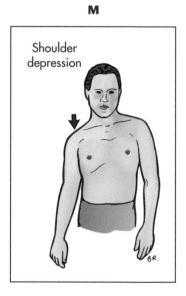

Shoulder depression

N

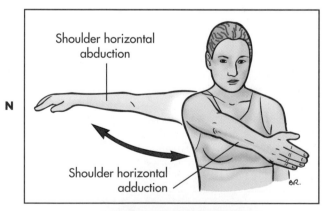

Shoulder horizontal abduction

Shoulder horizontal adduction

f i g . 9 - 2 6, cont'd

Joint movements.

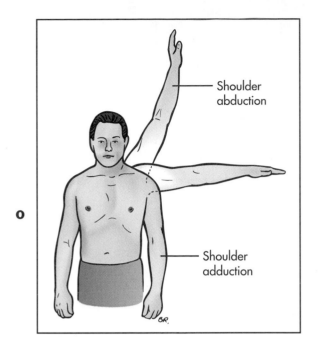

Shoulder abduction

Shoulder adduction

O

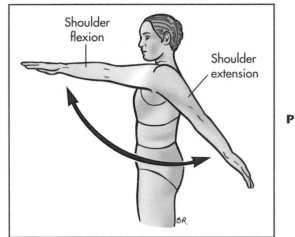

Shoulder flexion

Shoulder extension

P

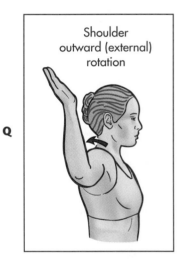

Shoulder outward (external) rotation

Q

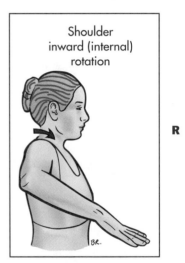

Shoulder inward (internal) rotation

R

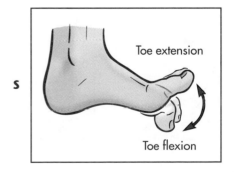

Toe extension

Toe flexion

S

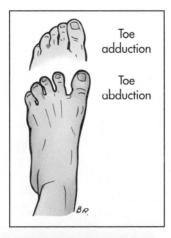

Toe adduction

Toe abduction

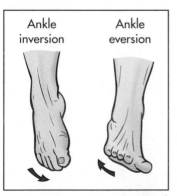

Ankle inversion

Ankle eversion

T, U

Continued.

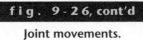

fig. 9-26, cont'd

Joint movements.

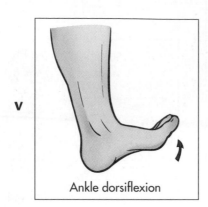

V   Ankle dorsiflexion

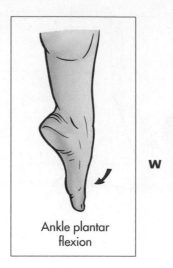

W   Ankle plantar flexion

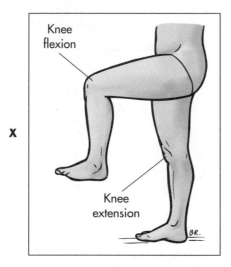

X   Knee flexion

Knee extension

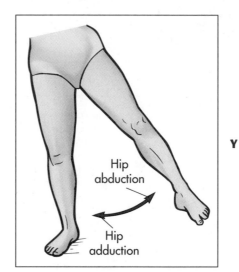

Y   Hip abduction

Hip adduction

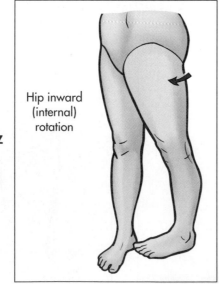

Z   Hip inward (internal) rotation

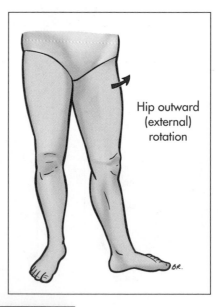

AA   Hip outward (external) rotation

fig. 9-26, cont'd

Joint movements.

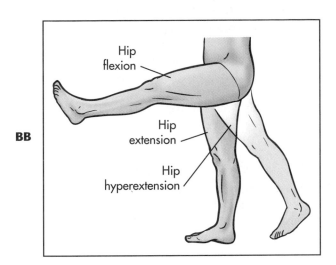

BB

Hip flexion

Hip extension

Hip hyperextension

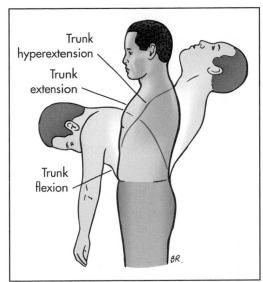

CC

Trunk hyperextension

Trunk extension

Trunk flexion

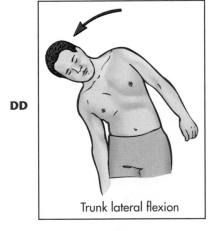

DD

Trunk lateral flexion

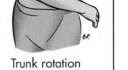

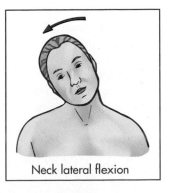

EE

Trunk rotation

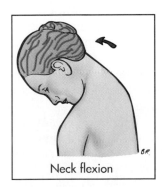

Neck flexion

FF

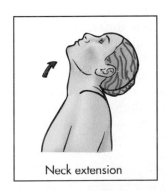

Neck extension

GG

Neck lateral flexion

HH

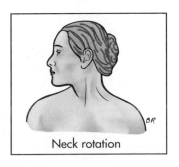

Neck rotation

II

f i g . 9 - 2 6, cont'd

Joint movements.

sively with movement of the joint and are not under voluntary control.

Comparison of a joint to a door hinge.

A good example of joint motion is found on a door. The hinge holds the door both to the casing and away from the casing. For the door to open and close efficiently *(osteokinematic movements)*, the space between the door and the door casing must be maintained and the fit must be correct. If the fit of the door in the door casing is incorrect or the space is not maintained, the door will not open and close correctly. In the body, ligaments act as the hinges.

The door hinge must be oiled. In the joint, the synovial membrane secretes synovial fluid, produced on demand from joint movement. If a joint does not move or is not moved, it will lock up like a rusty door hinge and movement will be restricted or lost.

If you look closely at a door hinge, you will notice the space around the pin in the hinge. If you move the hinge back and forth (not swing the door), the hinge and pin mechanism move a little *(arthrokinematic movements)*. This little movement can be likened to *joint play*. If the ligaments and connective tissue that make up the joint capsule are not firm enough to maintain joint space, the joint play is lost. If the capsule is too tight, joint play is lost as well. Muscles around a joint can spasm, pulling the bone ends together. Joint play will be affected.

If the ligaments and joint capsule are not pliable, flexibility is lost. If the ligaments and joint capsule do not support the joint, the fit is disrupted. Muscle contraction may pull the joint out of alignment. Muscle groups that flex and adduct the joints are about 30% stronger and have more mass than the extensors and abductors. If the body uses muscle contraction to stabilize a joint, the uneven pull between flexors and extensors and adductors and abductors will disturb the fit of the bones at the joint.

Limits to joint movement.

Joints have various degrees of range of motion. Anatomic, physiologic, and pathologic barriers to motion exist. **Anatomic barriers** are determined by the shape and fit of the bones at the joint. The anatomic barrier is seldom reached because the possibility of injury is greatest in this position. Instead the body protects the joint by establishing **physiologic barriers.**

Physiologic barriers are the result of the limits in range of motion imposed by protective nerve and sensory function to support optimal function. An adaptation in the physiologic barrier so that the protective function limits instead of supports optimal functioning is called a **pathologic barrier.** Pathologic barriers often display as stiffness, pain, or a "catch."

When using joint movement techniques, remain within the physiologic barriers. If a pathologic barrier exists that limits motion, use massage techniques to gently and slowly encourage the joint to increase the limits of the range of motion to the physiologic barrier.

Joint end-feel.

When a normal joint is taken to its physiologic limit, usually still a bit more movement is possible, a sort of springiness in the joint. This type of **joint end-feel** is called a *soft end-feel.*

When a joint is restricted or a muscle shortened with a pathologic barrier, thus reducing the range of motion, movement is always limited in some direction. As the limit is reached and exceeded, comfortable movement is no longer possible. In the case of abnormal restriction the limit does not have any spring as found at a physiologic barrier. However, similar to a jammed door or drawer, the joint is fixed at the barrier, and any attempt to take it further is uncomfortable and distinctly "binding" or jamming, rather than springy. This is called a *hard end-feel.*

Effects of Joint Movement Methods

Joint movement is effective because it provides a means of controlled stimulation to the joint mechanoreceptors. Movement initiates muscle tension readjustment through the reflex center of the spinal cord and lower brain centers. As positions change, the supported movement gives the nervous system an entirely different set of signals to process. It is possible for the joint sensory receptors to learn not to be so hypersensitive. As a result the protective spasm and movement restriction may lessen.

Joint movement also encourages lubrication of the joint and adds an important addition to the lymphatic and venous circulation enhancement systems. Much of the pumping action that moves these fluids in the vessels results from compression against the lymph and blood vessels during joint movement and muscle contraction. The tendons, ligaments, and joint capsule are warmed from the movement. This mechanical effect helps keep these tissues pliable.

Fig. 9-26 shows the direction and action of range of motion for each joint. Normal joint movements are often indicated by the degree of movement available. For example, the elbow is said to be able to flex 106 degrees and extend 180 degrees from neutral. The wrist flexion is 90 degrees and wrist extension is 70 degrees from neutral. The degrees of movement have been left off the chart so as to not create an expectation of what normal should be. Instead, each person will identify his or her "normal" range of motion for each joint. For additional study, consult a comprehensive anatomy and physiology book for the degrees of movement for joints.

Remember that each person is unique, and many factors influence available range of motion. Just because one does not have the textbook of range of motion does not mean what is displayed is abnormal. Abnormality is indicated by nonoptimal function. This can be either a limit or exaggeration in the "textbook normal" range of motion. Study Fig. 9-26 carefully, and use it as a guide to move each joint though its full range of motion, always being mindful to go slowly and stay within the comfort limits of each client.

Types of Joint Movement Methods

Joint movement involves moving the jointed areas within the physiologic limits of range of motion of the client. The two types of joint movement are active and passive.

Active joint movement means that the client moves the joint by active contraction of muscle groups. The two variations of active joint movement are as follows:

1. **Active assisted movement** occurs when both the client and massage practitioner move the area.
2. **Active resistive movement** occurs when the client actively moves the joint against a resistance provided by the massage practitioner.

Passive joint movement occurs when the client's muscles stay relaxed and the massage practitioner moves the joint with no assistance from the client. When doing passive joint movement, feel for the soft or hard end-feel of the joint range of motion. This is an important evaluation tool.

Whether active or passive, joint movements are always done within the comfortable limits of the range of motion of the client.

The client's body must always be stabilized, allowing only the joint being worked on to move. Occasionally the entire limb is moved to allow for coordinated interaction among all the joints of the area, but the rest of the body is still stabilized. It is essential to move slowly because quick changes or abrupt moves may cause the muscles to form protective contractions.

Nerves stimulate muscles to contract, moving the joints. Nerves respond to sensory stimulation. If the signal is not quite strong enough, the muscle may tense but not contract. This is called *facilitation*. A facilitated area responds to a lower-intensity sensory stimulation. If a threshold sensory signal does not occur, the nerve stays activated, waiting to contact the muscle and discharge the tension.

All massage professionals have had to deal with a leg or arm that is extremely stiff, even though the client thinks it is relaxed. Most practitioners will instruct the client to relax the muscles or use some other ineffective statement like, "Now just let me do it." It is important to recognize that the client cannot let go of the tension in the muscles because of the facilitation of the nerves.

Systems that incorporate progressive relaxation recognize that a muscle relaxes best if it contracts first. Active resisted range of motion provides a mechanism to contract muscles, discharge the nervous system, and then allow for the normal relaxation phase to take over. A good approach is to have the client use active joint movement, pressing the area to be moved against the stabilizing pressure of the massage practitioner. Then shake or rock the area to relax it.

Caution in Working with Joints

Joint-specific work, including any type of high-velocity manipulation, is beyond the scope of practice of the beginning massage professional. Because of the interplay between the joint proprioceptors, muscle tone, innervation of the joint, and surrounding muscles by the same nerve pattern, any damage to a joint can cause long-term problems. Working within the physiologic ranges of motion for each particular client is within the scope of practice of the massage professional. Specific corrective procedures for pathologic range of motion are best applied in a supervised heath care setting.

Joint Movement's Relationship to Lengthening and Stretching Methods

Joint movement becomes part of the application of muscle energy techniques to lengthen muscles and stretching methods to elongate connective tissues. Because of this the massage professional should concentrate on the ability to use joint movement efficiently and effectively.

How to Apply Joint Movement Methods

Hand placement with joint movement is very important. Make sure that the area is not squeezed, pinched, or restricted in its movement pattern. One hand should be placed close to the joint to be moved to act both as a stabilizer and for evaluation. The practitioner's other hand is placed at the distal end of the bone and is the hand that actually provides the movement. Proper use of body mechanics is essential when using joint movement. The stabilizing hand must remain in contact with the client and must be placed near the joint being affected.

Another method for placement of the stabilizing hand is to move the jointed area without stabilization and observe where the client's body moves most in response to the range of motion action. Place the stabilizing hand at this point.

Avoid working cross-body. Stand with thighs against the table while facing the client, positioned distal to the joint. Usually, the hand closest to the joint is the stabilizing hand. The actual movement comes from the massage practitioner's whole body, not from the shoulder, elbow, or wrist. The movements are rhythmic, smooth, slow, and controlled.

Before joint movement begins, the moving hand lifts and leans back to produce the slight traction necessary to put a small stretch on the joint capsule. If this is not done, the technique is much less effective. When tractioning is mastered and the joint is moved simultaneously, the size of the movement becomes smaller and effectiveness increases. It is not necessary or desirable to have the client's limbs flailing about in the air.

Active range of motion. In **active range of motion** the client moves the area without any type of interaction by the massage practitioner. This is a good assessment method and should be used before and after any type of joint work because it provides information about the limits of range of motion and the improvement after the work is completed. Active range of motion is also great to teach as a self-help tool. As mentioned previously, two variations of active range of motion methods exist: active assistive range of motion and active resisted range of motion.

Active assistive range of motion. Active assistive range of motion involves the client moving the joint though the range of motion and the massage practitioner helping or assisting the movement. This approach is very useful in cases of weakness or pain with movement. The action remains within the comfortable limits of movement for the client. The focus is to create movement within the joint capsule, encouraging synovial fluid movement to warm and soften connective tissue and support muscle function.

Active resisted range of motion. In active resisted range of motion the massage practitioner firmly grasps and holds the end of the bone just distal to the joint being addressed. The massage practitioner leans back slightly to place a small traction on the limb to take up the slack in the tissue. Then the practitioner instructs the client to push slowly against a stabilizing hand or arm while moving the joint through its entire range. A tap or light slap against the limb to begin the movement works well to focus the client's attention.

Another method is to stabilize the entire circumference of the limb and instruct the client to pull gently or move the area. The job of the massage practitioner is to maintain a gentle traction to prevent slack in the tissue, keep the movement slow, and give the client something to push or pull against, discharging the nervous system so the area can relax (Fig. 9-27). The counterforce applied by the massage practitioner does not exceed the pushing or pulling action of the client but instead matches it.

After a form of active range of motion is completed, the client's body is more apt to accept passive range of motion.

Passive range of motion. If a client is paralyzed or very ill, only **passive range of motion** or joint movement may be possible. Some clients do not wish to participate in active joint movement and prefer to take a very passive role during the massage. Client participation is not necessary.

Because the protective system of the joints does not like to be out of control, it takes time to prepare the body for passive range of motion. Shaking, rocking, and the active joint movement sequence previously described work well for this purpose.

To perform passive range of motion, instruct the client to relax the area by letting it lay heavy in your hands. Slowly and rhythmically move the joint though a comfortable range of motion for the jointed area. Repeat the action three or more times, increasing the limits of the range of motion as the muscles relax (Proficiency Exercise 9-10).

Suggested Sequence for Joint Movement Methods

When incorporating joint movement into the massage, follow these basic suggestions:

- If possible, do active joint movement first. Assess range of motion by having the client move the area without participation by the practitioner.
- Have the client move the area against a stabilizing force supplied by the practitioner to increase the intensity of the signals from the contracting muscles, which discharges the nervous system.
- Incorporate any or all of the previously discussed massage methods.
- After the tissue is warm and the nervous system relaxed, do the passive range of motion/joint movement.
- During a massage session, strive to move every joint approximately three times. Each time, take up any slack in the tissues and gently encourage an increase in the range of motion.

9-10

PROFICIENCY EXERCISE

1. Using Fig. 9-26 for reference, move each of your joints, with a variety of speeds, one at a time, through their normal range of motion. Notice the difference when you move slowly.
2. Pretend that a piece of plastic wrap is a joint. Hold one end tightly in your "stabilizing" hand. Now move the plastic wrap around, but do not stretch it or put drag on the "tissue." Use your "moving hand" to traction the plastic wrap. Pull on it as far as it will go without stretching the tissue. Pretend to assess range of motion from this point and feel the difference. Lastly, pull the plastic wrap just a little more. Feel the pliability and do the joint movement from this position. Feel for the difference in effect.
3. Design and perform a massage incorporating joint movement using each of the basic flow patterns.

Muscle Energy and Proprioceptive Neuromuscular Facilitation: Techniques to Lengthen Neurologic Shortened Muscles

Proprioceptive neuromuscular facilitation (PNF) techniques developed out of physical therapy during the 1950s. The first book on the subject, written by Margaret Knott and Dorothy Voss, was *Proprioceptive Neuromuscular Facilitation.*[7] The system was formalized as a rehabilitation

fig. 9-27

Examples of joint movement

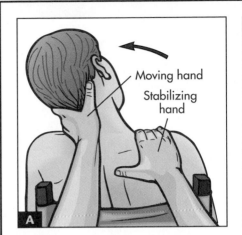

Moving hand
Stabilizing hand

A

Neck.

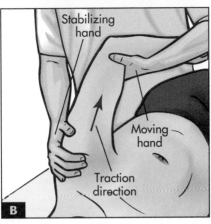

Stabilizing hand
Moving hand
Traction direction

B

Shoulder joint. Hand stabilizes at the shoulder joint.

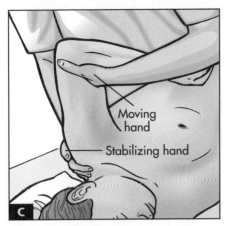

Moving hand
Stabilizing hand

C

Other hand produces a slight traction to the shoulder joint and moves shoulder through circumduction range of motion. (Circumduction—A circular movement of a jointed area.)

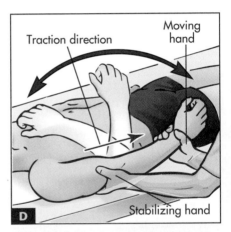

Traction direction
Moving hand
Stabilizing hand

D

Elbow joints. Stabilizing hand holds above elbow while moving hand produces a slight traction and moves joint through flexion and extension. Supination and pronation can also be achieved.

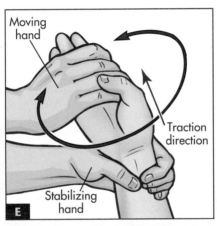

Moving hand
Traction direction
Stabilizing hand

E

Wrist joints. Stabilizing hand holds below wrist while moving hand produces a slight traction and moves joint through circumduction.

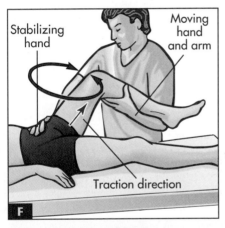

Stabilizing hand
Moving hand and arm
Traction direction

F

Hip joint. Stabilizing hand holds above hip, while moving hand and arm produces a slight traction and moves joint through circumduction.

Continued.

method for spinal cord injury and stroke. It used maximal contraction and rotary diagonal movement patterns to reeducate the nervous system. In recent years, massage professionals have begun to use pieces of the system to enhance muscle lengthening and stretching, primarily in athletes.

The diagonal movement patterns incorporate cross-body movement used in repatterning for children born with various types of damage to the motor areas of the brain. Popularized as *cross crawl,* the movements cause left and right brain hemispheres to function simultaneously by movement of one leg and the opposite arm into flexion and adduction to cross the midline of the body. The same movement is then repeated with the other leg and arm.

fig. 9-27, cont'd

Examples of joint movement

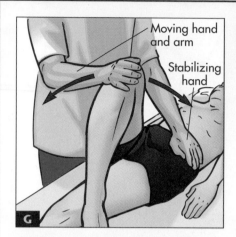

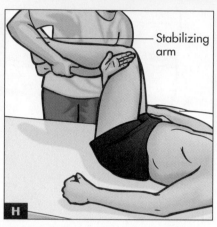

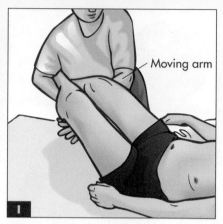

Hip joint alternate position. Stabilizing hand holds at opposite anterior superior iliac spine while moving hand moves hip through flexion and extension. No traction is produced in this position.

Pelvis. Stabilizing hand and arm holds legs at calf.

Moving arm and hand moves pelvis to a side-lying, "figure-eight" pattern.

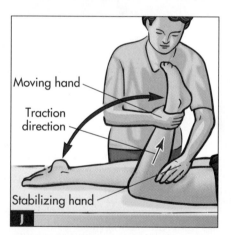

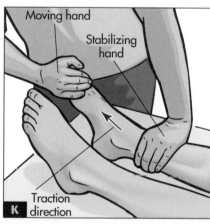

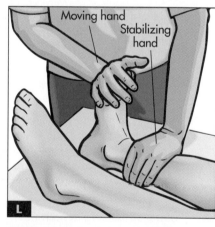

Knee. Stabilizing hand holds above knee while moving hand produces a slight traction and moves joint through flexion and extension.

Ankle. Stabilizing hand holds below above ankle.

Moving hand produces a slight traction and moves joint through circumduction.

These types of movements reflexively stimulate the gait or walking pattern and are a valuable addition to any massage system (Fig. 9-28).

Muscle energy methods emerged from the osteopathic profession. Dr. T. J. Ruddy developed a technique he called *resistive induction.* Dr. Fred K. Mitchell is acknowledged as the father of the system that is now called **muscle energy technique.** He built on Dr. Ruddy's method, turning it into a whole-body approach.[5] Dr. Karel Lewit, author of *Ma-nipulative Therapy in Rehabilitation of the Locomotor System,*[8] discusses the importance of methods that use postisometric relaxation. Dr. Leon Chaitow, author of many manual techniques textbooks, synthesized these gentle methods, which fall within the scope of practice of therapeutic massage when used for general body normalization.

Only those methods applicable to general massage are presented here, but the system has much to offer. The diligent student of therapeutic massage will seek out addi-

fig. 9-28

Cross crawl

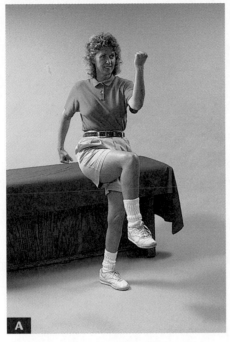

A

Demonstration of cross crawl.

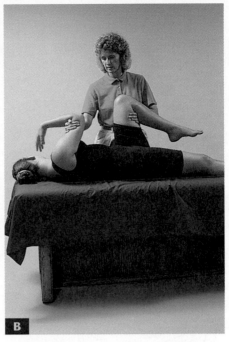

B

Application of cross crawl with client on the table.

tional training at more advanced levels. The majority of the information in this section is adapted from Dr. Chaitow's books and workshop notes.

The main differences between muscle energy and PNF are the origin of thought, the intensity of the muscle contraction, and the specificity of the approach. However, for the purposes of this textbook, muscle energy techniques and PNF can be thought of as the same thing.

Muscle Energy Techniques

Muscle energy techniques involve a voluntary contraction of the client's muscles in a specific and controlled direction, at varying levels of intensity, against a specific counterforce applied by the massage practitioner. Muscle energy procedures have a variety of applications and are considered active techniques in which the client contributes the corrective force. The amount of effort may vary from a small muscle twitch to a maximal muscle contraction. The duration may last from a fraction of a second to several seconds. All contractions are to begin and end slowly, gradually building to the desired intensity. No jerking is done in the movement.

The focus of muscle energy techniques is to stimulate

the nervous system to allow a more normal muscle resting length. To describe what happens, the term **lengthening** is used because lengthening is more of a neurologic response that allows the muscles to stop contracting and to relax. **Stretching** is more correctly defined as a mechanical force applied to the elongate connective tissue.

Muscle energy techniques are focused to specific muscles or muscle groups. It is important to be able to position muscles so that the origin and insertion are either close together or in a lengthening phase with the origin and insertion separated. Certain resources diagram specific positions for each muscle to assist in accomplishing this. An alternate approach is to study muscle charts and understand the configuration of the muscle patterns. Practice isolating as many muscles as possible, keeping in mind that proper positioning is very important. When practicing, make sure that the muscles can be isolated regardless of whether the client is in a supine, prone, side-lying, or seated position (Fig. 9-29).

Counterpressure is the force applied to an area that is designed to match the effort or force exactly (isometric contraction) or partially (isotonic contraction). This holding force can be applied with the hand(s) of the person

Text continued on p. 375.

fig. 9-29

Positions for muscle isolation.

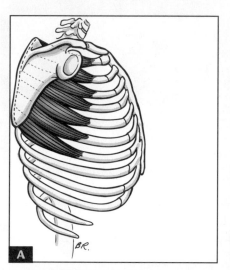

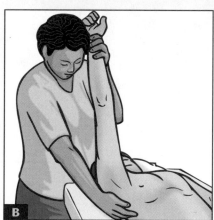

Serratus anterior.

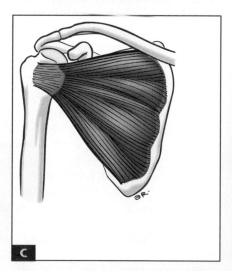

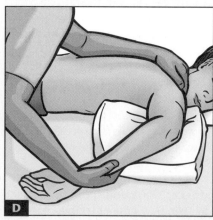

Subscapularis.

fig. 9-29, cont'd

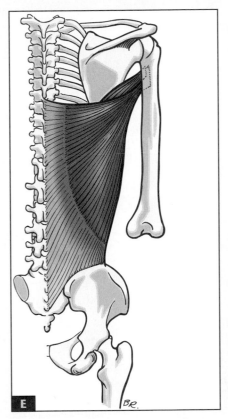

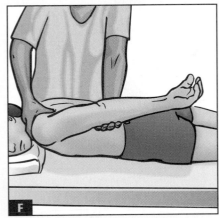

Latissimus dorsi.

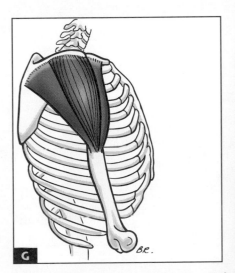

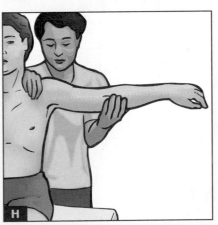

Deltoid.

Continued.

fig. 9-29, cont'd

Positions for muscle isolation

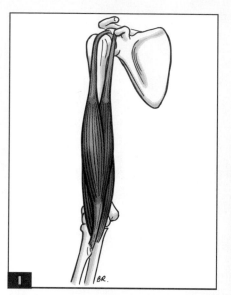

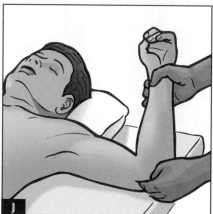

Biceps and brachialis.

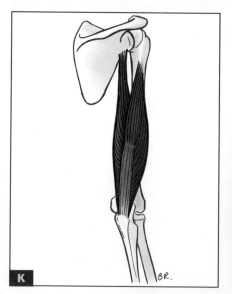

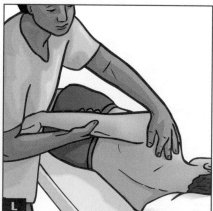

Triceps.

fig. 9-29, cont'd

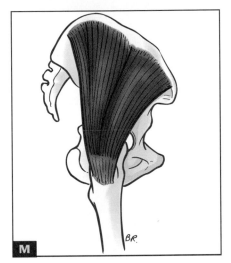

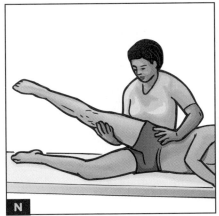

Gluteus medius.

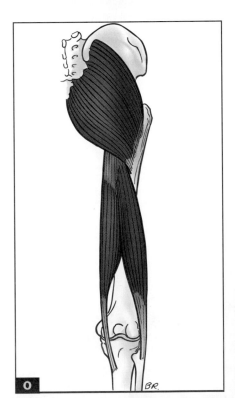

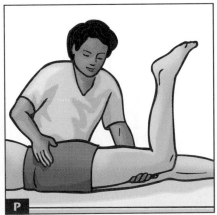

Gluteus maximus and hamstrings.

Continued.

fig. 9-29, cont'd

Positions for muscle isolation

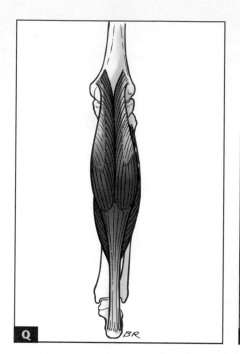

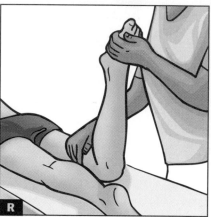

Gastrocnemius and soleus.

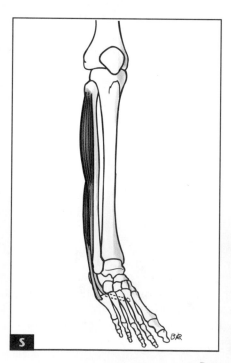

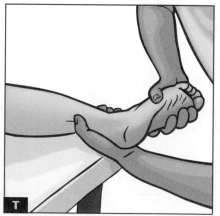

Peroneus.

doing the exercise (the massage practitioner) against an immovable object, or against gravity where appropriate. The response of the method is specific to a certain muscle or muscle group referred to as the **target muscle(s).**

Types of muscle contractions. The massage practitioner uses three different types of muscle contractions to activate muscle energy techniques: **isometric contraction, isotonic contraction,** and **multiple isotonic contractions.**

In an *isometric contraction,* the distance between the origin and insertion of the target muscle is maintained at a constant length. A fixed tension develops in the target muscle as the client contracts the muscle against an equal counterforce applied by the massage practitioner, preventing shortening of the muscle from the origin to the insertion. In this contraction the effort of the muscle, or group of muscles, is exactly matched by a counterpressure, so no movement occurs, only effort.

An *isotonic contraction* is one in which the effort of the target muscle or muscles is not quite matched by the counterpressure, allowing a degree of resisted movement to occur. With a **concentric isotonic contraction,** the massage practitioner applies a counterforce but allows the client to move the origin and insertion of the target muscle together against the pressure. In an **eccentric isotonic contraction,** the massage practitioner applies a counterforce but allows the client to move the jointed area, so origin and insertion of the target muscle separate as the muscle lengthens against the pressure.

Multiple isotonic contractions require the client to move the joint through a full range of motion, against partial resistance applied by the massage practitioner.

Muscle energy techniques usually do not use the full contraction strength of the client. With most isometric work, the contraction should start at about 25% of the strength of the muscle. Subsequent contractions can involve progressively greater degrees of effort but never more than 50% of the available strength.

Many experts use only about 10% of the available strength in muscles being treated in this way and find that they can increase effectiveness by using longer periods of contraction. Pulsed (a rapid series of repetitions) contractions using minimal strength are also effective.

The use of coordinated breathing to enhance particular directions of muscular effort is helpful. During massage, all muscular effort is enhanced by inhaling as the effort is made and exhaling on the lengthening phase.

Neurophysiologic principles and procedures. Two neurophysiologic principles explain the effect of the techniques as a result of physiologic laws being applied, not from mechanical force as in stretching. The principles are *postisometric relaxation* and *reciprocal inhibition.*

Postisometric relaxation. Postisometric relaxation (PIR, "tense and relax," "contact relax"), which occurs after an

isometric contraction of a muscle, results from the activity of the Golgi tendon bodies. It is in the brief latent period of 10 seconds or so after such a contraction that the muscle can be lengthened painlessly, further than it could before the contraction. After an isometric contraction (which will have loaded the Golgi tendon organs and the musculotendinous junction and reflexively inhibited the extrafusal fibers of the muscle spindles), the muscle is in a brief period during which nerve impulses to the target muscle are inhibited. This period is called the *refractory state;* it allows the target muscle to be lengthened passively to its comfort barrier. The **comfort barrier** is the first point of resistance short of the client perceiving any discomfort at either the physiologic or pathologic barrier. The isometric contraction involves minimal effort lasting 7 to 10 seconds. Repetitions continue until no further gain is noted.

The following is the procedure for PIR (Fig. 9-30):

1. Lengthen the target muscle to comfort barrier. Back off slightly.
2. Tense the target muscle for 7 to 10 seconds.
3. Stop contraction and lengthen the target muscle. Repeat steps 1 through 3 until normal full resting length is obtained.

Reciprocal inhibition. The second neurophysiologic principle is that of **reciprocal inhibition** (RI), which takes place when a muscle contracts, causing its antagonist to relax to allow for more normal movement. Generally, an isometric contraction of the antagonist of a shortened target muscle allows the muscle to relax and be taken to a new resting length. Such contractions usually begin in the mid-range rather than near the barrier of resistance and last 7 to 10 seconds. Reciprocal inhibition relaxes a target muscle as the tension increases in its antagonist. This response works through the central nervous system, which cannot allow both the prime movers and the antagonists to be tightening at the same time in this reflex arc pattern.

The following is the procedure for reciprocal inhibition (Fig. 9-31):

1. Isolate the target muscles by putting them in passive contraction (massage practitioner moves the origin and insertion of the muscles together using joint positioning).
2. Contract the antagonist muscle group (the muscle in extension).
3. Stop contraction and slowly bring the target muscle into a lengthened state, stopping at resistance.
4. Place the target muscle slightly into contraction again.
5. Repeat steps 2 through 4 until normal full resting length is obtained.

Reciprocal inhibition is a great way to soften a muscle so that it can be massaged at its deeper levels. Any massage practitioner knows what it is like to massage a hard and tense muscle, especially when trying to get to tissue

fig. 9-30

Procedure for postisometric relaxation (PIR)/tense and relax techniques

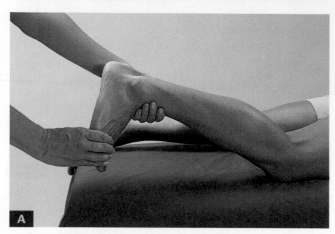

A

Step 1. Lengthen the target muscle (gastrocnemius/soleus) to comfort barrier.

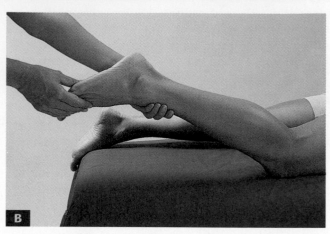

B

Back off slightly.

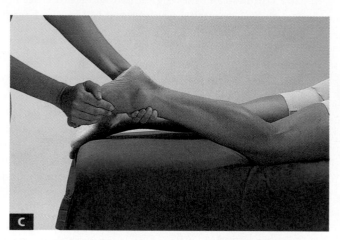

C

Step 2. Tense the target muscle for 7 to 10 seconds.

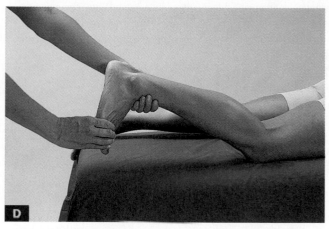

D

Step 3. Stop contraction and lengthen the target muscle.

Repeat steps 1 through 3 until normal full resting length is obtained.

under that muscle. The following procedure reflexively creates a soft muscle, which in turn makes massage much easier (Fig. 9-32):

1. Isolate a target muscle or muscle group identified to be made soft into passive contraction.
2. Place the hand that will massage the "soft muscle" on the target muscle. Place the other hand or other stabilizing object on the antagonist muscle group (the one that is stretched out at this point).
3. Have the client actively contract the antagonist muscles against the stabilization. The target muscle will be inhibited reciprocally and will become a "soft muscle."

It will be easier to massage, and the massage practitioner will be able to reach the deeper areas.

Combined methods: contract-relax-antagonist-contract. Tense and relax and reciprocal inhibition can be combined to enhance the lengthening effects. This method can be called *contract-relax-antagonist-contract.*

The following is the procedure for contract-relax-antagonist-contract:

1. Position the target muscles as in tense and relax procedures
2. Lengthen the target muscle to barrier. Back off slightly.

f i g . 9 - 3 1

Procedure for reciprocal inhibition

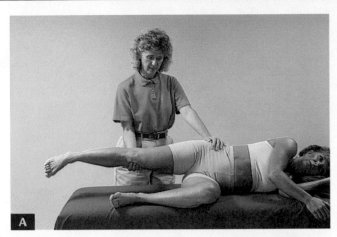

Step 1. Isolate the target muscles (adductors) by putting them in passive contraction (massage practitioner moves the origin and insertion of the muscles together using joint positioning.)

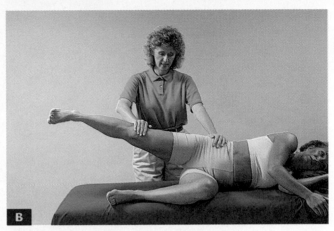

Step 2. Contract the antagonist muscle group (the muscle in extension).

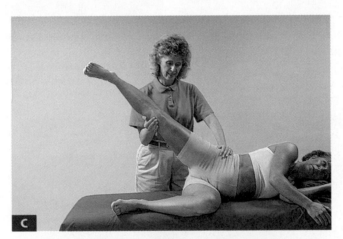

Step 3. Stop contraction and slowly bring target muscle into a lengthened state, stopping at resistance.

Step 4. Place the target muscle slightly into contraction again. Repeat steps 2 through 4 until normal full resting length is obtained.

3. Tense the target muscle for 7 to 10 seconds.
4. Contract the antagonist as in reciprocal inhibition.
5. Stop contraction of antagonist.
6. Lengthen the muscle to a more normal resting length.

Pulsed muscle energy. **Pulsed muscle energy** procedures involve engaging the comfort barrier and using small, resisted contractions (usually 20 in 10 seconds), which introduces mechanical pumping as well as PIR or RI depending on the muscles used.

The following is the procedure for pulsed muscle energy (Fig. 9-33):

1. Isolate the target muscle by putting it into a passive contraction.
2. Apply counterpressure for the contraction.
3. Instruct the client to contract the target muscle rapidly in very small movements for about 20 repetitions. Go to step 4 or use this variation: maintain the position, but switch the counterpressure location to the opposite

fig. 9-32

Procedure to make a soft muscle ("Make a soft muscle concept")

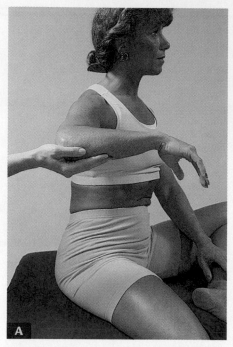

Step 1. Isolate target muscle (deltoid) or muscle group into passive contraction.

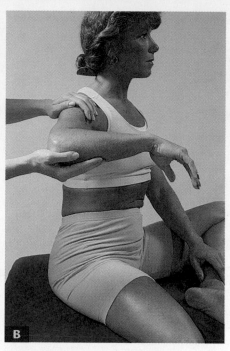

Step 2. Place the hand that will massage the "soft muscle" on the target (deltoid) muscle. Place the other hand or other stabilizing object on the antagonist muscle group (the ones that are stretched out at this point).

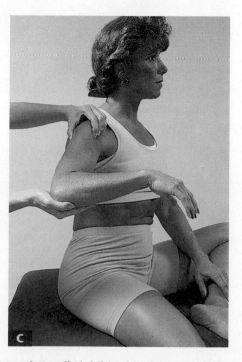

Step 3. Have the client actively contract the antagonist muscles against the stabilization.

The target muscle will be reciprocally inhibited and become a "soft muscle." It will be easier to massage, and the practitioner will be able to reach the deeper areas.

fig. 9-33

Procedure for pulsed muscle energy

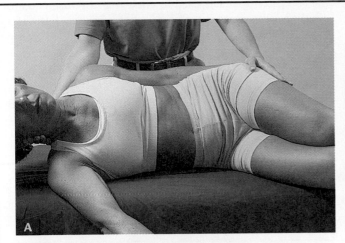

Step 1. Isolate the target muscle (abdominals) by putting it into a passive contraction.

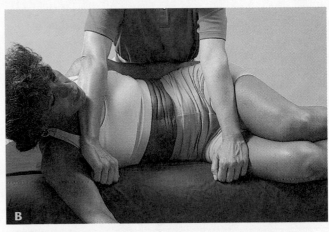

Step 2. Apply counterpressure for the contraction.

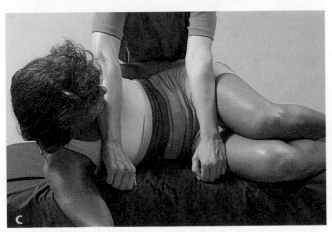

Step 3. Instruct the client to contract the target muscle rapidly in very small movements for about 20 repetitions.

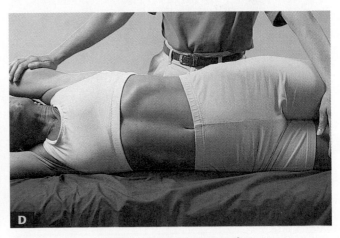

Step 4. Slowly lengthen the target muscle.

Repeat steps 2 through 4 until normal full resting length is obtained.

side and have the client contract the antagonist muscles for 20 repetitions.

4. Slowly lengthen the target muscle. Repeat steps 2 to 4 until normal full resting length is obtained.

NOTE: All contracting and resisting efforts should start and finish gently.

Direct applications. In some circumstances the client does not wish to or cannot participate actively in the massage. The principles of muscle energy techniques can still be used by direct manipulation of the spindle cells or Golgi tendons. Pushing muscle fibers together in the direction of the fibers in the belly of a muscle weakens the muscle by working with the spindle cells. As the fibers of the muscle are pushed together, the spindle cells (which sense muscle length) think that the muscle is too short. The proprioceptive response is to relax the muscle fibers so that the muscle can be comfortable in its chosen position. Pushing muscle fibers together in the belly of the muscle is a way to relieve a muscle cramp. This is sometimes called **approximation.**

Separating the muscle fibers in the belly of the muscle in the direction of the fibers strengthens the muscle.

When this occurs, the spindle cells "think" the muscle is too long; they signal the brain's proprioceptive intelligence to shorten the muscle so that the muscle can do the job it is supposed to do.

The same responses can be obtained by using the Golgi tendon organs, except that the manipulation of the proprioception signal cells is reversed. Manipulation of the Golgi tendon organs, is at the ends of the muscle where it joins the tendons. To weaken the muscle, pull apart on the tendon attachments of the target muscle. This tells the body's proprioception center that tension on the tendon is excessive and the muscle should loosen to be in balance. To strengthen the muscle, push the tendon attachments together. This signals the body that too little tension is on the tendon (in relation to the tension within the muscle belly). The muscle, in turn, contracts.

The pressure levels used to elicit the response need to be sufficient to contact the muscle fibers. Too light of a pressure will not access the proprioceptors. Excessive pressure will negate the response by activating protective reflexes. Moderate pressure where the muscle itself can be palpated is most effective.

The following is the procedure for direct manipulation of the spindle cells to initiate relaxation and lengthening response (Fig. 9-34):

---

fig. 9-34

Procedure for direct manipulation of spindle cells to initiate relaxation lengthening response

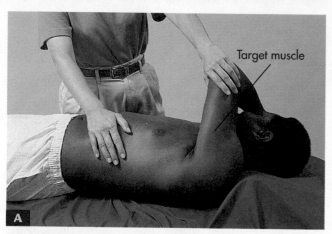

Step 1. Place the target muscle (triceps) in comfortable extension.

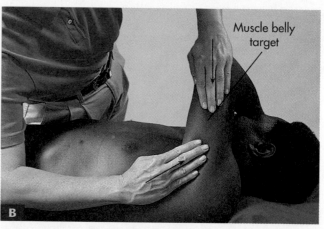

Step 2. Press the spindle cells together on the target muscle.

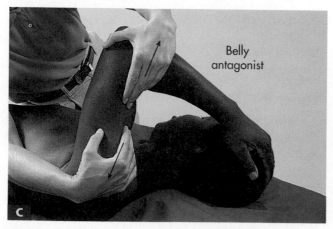

Step 3. Pull the spindle cells apart on the antagonist muscle.

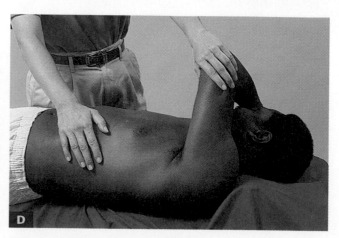

Step 4. Lengthen the target muscle.

Repeat steps 2 through 4 until normal full resting length is obtained.

1. Place the target muscle in comfortable extension.
2. Press the spindle cells together on the target muscle.
3. Pull the spindle cells apart on the antagonist muscle.
4. Lengthen the target muscle.
5. Repeat steps 2 through 4 until normal full resting length is obtained.

The following is the procedure for direct manipulation of the Golgi tendon organs to initiate the PIR response (Fig. 9-35):

1. Place the target muscle in comfortable extension.
2. Pull apart on the tendon attachments of the target muscle.

3. Push the tendon attachments together on the antagonist muscle.
4. Lengthen the target muscle.
5. Repeat steps 2 through 4 until normal full resting length is obtained.

Positional release/strain-counterstrain. **Strain-counterstrain** was formalized by Dr. Lawrence Jones and involves using tender points to guide the positioning of the body into a space where the muscle tension can release on its own. Orthobiotomy consists of similar concepts and grew from the foundation of strain-counterstrain.

Positional release is a more generic term to describe these methods. Positional release methods are used on

---

fig.9-35

Procedure for direct manipulation of the Golgi tendons to initiate PIR

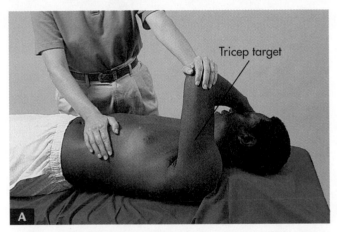

Tricep target

Step 1. Place the target muscle (triceps) in comfortable extension.

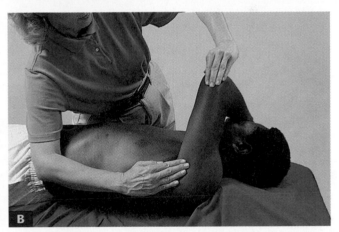

Step 2. Pull apart on the tendon attachments of the target muscle.

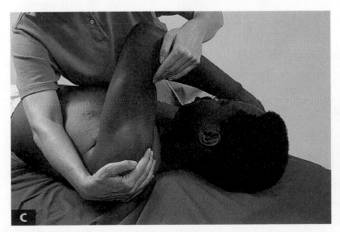

Step 3. Push the tendon attachments together on the antagonist muscle.

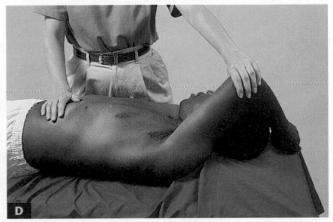

Step 4. Lengthen the target muscle.

Repeat steps 2 through 4 until normal full resting length is obtained.

painful areas, especially recent strains, either before, after, or instead of muscle energy methods. The tender points are often located in the antagonist of the tight muscle because of the diagonal balancing process the body uses to maintain an upright posture in gravity.

Repositioning of the body into the original strain (often the position of a prior injury) allows proprioceptors to reset and stop firing protective signals. By moving the body into the direction of ease (i.e., the way the body wants to go and out of the position that causes the pain), the propriocep-

tion is taken into a state of safety. By remaining in this state for a period of time, the neuromuscular mechanism is allowed to reset itself. The massage practitioner then gently and slowly repositions the area into neutral.

The positioning used during positional release is a full-body process. Remember, an injury or loss of balance is a full-body experience. For this reason, areas distant to the tender point must be considered during the positioning process. It is very possible that the position of the feet will have an effect on a tender point in the neck.

---

fig. 9-36

Procedure for generalized positional release

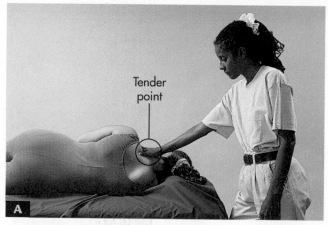

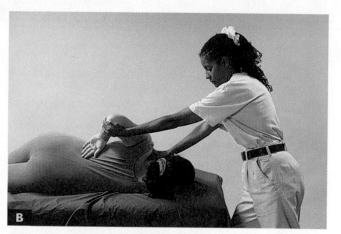

Step 1. Locate the tender point. Step 2. Gently initiate the pain response with direct pressure. Remember the sensation of pain is a guide.

Step 3. Slowly position the body until the pain subsides. Ease off the pressure. Step 4. Wait at least 30 seconds or longer until the client feels the release.

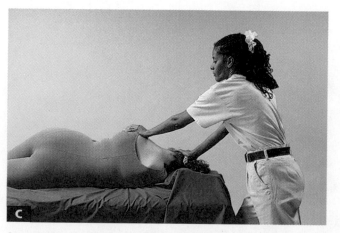

Step 5. Slowly reposition into extended position.

Step 4. Place the target muscle slightly into contraction again. Repeat steps 2 through 4 until normal full resting length is obtained.

The following is the procedure for positional release (Fig. 9-36):

1. Locate the tender point.
2. Gently initiate the pain response with direct pressure. Remember the sensation of pain is a guide.
3. Slowly position the body until the pain subsides.
4. Wait at least 30 seconds or longer until the client feels the release, lightly monitoring the tender point.
5. Slowly lengthen the muscle.
6. Repeat steps 1 through 5 until normal full resting length is obtained.

Positional release techniques are important because they gently allow the body to reposition and restore balance. They are also one of the most effective ways of dealing with tender areas regardless of the pathology. Sometimes it is impossible to know why the point is tender to the touch. However, if tenderness is present, a protective muscle spasm will surround it. Positional release is an excellent way to release these small areas of muscle spasm without inducing additional pain.

Integrated approach. Muscle energy methods can be used together or in sequence to enhance their effects. Muscle tension in one area of the body often indicates imbalance and compensation patterns in other areas of the body as well. Tension patterns can be self-perpetuating. Often using an integrated approach introduces the type of information the nervous system needs to self-correct. The procedure outlined here relies on the body's innate knowledge of what is out of balance and how to restore a more normal functioning pattern.

The following is the procedure for integrated approach (Proficiency Exercise 9-11). (Use the position from either Option A or Option B as the starting point for the rest of the process.)

OPTION A:

1. Identify the most obvious of the postural distortion symptoms.
2. Exaggerate the pattern by increasing the distortion, moving the body into ease. This position becomes the pattern of isolation of various muscles that will be addressed in the next part of the procedure (e.g., if the left shoulder is elevated and rotated forward, exaggerate and increase the elevation and rotation pattern).

OPTION B:

1. Identify a painful point.
2. Use positional release or move the body into ease until the point is substantially less tender to pressure. The position of ease found becomes the pattern of isolation of various muscles that will be addressed in the next part of the procedure.
3. Stabilize the client in as many different directions as possible.
4. Instruct the client to move out of the pattern. Be as vague as possible and do not guide the client because it is important for the client to identify the resistance pattern.
5. Provide resistance for the client to push or pull against.
6. Modify the resistance angle as necessary to achieve the most solid resistance pattern for the client.
7. After a few moments spent noticing when the breathing changes, continue to provide modified resistance but now allow the client to move through the pattern slowly against some resistance.
8. When the client has achieved as much extension as he can on his own, recognize that what he has achieved is the lengthen pattern.
9. Gently increase the lengthening. If additional elongation in this position is desired, connective tissue stretching can be achieved.
10. Pay attention to what body areas become involved besides the one being addressed. This is your guide to the next position.

Stretching

Stretching is a mechanical method of pulling connective tissue to reduce tensile stress and elongate areas of connective tissue shortening. Stretching affects the fiber component of connective tissue by elongating the fibers past the normal give of the fiber to enter the plastic range past the existing bind. This creates either a freeing and unraveling of fibers or a small therapeutic inflammatory response that signals for change in the fibers. The ground substance is also affected during stretching by being warmed and softened, increasing pliability.

9-11

PROFICIENCY EXERCISE

1. Design a progressive relaxation sequence for yourself using the concept of PIR.
2. Design a lengthening sequence for yourself using the pulsed muscle contraction.
3. Design a complete massage using pétrissage and compression on "soft muscles."
4. Experiment with positional release concepts to relax sore spots on your body.
5. Design a complete massage incorporating all of the muscle energy methods presented.

Because fascial sheaths provide structural support, it is important to work with a sense of three-dimensional awareness, realizing that shifts in structure have more than a localized effect. Because the body supports stability before mobility and compensation patterns are body-wide, changes in structure need to be balanced with either lengthening or strengthening activities that allow the body to maintain a sense of perpendicular orientation in gravity.

If the stability/mobility factor is not considered, the body's method of reacting to changes in structure is to increase muscle spasm and acute pain. This results in a decreased ability to adapt effectively to the changes introduced; it reduces the effectiveness of the methods.

How to Apply Stretching

Stretching and lengthening are different. Before any stretching, lengthening must be done or the muscles of the area may develop protective spasms because stretching often moves into pathologic barriers formed by connective tissue changes. The connective tissue component cannot be accessed until the muscle is lengthened. Without stretching, any neuromuscular lengthening may be restricted by shortened connective tissue. Although it is possible and often desirable to lengthen without stretching, it is always necessary to lengthen before stretching. During stretching the two methods work in conjunction with each other. Muscle energy techniques are used to prepare muscles to stretch by activating lengthening responses.

Longitudinal stretching pulls connective tissue in the direction of the fiber configuration. Cross-directional stretching pulls the connective tissue against the fiber direction. Both accomplish the same thing, but longitudinal stretching is done in conjunction with movement at the joint. If longitudinal stretching is not advisable, if it is ineffective in situations of hypermobility of a joint, or if the area to be stretched is not effectively stretched longitudinally, cross-directional stretching is a better choice. Cross-directional stretching is focused on the tissue itself and does not depend on joint movement.

NOTE: For the purposes of this textbook, the term *static stretching* refers to stretching a muscle with no previous preparation. A static stretch can fatigue the muscle, causing it to relax. It is the least effective method of muscle stretching.

The **direction of ease** is the way the body allows for postural changes and muscle shortening or weakening compensation patterns, depending on its balance in gravity. Although compensation patterns may be inefficient, the patterns developed serve a purpose and need to be respected. It may seem logical to locate a shortened muscle group or a rotated movement pattern and use direct methods to reverse the pattern. However, this may not be the best approach. Protective sensory receptors prevent any forced stretch out of a compensation pattern. Instead the pattern of compensation is respected and the body position is exaggerated and coaxed into a more efficient position.

For example, a client has shortened pectoralis muscles that pull the shoulders forward, giving a gorilla-like appearance. Instead of pulling the pectoralis muscles into a stretch by forcing the arms back, curl the shoulders and arms more into adduction, providing slack and space to the receptors in the pectoralis muscles. Begin corrective action from this point.

The following is the procedure for longitudinal stretching (Fig. 9-37):

1. Position the target muscle in the "direction of ease." Stabilize and isolate a muscle group.
2. Choose a method to prepare the target muscle to stretch (e.g., PIR, RI, pulsed muscle energy, direct application).
3. After the target muscle is prepared, stretch the muscle to its physiologic or pathologic barrier, or wherever protective contraction is engaged. Back off slightly to avoid muscle spasm. Stay in line with muscle fibers. Exert effort or movement with the inhalation. Stretch on the exhalation.

The following two approaches are used for the actual stretch phase:

1. Hold the position just off the physiologic or pathologic barrier for at least 10 seconds and up to 30 to 60 seconds to allow for the neurologic reset. This is the lengthening phase. Feel for secondary response (a small give in the muscle).
2. Take up slack and hold for 20 to 30 seconds to create longitudinal pull on the connective tissue. You must hold the muscle stretch as instructed to allow for changes in the connective tissue component of the muscle.

Alternate procedure for longitudinal stretching. If only a small section of muscle needs to be stretched, if the muscle does not lend itself to stretching with joint movement, or if the joints are so flexible that not enough pull is put on the muscles to achieve an effective stretch to the tissues, the following alternate procedure for longitudinal stretching should be used (Fig. 9-38):

1. Locate the fibers or muscle to be stretched.
2. Place hands, fingers, or forearms in the belly of the muscle or directly over the area to be stretched.
3. Contact muscle with sufficient pressure to reset the neuromuscular mechanism.
4. Separate fingers, hands, or forearms or lift tissue with pressure sufficient to stretch muscle. Take up all slack from lengthening, then increase the intensity slightly

---

fig. 9-37

Procedure for longitudinal stretching

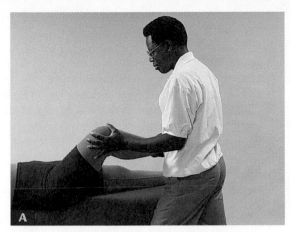

Step 1. Position target muscle (quadriceps group) in "direction of ease." Stabilize and isolate muscle group.

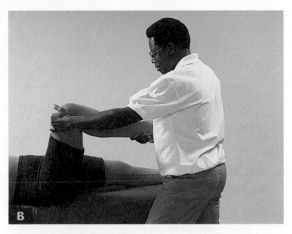

Step 2. Choose a method to prepare target muscle to stretch. (In this example, PIR is used with client contracting the quadriceps against the stabilizing force of the massage practitioner.)

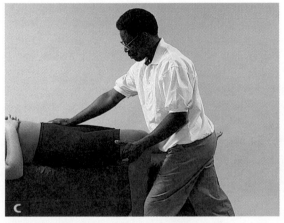

Step 3. After the muscle is prepared, stretch the muscle to physiologic or pathologic barrier or wherever protective contraction is engaged.

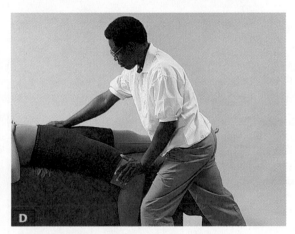

Stay in line with muscle fibers. Exert effort with one inhalation. Stretch on the exhalation.

---

and wait for the connective tissue component to respond (this may take as long as 30 seconds).

NOTE: All requirements for preparation of muscle and direction of stretch remain the same as described in the previous longitudinal stretching procedure.

The following is the procedure for active assisted longitudinal stretching:

1. Identify and isolate the muscle, making sure it is not working against gravity in this position. The client is reminded to exhale during the stretching phase of this technique.
2. The muscle is then lengthened to its physiologic or pathologic barrier, moved slightly beyond this point, and stretched gently for 1 to 2 seconds.
3. The muscle is then returned to its starting position, and this action is repeated in a rhythmic, pulselike fashion for 5 to 20 repetitions.
4. The client will benefit from doing a contraction with the antagonist while lengthening and then stretching the target muscle. As in all proper lengthening and

stretching movements, attention must be paid to the stretch reflex; bouncing is never done because it initiates this reflex.

Cross-directional tissue stretching uses a pull-and-twist component. The following is the procedure for cross-directional stretching (Fig. 9-39):

---

fig. 9-38

Alternate method for longitudinal stretching

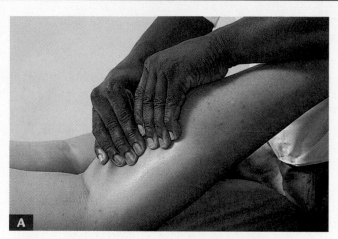

A

Step 1. Locate fibers or muscle to be stretched. Step 2. Place hands, fingers, or forearms in the belly of muscle or directly over area to be stretched. Step 3. Contact muscle with sufficient pressure to reset the neuromuscular mechanism.

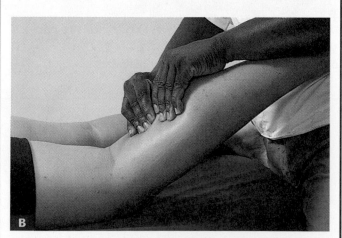

B

Step 4. Separate fingers, hands, or forearms, or lift tissue with pressure sufficient to stretch muscle. Take up all slack from lengthening first. Then increase intensity slightly and wait (this may take as long as 30 seconds) for connective tissue component to respond.

---

1. Access the area to be stretched by moving against the fiber direction.
2. Lift or deform the area slightly, and hold for 30 to 60 seconds until the area gets warm or seems to soften.

Use the following procedure for skin and superficial connective tissue:

1. Locate the area of restriction.
2. Lift and pull (like taffy), first moving into the restriction and then pulling and twisting out of it, keeping a constant tension on the tissue (remember the plastic wrap exercise). Go slow. Take up slack until the area warms and softens.

Use of cold applications and stretching. Dr. Janet Travell popularized the cold spray-and-stretch concepts. The reason the cold spray worked was that it stimulated cold receptors blocking other sensory signals, so the proprioceptors were inhibited momentarily, allowing the muscle to relax. The cold spray used was a type of refrigerant that is no longer available because it damages the ozone layer.

An ice pop (made by freezing water in a paper cup with a wooden stick inserted) can be used to create the same effect as cold spray. Move the ice pop on the skin from origin to insertion along the path of the muscle that is to be stretched. Move at a speed of about 1 inch per second and stretch the muscle.[11]

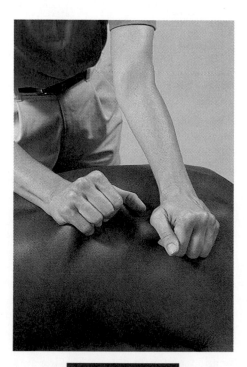

fig. 9-39

Cross-directional stretching.

Using tapotement with stretching. Using forms of tapotement on the skin over the muscle along the same pathway as the ice pop massage is effective in facilitating stretching. The skin is snapped quickly with a move like shooting marbles. If a tendon is tapped quickly, the muscle will contract.

Use this method to assist in stretching. Apply the tap to the antagonist muscles so that they contract reflexively. As a result, the muscle you wish to stretch is inhibited reciprocally, allowing for a relaxation response and the ability to stretch with reduced protective muscle spasm.

Stretching deep fascial planes. To access deep fascial planes it is necessary to have an understanding of the cranial sacral mechanisms and the deep structures involved. Entry-level training does not explore this advanced level of work. The approaches of cranial sacral therapy and advanced soft tissue systems such as myofascial release, deep tissue work, and soft tissue manipulation provide instruction in these very valuable methods. Chapter 11 expands on this information.

9-12

PROFICIENCY EXERCISE

1. Pétrissage (knead) extra flour into bread dough so that the consistency is quite firm. Practice stretching the dough. Feel for the give of the tissue as opposed to the tissue breaking.
2. Design a lengthening and stretching sequence for yourself that accesses the major muscle groups and connective tissue areas. Pay attention to the difference in the feel of neuromuscular lengthening with its quick release and connective tissue stretching with its softer, slower give.
3. Have a fellow student assume various stretch positions. Tell him or her to stretch as far as is comfortable and hold. Take the area and stretch it ⅛ inch further and hold it. Pay attention to the feeling, and talk with the student to get feedback.
4. Practice tapping antagonist tendons and using ice massage on a client as you position the body for various stretches.
5. Working with a partner, see how many massage manipulations and techniques you can combine and do at once (e.g., joint movement combined with compression, effleurage combined with a stretch, tapotement combined with a stretch, pétrissage combined with muscle energy methods—especially the "make a soft muscle" concept).
6. Design a massage for each of the basic flow patterns that combines at least two methods or techniques for every application.

It is important to realize that we have one body with all interconnecting parts. Therefore all stretching affects deep connective tissue. It is impossible to separate the body into layers. The only difference is the access point. A house may have three or four doors, each of which will let you into the house. Where you enter may be different, but after you are inside, you will have an influence on all the areas. Therefore effective stretching of the more superficial connective tissues as presented in this chapter indirectly affects the deeper connective tissue structures as well (Proficiency Exercise 9-12).

SEQUENCE AND FLOW

section objective

Using the information presented in this section, the student will be able to perform the following:

■ **Design a basic full-body massage**

The previous section presented massage manipulations and techniques. The next concern is how to combine the methods into a focused massage session. A million ways exist to give a massage, and the choices made each time a massage is given develop from an understanding of the principles and practice of therapeutic massage. Each massage is different because the client is different each time, even if that client has been seen for many massage sessions.

The focus of the session depends on the needs of the client. To understand what those needs are, the massage practitioner must be able to take a general history and do a basic assessment of the client. These procedures were presented in Chapter 3. Based on the information gathered in the history and assessment process, the therapeutic massage professional will then design the best massage for the individual client by picking and choosing what methods, rhythm, pacing, pressure, intensity, and amenities (such as music) to use. Refinement of the assessment process and criteria for decision making are addressed in the next chapter.

The Basic Full-Body General Massage

The basic full-body massage is a common approach in massage. The full-body general massage stimulates all the sensory nerve receptors, contacts all the layers and types of tissues, and moves all the major joints of the body.

The session lasts about 1 hour. The purpose of the massage is to affect the whole body using primarily effleurage, compression, tapotement, rocking, and range of motion to the joints, along with limited use of pétrissage, shaking, and general friction methods. The other manipulations and techniques are chosen as needed to address specific attention to problem areas if appropriate.

No matter the type of massage approach used, the first,

and maybe the most important massage manipulation to use is the resting position, or the first touch.

The next massage manipulations chosen are used for general, broad applications and to connect all the other methods during the massage session. Methods most commonly used for general broad applications are effleurage (gliding strokes), compression, rocking, and joint range of motion.

Effleurage, or gliding stroke, is effective for the following situations:

- Lubricant is used.
- A large surface area must be covered efficiently.
- Changes are made between manipulations.
- The practitioner is moving from one area to another.
- The client prefers a soothing massage with generalized body responses.

Compression is effective for the following situations:

- Lubricant is not used.
- People are hairy or ticklish.
- The client prefers a more stimulating massage.

Rocking is effective for the following situations:

- Lubricant is not used.
- Excessive rubbing or pressing on the skin or underlying tissue is not desirable.
- Clients desire a soothing massage with generalized body responses.

Joint range of motion is effective for the following situations:

- Lubricant is not used.
- People are hairy or ticklish.
- Excessive rubbing or pressing on the skin or underlying tissue is not desirable.
- The client desires a general increase in mobility.

It is beneficial to blend these four methods to provide the general base of the massage. The other massage manipulations and techniques provide uniqueness to the massage.

The full-body general massage has a sense of wholeness with a beginning point and an ending point. The basic flow patterns provided earlier in the chapter provide the basis for this sense of structure. The massage should have a general sense of continuity. In simple words, the massage needs to flow, to feel connected like one continuous experience made up of all the applications of the massage methods in response to the individual client's needs.

GENERAL MASSAGE SUGGESTIONS

section objectives

Using the information presented in this section, the student will be able to perform the following:

- ■ **Understand how to deal with difficult or unusual situations regarding body hair, skin problems, and avoidance of tickling**

- ■ **Make thoughtful decisions regarding application of massage techniques by body region**

Body Hair

Excessive body hair requires an alteration in the massage procedure. Gliding and kneading methods can pull the hair. A lubricant may feel uncomfortable. The use of compression, vibration, and rocking and shaking, coupled with lengthening and stretching procedures, is effective.

Skin Problems

People who have rashes, acne, psoriasis, and other skin problems require an alteration of massage procedures. The integrity of healthy skin prevents the transmission of pathogens. Physician referral and approval may be required. Massage can usually be provided by placing a clean, white bath towel over the affected area and using compression methods over the towel. Be very careful to avoid contact with any body fluids.

Working over a clean towel or sheet can be helpful for those who have sensitive skin and find the movement of massage irritating. Any method that does not glide on the skin can be used over a towel, sheet, or loose, nonrestrictive clothing. Using a towel to lift tissue, especially the tissue of the abdomen, proves helpful for an effective grip and is more comfortable.

Avoidance of Tickling

Tickling can usually be avoided by reducing the speed and increasing the pressure of the stroke. Also, because it is difficult to tickle oneself, placing the client's hand on the area that you wish to massage and massaging with it often solves the problem (Fig. 9-40). Tickling can often be avoided by working over a towel or sheet.

Considerations and Suggestions for Massage Applications by Body Region

Considerations and Suggestions for Head and Face Massage

- To avoid disturbing the client's hairstyle and makeup, always ask before massaging the head and face.
- Use lubricants carefully, keeping in mind the sensitivity of the facial skin. Avoid lubricant on the face if possible.
- Remember that the delicate nature of the facial skin and muscles requires a confident yet gentle touch.

The extensive motor/sensory sensitivly of the face enables massage to stimulate a large amount of nervous system activity that may be beneficial for relaxation and pain control.

The facial muscles create the expressions that reflect

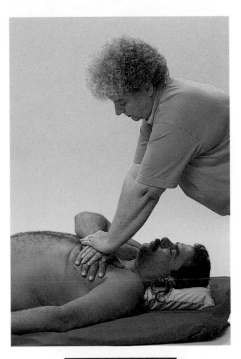

fig. 9-40

Use of client's hand to prevent tickling.

our mood and emotions. Changes in expression are processed in the emotional centers of the brain. Careful attention to massage of the face may gently interact with the way the recipient of the massage feels emotionally.

Always clean your hands before massaging the face. Pathogens can be easily spread though the mucous membranes of the eyes, nose, and mouth. Avoid direct contact with these areas.

Considerations and Suggestions for Neck Massage

- Keep in mind that side-lying is the most effective position for massage of the neck. The head is stabilized against the table, and the neck area is opened up for easy access.
- Always provide lengthening and stretching for the neck from the shoulder with the head stabilized. Injury may result if the neck is lengthened or stretched by moving the head.
- Avoid deep pressure into the anterior triangle of the neck (general area between the sternocleidomastoid muscle and the trachea). Damage to blood vessels and nerves located in this area can result.
- Use broad and generalized methods of massage using the forearm or the whole hand. This feels less invasive than using fingers and thumbs when massaging the neck.

The neck is a crowded and complex area. It can be affected by responses to stress and by chest and shoulder breathing, which can cause the neck muscles to become

rigid and hypertonic. Effective massage of the neck is necessary to provide for relaxed breathing and reduced stress perception.

Careful study of the anatomy of the neck shows that the direct soft tissue influence extends from the forehead to the second and third ribs, the middle thoracic vertebra, and the middle of the humerus. Because the neck area balances the head against gravity, postural distortion anywhere in the body is reflected in the neck. Massage to this area, in conjunction with an entire body approach, is most beneficial.

The brachial nerve plexus exits from the neck. It is helpful to think of most arm, wrist, and hand problems as beginning at the neck. Problems result from either a direct dysfunction of the neck or difficulties in the arm and hand, which often indirectly cause a neck problem.

Considerations and Suggestions for Shoulder Massage

- Keep in mind that the side-lying position is most effective for massage, range of motion, and lengthening and stretching of the shoulder.

The shoulder complex (scapula, clavicle, humerus, and associated muscles, ligaments, and tendons) floats on the trunk. It is constructed with a loose fit at the shoulder (glenohumeral) joint to provide for a wide range of motion. Soft tissue (muscles, tendons, ligaments, and fascia) connects the shoulder to the trunk with multidirectional forces coming from the back, chest, and neck. The practitioner should consider all these areas when providing massage to the shoulder.

The shoulder is stabilized at the iliac crest and sacrum by the latissimus dorsi muscle and the lumbar dorsal fascia. Any shoulder massage needs to consider massage application to the low back area.

The joint design reflects the fact that flexor (make a joint angle smaller) and adductor (pull toward the midline of the body) muscles exert more pull and are stronger than the extensors (increase the joint angle) and abductors (pull away form the midline). Joint fit may be compromised by an imbalance in these muscles' tone pattern. The practitioner should keep this in mind when working with the shoulder.

The brachial nerve plexus, which supplies the arm, may be affected by soft tissue dysfunction in the shoulder area. This is a very important consideration for clients who have arm pain and discomfort, often resulting from repetitive-use injury. Massaging the shoulder may help reduce muscle tension and soften connective tissue in the area, which may alleviate discomfort in the shoulder and arm.

Considerations and Suggestions for Arm Massage

- Positioning and stabilizing the arm for massage can be aided by massaging the arm in all the basic positions: supine, prone, and side-lying. Each offers advantages.

- Massage only the areas of the arm that are easily accessible in each position. Return to the arm as the client changes position.
- Massage the arm with the forearm stabilized against the massage table in the prone or supine position, or against the body in the side-lying position.
- Stabilize the arm between the trunk of the massage practitioner's body and the massage practitioner's upper arm, thus freeing both hands to massage the arm.
- The arm is often small enough in circumference to grasp with the hands and surround a bulk of the tissue. This approach provides a compressive effleurage to facilitate fluid movement. When massaging the arm, it is useful to remember that the fingers actually begin at the elbow and the shoulder mechanism extends to the elbow.

The elbow joint area is more complex than a hinge joint because of the pronation (palm down)/supination (palm up) action at the elbow. Flexion, extension, pronation, and supination movement patterns need to be considered when the practitioner massages the arm.

The nerves of the brachial nerve plexus run the entire length of the arm. Nerve impingement from soft tissue at the neck, shoulder, and elsewhere in the entire length of the arm needs to be considered if pain exists in the arm.

Considerations and Suggestions for Hand/Wrist Massage

- Because the hand is usually in a flexed position, opening and spreading the tissue of the palm is very beneficial.
- The use of compression to provide a pumping action on the palm of the hand stimulates the lymphatic plexus in the palm, which in turn encourages lymphatic flow. This can be very helpful for those whose hands swell.

The hand and wrist have an intricate and complex joint and soft tissue structure. Thorough attention to massage of these structures and range of motion of the hand and wrist requires time and a focus on detail.

Slow circumduction (moving in a circle) of the wrists, both passive and active against resistance, accesses the joint movement patterns of the wrist. The carpal and metacarpal (palm) joints of the hand can be addressed with a scissoring action. The phalangeal (finger) joints are hinge joints that respond well to active movement against resistance and passive range of motion.

The extensive motor/sensory sensitivity of the hand provides for intense neurologic stimulation through massage methods. The hand is an effective area for massage to initiate relaxation and pain control.

Massage of the hand can be a time of increased connection between the client and the massage practitioner. This is a result of the hand-in-hand position. The sense of intimacy created by the act of holding hands may shift the therapeutic focus from the client to the massage practitioner. Extra care is suggested to avoid transference/countertransference and professional boundary issues while not disturbing the closeness created at this time.

Considerations and Suggestions for Chest Massage

- The breast area of the female can pose difficulties in accessing the chest area. The side-lying position is effective because the breast tissue falls toward the table, allowing access to the side of the chest and axilla (armpit) area. Using the person's hand as a "buffer" between the practitioner's hand and the client, as when avoiding tickling, can be helpful when working around the clavicles and ribs.
- Broad compressive methods to the rib area in the side-lying position are effective in providing general range of motion to the ribs.
- Avoid the breast tissue and nipple area on both males and females. During general massage, no reason exists to massage this area and the tissue is often very sensitive to touch and can be easily irritated.
- Be extra attentive to changes in the tissue in the chest area. Without any alarm reaction, refer clients to their physician if you notice any lumps or tissue changes.

The intercostal muscles (between the ribs) are very important in respiratory function. Slow deliberate work between the ribs with the client in the side-lying position can be valuable in restoring mobility and breathing function.

The pectoralis muscles and associated connective tissue are involved in arm and shoulder movement. This large, soft tissue area is often shortened, not only affecting arm action but causing breathing difficulties as well. Effective massage, lengthening, and stretching are beneficial.

Considerations and Suggestions for Abdomen Massage

- The abdomen can be massaged in the supine or side-lying position. Side-lying on the left is the most effective position. During abdominal massage the knees are usually bent about 90 degrees to the trunk to tilt the pelvis and allow for more relaxed abdominal muscles.
- Because the abdomen contains no bony structure against which to apply pressure, much abdominal work is done with lateral pressure. The tissue is pushed against pressure from the massage practitioner's opposing hand or with kneading that lifts the tissue.

The abdomen has an expansive fascial system. Lifting methods to stretch this connective tissue can be beneficial. Using a towel to lift the abdominal tissue provides grip and protects against pinching.

The abdomen is often ticklish. This is a protective mechanism. Follow instructions for avoiding tickling.

Be careful of pressure down into the abdomen. Always move slowly, allowing the tissue to soften under the touch. If you feel a pulse or throbbing, immediately decrease the pressure.

Many times the abdomen is given only superficial attention during the massage. Avoid this tendency. This is an important area that deserves effective massage application.

Considerations and Suggestions for Back Massage

- Avoid spending excessive time on massage of the back. Often the reason for back pain or tightness is shortening and weakness of muscles in the chest and abdomen. The resulting change in posture is responsible for the back tension.
- The back is effectively massaged in the prone, side-lying, and seated positions.
- Use of the forearm is very effective for back massage. The lumbar dorsal fascia responds well to skin rolling (tissue lifting) and connective tissue stretching methods. Pressure over the spine is not appropriate. However, skin rolling techniques that lift the skin over the spine are effective.

The low back, including the deep quadratus lumborum muscle, is easily massaged in the side-lying position with the client's arm raised over the head to lift the ribcage away from the iliac crest. Deep, even pressure with the forearm often feels best to the client.

Gentle range of motion to provide for rotation of the spinal column is most effectively done in the side-lying position.

Nerve roots are located all along the spine. Massage close to, but not on, the spine is beneficial.

Considerations and Suggestions for Gluteal/Hip Massage

- Positioning for massage of the gluteals and hips is most effective in the side-lying or prone position. Lengthening and stretching methods are most easily done in the side-lying or supine position.
- This area is heavily muscled and reinforced with extensive ligament and tendon structures. The bones and joints in this area are large compared with other body areas. Deeper pressure, with increased duration, is often required to relax these tissues. Methods need to work slowly into the tissue. Avoid work with the hands and make extensive use of the forearm. Use of the forearm is often interpreted as less intimate and may be an important consideration when working with the gluteals and hips.

The sacroiliac joints are large joints that are not directly moved by muscular action. Range-of-motion actions are indirectly achieved through movement of the leg through a range-of-motion sequence.

The coxal articulations (hip joints) are massive joints with extensive ligament structure. The joint provides considerable range-of-motion, second only to the shoulder joint. When doing range of motion methods, include as many variations of flexion, extension, abduction, adduction, and internal and external rotation to involve all the soft tissue elements.

The lumbar and sacral plexuses both innervate this region. Nerve distribution patterns include the entire lower body. The largest nerve is the sciatic nerve. When using heavy pressure to address the soft tissue, avoid sustained deep pressure on the nerve tracts.

Considerations and Suggestions for Leg Massage

- Supine, prone, and side-lying are all effective positions for massage of the leg and are best used in combination to access all parts of the leg easily. For the most efficient use of time in the massage session, make sure that each area of the leg is massaged only once. For instance, if you massage the back of the leg in the prone position, it is not necessary to repeat the back of the leg again in the supine position unless a specific reason exists for doing so.
- The side-lying position offers the easiest access in the medial and lateral aspect of the leg. The supine position provides access to all aspects of the leg, whereas the prone position is the most limited.
- The soft tissue mass of the leg lends itself to massage with the forearm. Kneading is often uncomfortable on the leg because of body hair and the tight adherence of the skin and superficial fascia to the underlying tissue. Effleurage and compression are effective methods to use instead.
- Varicose veins most often occur in the leg, particularly in the saphenous veins. Thromboembolism and thrombophlebitis are serious conditions involving a blood clot in a vein. If the clot moves, it can lodge in the heart, lung, kidney, or brain and cause severe problems. Symptoms of deep vein thrombophlebitis in the legs are aching and cramping that can be mistaken for muscle pain. Massage of any type is contraindicated, and immediate referral is indicated for varicose veins, thromboembolism, and thrombophlebitis. Diagnosis is beyond the scope of practice for massage practitioners; therefore remain cautious of any leg pain and refer to the appropriate health care professional.
- Range of motion for the leg above the knee is hip range of motion. Make sure to effectively stabilize at the pelvis. Stabilizing pressure in this area can be uncomfortable. The use of a small pillow or folded towel over the stabilizing point provides comfort.

The knee is a complex joint influenced by muscles from above and below the joint. Knee instability is often compensated for by increased muscle tension in the leg muscles and thickening and shortening of the iliotibial tract (large connective tissue structure on the outside of the leg). This is resourceful compensation and the protective nature of the muscle and connective tissue tension must be considered. When massaging the leg of someone with a hypermobile knee, the practitioner can use the proper methods to reduce excessive muscle tension and connective tissue shortening, but he should not seek to remove the splinting action entirely. To do so may result in increased knee pain.

The lumbosacral plexus nerves supply the leg, with the sciatic nerve running the entire length of the leg. Impingement can occur anywhere along the nerve pathways. The distribution of leg pain can indicate the nerve portion affected. When located, the entire nerve tract needs to be searched above and below the impingement site for soft tissue restriction to provide soft tissue normalization around the nerves. Light stroking along the nerve tracks is very soothing.

Considerations and Suggestions for Foot/Ankle Massage

- The feet are often a safe place to begin a massage for a client who is nervous or in pain.
- Because of the number of joints in the foot and ankle, careful and deliberate range-of-motion work is beneficial in this area. Slow circumduction (circular movements), both passive and active against resistance, accesses the ankle movement patterns. The tarsal and metatarsal (main foot) joints can be accessed with a scissoring or bending movement of the foot. Phalangeal (toe) joints are hinge joints and benefit from

both active range of motion against resistance and passive range of motion.

The foot/ankle mechanism is a highly complex structure. It has many joints, muscles, and nerves that provide stability and neurologic positional information during walking and standing. An extensive connective tissue network provides stability. Any disruption of normal foot and ankle action often results in a compensatory pattern through the entire muscle/skeletal system.

Massage of the foot is one of the best ways to provide a high degree of nervous system input for relaxation and pain control. Many beneficial effects are obtained with foot massage because of the stimulation of parasympathetic activity, which results in the relaxation or quieting response.

The sole of the foot contains a vast lymphatic plexus that acts as a pump to move lymphatic fluid in the foot

9-13
PROFICIENCY EXERCISE

Design a 1-hour massage sequence on paper using a variety of methods and techniques from this chapter. Trade papers with another student and perform the other person's massage sequence on them. When you are finished, list what you learned from the experience and share the list with your partner in this exercise. Have your partner critique his or her massage design.

and legs. Compression used in a rhythmic pumping action is effective in stimulating the lymphatic system.

The tibial nerve, off the sciatic nerve, branches into the medial and lateral plantar nerve, which in turn branches to provide for an extensive nerve distribution in the foot. Sciatic nerve impingement can be felt into the foot. Nerve pain in the foot can indicate impingement anywhere along the nerve track from the lumbosacral plexus to the foot. Nerve pain in the foot needs to be addressed with massage of the entire leg, with the practitioner noticing which areas of restriction refer pain into the foot (Proficiency Exercise 9-13).

SUMMARY

In this chapter you have had the opportunity to design and give many different types of massage. Now that you have all the individual skills to give a great massage, your job is to practice using them in combination. It is common to be clumsy with massage applications at first. Skills will evolve with experience and practice. Very few people, if any, do something perfectly on their first attempt. Expertise is a never-ending process of learning, modification, and change. By working with a client-centered focus, allowing the client's needs to direct the massage, and not forcing any type of response, the client should experience beneficial results.

Massage manipulations and techniques can be combined to produce an infinite number of therapeutic massage applications. Give yourself permission to practice and improvise. As you practice, ask the client for feedback about how a particular application of a technique or massage manipulation feels and what its effects are. Always be open to innovation, and do not be afraid to experiment with new techniques.

REFERENCES

1. Anderson KE, Anderson LE, Glanze D, editors: *Mosby's medical, nursing, and allied health dictionary,* ed 4, St Louis, 1990, Mosby.
2. Baumgartner AJ: *Massage in athletics,* Minneapolis, 1947, Brugess Publishing.
3. Beard G: A history of massage technic, *Physical Ther Rev* 32:613, 1952.
4. Cyriax E: Some misconceptions concerning mechano-therapy, *Br J Physical Med* October 1938, 92-94.
5. Greenman PE: *Principles of manual medicine,* Baltimore, 1989, Williams and Wilkins.
6. Kellogg JH: *The art of massage,* Battle Creek, MI, 1929, Modern Medicine Publishing.
7. Knott M, Voss D: *Proprioceptive neuromuscular facilitation,* New York, 1956, Harper and Row.
8. Lewit K: *Manipulative therapy in rehabilitation of the locomotor system,* ed 2, Oxford, 1991, Butterworth-Heinemann Ltd.
9. McNaught AB, Callander R: *Illustrated physiology,* ed 4, New York, 1983, Churchill Livingstone.
10. Taylor GH: *An illustrated sketch of the movement cure: Its principal methods and effects,* New York, 1866, The Institute.
11. Travell JG, Simons DG: *Myofascial pain and dysfunction: the trigger point manual,* Baltimore, 1984, Williams and Wilkins.

WORKBOOK SECTION

Short Answer

1. What are the three effects of massage methods and techniques on the body? Explain each one.

_____

_____

_____

2. Which massage methods seem more mechanical?

_____

_____

_____

3. Which methods seem more reflexive?

_____

_____

_____

4. What are the seven aspects of quality of touch?

_____

_____

_____

5. What is the importance of variation of the quality of touch concepts as to variety in speed, rate, rhythm, and duration?

_____

_____

_____

6. What is the importance of a basic flow pattern?

_____

_____

_____

7. Why is the pattern for the abdominal massage always the same?

_____

_____

_____

8. Why do you think that similar trends, applications, and methods continue to make up the body of knowledge of therapeutic massage?

_____

_____

_____

9. What are the major differences between massage manipulations and massage techniques?

_____

_____

_____

10. What are the main uses for the resting position?

_____

_____

_____

11. How does the massage practitioner first approach the client?

_____

_____

_____

12. What is the distinguishing characteristic of effleurage?

_____

_____

_____

13. Why should deeper applications of effleurage/gliding always move slowly?

_____

_____

_____

14. What are some specific uses of the effleurage/gliding massage manipulation?

_____

_____

_____

WORKBOOK SECTION

15. What are the distinguishing qualities of pétrissage/kneading?

_____

_____

_____

16. Why should the massage professional use pétrissage sparingly?

_____

_____

_____

17. What conditions interfere with the use of pétrissage?

_____

_____

_____

18. What are the physiologic effects of compression?

_____

_____

_____

19. What are some things to remember to protect the massage practitioner's hands and arms while doing compression?

_____

_____

_____

20. What are the best anatomic locations to do vibration? Why?

_____

_____

_____

21. How is rocking different than shaking?

_____

_____

_____

22. What is the strongest physiologic effect of tapotement/percussion?

_____

_____

_____

23. Where does the movement for tapotement come from?

_____

_____

_____

24. What are the distinguishing characteristics of friction?

_____

_____

_____

25. How long does friction need to be done to accomplish the desired results?

_____

_____

_____

26. Describe two methods to apply friction.

_____

_____

_____

27. Why does the use of joint movement and muscle energy techniques make massage manipulations more effective?

_____

_____

_____

28. What are the three types of proprioceptors affected by movement techniques? What do they detect?

_____

_____

_____

WORKBOOK SECTION

29. What are the two different types of joint movement described in this text?

_____

_____

_____

30. What is the pathologic range-of-motion barrier?

_____

_____

_____

31. Explain hand placement for joint movement.

_____

_____

_____

32. What are the major uses of muscle energy techniques?

_____

_____

_____

33. Describe the concept of lengthening.

_____

_____

_____

34. What is the importance of positioning?

_____

_____

_____

35. What are the types of muscle contraction used for muscle energy techniques? Explain each one.

_____

_____

_____

36. What is postisometric relaxation (PIR)?

_____

_____

_____

37. What is reciprocal inhibition (RI)?

_____

_____

_____

38. How do pulsed muscle energy methods differ from the other methods described?

_____

_____

_____

39. What is the target muscle?

_____

_____

_____

40. How much strength is required during the contraction for the muscle energy method to work?

_____

_____

_____

41. When is direct manipulation of spindle cells and Golgi tendons used?

_____

_____

_____

42. When is positional release/strain-counterstrain used?

_____

_____

_____

WORKBOOK SECTION

43. Define stretching.

_____

_____

_____

44. Why must lengthening methods be used before stretching?

_____

_____

_____

45. When might stretching be an inappropriate method to use?

_____

_____

_____

46. What are the two basic types of stretch?

_____

_____

_____

47. What is direction of ease and why is it important?

_____

_____

_____

48. Explain the concept of the massage being a mixture.

_____

_____

_____

49. What is the goal of the general massage?

_____

_____

_____

50. Why are there a million ways to do a massage?

_____

_____

_____

WORKBOOK SECTION

Matching

Match the massage manipulation or technique with its description.

1. Active joint movement _____

2. Beating _____

3. Compression _____

4. Cross-directional stretching _____

5. Cupping _____

6. Effleurage (gliding stroke) _____

7. Friction _____

8. Hacking _____

9. Joint movement _____

10. Lengthening _____

11. Longitudinal stretching _____

12. Manipulation _____

13. Muscle energy techniques _____

14. Passive joint movement _____

15. Pétrissage (kneading) _____

16. Positional release _____

17. Postisometric relaxation _____

18. Proprioceptive neuromuscular facilitation (PNF) _____

19. Pulsed muscle energy _____

20. Reciprocal inhibition (RI) _____

21. Resting stroke _____

22. Rocking _____

23. Shaking _____

24. Skin-rolling _____

25. Slapping _____

26. Stretching _____

27. Stroke _____

28. Tapotement _____

29. Tapping _____

30. Techniques _____

31. Traction _____

32. Vibration _____

a. type of alternating tapotement that strikes the surface of the body with quick snapping movements.

b. the movement of the joint through its normal range of motion.

c. the assuming of a normal resting length by a muscle through the neuromuscular mechanism.

d. a stretch applied along the fiber direction of the connective tissues and muscles.

e. tissue stretching that pulls and twists connective tissue against its fiber direction.

f. by moving the body out of the position causing discomfort and into the direction it wants to go, the proprioception is taken into a state of safety and may stop signaling for protective spasm.

g. occurs after an isometric contraction of a muscle, resulting from the activity of minute neural reporting stations called the *Golgi tendon bodies*.

h. application of muscle energy techniques that combine muscle contractions with stretching and muscular pattern retraining.

i. rhythmic movement of the body.

j. body area is grasped and shaken in a quick loose movement. Sometimes classified as *rhythmic mobilization*.

k. a form of pétrissage that lifts skin.

l. the client produces the movement of a joint through its range of movement.

m. methods of therapeutic massage that provide sensory stimulation or mechanical alteration of the soft tissue of the body.

n. pressure into the body to spread tissue against underlying structures. This massage manipulation is sometimes classified with pétrissage.

o. gentle pull on the joint capsule to increase the joint space.

p. fine or coarse tremulous movement that creates reflexive responses.

q. a type of tapotement that uses a cupped hand; often used over the thorax.

WORKBOOK SECTION

r. horizontal strokes applied with the fingers, hand, or forearm that follow the fiber direction of the underlying muscle, fascial planes, or a dermatome pattern.

s. circular or transverse movements that are focused to the underlying tissue and do not glide on the skin.

t. procedures that involve engaging the barrier and using minute, resisted contractions (usually 20 in 10 seconds), which introduces mechanical pumping as well as PIR or RI (depending on the muscles used).

u. takes place when a muscle contracts, obliging its antagonist to relax to allow normal movement.

v. first stroke of the massage; the simple laying on of hands.

w. form of tapotement that uses a flat hand.

x. mechanical tension applied to lengthen the myofascial unit (muscles and fascia); two types exist: longitudinal and cross-directional.

y. a form of heavy tapotement that uses the fist.

z. a technique of therapeutic massage applied on the surface of the body, whether superficial or deep.

aa. springy, fast blows to the body to create rhythmic compression to the tissue. Also called *percussion*.

bb. type of tapotement done using the fingertips.

cc. skillful use of the hands in a therapeutic manner. Massage manipulations are focused to the soft tissues of the body and are not to be confused with joint manipulation using a high-velocity thrust.

dd. specific use of active contraction in individual or groups of muscles to initiate a relaxation response. Activation of the proprioceptors to facilitate muscle tone, relaxation, and stretching.

ee. the massage practitioner moves the jointed areas without the assistance of the client.

ff. rhythmic rolling, lifting, squeezing, and wringing of soft tissue.

Match the movement activity with its proper description.

1. Arthrokinematic movement _____

2. Concentric isotonic contraction _____

3. Counterpressure _____

4. Eccentric isotonic contraction _____

5. Isokinetic contraction _____

6. Isometric contraction _____

7. Osteokinematic movements _____

a. accessory movements that occur because of inherent laxity or joint play that exists in each joint. These essential movements occur passively with movement of the joint and are not under voluntary control.

b. during the contraction of a muscle, the massage practitioner applies a counterforce but allows the client to move, bringing the origin and insertion of the target muscle together against the pressure.

c. flexion, extension, abduction, adduction, and rotation. Also referred to as *physiologic movements*.

d. contraction in which the effort of the muscle, or group of muscles, is exactly matched by a counterpressure so that no movement occurs, only effort.

e. the client moves the joint through a full range of motion, using full muscle strength, against partial resistance supplied by the massage practitioner. This is therefore a multiple isotonic movement.

f. during the extension of a muscle, the massage practitioner applies a counterforce but allows the client to move it to let origin and insertion separate.

g. the force produced by the muscles of a specific area, which is designed to match the effort exactly (isometric contraction) or partially (isotonic contraction).

WORKBOOK SECTION

Match the term with the proper definition.

1. Antagonists _____

2. Barrier _____

3. Compressive force _____

4. Depth of pressure _____

5. Direction _____

6. Direction of ease _____

7. Drag _____

8. Facilitation _____

9. Golgi tendon receptors _____

10. Heavy pressure _____

11. Inhibition _____

12. Insertion _____

13. Joint kinesthetic receptors _____

14. Moderate pressure _____

15. Motor point _____

16. Neuromuscular mechanism _____

17. Origin _____

18. Positioning _____

19. Pressure _____

20. Prime movers _____

21. Proprioceptors _____

22. Range of motion _____

23. Refractory period _____

24. Reflex _____

25. Soft tissue _____

26. Spindle cells _____

27. Stabilization _____

28. Stimulation _____

29. Superficial fascia _____

a. a limitation in movement. Anatomic barriers are caused by the fit of the bones at the joint. Physiologic barriers are from the limits of range of motion from protective nerve and sensory function.

b. contact with no movement.

c. some sort of excitation that activates the sensory nerves.

d. connective tissue layer just under the skin.

e. a compressive pressure that can be light, moderate, deep, and variable.

f. the muscle or groups of muscles on which the response of the methods is specifically focused.

g. state of causing the muscle to contract or strengthen.

h. reflex that tones a muscle with stimulation through vibration methods at the tendon.

i. the amount of pull on the tissue.

j. the muscles that oppose the movement of the prime movers.

k. the state of a nerve when it is stimulated, but not to the point of threshold where it will transmit a nerve signal.

l. the body assumes postural changes and muscle shortening or weakening depending on the way in which it has balanced against gravity.

m. flow of massage strokes can be from the center of the body out (centrifugal), or from the extremities in toward the center of the body (centripetal). It can be from origin to insertion of the muscle following the muscle fibers, transverse to the tissue fibers, or in a circular motion.

n. compressive pressure that extends to the muscle layer but does not press the tissue against the underlying bone.

o. placing the body in such a way that specific joints of muscles are isolated.

p. compressive force.

WORKBOOK SECTION

30. Target muscles _____

31. Tone _____

32. Tonic vibration reflex _____

33. Touch _____

q. amount of pressure against the surface of the body to apply pressure to the deeper body structures.

r. the muscles responsible for a movement.

s. one of three types of sensory nerves in the joint that detect position and speed of movement.

t. point at which a motor nerve enters the muscle it innervates and will cause a muscle twitch if stimulated.

u. movement of joints.

v. response that depends on nervous system function. Reflexive methods work by causing a stimulation of the nervous system (sensory neurons) and the tissue changes in response to the body's adaptation to the neural stimulation.

w. holding the body in a fixed position during joint movement, lengthening, and stretching.

x. sensory receptors in the belly of the muscle that detect stretch.

y. the skin, fascia, muscles, tendons, joint capsules, and ligaments of the body.

z. amount of time that a muscle will be unable to contract after it has contracted.

aa. sensory receptors that detect joint and muscle activity.

bb. attachment point of a muscle at the fixed point during movement.

cc. the interplay and reflex connection between sensory and motor neurons and muscle function.

dd. receptors in the tendons that sense tension.

ee. compressive force that extends to the bone under the tissue.

ff. to decrease or cease a response or function.

gg. the muscle attachment point that is closest to the moving joint.

402 *Mosby's Fundamentals of Therapeutic Massage*

WORKBOOK SECTION

Problem-Solving Exercises

1. A client has tight leg muscles. She also has a history of varicose veins. This contraindicates direct massage of the area. What methods can be used to relax the legs?

   _____

   _____

   _____

   _____

   _____

2. A client has very sensitive skin and cannot have any type of lubricant used. What massage methods will you use?

   _____

   _____

   _____

   _____

   _____

3. A client's nose becomes stuffy and he gets a sinus headache when lying on his stomach. How will you give him a massage?

   _____

   _____

   _____

   _____

Professional Application

A massage professional finds that he becomes fatigued with the style of massage he tends to provide, which consists mostly of effleurage, pétrissage, and tapotement. He would like to be able to work more effectively. What recommendations can you provide?

   _____

   _____

   _____

   _____

   _____

ANSWER KEY
Short Answer

1. The three effects are mechanical, reflexive, and chemical. Mechanical effects in the tissue result directly from the application of the method. Reflexive effects add sensory stimulation and cause the nervous system to respond. Chemical effects cause release of chemicals either directly at the tissue worked with or through the endocrine system and nervous system. These responses are often classified as reflexive.
2. Methods that move through the skin to the underlying tissues.
3. Methods and techniques that stay within the skin or superficial fascial layer, move the body, or add heat or cold.
4. Depth of pressure, drag, direction, speed, rhythm, frequency, and duration.
5. The body will adapt to a repetitive sensory stimulation and stop responding to the sensory input. Varying the touch quality avoids the adaptation and continues to stimulate the body.
6. To be able to organize a systemic approach to the massage so that all the soft tissue is addressed and all the joints are moved.
7. To facilitate the natural flow and elimination pattern of the large intestine.
8. Regardless of when in history massage was used, it was applied to the same anatomy and physiology as it is today. Many approaches may be developed today, but they all tend to work for similar reasons.
9. Massage manipulations are based on Ling's and others' concept of passive movements. They involve the direct application of pressure or pulling of the soft tissue elements of skin, fascia, muscles, tendons, and ligaments. Massage techniques are based on gymnastics or movement-cure methods, as described by Ling, Taylor, and others. They use active involvement of the joints and movement patterns.
10. Initial contact, stillness, calling attention to an area of the body, addition of body heat, reestablishing contact.
11. With a slow, gradual, confident, secure approach, with a deliberate hesitation at the arms-length boundary, coupled with a verbal announcement that you will be touching.
12. It is applied horizontally in relation to the tissues.
13. The drag component of the heavier pressure works on a more mechanical level. It takes time for the tissues to warm and respond to the mechanical force. Going fast with a deep effleurage stroke is painful, causes spasm, and is ineffective.

WORKBOOK SECTION

14. Applying lubricant, warming the area with increasing pressure, connecting one area to another, evaluation, and abdominal massage.
15. The tissue is lifted, twisted, rolled, and squeezed. The stroke functions on the vertical lifting up.
16. It involves repetitive use of the massage professional's hands and wrists, which can cause overuse injury. It is better to substitute alternative methods to warm the tissue and use pétrissage only for a specific, deliberate purpose.
17. Tissue that will not lift, edema, excessive body hair, ticklish clients.
18. Superficial applications are reflexive, especially if applied over motor nerve points and nerve tracts. Moderate applications over arteries enhance arterial blood flow. Moderate to deep applications spread spindle cells, causing the muscle to contract and thereby toning the muscle. This small toning component is good for discharging the nervous system so that the muscle can relax. Deep applications affect the connective tissue by spreading it against the underlying bony structure and releasing histamine from the surrounding tissue. Compression that enters the tissue at 90 degrees and then shifts the angle to between 80 and 45 degrees, without slipping, will produce a drag on the tissue.
19. Avoid hyperextension of the wrist or finger joints. Avoid the use of the thumb. Use the tip or radial ulnar flat side of the elbow. Keep the hand and wrist relaxed when doing any work with the forearm. Change from palm to fist to forearm often.
20. At the tendon to affect the tonic vibration reflex, at motor points to stimulate nerves.
21. Shaking has a distinct snap at the end of the stroke, making the stroke irregular in its rhythm, whereas rocking is very rhythmic and regular. Shaking disrupts body rhythms, and rocking works to enhance them. Both inhibit muscle tone and relax, but for different reasons.
22. Activation of the tendon reflex when applied to the tendon. This causes the muscle to contract. As soon as one muscle contracts, its antagonist is reciprocally inhibited.
23. A relaxed wrist that moves in response to contraction and relaxation at the elbow joint.
24. Friction moves superficial tissue over deeper underlying tissue. Movement on the skin is avoided to prevent friction-type burns. To prevent sliding on the skin, no lubricant is used. The movements are applied to a specific location and are transverse to the grain of the tissue or are circular.
25. 30 seconds to 10 minutes.

26. (1) No lubricant is used. The braced fingers, hand, or elbow compresses the tissue to the depth required to access the tissue to be frictioned. The massage practitioner does not slide, but moves the tissues back and forth or around. (2) The practitioner applies compression over the area in which friction is to be used. Instead of moving the application hand, the practitioner moves the client's joint under the compression. The friction comes from the action of the underlying bone against the tissue.
27. These techniques warm the tissues, relax the nervous system, and relax and lengthen the muscles, thus reducing the need for repetitive massage manipulations.
28. (1) Joint kinesthetic receptors-position and rate of movement. (2) Spindle cells-stretch of muscle. (3) Golgi tendon organs-muscle tension at the tendon.
29. (1) Active: produced by the client. (2) Passive: produced by the massage professional.
30. The point at which motion causes a bind, catch, or pain.
31. One hand should be placed close to the joint to be moved. This hand acts both as a stabilizer and for evaluation. The other hand is placed at the distal end of the bone and is the hand that actually provides the movement.
32. Muscle lengthening, reducing spasm, strengthening weak muscles, reducing local edema, and as preparation for stretching.
33. Lengthening is a neurologic response that allows muscles to assume a normal resting length.
34. Muscle energy methods are focused to specific muscles and resultant joint function. To access the muscles for the proper contraction, the muscles must be positioned in such a way that the origin and insertion are as close together as possible for contraction, whether active or passive, and lengthening (extended) with origin and insertion separated.
35. Isometric: No movement, only effort.
    Isotonic: Movement against resistance. There are three types:
    Concentric isotonic: origin and insertion come together against resistance.
    Eccentric isotonic: origin and insertion separate against resistance.
    Multiple isotonic: combination of concentric and eccentric contraction against resistance for a full range of movement for a joint.
36. A muscle relaxation after a contraction.
37. When a muscle contracts, its antagonist must relax.
38. Instead of one strong contraction, small, light, rapid

WORKBOOK SECTION

contractions of the muscles are used to activate the receptors and the reflexive movement.

39. The target muscle is the muscle or muscle group on which the massage practitioner is specifically focusing a particular response.

40. Usually no more than 25% of muscle strength is required. The exception to this is strengthening weak muscles. In this case, a stronger contraction or repeated contraction may be required.

41. To replace the active contraction portion of muscle energy techniques when the client cannot or does not wish to participate in the massage.

42. When specific tender points are found, or if the client is in pain. It is a good method for gentle, painless release of all specific sore spots regardless of pathology (what is wrong). The tender point is the guide to the proper positioning of the clients. Use a full-body approach in positioning, and do not focus solely on the area around the tender point.

43. Stretching is a mechanical method that pulls connective tissue to elongate it.

44. To avoid protective spasm of the muscles in the area to be stretched.

45. Stretching is not used in acute situations. If the connective tissue is normal in an area and the problem is recent, only lengthening needs to be used. Stretching does need to be done in most chronic conditions.

46. Longitudinal stretching, which pulls tissue in the fiber direction, and cross-directional stretching, which pulls tissue against the fiber direction, often with a twisting component.

47. Direction of ease is the position and postural change that the body has assumed to adjust to pain, repetitive movement, or structural distortion. The massage professional must not directly pull a client out of the ease pattern, but instead increase the positioning, allowing for the protective sensory receptors to "relax," and then gently coax with lengthening and stretching the body into a more efficient pattern.

48. The massage needs a base of general, broad application methods to form the structure of the massage. The methods most commonly used are effleurage/gliding stroke, compression, and rocking.

49. Stimulation of all the sensory receptors, touching all the layers and types of tissue, and moving all the major joints of the body.

50. Subtle shifts and changes in pressure, intensity, methods used, positioning, sequence, and focus allow for each massage to be different. A musical scale contains only 12 notes, yet all the music comes from combinations of the notes. Massage is the same. Each client is different, and therefore each massage is different.

Matching

1. l	9. b	17. g	25. w
2. y	10. c	18. h	26. x
3. n	11. d	19. t	27. z
4. e	12. cc	20. u	28. aa
5. q	13. dd	21. v	29. bb
6. r	14. ee	22. I	30. m
7. s	15. ff	23. j	31. o
8. a	16. f	24. k	32. p

1. a	5. e
2. b	6. d
3. g	7. c
4. f	

1. j	10. ee	18. o	26. x
2. a	11. ff	19. p	27. w
3. q	12. gg	20. r	28. c
4. e	13. s	21. aa	29. d
5. m	14. n	22. u	30. f
6. l	15. t	23. z	31. g
7. i	16. cc	24. v	32. h
8. k	17. bb	25. y	33. b
9. dd			

Problem-Solving Exercises

1. Muscle energy methods to produce lengthening, relax the muscle. Rocking of the body may relax the muscles.

2. Do compression and tapotement over a towel or sheet. The resting stroke can be used as can shaking, rocking, and all massage techniques of joint movement, muscle energy, positional release, and lengthening and stretching approaches.

3. The entire body can be accessed in the other positions of supine, side-lying, and seated.

Professional Application

Reduce the amount of pétrissage and tapotement, and use it only when there is a specific purpose. Increase the muscle energy methods and lengthening. Increase the shaking and rocking methods. He should make sure that he is centered before giving the massage and stretch his body afterward. He should check to see that he is applying strokes with the correct body mechanics and making minimal use of his hands.

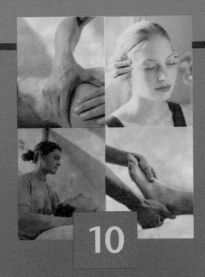

10

ASSESSMENT PROCEDURES FOR DEVELOPING A CARE PLAN

o b j e c t i v e s

After completing this chapter, the student will be able to perform the following:

- Conduct an effective client interview
- Perform a basic physical assessment
- Interpret assessment information and develop a care/treatment plan

As the learning process begins, it is important that the student understand the value of the sequence and general flow of the massage pattern. Although modeling precise massage routines is a valuable learning exercise, after the student grasps the concepts, the routine must evolve to meet the unique needs of the individual client. If the student knows how to perform a certain massage routine but does not understand how to modify and alter the application of therapeutic massage, her ability to serve the client will be limited. People do not fit neatly into a routine sequence of massage techniques. For the best results, the concepts learned from performing the routines must be designed to fit the client's individual needs, rather than trying to make the client fit the routine.

Rather than providing the structure of a precise, step-by-step routine, this chapter teaches the student to perform an assessment and develop an individual care plan.

The assessment process can be as simple as ruling out contraindications for a one-time session in a personal service environment (e.g., day spa, cruise ship, resort) or as comprehensive as determining a client's needs for therapeutic massage provided as a health care component (e.g., as part of a rehabilitation or pain management program or in the development of coping strategies for anxiety disorder).

Treatment/care plans also can be as simple as providing a 1-hour vacation from daily stress, a present for Mother's Day or Father's Day, or a session of pleasure and pampering for a client. They also can be complex, as would be required for the use of massage as a management tool in asthma, depression, stroke rehabilitation, symptoms caused by chemotherapy, and sports training protocols.

This chapter presents the assessment skills a practitioner needs to function with supervision in a health care setting, providing massage as part of a comprehensive treatment plan. The massage professional should be able to participate in this process by providing reliable information to be considered in the development of the treatment plan. These skills exceed those usually required in the personal service setting; however, as more employment opportunities open in the health care setting, it is important to be able to function as part of a multidisciplinary health care team. The ability to reason clinically at this level supports the effectiveness of all massage interactions, be it for relaxation and pleasure outcomes or for the management of complex conditions.

For the professional, it is better to have the skill and not need it than to need a skill and not have it. Because most of the physiologic changes and benefits of massage arise from the most basic of technical skills, expertise comes from the decisions made in applying those skills. The practitioner's ability to make those decisions depends on his ability to gather the client's history data, perform assessment analysis, and interpret the information. Then, with the information gathered and the client outcomes determined, the massage methods and approaches to achieve the agreed-on goals are chosen and the plan developed.

ASSESSMENT

section objectives

Using the information presented in this section, the student will be able to perform the following:

- Interview a client effectively
- Complete a basic physical assessment, a gait assessment, a 14-level palpation assessment, and a muscle testing assessment

Assessment is a learned skill. The ability to incorporate this skill into massage sessions enhances the quality of treatment given by the massage professional. **Assessment** is the collection and interpretation of information provided by the client, the client's consent advocates (parent or guardian), and the referring medical professionals, as well as information gathered by the massage practitioner. In a growing number of clinical health care settings, the massage professional's assessment is considered in the treatment plan developed by the multidisciplinary health care team. Therefore the massage practitioner must understand and practice standard assessment and charting procedures. Chapter 3 introduced these concepts. This chapter refines and synthesizes them. Although the massage professional observes, interprets, and makes decisions based on information gathered during assessment procedures, it is important to remember that the massage professional is not equipped to diagnose or treat any specific medical condition except under the direct supervision of a licensed medical professional. Interpretation of information gathered during a premassage assessment has three purposes:

- To determine whether the client should be referred to a medical professional
- To obtain input from the client that is used in developing the massage care/treatment plan
- To design the best massage for the client

In reality, the assessment and the application of massage technique are almost the same thing. It is not uncommon during a massage to use massage manipulations and techniques to evaluate and assess the tissue and then use the same manipulations and techniques, altered slightly in intensity, to normalize the situation (adaptation).

For teaching purposes, the two approaches have been separated. One of the truly difficult concepts to teach and learn is pure assessment. Students typically rush into adaptation techniques without taking the time to discover the pattern the client is presenting. *Assessment does not change a condition; rather it is an attempt to understand it.* Interventions cause change. To understand the results of the massage session, the student must learn to separate assessment information obtained before, during, and after the massage from methods of intervention.

Establishing Rapport

The client is the most important resource involved in the assessment process. The skills a massage professional requires for this process are an ability to establish rapport, keen observation, successful interviewing methods, and active listening.

Rapport is the development of a relationship based on mutual trust and harmony. It is the responsibility of the massage professional to establish a sense of rapport with clients.

The best way to begin establishing rapport is to learn and use the client's name. The massage practitioner needs to show a genuine interest in the person that goes beyond the problems and goals the person presents. What happens to a person affects the whole being.

Many people need time to sort out their thoughts and feelings and develop their statements. The conversation should proceed slowly, and the client should never be rushed. By giving the person full attention and by observing what makes the client most comfortable, it is easier to resist the urge to treat everyone in the same manner. Rapport is enhanced if the massage professional uses words, a voice tone, and body language similar to those of the client.

How to Observe

Attention to detail and the needs of the client provides a sensitive, well-trained therapist with essential information. Clients notice the difference between a massage professional who takes the time to honor the client's space and adjust to it and one who tries to make the client fit into a routine method of massage application. During the initial conversation, it is important to pay very close attention to the client visually. If the practitioner has a visual impairment, information gathered from the interview and physical assessment replaces visual assessment. An effective therapist uses all the senses—hearing, sight, smell, touch, and intuition—in the assessment of the client.

At this point information is only gathered, not interpreted; resist the urge to try to understand what all the information means. Interpretation comes after *all* the information has been gathered. This may take several sessions.

At the beginning of each session the practitioner gets a sense of the client's general presence. How well does the client move and breathe? Does the client's presence suggest sympathetic or parasympathetic activation? Sympathetic activation is the display of restlessness, anxiety, fear, anger, agitation, elation, or exuberance. Parasympathetic activation is indicated by a generally relaxed appearance, contentment, slowness, or depression. Because therapeutic massage can either stimulate or relax, this needs to be considered when designing the massage.

If a client is active and exuberant (sympathetic activation), the initial massage approach and the massage practitioner's energy level need to match the client's energy level. If the focus of the session is to calm the client, the therapist begins to slow down as the massage progresses and may introduce appropriate rhythmic entrainment approaches to provide a calming effect.

If the client is tired or moderately depressed, the therapist should proceed slowly in the initial pace of the massage. During the session, the energy and activity level of the massage practitioner and the methods used can be increased as the client's energy increases.

The practitioner pays attention to where and how a client indicates a problem on his or her body. These gestures often reveal whether a client has a muscle, joint, or visceral problem. (The section Interpretation and Analysis of Assessment Information, below, explains this in greater detail.) It also is important for the therapist to observe the client's body language and nonverbal responses while discussing various topics. Everything the person does is important. Everyone's behavior has a pattern, and all the bits of information combine to reveal that pattern (Proficiency Exercise 10-1).

Interviewing and Listening: the Subjective Aspect of Assessment

Communication skills first were presented in Chapter 2. These skills are used during interviewing sessions and throughout client/practitioner interactions. Open-ended questions encourage conversation. It is important to avoid questions that can be answered with only one word. The point of the interview is to help the client communicate his health history and to reveal the reason for the massage. The question, "Have you ever had a professional massage before?" requires only the client answer "Yes" or "No." A better question would be, "What is your experience with therapeutic massage?" This question requires the client to give more detail in answering. When the client provides information, it is important for the practitioner to restate what the client has said. The client then has the opportunity to correct any information and is reassured that the therapist was listening.

When speaking to a client, it is important to use words she can understand. Although professionalism is important, medical terminology need not be used. If the client

---

10-1
PROFICIENCY EXERCISE

1. Watch people in a public place such as a mall or an airport. Is the general presence of each person observed sympathetic or parasympathetic in nature?
2. Ask 10 people to explain a physical ache or pain to you. Watch their gestures carefully. What similarities do you notice in their explanations?

uses a word that is unclear, the therapist should ask what she means. Asking for clarification enhances knowledge and understanding of the information obtained from the client.

Certain specific information must be obtained from the client. When encouraging conversation, it is easy to forget to ask the important questions. A client information form (see Box 3-1, p. 121) provides a framework for obtaining necessary and important information during the interview.

When listening, it is important to do nothing but listen. You cannot listen while thinking about what is going to be said, writing, or interpreting information. An active listener nods or shows other signs of interest to encourage the person to continue to speak.

The client must be allowed to finish a sentence and must not be rushed or interrupted. Some people rehearse what they say internally before speaking. They speak with pauses between statements, and the practitioner must wait for the client to complete her thoughts. If interrupted, the client often forgets what she was going to tell you. Other clients talk nonstop. They may need to sort through their information by saying it aloud.

When the client has completed a thought and verbalized it, it is important for the massage therapist to summarize and restate the information to ensure that she understood it. It is amazing how often information is misinterpreted. A competent professional is very careful of any preconceived ideas and keeps an open mind while the assessment is in progress (Proficiency Exercise 10-2).

Physical Assessment: the Objective Aspect of Assessment

After the subjective assessment has been completed, the massage practitioner may choose to do a physical assessment before beginning the massage. For a single-session general massage, the physical assessment usually is limited to having the client show the massage technician any movements that feel restricted or may be causing pain. It is important to ask the client to point out any bruises, varicose veins, or areas of inflammation in order to avoid working over these areas. The massage technician must ask the question, "Are there any areas that you feel I should avoid?" Be sure the information is indicated on the

---

10-2

PROFICIENCY EXERCISE

1. With a partner, practice asking three open-ended questions that you might use during an interview.
2. Hold conversations with 10 different people. Practice restating information given to you in response to a question you asked.

---

client information form and that these areas are then avoided.

Assessment for a basic therapeutic massage with treatment plan development and agreed outcomes for the massage includes a general evaluation of the client's posture and gait (walking pattern). For the physical assessment, the main considerations are body balance, efficient function, and basic symmetry.

People are not perfectly symmetric, but the right and left halves of the body should be similar in shape, range of motion, and ability to function. The greater the discrepancy in symmetry, the greater the potential for soft tissue dysfunction. The ear, shoulder, hip, and ankle should be in a vertical line.

Disruption of the gate reflexes creates the potential for many problems. Common gait problems include a functional short leg caused by muscle shortening, tight neck and shoulder muscles, aching feet, and fatigue. The massage therapist must understand basic biomechanics, including posture, interaction of joint functions, and gait.

Posture Assessment: Standing Position

Three major factors influence posture: heredity, disease, and habit. These factors must be considered when evaluating posture. The easiest influence to adjust is habit. By normalizing the soft tissue and teaching balancing exercises, the massage practitioner can play a very beneficial role in helping clients overcome habitual postural distortion. Effects may arise from occupational habits (e.g., a shoulder raised from talking on the phone) and recreational habits (e.g., a forward-shoulder position in a bike rider), or they may be sleep related.

Clothing, shoes, and furniture affect the way a person uses his or her body. Tight collars or ties restrict breathing and contribute to neck and shoulder problems. Restrictive belts, control top undergarments, or tight pants also limit breathing and affect the neck, shoulders, and mid-back. Shoes with high heels or those that do not fit the feet comfortably interfere with postural muscles. Shoes with worn soles imprint the old postural pattern, and the client's body assumes the dysfunctional pattern if she puts them back on after the massage. If postural changes are to be maintained, it is important to change to shoes that do not have a worn sole. Sleep positions can contribute to a wide range of problems. Furniture that does not support the back or that is too high or too low perpetuates muscular tension.

When assessing posture, it is important for the massage practitioner to notice the complete postural pattern. Every action has a reaction. Most compensatory patterns (reactions) respond to gravitational forces. The body makes countless compensatory changes daily. This is normal, and if other pathologic conditions are not present, they seldom become problematic. However, if the client has had an injury, maintains a certain position for a prolonged period, or overuses a body area, the body may not be able to return to a normal dynamic balance efficiently. The balance of the body against the force of gravity is the fundamental determining factor in a person's posture or upright position. Even subtle shifts in posture demand a whole-body compensatory pattern (Fig. 10-1).

The cervical, thoracic, lumbar, and sacral curves develop because of the need to maintain an upright position against gravity (Fig. 10-2). In adults the cervical vertebrae viewed laterally form a symmetric anterior convex curve.

The thoracic vertebrae curve posteriorly, and the lumbar vertebrae reverse and curve in the anterior direction, with a posterior curve of the sacrum. The sharp angulation above C1, the atlas that allows the head to be on a level, horizontal plane, has also been considered a curve. Changes in the normal spinal curves result in scoliosis, lordosis, and kyphosis.

Mechanical balance. A mechanically balanced, weight-bearing joint must be in the gravitational line of the mass it supports and fall exactly through the axis of rotation. Placement of the feet influences the stability of the standing position by providing a base of support. The most common position is one leg in front of the other, with external rotation of the forward leg. It is common for people

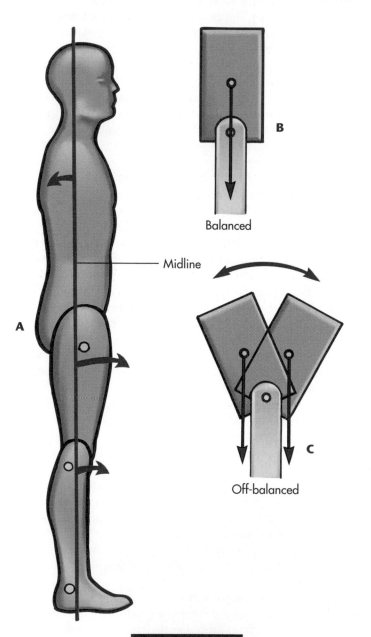

fig. 10-1

A, In normal relaxed standing, the leg and trunk tend to rotate slightly off the midline of the body but maintain a counterbalance force. Balance is achieved in **B** but not in **C.** Any time the trunk moves off this midline balance point, the body must compensate.

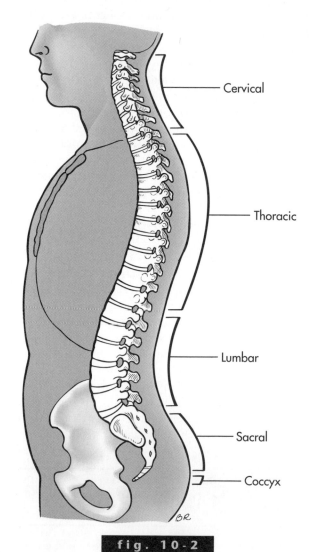

fig. 10-2

Normal spinal curves.

to have a functionally long and short leg. When standing, the long leg often is the front one. When seated with the legs crossed, the long leg often is on top.

The standing posture requires various segments of the body to cooperate mechanically as a whole. Passive tension of ligaments, fascia, and the connective tissue elements of the muscles supports the skeleton. Muscle activity plays a small but important role. Postural muscles maintain small amounts of contraction that stabilize the body upright in gravity by continually repositioning the body weight over the mechanical balance point.

In relaxed symmetric standing, both the hip and the knee joints assume a position of full extension to provide for the most efficient weight-bearing position. The knee joint has an additional stabilizing element in its "screw home" mechanism. The femur rides backward on its medial condyle and rotates medially about its vertical axis to lock the joint for weight bearing. This happens only in the final phase of extension. The normal "screw home" extension pattern of the knee is not hyperextension, which causes a strain on the knee. The hamstrings are the major muscles that resist the force of gravity at the knee.[4,5]

At the ankle joint, bones and ligaments do little to limit motion. Passive tension of the two-joint gastrocnemius muscle (i.e., the muscle crosses two joints) becomes an important factor. This stabilizing force is diminished if high-heeled shoes are worn. The heel of the shoe puts the gastrocnemius on a slack. If these heels are worn constantly, the muscle and the Achilles tendon shorten.

Body sway is limited by intermittent action of appropriate antigravitational postural muscles. During prolonged standing, the average person shifts position frequently. The two basic positions used are the symmetric stance, with the weight distributed equally on both feet, and the asymmetric stance, in which nearly all the weight rests on one foot. The asymmetric stance is the most common, with the weight shifted back and forth between the two feet. This allows for rest periods and shifting of the gravitational forces (Fig. 10-3).

Assessment procedures for the standing position. When assessing the posture of a client who is in the standing position, it is important that the client use the symmetric stance. The feet are about shoulder width apart, and the eyes are closed. With the eyes closed, most of the client's postural patterns are exaggerated because the client is unable to orient the body visually. Often the client will tip his head or rotate it slightly to feel balanced. This information indicates muscular imbalance and internal postural imbalances from positional receptors. Box 10-1 presents a list of indicators of lack of symmetry. The physical assessment form in Box 3-2, p. 122, is a helpful tool for the physical assessment.

Gait Assessment

Understanding the basic body movements of walking helps the massage practitioner recognize dysfunctional and inefficient gait patterns. To begin, the therapist should do a visual observation of the client when walking, noticing the heel-to-toe foot placement. The toes should point directly forward with each step (Fig. 10-4).

Observe the upper body. It should be relaxed and fairly symmetric. There is a natural arm swing that is opposite to the leg swing. The arm swing begins at the shoulder joint. On each step the left arm moves forward as the right leg moves forward and then vice versa. This pattern provides balance. The rhythm and pace of the arm and leg swing should be similar. Walking speed increases the speed of

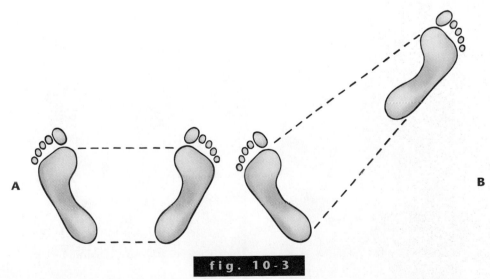

fig. 10-3

A, Symmetric stance. **B,** Asymmetric stance. The asymmetric stance, with the weight shifted from foot to foot, is the most efficient standing position.

box 10-1

LANDMARKS THAT HELP IDENTIFY LACK OF SYMMETRY

The following landmarks can be used for comparison. Be sure to observe the client from the back, the front, and the left and right sides.

- The middle of the chin should sit directly under the tip of the nose. Check the chin alignment with the sternal notch. These two landmarks should be in a direct line.
- The shoulders and clavicles should be level with each other. The shoulders should not roll forward or backward.
- The arms should hang freely and at the same rotation out of the glenohumeral (shoulder) joint.
- The elbows, wrists, and fingertips should be in the same plane.
- The skin of the thorax (chest and back) should be even and should not look as if it pulls or is puffy.
- The navel, located on the same line as the nose, chin, and sternal notch, should not look pulled.
- The ribs should be even and springy.
- The abdomen should be firm but relaxed and slightly rounded.
- The curves at the waist should be even on both sides.
- The spine should be in a direct line from the base of the skull and on the same plane as the line connecting the nose and navel. The curves of the spine should not be exaggerated.
- The scapulae should appear even and should move freely. You should be able to draw an imaginary straight line between the tips of the scapulae.
- The gluteal muscle mass should be even.
- The tops of the iliac crests should be even.
- The greater trochanter, knees, and ankles should be level.
- The circumferences of the thigh and calf should be similar on the left and right sides.
- The legs should rotate out of the acetabulum (hip joint) evenly in a slight external rotation.
- The knees should be locked in the standing position but should not be hyperextended. The patellae (kneecaps) should be level and pointed slightly laterally.
- A line dropped from the nose should fall through the sternum and navel and be spaced evenly between the knees, ankles, and feet.
- The ankles should sit squarely over the feet without falling in or out.
- The feet should have even arches that are not overly exaggerated or flattened.
- The toes should contact but not grip the floor.

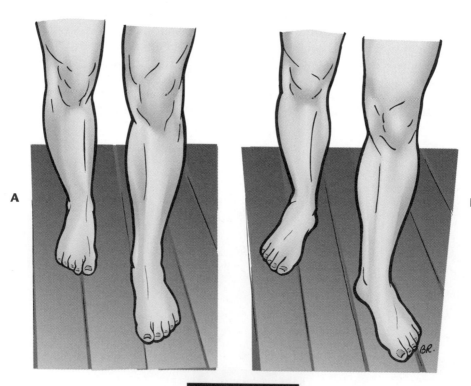

fig. 10-4

Proper (A) and improper (B) foot position in walking.

the arm swing. The length of the stride determines the arc of the arm swing (Fig. 10-5).

Observe the client walking, and notice her general appearance. The optimal walking pattern is as follows:

1. The head and trunk are vertical, with the shoulders level and perpendicular to the vertical line.
2. The arms swing freely opposite the leg swing.
3. Step length and timing are even.
4. The body oscillates vertically with each step.
5. The entire body moves rhythmically with each step.
6. At the heel strike, the foot is approximately at a right angle to the leg.
7. The knee is extended, not locked, in slight flexion.
8. The body weight is shifted forward into the stance phase.
9. At push-off, the foot is strongly plantar flexed, with defined hyperextension of the metatarsophalangeal joints of the toes.
10. During the leg swing, the foot easily clears the floor with good alignment and the rhythm of movement remains unchanged.
11. The heel contacts the floor first.
12. The weight then rolls to the outside of the arch.
13. The arch flattens slightly in response to the weight load.
14. The weight then is shifted to the ball of the foot in preparation for the spring-off from the toes and the shifting of the weight to the other foot.

During walking, the pelvis moves slightly in a side-lying figure-eight pattern. The movements that make up this sequence are transverse, medial, and lateral rotation. The stability and mobility of the sacroiliac joints play very important roles in this alternating side figure-eight movement. If these joints are not functioning properly, the entire gait is disrupted. The sacroiliac joint is one of the few joints in the body that is not directly affected by muscles that cross the joint. It is a large joint, and the bony contact between the sacrum and ilium is broad. It is common for the rocking of this joint to be disrupted (Fig. 10-6).

The hips rotate in a slightly oval pattern beginning with a medial rotation during the leg swing and heel strike, followed by a lateral rotation through the push-off. The knees move in a flexion and extension pattern opposite each other. The extension phase never reaches enough extension to initiate the normal knee lock pattern that is used in standing. The ankles rotate in an arc around the heel at heel strike and around a center in the forefoot at push-off. Maximal dorsiflexion at the end of the stance phase and maximal plantar flexion at the end of push-off are necessary.

Procedures for assessing gait. Observing which areas of the body do not move efficiently during walking provides a good indicator of dysfunctional areas. Pain causes the body to tighten and alters the normal relaxed flow of walking. Muscle weakness and shortening interfere with the neurologic control of the agonist (prime mover) and antagonist muscle action. Limitation of joint movement results in protective muscle spasm. If the situation becomes chronic, both muscle shortening and muscle weakness result. Changes in the soft tissue, including all the connective tissue elements of the tendons, ligaments, and fascial sheaths, restrict the normal action of muscles. Connective tissue usually shortens and becomes less pliable.

Amputation disrupts the body's normal diagonal balance. Any amputation of the leg disturbs the walking pattern. What is not so obvious is that amputation of any part of the arm affects the counterbalance movement of the arm swing during walking. The rest of the body must compensate for the loss. Loss of any of the toes greatly affects the postural information sent to the brain from the feet. So often these details are overlooked, when in fact

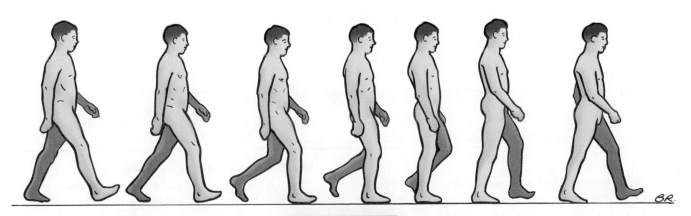

fig. 10-5

Efficient gait position.

they may be major contributing factors in posture and gait problems.

It is possible to have soft tissue dysfunction without joint involvement. Any change in the tissue around a joint has a direct effect on the joint function. Changes in joint function eventually cause problems with the joint. Any dysfunction with the joint immediately involves the surrounding muscles and other soft tissue.

Any disruption of the gait demands that the body compensate by shifting movement patterns and posture. Because of this, all dysfunctional patterns are whole-body phenomena. Working only on the symptomatic area is ineffective and offers limited relief. Therapeutic massage with a whole-body focus is extremely valuable in dealing with gait dysfunction (Proficiency Exercise 10-3).

Assessment by Palpation

Palpation is the use of the hands or fingers to examine. Our hands are our most versatile and exquisite assessment tool. Technology does not come close to the sensitivity and accuracy of a trained assessing hand. Our hands need

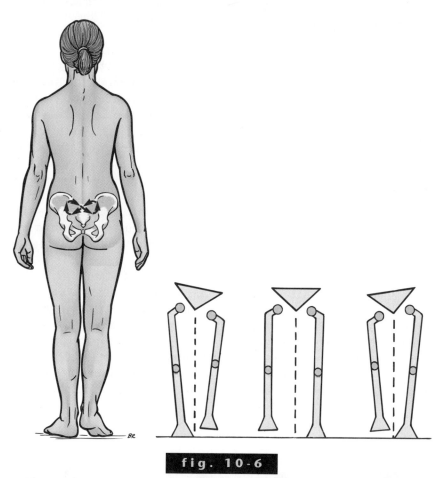

fig. 10-6

The mechanism of the slight rocking movement of the sacroiliac joint.

10-3
PROFICIENCY EXERCISE

1. Watch people walk.
2. Pay attention to yourself when walking. Put on two different shoes and notice what happens when you walk. Tie one arm to your leg and pay attention to what happens when you walk.
3. Place your thumbs on a person's sacroiliac joints and walk behind as the person walks. Feel for the movement. Notice if the figure-eight pattern is even or lopsided.
4. Using the information just presented and the form provided in Box 3-2 (p. 122), do a physical assessment of 10 people.

to be trained to interpret what they perceive accurately. For the therapeutic massage professional, palpation is an essential and continuous process, and the hands become skilled with experience. This section provides structure to facilitate learning palpation assessment.

When dealing with palpation assessment, the main considerations for basic massage are the ability to differentiate between different types of tissue and the ability to distinguish differences of tissue texture within the same tissue types. Palpation includes assessment for hot and cold and observation of skin color and general skin condition. Palpation also assesses various body rhythms, including breathing patterns and pulses.

The tissues that the massage therapist should be concerned with and should be able to distinguish are skin, superficial fascia, fascial sheaths, tendons, ligaments, blood vessels, muscles, and bone.

Mechanisms of Palpation

Before discussing actual palpation skills, it is important to understand what mechanism is being used to make palpation an effective assessment tool. The proprioceptors and mechanoreceptors of the hand receive stimulation from the tissue being palpated. This is the reception phase. These impulses are then transmitted through the peripheral and central nervous systems to the brain, where they are interpreted.

The somatosensory area of the brain that interprets this sensory information devotes a massive area to the hand. The refined discriminatory sense of the hand can perceive very subtle shifts and changes. The interpretation ability usually is a sense of comparison. This tissue is softer than that tissue, or this feels rougher than that. Because comparison is a necessity, the practitioner must be careful to compare apples with apples; for example, it is not logical to compare skin on the back with skin on the feet.

It is this same mechanism that makes self-massage less effective. It is difficult for the brain to decide which signals to pay attention to when the hand is doing the massage and trying to send sensory information, and the body area being massaged is also trying to decide what is happening. Because the hand sensory and motor areas in the brain are so large, it is possible that the information from the hand supersedes the information coming from the part of the body being self-massaged. The body seems to respond to the strongest set of signals. The result is that the brain pays attention to the hand and does not focus enough motor response to the area being massaged. The same area being massaged by another person can respond without conflicting sensory input.

It is important not to limit a palpation sense only to the hand. Movement, heat, and other sensations can be felt with the entire body. It is essential that the massage therapist's entire self become sensitive to subtle differences in the client's body. This is especially true with palpation skills. With palpation, what is going on must be felt and not thought about.

How to Palpate

Palpation can begin many different ways. After the skills have been learned, the particular protocol presented in this text need not be followed. It is best to begin with the lightest palpation and move to the deepest levels because after the hands have been used for deep compression, the light-touch sensors momentarily decrease in sensitivity.

During palpation varying depths of pressure must be used to reach all the tissue types and layers. Do not stay in one area too long or concentrate on a particular spot. The receptors in the practitioner's hand or body adapt, and what is subsequently felt or perceived is then lost. The practitioner's first impression should be trusted; if the area feels hot, it probably is.

Near-touch palpation. The first application of palpation does not include touching the body. It detects hot and cold areas. This is done best just off the skin using the back of the hand because the back of the hand is very sensitive to heat. The general temperature of the area and any variations should be noted. It is important to move fairly quickly in a sweeping motion over the areas being assessed because heat receptors adapt quickly.

Very sensitive cutaneous (skin) sensory receptors also detect changes in air pressure and currents and movement of the air. This is one reason we can feel someone come up behind us when we cannot see him. The movement and change in the surrounding air pressure alert us; this is a protective survival mechanism. Being able consciously to detect subtle sensations is an invaluable assessment tool. It is important to realize from where the information comes and why it can be sensed to avoid any idea that this ability is of an "extrasensory" origin. We are subconsciously aware of all the sensory stimulation that we have receptor mechanisms to detect. It is possible, with practice, to become consciously aware of these more subtle sensory experiences. Sensitivity or intuition is the ability to work with this information on a conscious level.

The information received from near-touch assessment just above the skin feels somewhat similar to putting two poles of a magnet together: a very subtle resistance occurs. Areas that seem thick, dense, or bumpy, or those that tend to push the therapist away are hyperactive. Deeper palpation often reveals muscular hyperactivity or hot spots. Areas that seem thin or feel as though holes are present usually are underactive.

Palpation of the surface of the skin. The second application of palpation is very light surface stroking of the skin. First, determine whether the skin is dry or damp. Damp areas feel a little sticky, or the fingers drag. This light stroking also causes the root hair plexus that senses light touch to respond. It is important to notice whether an area gets more goose bumps than other areas (pilomotor reflex). This is a good time to observe for color, especially blue or yellow coloration. The practitioner also should note and keep track of all moles and surface skin

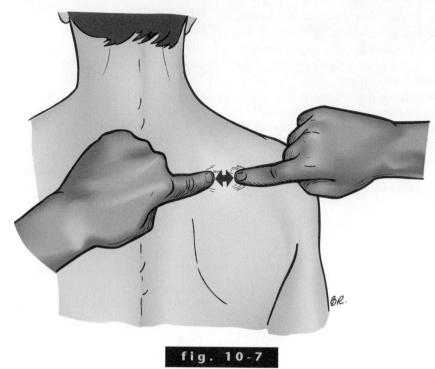

fig. 10-7

Skin stretching used to assess for elasticity. Skin that seems tight compared with surrounding skin may indicate dysfunctional areas.

growths, pay attention to the quality and texture of the hair, and observe the shape and condition of the nails.

Palpation of the skin. The third level of palpation is the skin itself. This is done through gentle, small stretching of the skin in all directions, comparing the elasticity of these areas. The skin also can be palpated for surface texture. By applying light pressure to the skin surface, roughness or smoothness can be felt (Fig. 10-7).

Palpation of the skin and superficial connective tissue. The fourth application of assessment is a combination of skin and superficial connective tissue. A method such as *pétrissage*, or skin rolling, is used to further assess the texture of the skin by lifting it from the underlying fascial sheath. The skin should move evenly and glide on the underlying tissues. Areas that are stuck, restricted, or too loose should be noted (Fig. 10-8). Any areas of the skin that become redder in comparison with surrounding areas are to be noted as well.

Palpation of the superficial connective tissue. The fifth application of palpation is the superficial connective tissue, which separates and connects the skin and muscle tissue. It allows the skin to glide over the muscles during movement. This layer of tissue is found by using compression until the fibers of the underlying muscle are felt. The pressure then should be lightened so that the muscle cannot be felt, but if the hand is moved, the skin also

moves. This area feels a little like a very thin water balloon. The tissue should feel resilient and springy, like gelatin. Superficial fascia holds fluid. If surface edema is present, it is in the superficial fascia. This water-binding quality gives this area the feel of a water balloon, but it should not feel boggy or soggy or show pitting edema (i.e., the dent from the pressure stays in the skin).

Palpation of vessels and lymph nodes. The sixth application of palpation involves circulatory vessels and lymph nodes. Just above the muscle and still in the superficial connective tissue lie the more superficial blood vessels. The vessels are distinct and feel like soft tubes. Pulses can be palpated, but if pressure is too intense, the feel of the pulse is lost. Feeling for pulses helps detect this layer of tissue.

In this same area are the more superficial lymph vessels and lymph nodes. Lymph nodes usually are located in joint areas and feel like small, soft gelcaps. The compression of the joint action assists in lymphatic flow. A client with enlarged lymph nodes should be referred to a medical professional for diagnosis. Very light, gentle palpation of lymph nodes and vessels is indicated in this circumstance.

Palpation of muscles. The seventh application is skeletal muscle. Muscle has a distinct fiber direction that can be felt. This texture feels somewhat like corded fabric or fine rope. Muscle is made up of contractile fibers embedded in

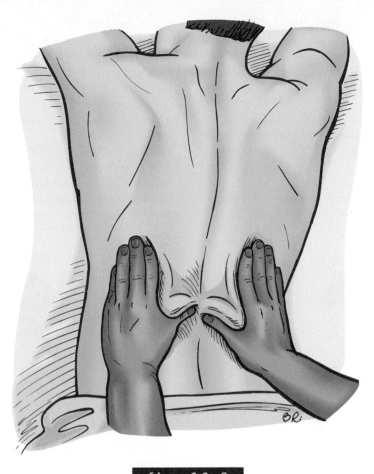

fig. 10-8

Use of pétrissage (skin rolling) to assess the skin and superficial connective tissues by lifting the tissues.

connective tissue. Where the muscle fibers end and the connective tissue continues, the tendon develops. This is called the *musculotendinous junction*. It is a good practice activity to locate this area for all surface muscles and as many underlying ones as possible. Almost all muscular dysfunctions, such as trigger points or microscarring from minute muscle tears, are found at the musculotendinous junction. Most acupressure points, often classified as motor points, also are located in these areas.

Often three or more layers of muscle are present in an area. Compressing systematically through each layer until the bone is felt is important. The layers usually run crossgrain to each other. The best example of this is the abdominal muscle group. Even in the arm and leg, where all the muscles seem to run in the same direction, a diagonal crossing and spiraling of the muscle groups is evident.

Palpation of tendons. The eighth application of palpation is the tendons. Tendons have a higher concentration of collagen fibers and feel more pliable and less ribbed than muscle. Tendons feel like duct tape. Tendons attach muscles to bones. These attachments can be directly on

the bone, but it is just as common to find tendons attaching to ligaments, other tendons, and fascial sheaths for indirect attachment to the bone. The important thing to remember is that these attachment areas are made of various types of connective tissue. The difference in the connective tissue is the ratio of collagen, elastin, and water. Under many tendons is a fluid-filled bursa cushion that assists the movement of the bone under the tendon. Bursae feel like little water balloons or bubbles.

Palpation of fascial sheaths. The ninth application of palpation is fascial sheaths. Fascial sheaths feel like plastic wrap. Fascial sheaths separate muscles and expand the connective tissue area of bone for muscular attachment. Some, such as the lumbodorsal fascia, the abdominal fascia, and the iliotibial band, run on the surface of the body. Others, such as the linea alba and the nuchal ligament, run perpendicular to the surface of the body and the bone. Still others run horizontal through the body. The horizontal pattern occurs at joints, the diaphragm muscle (which is mostly connective tissue), and the pelvic floor. Fascial sheaths separate muscle groups.

The larger nerves and blood vessels lie in grooves created by the fascial separations. Careful comparison reveals that the location of the traditional acupuncture meridians corresponds to these nerve and blood vessel tracts, as do the motor points that correspond to the acupuncture points. The layers can be separated by palpating with the fingers. With sufficient pressure, the fingers tend to fall into these grooves, and then they can be followed. These areas need to be resilient but distinct. They serve both as stabilizers and separators (Fig. 10-9).

Palpation of ligaments. The tenth application of palpation is the ligaments. Ligaments, which are found around joints, are high in elastin and somewhat stretchy. They feel like bungee cords. Some are flat. Ligaments hold joints together and maintain joint space in synovial joints by keeping the joint apart. Ligaments should be flexible enough to allow the joint to move, yet stable enough to restrict movement. It is important to be able to recognize a ligament and not mistake it for a tendon.

Palpation of joints. The eleventh application of palpation is the joints. Joints are found where two bones come together. Careful palpation should reveal the space between the synovial joint ends. Joints often feel like hinges. Most assessment, at the basic massage level, is with active

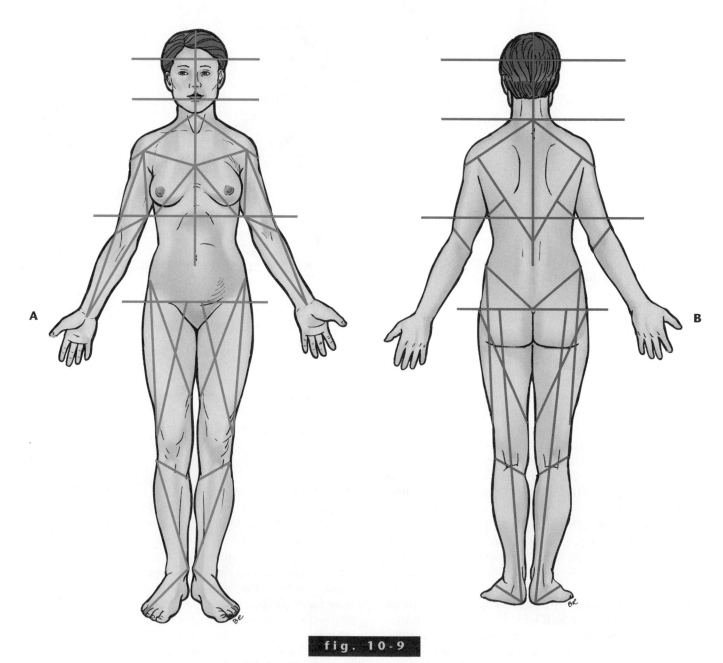

fig. 10-9

Fascial sheaths. A, Anterior view. **B,** Posterior view.

and passive joint movements. An added source of information is palpation of the joint while it is in motion. The sense should be a stable, supported, resilient, and unrestricted range of motion. Box 10-2 presents a summary of joint function.

With the joint movements, it is important to assess for **end-feel.** End-feel is the perception of the joint at the limit of its range of motion. The end-feel is either soft or hard. In most joints it should feel soft. This means that the body is unable to move any more through muscular contraction, but a small additional move by the therapist still produces some give. A hard end-feel is what the bony stabilization of the elbow feels like on extension. No more active movement is possible, and passive movement is restricted by bone.

Palpation of bones. The twelfth application of palpation is the bones. Those who have developed their palpation skills find a firm but detectable pliability to bone. Bones feel like young sapling tree trunks and branches.

For the massage practitioner, it is important to be able to palpate the bony landmarks that indicate the tendinous attachment points for the muscles and trace the bone's shape.

Palpation of abdominal viscera. The thirteenth application of palpation is the viscera. The abdomen contains the viscera, or internal organs of the body. It is important for the massage professional to be able to locate and know the layering of the organs in the abdominal cavity. A good anatomy text can help with this information. The mas-

---

box 10-2

JOINT FUNCTION

For the most part, massage practitioners work with synovial (freely movable) joints. The focus of this text is on the synovial joints; however, all joints are basically the same. The amount of joint movement depends on the bone structure, supportive elements of the ligaments, and arrangement of the muscles. Almost all joint movement is based on the basic flexion-extension concept. Flexion decreases the angle of a joint, and extension increases the angle of a joint. Circumduction is a combination of flexion-extension and adduction-abduction movements.

In order for a joint to move, the muscular elements must be functioning properly and the joint structure, including the cartilage, must also be functional. Joints are designed to fit together in a specific way. For a joint to be able to move, there must be a space between the bone ends. This space must be smooth and lubricated to avoid friction. Anything that interferes with these key elements interferes with joint function.

Balance is another key element in joint function. If the positional receptors in a joint relay information to the central nervous system indicating that damage to the joint may occur, the motor activity (muscles) are affected.

The basic configuration of muscles around a joint is a one-joint muscle and a two-joint muscle. One-joint muscles consist of short levers and long levers (Fig. 10-10). Short levers initiate and stabilize movement. They often have the best mechanical advantage in joint movement. They usually are located deep to the long levers. Long levers have the strength to carry out the full range of motion of the joint pattern. They are superficial to the short levers and deep to the two-jointed muscles. Two-joint muscles are muscles that cross two joints and coordinate movement patterns. They usually are the most superficial of the muscles. A noted exception to this is the psoas muscle.

When evaluating joint function, the massage professional is most concerned with pain-free, symmetric range

of motion. It is difficult to tell whether pain on movement is a muscle or tendon problem or a ligament or joint problem. Therapeutic massage can deal with nonspecific soft tissue dysfunction. Joint dysfunction is out of the scope of practice for the massage professional unless specifically supervised by a chiropractor, physician, or physical therapist.

It is important to be able to distinguish between the muscle and tendon components and the ligament and joint components in a restricted movement pattern. When in doubt, *always* refer suspected joint problems to a medical professional.

The following two means of distinguishing between the muscle and tendon components and the ligament and joint components are recommended:

1. Pain on gentle traction usually is a muscle or tendon problem. Pain on gentle compression usually is a problem with the ligament or joint.
2. If active range of motion produces pain and passive range of motion does not, it usually is a muscle or tendon problem. If both passive and active ranges of motion produce pain, the problem usually is a ligament or joint.

When working with joints, it is important to distinguish between the anatomic barrier and the physiologic barrier. The anatomic barrier is the bone contour and soft tissue, especially the ligaments, that serves as the final limit to motion in a joint. Beyond this motion limit, tissue damage occurs. The physiologic barrier is more of a nervous system protective barrier that prevents access to the anatomic barrier when damage to the joint could occur. It is important for the massage therapist to stay within the limits of the physiologic barrier to avoid possible hypermovement of a joint. Therapeutic massage may increase the range of motion of a jointed area by resetting the confines of the pathologic barrier of the joint.

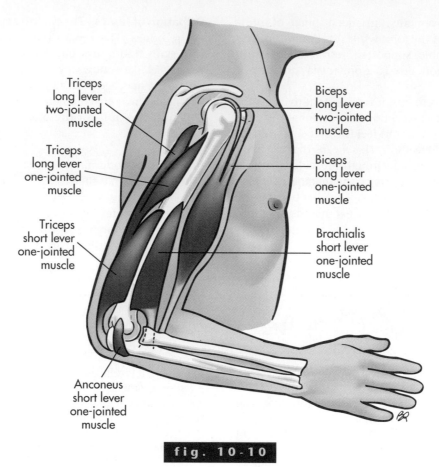

Triceps
long lever
two-jointed
muscle

Triceps
long lever
one-jointed
muscle

Triceps
short lever
one-jointed
muscle

Anconeus
short lever
one-jointed
muscle

Biceps
long lever
two-jointed
muscle

Biceps
long lever
one-jointed
muscle

Brachialis
short lever
one-jointed
muscle

fig. 10-10

One- and two-joint muscles. Functional short- and long-lever muscles.

sage therapist should be able to palpate the distinct firmness of the liver and the large intestine. Although deep massage to the abdomen is not suggested for those trained in basic massage, light to moderate stroking of nthe abdomen is beneficial for the large intestine. The massage therapist should be able to locate and palpate this organ.

Palpation of body rhythms. The fourteenth application of palpation is the body rhythms. Body rhythms are felt as even pulsations. Body rhythms, those mentioned and not mentioned, are designed to operate in a coordinated balanced and synchronized manner. In the body the rhythms all entrain. When palpating body rhythms the practitioner should get a sense of this harmony. Although the trained hand can pick out some of the individual rhythms, just as one can hear individual notes in a song, it is the whole connected effect that is important. When a person feels "off" or "out of sync," often he or she is speaking of disruption in the entrainment process of body rhythms.

The three basic rhythms are the respiration, circulation, and craniosacral rhythms.

Respiration. The breath is easy to feel. It should be even and should follow good principles of inhalation and exhalation (see Chapter 13). Palpation of the breath is done by placing the hands over the ribs and allowing the body to go through three or more cycles as the practitioner evaluates the evenness and fullness of the breath.

Circulation. The movement of the blood is felt at the major pulse points. The pulses should be balanced on the two sides. Basic palpation of the movement of the blood is done by placing the fingertips over pulse points on both sides of the body and comparing for evenness (Fig. 10-11).

Craniosacral rhythm. The craniosacral rhythm, sometimes called the *primary respiratory mechanism,* and related cranial rhythmic impulse is a subtle but detectable widening and narrowing movement of the cranial bones. A to-and-fro oscillation of the sacrum should be noted.[3] Specific training for craniosacral therapy focuses on this mechanism. Basic palpation of the craniosacral rhythm is done by lightly placing the hands on either side of the head and sensing

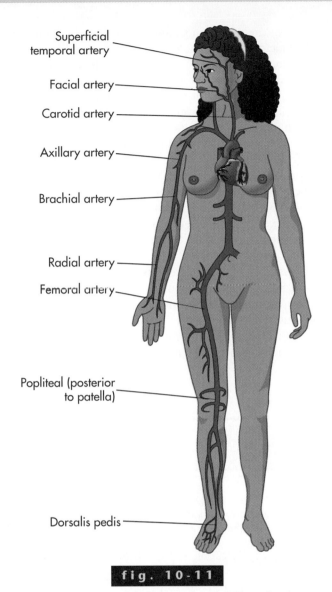

Superficial temporal artery

Facial artery

Carotid artery

Axillary artery

Brachial artery

Radial artery

Femoral artery

Popliteal (posterior to patella)

Dorsalis pedis

f i g .   1 0 - 1 1

Pulse points. Each pulse point is named after the artery with which it is associated. (From Thibodeau GA, Patton KT: *The human body in health and disease,* ed 2, St Louis, 1997, Mosby.)

for the widening and narrowing of the skull. Also, place a hand over the sacrum and feel for the to-and-fro (back-and-forth) movement. These sensations normally occur at a rate of 10 to 14 times per minute.[3] The movement of the cranium and sacrum should feel coordinated and even (Proficiency Exercise 10-4).

Assessment Procedures for Muscle Testing

Muscle testing procedures are used for different purposes. The purpose of **strength testing** is to discover whether the muscle is responding with sufficient strength to perform

the required body functions. The purpose of **neurologic muscle testing** is to discover whether the neurologic interaction of the muscles is working smoothly. The third type of muscle testing, which is used in **applied kinesiology,** relies on muscle strength or weakness as an indicator of body function. It is somewhat like a body biofeedback mechanism. The system itself is too complex to cover in this book, but it is important to identify applied kinesiologic muscle testing procedures as a method of assessment and evaluation.

Strength Testing

In general, the purpose of strength testing is to determine whether the muscle or muscle groups are able to respond with adequate force to a demand without excessive recruitment of other muscles, and whether the muscle strength patterns are similar on both sides of the body.

Strength testing determines a muscle's force of contraction. The preferred method is to isolate the muscle or muscle group by positioning the muscle with its attachment points as close together as possible. The muscle or muscle group being tested should be isolated as specifically as possible. Many good kinesiology manuals are available that provide instruction on ways to isolate a specific muscle or muscle group. The client holds or maintains the contracted position of the muscle isolation while the therapist slowly and evenly applies a counterpressure to pull the muscle out of its isolated position. The massage therapist must use sufficient force to recruit a full response by the muscles being tested but not enough to recruit other muscles in the body. If strength testing is done this way, there is little chance the therapist will injure the client. As with palpation, it is necessary to compare the muscle test with a similar area, usually the same muscle group on the opposite side.

Testing the coordination of the agonist and antagonist interaction. Another testing method is to compare a muscle group's strength with its antagonist pattern. The body is designed so that the flexor and adductor muscles are about 25% to 30% stronger than the extensors and abductors. It is also designed so that flexors and adductors usually work against gravity to move a joint. The main purposes of extensors and abductors are to balance the flexor and adductor movement and return the joint to a neutral position. Less strength is required because gravity is assisting the function.

Strength testing should reveal a difference in the pattern between flexors and abductors and extensors and adductors in an agonist/antagonist pattern. These groups should not be equally strong. Flexors and adductors should show more muscle strength than extensors and abductors.

Muscle testing and gait patterns. It also is important to consider the pattern of muscle interactions that occurs with walking. Remember that gait has a certain pattern for efficient movement.

For example, if the left leg is extended for the heel strike, the right arm also is extended. This results in activation of the flexors of both the arm and leg and inhibition of the extensors. It is common to find a strength imbalance in this gait pattern. One muscle out of sequence with the others can set up tense or inhibited muscle imbalances. Whenever a muscle contracts with too much force, it overpowers the antagonist group, resulting in inhibited muscle function. The imbalances can occur anywhere in the pattern.

Strength muscle testing should reveal that the flexor and adductor muscles of the right arm should activate, facilitate, and coordinate with the flexors and adductors of the left leg. The opposite is also true: left arm flexors and adductors activate and facilitate the right leg flexors and adductors. Extensors and abductors in the limbs coordinate in a similar fashion.

This being the case, if the flexors of the left leg are activated, as occurs during strength testing, the flexors and ad-

ductors of the right arm should be facilitated. The flexors and adductors of the right leg and left arm should be inhibited. Also, the extensor and abductors in the right arm and left leg should be inhibited. All associated patterns follow suit (i.e., activation of the right arm flexor pattern facilitates the left leg flexor pattern and inhibits left arm and right leg flexor muscles while facilitating extensors and abductors). In a similar way, activation of the adductors of the right leg facilitates the adductors of the left arm and inhibits the abductors of the left leg and right arm. The other adductor/abductor patterns follow the same interaction pattern.

All these pattern are associated with gait mechanisms and reflexes. If any pattern is out of sync, gait, posture, and efficient function are disrupted.

Gait muscle testing as an intervention tool. An understanding of gait provides a powerful intervention tool. For example, a person trips and strains the left leg extensor muscles. Gait muscle testing reveals the imbalanced pattern by showing that the left leg extensor muscles are weak, whereas the flexors in the left leg and right arm are overly tense. The leg

---

10-4

PROFICIENCY EXERCISE

1. Palpate several objects with different textures. Then palpate the same objects through a sheet, towel, blanket, and foam. See how many you can recognize.
2. Have people walk up to you while you are blindfolded. Pay attention to when you sense the person's presence.
3. Feel heat radiating off various objects. How far away can you get from the object before you cannot feel the heat?
4. Feel appliances or machinery as the motor runs. Pay attention to the vibrations. How far away can you get and still feel the vibrations?
5. Put a dime in a phone book under two pages. Locate the dime. Keep increasing the number of pages over the dime until you cannot feel it.
6. Get two magnets and play with them. Feel for the "force field."
7. Using the following list, palpate and observe all the following on five clients. Compare with related areas.
   - Heat and cold
   - Air pressure and current shifts
   - Damp or dry skin
   - Goose bumps
   - Color
   - Hair
   - Nails

- Skin texture
- Skin roughness or smoothness
- Skin and superficial connective tissue connection
- Superficial connective tissue
- Blood vessels
- Pulses
- Lymph nodes
- Direction of skeletal muscle fiber
- Musculotendinous junction
- Motor points
- Muscle layers
- Tendons
- Fascial sheaths
- Ligaments
- Bursae
- Joints
- Joint space
- Joint movement
- Joint movement end-feel
- Bone
- Bony landmarks
- Bone shape
- Viscera
- Craniosacral rhythms
- Breathing

is sore and cannot be used for work, but the arm muscles are fine. By activating the extensors in the right arm, the left leg extensor muscles can be facilitated. By activating the flexors of the left arm, the flexors of the left leg are inhibited. This process may restore balance in the gait pattern. Many combinations are possible based on the gait pattern and reflexes. Gait muscle testing provides the means of identifying these interactions.

Careful study of this interaction is important for work with individuals such as athletes or dancers. An understanding of this interaction also is helpful in working with people who have various forms of spastic paralysis and spastic muscle conditions. For example, a child with a head injury that causes flexor spasms in the right arm may be helped temporarily by a reduction in the spasm pattern through activation of left leg extensor patterns, especially if the child has more coordination in that area. All other possible interactions follow suit. If voluntary activation of the muscles is not possible, tapotement at the tendons of the muscle required to contract usually provides the appropriate neurologic signal.

Neurologic Muscle Testing

Neurologic muscle testing focuses more on the patterns of muscle communication. A small force is used for testing because only the nervous system is activated. An efficient pattern is one in which the muscles contract evenly, without jerking and without a lot of synergistic (helper muscle) activity. The same isolation of muscle groups is used as in strength testing. The client holds the contraction, and the massage therapist provides moderately light pressure against the muscle. As always, the goal is to locate the muscle interaction pattern, not only for the muscle directly tested but also for all other muscles linked through gait and postural reflexes.

When testing neuromuscular activity, it is important to notice what the rest of the body does when the isolated muscle group is tested. For example, if testing of the neck flexor muscles causes the left leg to roll in, a pattern of interaction has shown itself. These patterns may be natural, such as the gait reflexes, but often are a mixed-up set of signals that cause the body to respond inappropriately. Inefficient patterns cause some muscles to contract more than is necessary. Muscles may not be able to stop contracting and thus maintain tension patterns. Whenever a pattern of overly tight muscles exists, there is a pattern of inhibited and weak muscles. These imbalances use energy and contribute to fatigue and pain in the client.

Muscle group interactions. Remember from the discussion on joints that the body has one-jointed muscles and two-jointed muscles for most joints. Muscles are tested in groups because it is almost impossible to isolate just one muscle. The brain does not process this type of infor-

mation. It is more important to work with muscles in patterns of flexion and extension, adduction and abduction, or elevation and depression than to be concerned with the function of individual muscles. The movement pattern of each synovial joint is based on the flexion and extension principle. To move in gravity, each joint must be stabilized by some sort of diagonal pattern as a counterbalance. Therefore the entire body is involved in all movement patterns.

Postural and phasic muscles. The two basic types of muscles are those that support the body in gravity and those that move it through gravity. Those that support the body in gravity are called **postural muscles.** Those that move the body are called **phasic muscles** (Box 10-3).[1]

The two muscle types consist of different types of muscle fibers. Postural muscles have a higher percentage of slow-twitch red fibers, which can hold a contraction for a long time before fatiguing. Phasic muscles have a higher percentage of fast-twitch red fibers, which contract quickly but tire easily.

---

box 10-3

MAJOR POSTURAL AND PHASIC MUSCLES

Main postural muscles	*Main phasic muscles*
Gastrocnemius	Neck flexors
Soleus	Deltoid
Adductors	Biceps
Medial hamstrings	Triceps
Psoas	Brachioradialis
Abdominal	Quadriceps
Rectus femoris	Hamstring
Tensor fascia lata	Gluteus maximus
Piriformis	Anterior tibialis
Quadratus lumborum	
Erector spinae group	
Pectoral	
Latissimus dorsi	
Neck extensors	
Trapezius	
Scalene	
Sternocleidomastoid	
Levator scapula	

These two types of muscle are tested differently and develop different types of dysfunction.

Postural muscles. Postural muscles are relatively slow to respond compared with phasic muscles. They do not produce bursts of strength if asked to respond quickly, and they may cramp. They are the deliberate, slow, steady muscles that require time to respond. If compared with the story about the tortoise and the hare, these muscles are the tortoise. Inefficient neurologic patterns, muscle tension, reorganization of connective tissue with fibrotic changes, and trigger points are common in postural muscles.[1]

If posture is not balanced, postural muscles must function more like ligaments and bones. When this happens, additional connective tissue develops in the muscle to provide the ability to stabilize the body in gravity. The problem is that the connective tissue freezes the body in the position because, unlike muscle, which can contract and lengthen, connective tissue is static tissue.

Postural muscles tend to shorten and increase in tension when under strain. This information is important when attempting to assess which muscles are tense and therefore in need of lengthening and which groups of muscle are apt to develop connective tissue changes and require stretching. Connective tissue shortening is dealt with mechanically through forms of stretch. Hypertension of muscles is dealt with through reflexive lengthening procedures (see Chapter 9).

Phasic muscles. Phasic muscles jump into action quickly and tire quickly. It is more common to find musculotendinous junction problems in phasic muscles. The four

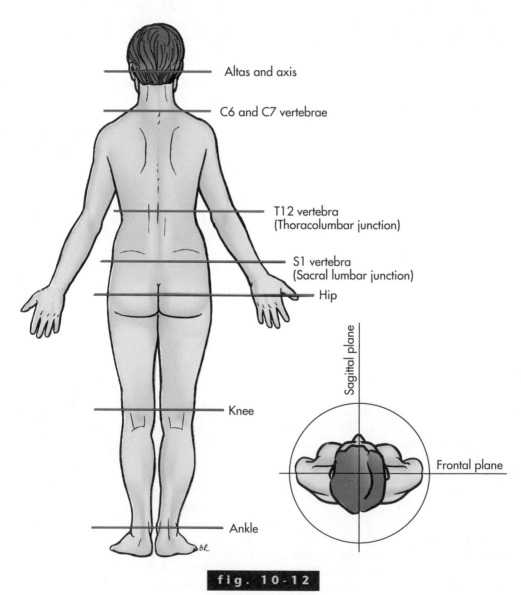

fig. 10-12

Quadrants and movement segments.

most common problems are microtearing of the muscle fibers at the tendon, inflamed tendons (tendinitis), tendons adhering to underlying tissue, and bursitis.

Phasic muscles usually weaken in response to postural muscle shortening. Sometimes the weakened muscles also shorten. This shortening allows the weak muscle the same contraction power on the joint. It is important not to confuse this condition with hypertense muscles. These muscles are inhibited and weak.

Phasic muscles occasionally become overly tense. This almost always results from some sort of repetitive behavior and is a common problem of athletes. Phasic muscles also become tense in response to a sudden posture change that causes the muscles to assist the postural muscles in maintaining balance. These common, inappropriate muscle patterns often result from an unexpected fall or near fall, an automobile accident, or some other trauma. Basic massage methods discussed in this text can be used to reset and retrain out-of-sync muscles.

Neurologic interaction patterns and mechanisms of dysfunction. No set system exists for figuring out neuromuscular patterns. These patterns are activated in response to a disruption of balance in gravity, as in a fall. A general pattern can be detected, and then modification for the individual client can be initiated. Gait patterns have a powerful influence. Additional powerful determinants are righting reflexes in the neck that, coordinated with the eyes, keep the body oriented perpendicular to a horizontal plane. Balance mechanisms of the inner ear also are a factor. Any inner-ear difficulties or visual distortion affects neuromuscular interactions and postural balance patterns.

A common and often undiagnosed eye/ear problem is benign paroxysmal (sometimes called *vestibular*) positional vertigo. This condition exists when otolith crystals in the inner ear become displaced and send erroneous positional information to the lower brain balance and muscle coordination centers. The eyes are linked through the righting reflex mechanism. Various muscle tension patterns can be linked to this and other similar conditions. Referral to the appropriate health care professional is important for proper diagnosis.

Postural influence. The body is a circular form divided into four quadrants: a front, a back, a right side, and a left side. With divisions on the sagittal and frontal planes, the body must be balanced in three dimensions to withstand the forces of gravity.

The body moves and is balanced in the following skeletal areas: the atlas; the C6 and C7 vertebrae; the T12 and L1 vertebrae (the thoracolumbar junction); the L4, L5, and S1 vertebrae (the sacrolumbar junction); and at the hips, knees, and ankles, with stabilization at the shoulder (Fig. 10-12). If a postural distortion exists in any of the four quadrants or within one of the jointed areas, the entire balance mechanism must be adjusted. This occurs in a

pinball-like effect that jumps front to back and side to side at the movement lines.

To gain an understanding of postural balance, locate a pole of some type (a broom handle without the broom portion will work). Tie a string around the pole.

Now, try to balance the pole on its end using the string. Note that you work opposite of the fall pattern in trying to counter the fall pattern of the pole. If the pole tends to fall forward and to the left, you apply a counterforce back and to the right.

This is what the body does as well if part of the body moves off the balance line. The body is made up of many different poles stacked on top of one another. The poles stack at each of the movement segments. Muscles between the movement segments must be three-dimensionally balanced in all four quadrants to support the pole in that area.

Each area needs to be balanced. If one pole area tips a bit to the right, the body compensates by tipping the adjacent pole areas to the left. If a pole area is tipped forward, adjacent poles are tipped back. A chain reaction occurs, such that when compensating poles tip back, their adjacent areas must counterbalance the action by tipping forward. This is how the body-wide compensation pattern is set up.

Whether the pole areas sit nicely on top of each other with evenly distributed muscle action or whether they are tipped in various positions and counterbalanced by compensatory muscle actions, the body remains balanced in gravity. However, the "tippy pole" pattern is much more inefficient than the balanced pole pattern (Fig 10-13).

Intervention plans attempt to normalize the balance process by relaxing the tension pattern in overly tight areas, strengthening muscles in corresponding weak areas, and allowing the poles to straighten out. If a pole is permanently tippy, such as with scoliosis or kyphosis, intervention plans attempt to support the appropriate compensation patterns and prevent them from increasing beyond what is necessary for postural balance (Proficiency Exercise 10-5).

10-5

PROFICIENCY EXERCISE

1. Have three other students do a muscle testing assessment of you. Include all the postural and phasic muscles listed for both strength and neuromuscular function. Compare the information they gather with what you gathered. As a group, compare the information gathered for similarities and differences. Rotate so that each student is assessed.
2. Do a complete physical assessment of 10 different people.

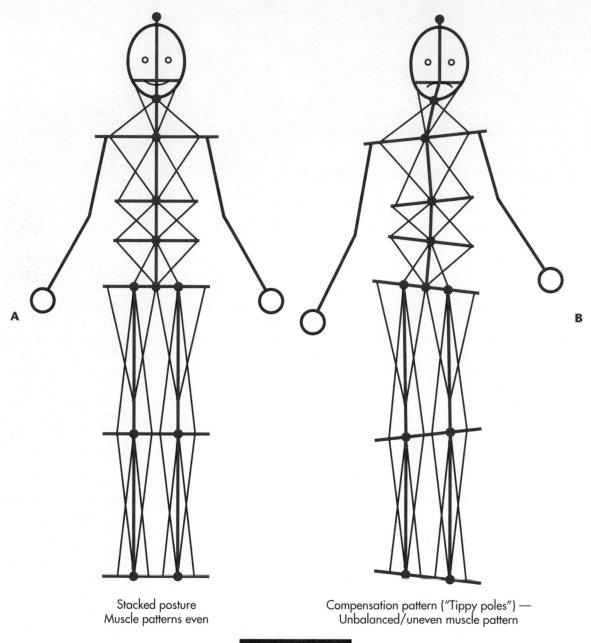

Stacked posture
Muscle patterns even

Compensation pattern ("Tippy poles") —
Unbalanced/uneven muscle pattern

fig. 10-13

Stacked pole **(A)** versus tippy pole **(B)** postural influences on the body.

INTERPRETATION AND ANALYSIS OF ASSESSMENT INFORMATION

section objectives

Using the information presented in this section, the student will be able to perform the following:

■ Interpret assessment information to design a basic full-body massage session that focuses on the specific outcome desired by the client

■ Refer clients for care when the assessment information indicates the need for specific diagnosis and treatment

■ Use the clinical reasoning model to choose specific massage approaches to serve as intervention methods during the massage session

After information has been gathered, it is time to connect all the pieces in an interpretation and analysis process to develop the best massage plan for the individual client. This requires clinical reasoning and problem-solving skills. The main purpose of intervention is to help the body regain symmetry. Therefore, when observing gait or posture, the practitioner notes areas that seem pulled, twisted, or dropped. The massage practitioner's job is to use all massage methods to lengthen shortened areas, untwist twisted areas, raise dropped areas, soften hard areas, firm soft areas, warm cold areas, and cool hot areas.

After rapport has been established, the client will be comfortable and will trust the practitioner enough to let her guard down. She will communicate a variety of information during the discussion or the massage session. The practitioner should listen for repeated phrases, such as "It is a real pain in the neck" or "I can hardly stand up to it." The practitioner should not counsel or explain the ramifications of the information, only notice the pattern and keep general clinical notes.

Careful attention should be paid to the order of priority in which the client relays the information. If the headache is mentioned first, the knee ache second, and the tight elbow last, then the areas should be dealt with in that order, if possible, in the massage flow.

The importance of listening to understand is paramount. Many experienced professionals have learned that if we listen to our clients, they will tell us what is wrong and how to help them restore balance. Slow down, do not jump to conclusions, pay attention, and let the information unfold. Realize that each client is the expert about himself. Clients are your teachers about themselves, and in teaching you they often begin to understand themselves better. Every session, approach each client with fascination about what you will learn from her. *No textbook, class, or instructor can equal the teaching provided by careful attention to the client.*

General Presence

In general, excessive sympathetic activation would be balanced by a relaxing massage, and excessive parasympathetic activation would be balanced by a stimulating massage. However, it is not quite that easy. In the discussion of rapport, the author recommended that the practitioner work with a client by meeting the client's current state. This is also very true in deciding whether the general massage approach will be stimulation or relaxation.

If the client is functioning from sympathetic nervous system dominance and relaxation methods such as rocking and slow effleurage are used initially, the work often seems irritating to the client. If the session is begun with a more stimulating approach, using such strokes as rapid compression, muscle energy methods, lengthening, and tapotement, the design of the massage fits the physiologic level of the client. After some of the nervous energy has been discharged, the client is ready for the more relaxing methods.

The same is true with parasympathetic dominant patterns. If the client is "down" that day, beginning with a stimulation approach may feel like an attack. It is better to begin with the more subtle relaxation methods and progress slowly into the stimulation approaches to encourage balance.

If the client seems "out of sorts," operating more as a collection of parts than the sum of the parts, entrainment processes may be off. The centered, coordinated presence of the professional providing a harmonized approach to the massage is beneficial.

Gesturing

The general guidelines for gestures listed are not written in stone. Professional experience indicates that those listed in this text are fairly dependable starting points until the student is more experienced with interpreting an individual's body language.

People tend to be consistent with their gestures and word phrases within their own internal body language system. However, body language is as individual as the person. Particular gestures or styles of body language cannot be generalized to mean one specific thing. It is the professional's responsibility to understand what a gesture means for a particular individual.

Because of nervous system patterns and basic universal body language connected with survival emotions such as fear, anger, distress, and happiness, some body language is fairly consistent from person to person. But it cannot be assumed that a certain gesture always means the same thing with every person. It takes time and careful observation to decipher an individual's body language code. This is done by watching for repetitive body language of a client and connecting the particular gesture or posture to the mood, state, and content of the conversation. Eventually the client repeats the body language patterns enough so that the individual pattern is evident.

The following are common gestures:

- A finger pointing to a specific area suggests an acupressure or motor point hyperactivity or a joint problem. What the pointing means depends on the area indicated.
- If the finger is pointed to a specific area but then the hand swipes in a certain direction, it may be a trigger point problem.
- If the area is grabbed, pulled, or held and moved as if being stretched, this often indicates muscle or fascial shortening.
- If movement is needed to show the area of tightness, the area may need muscle lengthening combined with muscle energy work to prepare for the stretch and reset of neuromuscular patterns.
- If the client moves into a position and then acts as if stuck, the area may need connective tissue stretching.
- If the client draws lines on his body, it may indicate nerve entrapment in the fascial planes or grooves.

Posture Assessment

The focus is symmetry. When applying the techniques, the massage practitioner should honor what the body is doing. This can be done by creating a slight exaggeration of the asymmetric pattern found and then slowly encouraging the body to shift to a more symmetric pattern.

Misalignment of body areas can be caused by muscles that pull or do not stabilize, connective tissue shortening or laxity, or, more likely, a combination of these. It is best to follow the lead provided by the client's body. It may be hard to tell if one shoulder is too high or the other one is dropped. Instead, the bodyworker should exaggerate the pattern and have the client push or pull out of the stabilizing pressure (the integrated muscle energy approach explained in Chapter 9, p. 383, is effective in these situations). Attention should be paid to the pattern in which the client uses the most effort when pushing or pulling. This indicates where to look for further dysfunction.

For example, a client has a long left leg with an externally rotated foot. As part of the massage, a good approach is to pull on the long leg to increase the pattern and externally rotate the foot even more. Then the corrective pattern can be encouraged by having the client pull and rotate the leg in the opposite direction against stabilizing pressure. As the client finishes this move, the lengthening and stretch should be continued in the same direction as the client's pulling force. All the shortened areas should then be massaged and the overstretched areas stimulated.

The method just described works well for neuromuscular problems. It is not as effective for altering connective tissue dysfunction but does prepare the body for connective tissue work.

If the areas of contracted and shortened connective tissue are stretched without this preparation, the body may respond with protective spasms. Working with connective tissue often requires slow, sustained stretching that puts a sufficient pull into the connective tissue and specific application of friction massage manipulations. Connective tissue approaches normalize the twists and pulls of shortened connective tissue.

Asymmetry usually results when overly tense muscles or shortened connective tissue pulls the body out of alignment. Direct trauma pushes joints out of alignment. Weak stabilizing mechanisms, such as overstretched ligaments or inhibited antagonist muscles, contribute to the problem. In these situations a chiropractor, an osteopath, or another trained medical professional skilled in skeletal manipulation is needed. Often a multidisciplinary approach to client care is necessary.

Gait Assessment

When interpreting the information gathered from gait assessment, the focus should be on areas that do not move easily when the client walks and areas that move too much. Areas that do not move are restricted; areas that move too much are compensating for inefficient function. By releasing the restrictions through massage and reeducating the re-

flexes through neuromuscular work and exercise, the practitioner can help the client improve the gait pattern.

The techniques followed are similar to those for postural corrections. The shortened and restricted areas are softened with massage, then the neuromuscular mechanism is reset with muscle energy techniques, muscle lengthening, and stretches.

The client should be taught slow lengthening and stretching procedures. After stimulating the muscles in weakened areas, the practitioner can teach the client strengthening exercises. The therapist must be sure the adaptation methods are built into the context of a complete massage rather than spot work on isolated parts of the body. Suggestions could be made to the client to evaluate factors that may contribute to these adaptations, such as posture, foot care, chairs, tables, beds, clothing, shoes, work stations, physical tasks (e.g., shoveling), and repetitive exercise patterns.

Proper functioning of the sacroiliac joint is an important factor in walking patterns. Because sacroiliac joint movement has no direct muscular component, it is difficult to use any kind of muscle energy lengthening when working with this joint. The joint is embedded deep in supporting ligaments. To keep the surrounding ligaments pliable, direct and specific connective tissue techniques are indicated unless the joint is hypermobile. If that is the case, external bracing combined with rehabilitative movement may be indicated. Sometimes the ligaments restabilize the area. Stabilization of the jointed area should be interspersed with massage and gentle stretching to ensure that the ligaments remain pliable and do not adhere to each other. This process takes time.

The diagnosis of specific joint problems and fitting for external bracing is outside the scope of practice for therapeutic massage, and the client must be referred to the appropriate professional.

Palpation Assessment

Palpation assessment becomes part of the massage. In any given massage, about 90% of the touching is also assessment developed as part of effleurage, pétrissage, or joint movement. Palpation assessment meets tissue but does not override it or encourage it to change. This type of work generally relaxes or stimulates the client, depending on the type of strokes used.

Hot and Cold Areas

Hot areas may be caused by inflammation, muscle spasm, hyperactivity, or increased surface circulation. When the focus of intervention is to cool down the hot areas, one method to use is application of ice (see section on hydrotherapy in Chapter 11). Another way to cool an area is to reduce the muscle spasm and encourage more efficient blood flow in the surrounding areas.

Cold areas often are areas of diminished blood flow, increased connective tissue formation, or muscle flaccidity. The cold areas may have heat applied to them. Stimulation massage techniques increase muscle activity, thus heating up the area. Connective tissue approaches soften connective tissue, help to restore space around the capillaries, and release histamine, a vasodilator, to increase circulation. These approaches can warm a cold area.

Skin

Skin should be contained, resilient, elastic, and even, with rich coloring. It should have no blue, yellow, or red tinges. Blue coloration suggests lack of oxygen, yellow indicates liver problems such as jaundice, and redness suggests fever, alcohol intake, trauma, or inflammation. Color changes are most noticeable in the lips, around the eyes, and under the nails.

Bruises are to be noted and avoided during massage. If a client displays any hot redness or red streaking, she should be referred to a physician immediately. This is especially important in the lower leg because of the possibility of deep vein thrombosis (blood clot).

The skin should be watched carefully for changes in any moles or lumps. As massage professionals, we often spend more time touching and observing a person's skin than anyone else, including the person. If we keep a keen eye for changes and refer clients to physicians early, many skin problems can be treated before they become serious.

Depending on the area, the skin may be thick or thin. The skin of the face is thinner than the skin of the lower back. The skin in each particular area, however, should be similar. The skin loses its resilience and elasticity over areas of dysfunction. It is important to know visceral referred areas to the skin. If changes occur to the skin in these areas, refer to a physician (see Chapter 5, p. 202).

The skin is a blood reservoir. At any given time it can hold 10% of available blood in the body. The connective tissue in the skin must be soft to allow the capillary system to expand to hold the blood. Histamine, which is released from mast cells found in the connective tissue of the superficial fascial layer, dilates the blood vessels. Histamine is also responsible for the client's reported sense of "warming and itching" in an area that has been massaged.

Damp areas on the skin are indications that the nervous system has been activated in that area. This small amount of perspiration is part of a sympathetic activation called a *facilitated segment*.

Surface stroking with enough pressure to drag over the skin elicits a red response over the area of a hyperactive muscle. Deeper palpation of the area usually elicits a tender response.

The small erector pili muscles attached to each hair also are under the control of the sympathetic autonomic nervous system. Light fingertip stroking produces goose bumps over areas of nerve hyperactivity.

Hair and Nails

The hair and nails are part of the integumentary system and can reflect health conditions.

The hair should be resilient and secure; hair loss should not be excessive when massaging the scalp.

The nails should be smooth. Vertical ridges can indicate nutritional difficulties, and horizontal ridges can be signs of stress caused by changes in circulation that affect nail growth. Clubbed nails may also indicate circulation problems. The skin around the nails should be soft and free of hangnails.

During times of stress, the epithelial tissues are affected first. Hangnails, split skin around the lips and nails, mouth sores, hair loss, dry scaly skin, and excessively oily skin are all signs of prolonged stress, medication side effects, or other pathologic conditions. Only a physician can diagnose the cause of the condition (refer to the contraindications in Appendix A for more information).

Superficial Connective Tissue

Methods of palpation that lift the skin, such as pétrissage and skin rolling, provide much information. Depending on the area of the body and the concentration of underlying connective tissue, the skin should lift and roll easily. Loosening these areas is very beneficial and can be done by being more deliberate and slow with the assessment methods to allow for a shift in the tissues. A constant drag should be kept on the tissues because both the skin and superficial connective tissue are affected.

Any areas that become redder than the surrounding tissue or that stay red longer than other areas are suspect for connective tissue changes. Usually lifting and stretching of the reddened tissue or use of the myofascial approaches presented in Chapter 11 normalize these areas.

Vessels, Pulses, and Lymph Nodes

Vessels should feel firm but pliable and supported. If any areas of bulging, mushiness, or constriction are noted, the practitioner should refer the client to a physician.

Pulses should be compared by feeling for a strong, even, full-pumping action on both sides of the body. If differences are perceived, the practitioner should refer the client to a physician. Sometimes the differences in the pulses can be attributed to soft tissue restriction of the artery or a more serious condition that can be diagnosed by the physician.

Enlarged lymph nodes may indicate local or systemic infection or more serious conditions. The client should be referred to a physician immediately.

Skeletal Muscle

Skeletal muscle is assessed both for texture and for function. It should be firm and pliable. Soft, spongy muscle or hard, dense muscle indicates connective tissue dysfunction. Muscle atrophy makes the muscle feel smaller than normal. Hypertrophy makes the muscle feel larger than normal. Application of the appropriate techniques can normalize the connective tissue component of the muscle. Excessively strong or weak muscles can be caused by problems with neuromuscular control or imbalanced work or exercise demand. Weak muscle can be a result of wasting (atrophy) of the muscle fibers.

It is amazing what sorts itself out during a thorough generalized massage when the entire body is addressed. Do not discount the effectiveness of this type of massage when skeletal muscle imbalances are detected.

Spot work on isolated areas is seldom effective. Muscle imbalances are linked by reflex patterns, most notably the gait reflexes and the interaction between postural and phasic muscles.

Tendons

Tendons should feel elastic and mobile. If a tendon has been torn, it may adhere to the underlying bone during the healing process. Some tendons such as the tendons of the fingers and toes are enclosed in a sheath and must be able to glide within the sheath. If they cannot glide, inflammation builds, and the result is tendinitis. Overuse also can cause inflammation. Inflammation signals the formation of connective tissue, which can interfere with movement and cause the tendons to adhere to surrounding tissue. Frictioning techniques help these conditions.

An important area is the musculotendinous junction, where the nerve usually enters the muscle. As was pointed out earlier, motor points cause a muscle contraction with a small stimulus, somewhat like a pilot light for a gas stove. Disruption of sensory signals at the motor point causes many problems, including trigger points and referred pain (Chapter 11), hypersensitive acupressure points (Chapter 11), and restrictive movement patterns caused by the increase in the physiologic barrier and development of pathologic barriers.

The condition that develops depends on the person's heredity, activity level, and general health. It would be nice to give suggestions on how to proceed, but in this case, careful assessment of the entire pattern, use of clinical reasoning and problem-solving skills, and good general massage that addresses all tissue components are the best recommendations.

Fascial Sheaths

Fascial sheaths should be pliable, but because they are stabilizers they may be more dense than tendons in some areas. Problems arise if the tissues these sheaths separate or stabilize become stuck to the sheath.

Myofascial and craniosacral approaches are best suited to dealing with the fascial sheaths. This type of bodywork is not usually included in basic massage training, but an introduction to the methods is provided in Chapter 11.

Mechanical work, such as slow, sustained stretching, and methods that pull and drag on the tissue are used to soften the sheaths. Because it often is uncomfortable, the work should not be done unless the client is committed to regular appointments until the area is normalized. This may take 6 months to 1 year.

Chronic health conditions almost always show dysfunction with the connective tissue and fascial sheaths. Any techniques discussed as connective tissue approaches are effective as long as the practitioner proceeds slowly and follows the tissue pattern. The massage therapist should not override the tissue or force the tissue into a corrective pattern. Instead, the tissue must be untangled or unwound gradually.

Fascial separations between muscles create pathways for the nerves and blood vessels. When palpated, these pathways feel like grooves running between muscles. If these areas become narrow or restricted, blood vessels may be constricted and nerves impinged. A slow, specific, stripping effleurage along these pathways can be beneficial. The nerves run in these fascial pathways, and the nerve trunks correlate with the traditional meridian system. Therefore most meridian and acupressure work takes place along these fascial grooves.

Water is an important element of connective tissue. To keep connective tissue soft, the client must rehydrate the body by drinking a minimum of eight 8-ounce glasses of clean, pure water daily, as recommend by nutritionists and physicians.

Highly developed assessment and palpation skills are a must for working with connective tissue dysfunction specifically. General massage methods that are applied slowly and gently to pull the tissue are the best recommendations until more specific training is obtained.

When an emotional component is involved in the client's physical pattern, that component often surfaces while the practitioner is dealing specifically with the connective tissues. It seems that emotional chemicals and residue from trauma, addictions, and toxicity are stored in this tissue. Because of this, the effects of connective tissue work can influence emotional states. Mental health support often is indicated. In these situations refer, but do not attempt to intervene.

Ligaments, Joints, and Bones

Moving the joints through comfortable ranges of motion can be used as an evaluation method. Comparison of the symmetry of range motion (e.g., comparing the circumduction pattern of one arm against the other) is effective in detecting limitations of a particular movement.

Muscle energy methods, as well as all massage manipulations, can be used to support symmetric range-of-motion functions.

Dealing specifically with ligaments, joints, and bone is out of the scope of practice of basic massage therapy as presented in this text. With additional education, such as that found in Ontario, British Columbia, and other advanced-level therapeutic massage training programs, a massage practitioner can learn applications that are beneficial for ligaments, joints, and bones.

All these tissues and structures are supported by general massage applications that effect increased circulation, unrestricted soft tissue, and normalized neuromuscular patterns.

Massage can positively affect the normal limits of the physiologic barrier. When joints are traumatized, the surrounding tissue becomes "scared," almost as if saying, "This joint will never get in that position again." When this happens, all the proprioceptive mechanisms reset to limit the range of motion. Massage and appropriate muscle lengthening and general stretching, combined with muscle energy techniques and self-help, can affect ligaments, joint function, and bone health.

These tissues are relatively slow to regenerate, and it takes time to notice prolonged improvement.

Abdomen

Refer the client to a physician if any hard, rigid, stiff, or tense areas are noted in the abdomen. Close attention must be paid to the visceral referred pain areas (see Chapter 5, p. 202). If tissue changes are noted, the practitioner must refer the client to a physician.

The skin often is tighter in areas of visceral referred pain. As a result of cutaneous/visceral reflexes, benefit may be obtained by stretching the skin in these areas. There is some indication that normalizing the skin over these areas has a positive effect on the functioning of the organ. If nothing else, circulation is increased and peristalsis (intestinal movement) may be stimulated.

In accordance with the recommendations for colon massage (see Chapter 9, p. 335), repetitive stroking in the proper directions may stimulate smooth muscle contraction and can improve elimination problems and intestinal gas. An understanding practitioner is prepared for the results and will point the way to the restroom.

Body Rhythms

The body rhythms are assessed before and after the massage. An improvement in stability, rate, and evenness should be noticed after the massage. Massage offered by a centered practitioner with a focused, rhythmic intent provides patterns for the client's body to use to entrain its own rhythms. The massage practitioner must remain focused on the natural rhythm of the client. Although the entrainment pattern of the practitioner and the massage provides a pattern for the client, it should not superimpose an unnatural rhythm on the client. Any foreign patterns ultimately will be rejected by the client's body. Instead, the practitioner should support the client in reestablishing her innate entrainment rhythm. Supported by rocking methods and a rhythmic approach to the massage, the body can reestablish synchronized rhythmic function.

Breathing. Improved breathing function helps the entire body. The muscular mechanism for inhalation and exhalation of air is designed like a simple bellows system and depends on unrestricted movement of the musculoskeletal components of the thorax. The muscles of respiration include the scalenes, intercostals, anterior serratus, diaphragm, abdominals, and pelvic floor muscles. If hyperventilation syndrome (Chapter 4, p. 167) is a factor and the person is prone to anxiety, intervention softens and normalizes the upper body and breathing mechanism.

Because of the whole-body interplay between muscle groups in all actions, it is not uncommon to find tight lower leg and foot muscles interfering with breathing. By contracting the lower legs and feet and taking a deep breath, a person can discover for himself that breathing is a whole-body function.

Disruption of function in any of these muscle groups inhibits full and easy breathing. For additional breathing information, see Chapter 13.

General relaxation massage and stress reduction methods seem to help breathing the most. The client can be taught slow lengthening and stretching methods and the breathing retraining pattern found in Chapter 13. The client also can be advised not to wear restrictive clothing or hold in the stomach.

Muscular Imbalance

Muscle imbalance, discovered through muscle testing procedures, often indicates how the body is compensating for postural imbalances. Muscle testing also can locate the main muscle problems. When the primary dysfunctional group of muscles is tested, the main compensatory patterns are activated, and the other body compensation patterns activate and exaggerate. The massage professional must become a detective, looking for clues to unwind the pattern. By concentrating on methods that restore symmetry of function, the practitioner helps the client's body work out the details.

A major muscle problem is overly tense muscles. If these muscles can be relaxed, lengthened, and, if necessary, stretched, the rest of the dysfunctional pattern often resolves.

If the extensors and abductors are stronger than the flexors and adductors, major postural imbalance and postural distortion result. Similarly, if the extensors and abductors are too weak to balance the other movement patterns, the body curls into itself, and nothing works properly.

If gait patterns are inefficient, more energy is required for movement, and fatigue and pain can result.

Shortened postural muscles must be lengthened and

then stretched. This takes time and uses all the massage practitioner's technical skills. Because of the fiber configuration of the muscle tissue (red or white twitch fibers), techniques must be sufficiently intense and must be applied long enough to allow the muscle to respond.

Shortened and weak phasic muscles must first be lengthened and stretched. Eventually, strengthening techniques and exercises will be needed.

If the hypertense phasic muscle pattern is caused by repetitive use, the muscles can be normalized with muscle energy techniques and then lengthened. Overly tense muscles often increase in size (hypertrophy). The client must reduce the activity of that muscle group until balance is restored, which usually takes about 4 weeks. Muscle tissue that has undergone hypertrophy begins to return to normal if it is not used for the activity during that time. Athletes often display this pattern and very likely will resist complete inactivity. A reduced activity level and a more balanced exercise program, combined with flexibility training, can be beneficial for them. Refer these individuals to appropriate training and coaching professionals if indicated.

Compensation Patterns

Years of clinical experience have taught many therapists that most symptoms and dysfunctional patterns are compensatory patterns. Some problems are recent, and some qualify for archaeologic exploration, having developed in early life and having been compounded through time.

Compensatory patterns often are complex, but the client's body frequently can show us the way if we can listen to the story it tells.

The importance of compensation must be considered. There are many instances of **resourceful compensation,** a term used for the adjustments the body makes to manage a permanent or chronic dysfunction. Protective muscle spasm around a compressed disk is an example. The splinting action of the spasms protects the nerves and provides additional stability in the area.

Decisions must be made regarding how and to what degree the compensatory pattern should be altered. It seems prudent to assume the body knows what it is doing. The wise therapist spends time coming to understand the reasons for the compensatory patterns presented by the body.

When resourceful compensation is present, therapeutic massage methods are used to support the altered pattern and prevent any more increase in postural distortion than is necessary to support the body change (compensation).

Some compensatory patterns are also set up for short-term situations that do not require permanent adaptation. Having a leg in a cast and walking on crutches for a period of time is a classic example. The body catching itself during an "almost" fall is another classic set-up pattern. Unfortunately, the body often habituates these patterns and maintains them well beyond their usefulness. Over

time the body begins to show symptoms of pain, inefficient function, or both.

Many compensatory patterns develop to maintain a balanced posture, and even though the posture becomes distorted during compensation, the overall result is a balanced body in a gravitational line. It also is important to consider the pattern of muscle interactions, such as the ones that occur when walking, and to recognize that gait has a certain pattern for the most efficient movement that the body can manage.

Whenever a pattern of tight muscles exists, a pattern of weak muscles also is present. These imbalances are inefficient, use excessive energy, and contribute to fatigue and pain in the client.

Inefficient compensatory patterns often are set up by an unexpected fall or "almost" fall, car accident, or other trauma. They are activated in response to some sort of disruption in balance against gravity, repetitive activity, or learned behavior such as "pull in that stomach" or "sit still." There is no set system for figuring out the compensatory patterns. All these factors must be considered in a plan that best serves the client.

Dysfunction as a Solution

No education on assessment is complete without a discussion of whether the pattern discovered is a problem or a solution. The previous section defined resourceful compensation as the best that can be expected under the circumstances. The concept of dysfunction as a solution is similar to the patterns of resourceful compensation. If all the information gathered during assessment can be viewed as *an attempt at a solution,* a broader perspective in the decision making required for effective massage care plans is created. As discussed in Chapter 5, it is important to consider the client's whole situation in determining whether a condition is a dysfunction or solution:

- A workaholic client has continual tension headaches. When the client has a headache, she tends to slow her pace and work fewer hours. Is the headache a problem or a solution?
- A massage therapist who regularly provides massage sessions for 30 to 40 clients a week develops a low back condition that prevents her from working with more that 10 clients a week. Management of the low back condition requires the massage professional to receive regular massage, exercise regularly, and manage stress. She has to cut her workload, which opens time for teaching and community service. Is the low back dysfunction a problem or a solution?

Understanding the bigger picture when analyzing assessment information adds a very important dimension for the development of essential and appropriate massage care plans. If you can view each pattern as a solution and realize that problems are solutions that no longer provide benefit, a respect for the adaptable human being evolves. Solutions are to be supported. Problems must be understood and other possibilities offered for solution. Massage effectively provides both for the body.

CLINICAL REASONING AND PROBLEM SOLVING TO CREATE MASSAGE CARE/TREATMENT PLANS

section objective

Using the information presented in this section, the student will be able to perform the following:

■ **Use the clinical reasoning model as a decision-making tool in the development of massage care/treatment plans**

Specific protocols or recipes for therapeutic intervention seldom work without modification because each person is different. Protocols provide a model of how to begin a therapeutic process, but the massage professional must modify applications of methods based on the client's individual needs and circumstances. The ability to process information effectively in the development of a therapeutic plan is based on a clinical reasoning approach rather than protocols.

The ability to apply what is learned comes from a reasoning/problem-solving process. Effective work with clients becomes a continual learning process of assessment, determining intervention procedures, analysis of their effectiveness by a postassessment process, and recognition of progress made from session to session. Even in the most basic sessions with a client, when the goals are pleasure and relaxation, decisions must be made about the best way to encourage the body to respond to meet the particular client's goals.

After a history has been completed and an assessment done, the information gathered is analyzed and interpreted. The next step is to make decisions about what to do and how to develop the process into a coordinated, effective plan for achieving the client's goals. This information was first presented in Chapter 3; now we put it all together.

Effective assessment, analysis, and decision making are essential to meet the needs of each individual client. Routines or recipe-type applications of soft tissue and movement methods often are limited and ineffective in attempts to individualize sessions for clients because each person has a different set of presenting circumstances and outcome goals. The mark of an experienced professional is the ability to use clinical reasoning effectively.

As noted in Chapter 3, sessions with massage professionals are goal oriented. Goals describe desired outcomes. A primary reason for developing treatment/care plans is to set achievable goals and outline a general plan for reaching them. It is important to develop measurable, activity-based (functional) goals that are meaningful to the client. Goals must be *quantifiable* and *qualifiable*.

The database developed in history taking and assessment procedures, combined with any heath care treatment orders from other professionals, provides the foundation for clinical reasoning and decision making. Decisions are based on an analysis of the database information. The analysis process has been presented in many ways throughout this text. Again, the steps in the analysis process are as follows:

1. Review the facts and information collected.
   Questions that can help with this process are the following:
   • What are the facts?
   • What is considered normal or balanced function?
   • What has happened? *(spell out events)*
   • What caused the imbalance? *(can it be identified?)*
   • What was done or is being done?
   • What has worked or not worked?
2. Brainstorm the possibilities.
   Questions that can help with this process are the following:
   • What are the possibilities? *(what could it all mean?)*
   • What is my intuition suggesting?
   • What are the possible patterns of dysfunction?
   • What are the possible contributing factors?
   • What are possible interventions?
   • What might work?
   • What are other ways to look at the situation?
   • What do the data suggest?
3. Consider the logical outcome of each possibility.
   Questions that can help with this process are the following:
   • What is the logical progression of the symptom pattern, contributing factors, and current behaviors?
   • What is the logical cause and effect of each intervention identified?
   • What are the pros and cons of each intervention suggested? *(remember to look at both sides of the issue)*
   • What are the consequences of not acting?
   • What are the consequences of acting?
4. Consider how people would be affected by each possibility.
   Questions that can help with this process are the following:
   • In terms of each intervention being considered, what is the impact on the people involved: client, practitioner, and other professionals working with the client?
   • How does each person involved feel about the possible interventions?
   • Is the practitioner within his/her scope of practice to work with such situations?

- Is the practitioner qualified to work with such situations?
- Does the practitioner feel qualified to work with such situations?
- Is there a feeling of cooperation and agreement between all parties involved?

Care or Treatment Plan

The development of a care or treatment plan is based on the four-part analysis of the information. After the analysis has been completed, the practitioner can make a decision about what will be involved in the care or treatment plan. Methods are chosen to achieve the agreed goals for the session. The plan is not an exact protocol set in stone, but rather a guideline. The care/treatment plan may evolve over the first three or four sessions and be altered if a change occurs in the therapeutic goals or the client's status.

Decision making becomes a part of each session. As the care/treatment plan unfolds with each successive session, an update on effects, progress, and setbacks is discussed with the client before beginning the massage. An updated assessment is done, and clinical reasoning and problem solving are used to choose the most effective methods for achieving the best results for the current session. As the

plan is implemented, it is recorded sequentially, session by session, in some form of charting process (e.g., SOAP notes [Chapter 3]).

An analysis of the effectiveness (or lack of effectiveness) of intervention procedures is compared with previous sessions. Review of the charting notes from previous sessions becomes the foundation for this analysis. The plan is refined, reevaluated, and adjusted as necessary as the sessions progress (Proficiency Exercise 10-6).

Reassessment

During the massage, assessment and intervention intermingle. Unless one watches carefully, it is difficult to distinguish assessment from intervention. For the experienced massage professional, assessment and intervention dance with each other in the context of the massage session. An area of imbalance is discovered through various methods of palpation and passive and active range of motion. Assessment leads into intervention—often simply by gently increasing the intensity or duration of the original evaluation method and repeating the methods three or four times.

After the massage is complete, it is a good idea to do a quick reassessment to see what changes the body has made. This can be done quickly by targeting a few major

Text continued on p. 444.

10-6

PROFICIENCY EXERCISE

The following case studies will help the student begin to make decisions about what the information gathered during assessment procedures might mean and how to make decisions on ways to achieve the client's goals. Remember, decision making is always a process. There are no right answers for this activity; effective applications are those that benefit the client.

This decision-making process should feel familiar by now. It was first introduced in Chapter 2 to help the student learn ethical decision making, and it is a thread that winds throughout the text. The same process is used to make intervention decisions on ways to proceed with the application of the best approach for a massage session.

Case Study #1

A 54-year-old man seeks massage to deal with a nagging catch in his low back. No medical reason for the problem has been identified, and the physician indicated age, an old injury, and flat feet as the probable culprits. The client

was fitted with orthopedic shoes, and massage was suggested as an adjunct strategy.

The client's history revealed that the problem has been increasing over the past 2 years. The client played many high school and college sports, particularly football, and had many injuries that he did not allow to heal before playing again. He was an Air Force jet pilot for many years, which required long periods of sitting in confined areas and body positioning to accommodate for the gravitational forces of aerial combat maneuvers.

The client's current profession requires long hours of sitting and being attentive to people. Because of a change in physical activity, he gained 40 pounds over the past 4 years, and he has practically eliminated any physical exercise program. However, in the past 6 months he has lost the weight and begun exercising regularly.

The client had broken his foot 6 years ago, and 4 years ago had it rebroken and pinned to correct difficulties with the original healing process.

He has been under increased emotional stress for both professional and personal reasons. His sleep has been disrupted off and on for the past 2 years.

10-6

PROFICIENCY EXERCISE—CONT'D

The client manifests symptoms of adult attention deficit disorder but chooses not to use medication to treat it.

He has no other health concerns. His last physical examination indicated normal functioning.

During the interview the client poked at his low back on the right, pulled at his neck, moved his left shoulder around, and pointed to the glenohumeral joint numerous times.

Physical assessment indicated the following:

- The head is held in a forward position, with the chin elevated and the posterior neck area shortened.
- The shoulders are rolled forward, more so on the left.
- A slight lordosis is present.
- The most notable deviation is flat feet and a rolling to the outside of the heel of the foot, more so on the left.

Gait assessment indicated reduced arm and leg movement on the left side. The entire right side of the body seemed to lunge forward during walking. It also revealed the following:

- The sacroiliac joint was more fixed on the right side.
- The weight is carried mostly on the heels and to the outside of the foot.
- The shoes indicate an uneven wear pattern.

Palpation indicated areas of cold on the back of the neck and a thickened skin texture, as well as the following:

- The right lumbar area was warmer than surrounding tissue, with a damp area and exaggerated reddening just below the last rib.
- Superficial connective tissue all seemed tight, and it was difficult to lift the skin in any area.
- The muscle mass in the legs seemed overdeveloped in relation to the muscle mass of the upper body.
- The left shoulder had restricted range of motion and a hard end-feel in all directions.
- The left foot and ankle were restricted and had limited range of motion compared with the right foot and ankle.
- The breath was even but seemed out of sync with the rest of the rhythms.

Muscle testing indicated bodywide imbalance in adduction/abduction patterns, with adductors very tense and abductors weak and shortened.

The client seemed edgy and spoke rapidly. He seemed impatient with the pain in his back. He kept saying that he was too busy to deal with this and he wished he could ignore it.

Using this information, complete the clinical reasoning process and develop a series of massage interventions and referrals to help this client. It can be helpful to puzzle through the information individually and then work together in groups to compare analysis processes and decisions.

1. Review the facts and information collected.
   Questions that can help with this process are the following:
   - What are the facts?

   - What is considered normal or balanced function?

   - What has happened? *(spell out events)*

   - What caused the imbalance? *(can it be identified?)*

   - What was done or is being done?

Continued.

10-6
PROFICIENCY EXERCISE—CONT'D

- What has worked or not worked?

- What might work?

2. Brainstorm the possibilities.
   Questions that can help with this process are the following:
   - What are the possibilities? *(what could it all mean?)*

- What are other ways to look at the situation?

- What do the data suggest?

- What is my intuition suggesting?

3. Consider the logical outcome of each possibility.
   Questions that can help with this process are the following:
   - What is the logical progression of the symptom pattern, contributing factors, and current behaviors?

- What are the possible patterns of dysfunction?

- What are the possible contributing factors?

- What is the logical cause and effect of each intervention identified?

- What are possible interventions?

- What are the pros and cons of each intervention suggested? *(remember to look at both sides of the issue)*

PROFICIENCY EXERCISE—CONT'D

- What are the consequences of not acting?

- What are the consequences of acting?

4. Consider how people would be affected by each possibility.
   Questions that can help with this process are the following:
   - In terms of each intervention being considered, what is the impact on the people involved: client, practitioner, and other professionals working with the client?

- How does each person involved feel about the possible interventions?

- Is the practitioner within his/her scope of practice to work with such situations?

- Is the practitioner qualified to work with such situations?

- Does the practitioner feel qualified to work with such situations?

- Is there a feeling of cooperation and agreement between all parties involved?

Based on the analysis, answer the following questions:

1. Does the client need referral, and if so, to which professionals?

2. What are the measurable function goals for the care/treatment plan?

Continued.

10-6

PROFICIENCY EXERCISE—CONT'D

3. What interventions would you choose to achieve those goals?

4. How would you use them to address the various imbalances?

5. What results do you expect?

6. How long do you think it will take to achieve the goals?

Case Study #2

The client, a 16-year-old young woman, displays atypical seizure patterns daily, but neurologic tests do not indicate an abnormality. The neurologist referred the patient to a mental health professional, suggesting stress as the causal factor. Physiologic evaluation indicates several emotional stressors, including the life-threatening illness of a family member, the recent relocation of a special friend, relationship problems, learning difficulties, and a tendency toward obsessive-compulsive behavior. Hyperventilation syndrome is evident. Self-esteem is low.

In the past 2 years the client has had two car accidents. The client is taking several medications to try to control the seizure activity. Her diet is low in vitamins and minerals, and medications and counseling have had minimal benefit. A mental health professional referred the client for massage as part of the comprehensive treatment plan monitored by the neurologist.

The physical assessment indicated restricted breathing with primarily an upper-chest pattern, shortened muscles, and an elevated scapula on the left, with trigger points that generate the suspected seizure activity when palpated. No other obvious indications are evident with physical or gait assessment.

The client seems cooperative during assessment procedures, but distant and distracted. The client's mother was supportive but overwhelmed. Both seem somewhat desperate for an answer to what was happening.

Using this information, complete the clinical reasoning process and develop a series of massage interventions and referrals to help this client. It can be *helpful to puzzle through the information individually and then work together in groups to compare analysis processes and decisions.*

1. Review the facts and information collected.
   Questions that can help with this process are the following:
   • What are the facts?

   • What is considered normal or balanced function?

   • What has happened? *(spell out events)*

   • What caused the imbalance? *(can it be identified?)*

   • What was done or is being done?

   • What has worked or not worked?

2. Brainstorm the possibilities.
   Questions that can help with this process are the following:
   • What are the possibilities? *(what could it all mean?)*

   • What is my intuition suggesting?

   • What are the possible patterns of dysfunction?

- What are the possible contributing factors?

- What are possible interventions?

- What might work?

- What are other ways to look at the situation?

- What do the data suggest?

3. Consider the logical outcome of each possibility.
   Questions that can help with this process are the following:
   - What is the logical progression of the symptom pattern, contributing factors, and current behaviors?

- What is the logical cause and effect of each intervention identified?

- What are the pros and cons of each intervention suggested? *(remember to look at both sides of the issue)*

- What are the consequences of not acting?

- What are the consequences of acting?

4. Consider how people would be affected by each possibility.
   Questions that can help with this process are the following:
   - In terms of each intervention being considered, what is the impact on the people involved: client, practitioner, and other professionals working with the client?

Continued.

PROFICIENCY EXERCISE—CONT'D

- How does each person involved feel about the possible interventions?

- Is the practitioner within his/her scope of practice to work with such situations?

- Is the practitioner qualified to work with such situations?

- Does the practitioner feel qualified to work with such situations?

- Is there a feeling of cooperation and agreement between all parties involved?

Based on the analysis, answer the following questions:

1. Does the client need referral, and if so, to which professionals?

2. What are the measurable function goals for the care/treatment plan?

3. What interventions would you choose to achieve those goals?

4. How would you use them to address the various imbalances?

5. What results do you expect?

6. How long do you think it will take to achieve the goals?

10-6

PROFICIENCY EXERCISE—CONT'D

Case Study #3

The client is a 40-year-old woman. Today is her birthday, and she received a gift certificate for a massage from her daughter. Her history does not indicate any contraindications. The client has no particular goals for the session and is not sure whether she will have any other massage sessions. The physical assessment does not reveal any major deviations of symmetry.

Using this information, complete the clinical reasoning process and develop a series of massage interventions and referrals to help this client. It can be helpful to puzzle through the information individually and then work together in groups to compare analysis processes and decisions.

1. Review the facts and information collected.
   Questions that can help with this process are the following:
   • What are the facts?

   • What is considered normal or balanced function?

   • What has happened? *(spell out events)*

   • What caused the imbalance? *(can it be identified?)*

• What was done or is being done?

• What has worked or not worked?

2. Brainstorm the possibilities.
   Questions that can help with this process are the following:

   • What are the possibilities? *(what could it all mean?)*

   • What is my intuition suggesting?

   • What are the possible patterns of dysfunction?

PROFICIENCY EXERCISE—CONT'D

- What are the possible contributing factors?

- What are possible interventions?

- What might work?

- What are other ways to look at the situation?

- What do the data suggest?

3. Consider the logical outcome of each possibility.
   Questions that can help with this process are the following:
   - What is the logical progression of the symptom pattern, contributing factors, and current behaviors?

- What is the logical cause and effect of each intervention identified?

- What are the pros and cons of each intervention suggested? *(remember to look at both sides of the issue)*

- What are the consequences of not acting?

- What are the consequences of acting?

4. Consider how people would be affected by each possibility.
   Questions that can help with this process are the following:
   - In terms of each intervention being considered, what is the impact on the people involved: client, practitioner, and other professionals working with the client?

PROFICIENCY EXERCISE—CONT'D

- How does each person involved feel about the possible interventions?

- Is the practitioner within his/her scope of practice to work with such situations?

- Is the practitioner qualified to work with such situations?

- Does the practitioner feel qualified to work with such situations?

- Is there a feeling of cooperation and agreement between all parties involved?

Based on the analysis, answer the following questions:

1. Does the client need referral, and if so, to which professionals?

2. What are the measurable function goals for the care/treatment plan?

3. What interventions would you choose to achieve those goals?

4. How would you use them to address the various imbalances?

5. What results do you expect?

6. How long do you think it will take to achieve the goals?

areas that were the core focus of the massage. The reassessment process helps the client integrate the body changes. The before-and-after awareness also is a reinforcing factor for the client regarding the benefits of massage.

The entire process of massage is an assessment, an intervention for adaptation, and then a reassessment to see whether the approach was beneficial. This takes practice. During the learning process, assessment and reassessment can feel choppy. The skilled massage professional learns through practice to flow between the three steps of assessment, intervention/adaptation, and reassessment during the massage, providing a sense of continuity and fluidity to the session (Proficiency Exercise 10-7).

SUMMARY

Massage is a whole-body discipline. Assessment skills are the basis for developing intuition through learning to pay closer attention and becoming more skilled in the interpretation of the assessment information. With practice and experience, these skills become almost second nature.

A trained massage professional modifies intensity and method to best address the client's needs. The professional does not perform massage "routines." Massage methods are simple, but when they are applied with the right intensity and in the right location, the body recognizes the stimulation and can respond resourcefully. This learning is continuous; the client never stops teaching the therapist.

The more reliable the assessment information, the more likely the interpretation of it will be accurate. The more accurate the interpretation, the more specific the application of massage methods. Massage and bodywork techniques are relatively basic. Soft tissue can be pushed, pulled, shaken, stretched, and pounded, regardless of the bodywork system. The only variables are the location of the application, intensity, and duration. The detective work and skills required to assist the client in figuring out each individual pattern prevents massage from becoming boring.

After completing 1000 massage sessions, the massage professional begins to own the information learned in school. After 5000 massage sessions, the massage professional has enough experience to begin to trust the process of massage. After 10,000 massages, the massage therapist allows the massage to happen. A master of massage has

learned to respect the client and follow the client's lead. This takes years of practice.

The bottom line is that the client knows his or her body best. It is the practitioner's job to understand what the client says verbally, visually, through body language, and in the tissues and movement patterns. Each person's body language is unique. It takes time to learn it. Only through listening, observing, and touching and then using effective clinical reasoning skills do the patterns begin to emerge, allowing solutions to be found for the individual.

The therapist should not hesitate to ask for help and should refer a client when the problem is beyond the professional skills determined by the scope of practice for massage therapy. By joining in the team approach with other health professionals, the massage practitioner can help massage, in some form, become an important part of the client's treatment.

Practice enables the massage professional's skills to grow. The student will be surprised at how perceptive and sensitive the body actually is once we learn to pay attention.

Robert Fulghum tells a story about hiccups that epitomizes massage[2]:

The reason most cures work, at some time on some people, is that hiccups usually last from between seven and 63 hicks before stopping of their own accord. Whatever you do to pass the time while the episode runs its course seems to qualify as a cure, so the more entertaining the cure is, the better . . . The hiccuper will be treated with great solicitation while in the throes of these miniconvulsions, and the shaman who has come up with the winning cure will be looked upon with respect.

Applications of therapeutic massage certainly are "entertaining" for the body, and conditions often do improve with therapeutic massage.

When massage intervention allows more efficient functioning for the client, the massage professional must be mindful that he or she is not a "shaman"; rather, the professional should focus on educating the client about the body's responses so that the client begins to experience personal empowerment and recognizes the body's own healing potential. We also must learn not to judge ourselves according to the "success" of the client's outcome. Instead, continual analysis of our own professional growth provides more accurate information for self-assessment.

10-7

PROFICIENCY EXERCISE

Design and conduct five massage sessions, following the assessment guidelines in this chapter.

REFERENCES

1. Chaitow L: *Soft tissue manipulation,* Rochester, Vt, 1988, Healing Arts Press.
2. Fulghum R: *Uh-oh,* New York, 1991, Villard Books.
3. Greenman PE: *Principles of manual medicine,* ed 2, Baltimore, 1996, Williams & Wilkins.
4. Norkin CC, Levangie PK: *Joint structure and function: a comprehensive analysis,* ed 2, Philadelphia, 1992, FA Davis.
5. Smith LK, Weiss E, Lehmkuhl L: *Brunnstrom's clinical kinesiology,* ed 5, Philadelphia, 1996, FA Davis.

WORKBOOK SECTION

Short Answer

1. What is an assessment?

2. Why does the massage practitioner perform an assessment?

3. What or who is the most important source of information during the assessment process?

4. What is rapport?

5. What is considered when observing the general presence of the client?

6. What information can be gathered by watching a person's gestures?

7. What is the importance of patterns?

8. What is the importance of open-ended questions?

9. Why is it important to repeat what the client has told you?

10. What interferes with the ability to listen?

11. What are the three factors that influence posture, and which one is easiest to affect?

12. What is the essence of mechanical balance?

WORKBOOK SECTION

13. What is required to stand?

_____

_____

_____

_____

14. What is the "screw home" mechanism of the knee?

_____

_____

_____

_____

15. What is the position of the client during assessment of the standing position?

_____

_____

_____

_____

16. What is the importance of bony landmarks in the assessment process?

_____

_____

_____

_____

17. Why assess for efficient gait patterns?

_____

_____

_____

18. What is the importance of the sacroiliac joint during walking?

_____

_____

_____

19. What are the two main factors to look for during the assessment of gait?

_____

_____

_____

_____

20. What are the most common reasons for dysfunctional walking patterns?

_____

_____

_____

_____

21. Why is full-body massage beneficial for efficient gait patterns?

_____

_____

_____

_____

22. What is palpation?

_____

_____

_____

_____

23. Why is the hand such an effective assessment tool?

_____

_____

_____

_____

24. Are palpation skills limited to the hand?

_____

_____

_____

_____

WORKBOOK SECTION

25. Why is it important to trust first impressions during palpation?

_____

_____

_____

_____

26. Why can we feel something that does not touch us?

_____

_____

_____

27. What is intuition?

_____

_____

_____

_____

28. What type of information is gathered with near touch, or palpation that does not actually touch the body?

_____

_____

_____

_____

29. What types of things are noticed when palpating the skin?

_____

_____

_____

_____

30. What does the superficial connective tissue layer feel like?

_____

_____

_____

_____

31. Where are the superficial blood and lymph vessels located?

_____

_____

_____

_____

32. Why refer clients with enlarged lymph nodes to a physician?

_____

_____

_____

_____

33. How can you tell if you are feeling skeletal muscle?

_____

_____

_____

_____

34. What is the importance of the musculotendinous junction?

_____

_____

_____

_____

35. Do tendons attach only to bone?

_____

_____

_____

_____

36. What is the function of fascial sheaths?

_____

_____

_____

_____

WORKBOOK SECTION

37. Why is it important for the massage therapist to be able to palpate and recognize a ligament?

_____

_____

_____

_____

38. What is joint end-feel?

_____

_____

_____

_____

39. What should a joint feel like?

_____

_____

_____

40. What is the basic configuration of muscles around a joint?

_____

_____

_____

_____

41. What would pull the alignment of a joint out of its anatomic position?

_____

_____

_____

_____

42. Why is it important to differentiate between joint and soft tissue dysfunction?

_____

_____

_____

_____

43. Explain why you palpate bone.

_____

_____

_____

_____

44. What are the important things to look for when palpating the abdomen?

_____

_____

_____

_____

45. What are body rhythms?

_____

_____

_____

_____

46. What are the three basic types of muscle testing?

_____

_____

_____

_____

47. What is the difference between strength testing and neurologic muscle testing?

_____

_____

_____

_____

48. When evaluating muscles both for strength and neurologic function, what is the importance of the pattern?

_____

_____

_____

_____

WORKBOOK SECTION

49. What are the two basic types of muscles?

_____
_____
_____
_____

50. Typically, how do muscle imbalances set up patterns?

_____
_____
_____
_____

51. When is the information from the assessment interpreted?

_____
_____
_____
_____

52. What are some key elements in designing a massage?

_____
_____
_____
_____

53. What is the purpose of the design of the massage?

_____
_____
_____
_____

54. How does the massage therapist decide which method to use?

_____
_____
_____
_____

55. What is the importance of reassessment?

_____
_____
_____
_____

56. How does the quote from Robert Fulghum on p. 444 pertain to massage?

_____
_____
_____
_____

Additional Activity

Doing the paperwork

The following is a simulation of a massage session from initial interview to completion of the massage. Read the information given and then follow the instructions.

Sue Williams, a 37-year-old client, is coming in for her first massage with you. She had received bodywork previously while a member of a health spa. She indicates that the massages were light and relaxing. At work she is a middle-management supervisor for a local manufacturing company. Her job requires time on the phone and many hours of meetings. The company is in the process of downsizing. She has been experiencing tingling in her arms and headaches (usually a 6 to 8 on a 1 to 10 pain scale), mainly at the back of her head. You notice that she squeezes the occipital area and pulls her hair in that location as she explains the headache. She has had some shortness of breath and lately has not been sleeping well. She has had a full physical checkup in which nothing was found. Her physician indicated that she was stressed and needed to find some ways to relax. Massage and exercise were given as options. She is in a long-term relationship and has two children, a 16-year-old and a 9-year-old. She was in a car accident 4 years ago and suffered minor head trauma and whiplash. She broke her left ankle while cheerleading in high school and tends to walk on the outside of that foot.

You notice that she also tends to roll her shoulders while breathing and that she sighs a lot. During the physical assessment you find that she swings her left leg far-

WORKBOOK SECTION

ther than the right leg when walking and that her right shoulder is high. She definitely is using shoulder muscles when she breathes. Her head is tilted toward her right shoulder. She has a very mild kyphosis and is pulled forward in the chest area, more so on the right, so that a rotation is present at the thoracolumbar junction. There is limited movement in her right scapula and the right side of her rib cage. Palpation and muscle testing reveal that the upper thorax is tight and restricted. Her lower leg muscles are tight, and her abdominals are weak.

You give a general massage using muscle energy methods to lengthen the shoulders, lower legs, and upper posterior neck. You explain to Sue that there is some connective tissue shortening in the upper chest, low back, and posterior neck areas. You teach her lengthening exercises for the shoulders and lower leg. You also suggest weekly massage sessions for about 6 weeks and then a reevaluation.

Sue agrees and says after the session that her headache is better but not entirely gone, and she thinks she can breathe better. Overall she feels more relaxed and wants to go home and take a nap.

After Sue leaves, you review her chart and wonder about the pattern between the broken ankle, the whiplash, and the tight lower legs, shoulders, chest, and neck. You also wonder whether her wearing high heels may have something to do with the pattern, as well as excessive sitting in meetings and talking on the phone.

Instructions

Using this case study, complete the following Physical Assessment Form (Box 10-4). It helps if you assume the different postures as indicated in the information above and then assess yourself in a mirror. Next, complete the Care/Treatment Plan Form (Box 10-5). Finally, complete the SOAP Notes Form (Box 10-6), using only the information given. Remember that much of this information is recorded on the client history form. Record only the information relevant for SOAP notes.

Problem-Solving Exercises

1. A client is obviously tense after a traffic tie-up on the freeway. She is pacing and talking loud and fast. How would you begin the massage?

   _____

   _____

   _____

   _____

2. A client is complaining about a leg problem and showing you a spot on his knee. He keeps pointing to a particular area and drilling into the spot. What kinds of problems could be going on in that area?

   _____

   _____

   _____

   _____

3. A client has a damp area by her scapula that gets goose bumps when it is lightly touched. It also gets very red when massaged. What could be happening to cause these signs?

   _____

   _____

   _____

   _____

4. In comparing pulses in the foot, you notice that the right side is not as strong as the left side. The client says his right leg has been tingling. What should you do?

   _____

   _____

   _____

   _____

5. A factory worker has very tight trapezius and pectoralis muscles on the right side. His left hip recently has begun to ache and spasm. What might be going on?

   _____

   _____

   _____

   _____

Professional Application

You are being considered for a massage position with a chiropractor. The chiropractor wants to expand the wellness program that her office currently has and feels that massage would be a wonderful health service to offer. One of the major concerns of all the current staff members is the ability of another person to work effectively as part of

Text continued on p. 457.

WORKBOOK SECTION

box 10-4

PHYSICAL ASSESSMENT FORM

NOTE: It is helpful to stand and walk in front of a full-length mirror in a swimsuit or similar clothing while completing this form.

Client Name:_____

Date: _____

PHYSICAL

ALIGNMENT:

___ Chin in line with nose, sternal notch, navel   ___ Other _____

HEAD:

___ Tilted left   ___ Tilted right   ___ Rotated left   ___ Rotated right

EYES:

___ Level   ___ Equally set in socket   ___ Other _____

EARS:

___ Level   ___ Other _____

SHOULDERS:

___ Level   ___ Right high/Left low   ___ Left high/ Right low

___ Left rounded forward   ___ Right rounded forward   ___ Muscle development even

___ Other_____

CLAVICLES:

___ Level   ___ Other_____

ARMS:

___ Hang evenly   ___ Left rotated: ___ medial   ___ lateral   ___ Right rotated: ___ medial   ___ lateral

___ Other _____

ELBOWS:

___ Even   ___ Other _____

WRISTS:

___ Even   ___ Other_____

FINGERTIPS:

___ Even   ___ Other _____

RIBS:

___ Even   ___ Other _____

___ Springy   ___ Other _____

Continued.

WORKBOOK SECTION

box 10-4

PHYSICAL ASSESSMENT FORM—CONT'D

SCAPULA:

___ Even   ___ Other _____

___ Move freely   ___ Other_____

ABDOMEN:

___ Firm   ___ Other _____

___ Hard areas: Describe _____

WAIST:

___ Level   ___ Other _____

SPINE CURVES:

___ Normal   ___ Other _____

GLUTEAL MUSCLE MASS:

___ Even   ___ Other _____

ILAIC CREST:

___ Even   ___ Other_____

KNEES:

___ Even   ___ Other_____

PATELLA:

___ Left movable   ___ rigid

___ Right movable   ___ rigid

ANKLES:

___ Even   ___ Other _____

FEET:

___ Relaxed   ___ Other_____

ARCHES:

___ Even   ___ High   ___ Flat   ___ Other_____

TOES:

___ Straight   ___ Other_____

SKIN:

___ Moves freely   ___ Pulls   ___ Puffy   ___ Other _____

WORKBOOK SECTION

box 10-4

PHYSICAL ASSESSMENT FORM—CONT'D

SOFT TISSUE:

___ Normal   ___ Tender   ___ Restricted   ___ Flaccid   ___ Hot   ___ Cold

___ Other _____

Location(s) of Tissue Change(s): _____

FUNCTIONAL MOBILITY:

___ Normal   ___ Restricted   ___ Exaggerated   ___ Painful

___ Other _____

Location(s) of Mobility Change(s): _____

GAIT

HEAD:

___ Remains steady   ___ Other_____

TRUNK:

___ Remains vertical   ___ Other_____

SHOULDERS:

___ Remain level   ___ Other _____

ARMS:

___ Motion is opposite leg swing   ___ Motion is even left and right

___ Other _____

___ Left swings freely   ___ Right swings freely   ___ Other _____

HIPS:

___ Remain level   ___ Twist during walking   ___ Other _____

LEGS:

___ Swing freely at hip ___ Other _____

KNEES:

___ Flex and extend freely through stance and swing   ___ Other _____

FEET:

___ Heel strikes first at start of stance   ___ Plantar flexed at push-off   ___ Foot clears floor during swing phase

___ Other _____

STEP:

___ Length is even   ___ Timing is even   ___ Other _____

OVERALL:

___ Rhythmic motion ___ Other_____

WORKBOOK SECTION

box 10-5

TREATMENT PLAN FORM

Client Name:_____

Date: _____

Choose One: Original plan   Reassessment (original dated _____)

Short-Term Client Goals:

_____

_____

Long-Term Client Goals:

_____

Therapist Objectives:

_____

_____

Frequency, Length, and Duration of Visits:

_____

Progress Measurements To Be Used:

_____

Dates of Reassessment:

_____

Massage Methods To Be Used:

_____

_____

Additional Notes:

_____

_____

_____

_____

Client Signature: _____

Date: _____

Therapist Signature: _____

Date: _____

WORKBOOK SECTION

box 10-6

SOAP CHART FORM

Client Name:_____

Date: _____

S: SUBJECTIVE
Client States:

_____

_____

_____

_____

_____

O: OBJECTIVE
I Observed from Assessment Procedures:

_____

_____

_____

_____

_____

_____

What I Did This Session:

_____

_____

_____

_____

Continued.

WORKBOOK SECTION

box 10-6

SOAP CHART FORM—CONT'D

A: ANALYSIS (ASSESSMENT OF EFFECTIVENESS)
The Results: What Worked/What Didn't:

_____
_____
_____
_____
_____
_____
_____
_____

P: PLAN
Plans for Next Session, What Client Will Work On:

_____
_____
_____
_____

WORKBOOK SECTION

the team. How will assessment skills be a major influencing factor for this job?

_____

_____

_____

_____

ANSWER KEY
Short Answer

1. The collection and interpretation of information provided by the client, the massage practitioner, and referring medical professionals.
2. To decide whether the client should be referred to a medical professional and to gather information to be used in designing a massage that meets the individual's specific needs.
3. The client. If you watch and listen long enough, the client will tell you what is wrong and what needs to be done to restore balance.
4. The development of a relationship based on mutual trust and harmony. It is the responsibility of the massage professional to create an environment that supports rapport. This is done by following the client's lead.
5. Look for efficiency of movement, breathing patterns, and the general state of sympathetic or parasympathetic activation.
6. The way a person points and touches the body during conversation can give clues as to whether the problem is muscular, joint related, or visceral.
7. Nothing occurs randomly; the body is connected in all its functions. Seemingly unconnected responses, behavior, words, and sensations fit together like pieces of a puzzle.
8. They encourage the client to discuss all situations and provide more information than questions that can be answered with "Yes" or "No."
9. To confirm the information and make sure that you understood everything that was said.
10. Thinking about what you are going to say, writing something down, interpreting information, interrupting people, finishing people's sentences, sorting through many words that express a single thought, and preconceived ideas.
11. Heredity, disease, and habit. Habit is the easiest to adjust. Habitual patterns are occupational, recreational, and sleep related.

12. The gravitational line must fall through the axis of the weight-bearing joint. If it does not, extra effort is required of the muscles to maintain the upright position.
13. The various segments of the body must cooperate. Passive tension of ligaments, fascia, and the connective tissue elements of the muscles support the skeleton. Muscle plays a small part, through the activity of the postural muscles, by continually repositioning the body over the mechanical balance point. If the mechanical balance is disputed, the postural muscles struggle with this function.
14. This is the normal knee position of the femur as it rides back on the medial condyle and rotates medially about its vertical axis to lock the joint for the weight bearing used in standing. The design of the knee stabilizes the body in the standing position and makes that position less fatiguing.
15. A symmetric stance, with eyes focused forward and closed.
16. Bony landmarks provide markers for checking levelness and symmetry.
17. Walking is something that we do every day. If this pattern is inefficient, more energy is used than is necessary for the activity. This can translate into fatigue and possibly pain during walking.
18. It moves in an alternating-side figure-eight pattern. If the joint is limited in this very important function, the entire gait pattern is disrupted.
19. Watch for areas that move too much, as well as those that do not move during walking. It is important to consider the entire body when looking for these patterns because the activity of the arms provides a counterbalance to the legs.
20. Pain, muscle weakness, muscle shortening, limitation of joint movement, and changes in bone or soft tissue.
21. Walking is a full-body experience that demands many coordinated activities of the arms and legs, neck and trunk, and eyes and ears. Almost every joint, muscle, and bone is involved with every step taken. Walking is one of the most important survival activities. The body expends a lot of energy to walk. Full-body massage restores balance and efficiency to the walking pattern.
22. Touch assessment that differentiates between tissue textures within the same tissue types. Palpation is a way to compare tissue to tissue and check for heat and cold. Palpation is a good time to observe skin color and the state of the hair and nails.
23. The proprioceptors and mechanoreceptors of the hand receive stimulation from the tissue palpated.

WORKBOOK SECTION

The brain devotes a large sensory area to the hand. The refined discriminatory sense of the hand can perceive subtle sensory shifts.

24. No. The whole body can be used to pick up sensory information. The areas most sensitive to posture shift and movement changes are the massage therapist's joints. This is because of the large concentration of positional receptors found in and around joint capsules. Therefore the hip, elbow, and knee, when placed against the client, also can detect sensory data about client movement.

25. The sensory receptors in the massage practitioner's hand adapt quickly and will not respond as well to prolonged stimulation; you simply do not feel it the second time you try. Thinking about what you are feeling also interferes with perception of the sensory data. Do not think until after you have felt.

26. The skin sensory receptors are designed to detect subtle changes in heat, air pressure, and air movement. This survival mechanism becomes most sensitive at a distance of about an arm's length from the person or object.

27. We are subconsciously aware of all the sensory stimulation that we have receptor mechanisms to detect. Sensitivity, or intuition, is the ability to work with this information on a conscious level. It does not depend on extrasensory skills but rather on conscious awareness of everything.

28. Heat and cold, as well as areas of not enough or too much sensitivity to air pressure changes. Sometimes this sensation feels like the repelling action between magnets with the north poles together. There is a subtle sense of resistance or of a force field.

29. Whether the skin is damp or dry; whether there are goose bumps, moles, or surface growths; the elasticity of the skin; the surface texture; and the mobility of the skin against the superficial connective tissue.

30. This area is a thin, gelatinous layer that feels like a thin water balloon. It can get waterlogged with surface edema.

31. In the superficial connective tissue; these vessels feel like soft tubes. Any changes in the superficial connective tissue affect circulation. You can feel pulses in the arteries, but if you press too hard you lose the pulse. This may give some idea of how to locate the superficial connective tissue layer.

32. The lymph nodes can be indicators of many different conditions, from a minor local infection to a life-threatening condition. Only a physician is equipped to make that determination.

33. Skeletal muscle has a distinct, ribbed feeling created by the fiber direction. It should feel firm and resilient without feeling stringy. There are usually three and sometimes more layers to skeletal muscle, and these layers crisscross over each other. It is important to feel through all the layers.

34. This is the transition area between muscle and tendons. For this reason the area is the site of the most strain and therefore the most injury. In addition, this is the area where the nerves often enter, and it is the location of the motor points that activate the muscle. Most muscle dysfunction arises at the musculotendinous junction.

35. No. Tendons are just as likely to adhere to all surrounding connective tissue. The fascial sheaths, ligaments, and other tendons, as well as bone, serve as attachment points. During palpation, it is important to be able to trace the tendon, rather than rely on the bony attachment sites shown in diagrams.

36. Fascial sheaths separate muscles, expand the skeleton, and provide stability. They provide grooves in which the nerves, blood, and lymph vessels lie. Fascial sheaths run primarily horizontally and vertically through the body. They must be pliable and distinct to serve these important functions.

37. Ligaments support and connect joints. Connection and separation of the joint is very important for posture because of the positional receptors in the joint. If the function of the ligaments is disrupted, postural distortion develops. Because of their limited blood supply, ligaments do not heal well if injured. Unless specifically trained in methods to work with ligaments, the massage therapist should avoid any direct work with them.

38. End-feel is the perception of the joint at the limit of its range of motion. It is either hard or soft. End-feel is perceived at the anatomic barrier if range of motion is unrestricted and at the physiologic barrier if the area is dysfunctional in any way.

39. Stable, supported, resilient, and unrestricted. The joint space should be able to be palpated. Much information can be obtained by palpating the joint while it is in motion.

40. With a short lever, one-jointed muscle initiates and stabilizes the joint movement. With a long lever, one-jointed muscle provides for full range of movement and power in the movement. A two-jointed muscle coordinates the movement with either the joint above or the joint below and assists the long-lever muscle.

41. Hypertonic muscles and shortened connective tissue. Usually the flexor and adductor muscles are the mus-

WORKBOOK SECTION

cles that pull the joint out of alignment because they are approximately 30% stronger than the extensor and abductor muscles. Trauma also may push a joint out of alignment.

42. Joint dysfunction is out of the scope of practice for massage. The two ways to determine this are as follows: (1) pain on traction usually is soft tissue dysfunction; (2) pain on compression usually is joint dysfunction. If active range of motion produces pain and passive range of motion does not, the problem usually is a soft-tissue problem. If both cause pain, the problem usually is a joint problem. Always refer suspected joint problems to a physician.

43. To locate bony landmarks for palpation and comparison.

44. Hard and spongy areas, referred pain patterns, and the location of the liver and large intestine. If any unusual areas are noted, refer the patient for diagnosis.

45. The three primary body rhythms are respiration, blood and lymph circulation, and craniosacral rhythm. These rhythms ebb and flow in an undulating fashion. The breath is particularly important. Massage tends to stabilize and even out these rhythms. The craniosacral rhythm is the most subtle and requires practice to feel.

46. *Strength muscle testing* seeks to discover whether the muscle being tested is responding with sufficient strength. *Neurologic muscle testing* evaluates the ability of the nerves to respond appropriately to a signal. *Applied kinesiologic muscle testing* is used as a biofeedback monitor of body function.

47. With strength testing, the muscle to be isolated is placed in contraction and the client holds it in place with a stabilizing force while the massage practitioner attempts to pull or push the muscle from its contracted position without recruiting other muscles. Strength patterns must be compared against a similar area, such as the same muscle on the other side, or against antagonist patterns. Neurologic muscle testing uses the same isolation of muscles, and the client holds the stabilizing force. The massage therapist provides a light pressure to evaluate the response of the muscle.

48. Because all muscles are linked neurologically, especially for the walking pattern, overly strong or weak muscles affect the entire pattern because they do not respond correctly to neurologic signals.

49. Postural muscles are made up of slow-twitch red fibers that can maintain a sustained contraction; these muscles are used to keep the body balanced against gravity. When stressed, they tend to shorten. Phasic muscles are primarily used for movement and are made up of fast-twitch red fibers that contract quickly but fatigue easily. They tend to weaken in response to postural muscle shortening. A muscle can serve a dual role and have a mixed fiber configuration.

50. The body moves in segments. These areas counterbalance each other against gravity and during movement. A typical muscle imbalance pattern bounces front to back and side to side at the segments.

51. Interpretation is done after the assessment. With experience, the two are not separated. When learning the process, it is easy to jump to conclusions if all the information is not gathered first. Interpretation is the process of piecing together all the information and then designing the best massage for the client.

52. Noting the client's general presence and the sequence that the client uses in gesturing and explaining. Also to be considered are symmetry of posture, efficiency of movement, tissue texture and condition, and areas that are hot or cold and overactive or underactive.

53. To provide balance by respecting current patterns and providing stimulation to encourage a more efficient function. Put simply, the purpose of the design of the massage is to cool down the hot spots, warm up the cold spots, lengthen the short areas, strengthen the weak areas, "unstick the stuck spots," and so forth.

54. All the information discussed regarding the physiologic effects of each massage method determines the methods chosen. When all is said and done, you can only push on it or pull on it, shake it, stretch it, and so on. What varies is the location of application, intensity, and duration of the methods used.

55. Reassessment allows both the massage practitioner and the client to determine what was successful during the massage process. Information given before and after the massage reinforces the benefits of massage for the client.

56. Most conditions with which the massage professional deals are chronic or self-limiting problems. Symptomatic relief, combined with activity to pass the time while the body heals itself, goes a long way toward assisting clients with this type of difficulty. Massage provides the hope that the body may not always feel like this, and the physiologic effects stimulate the body to reorganize toward a more efficient pattern. This takes time, and distracting the body from the current situation for a while is extremely helpful. Massage is simple, repetitive, and humble work. Be proud that you are studying to become part of this profession.

Text continued on p. 466.

WORKBOOK SECTION

Additional Activity

box 10-7

COMPLETED PHYSICAL ASSESSMENT FORM

Client Name: *Sue Williams*

Date: *00-00-00*

PHYSICAL

ALIGNMENT:

___ Chin in line with nose, sternal notch, navel   ✓ Other *Tilted to right*

HEAD:

___ Tilted left   ✓ Tilted right   ___ Rotated left   ___ Rotated right

EYES:

___ Level   ___ Equally set in socket   ✓ Other *Left eye higher*

EARS:

___ Level   ✓ Other *Left ear higher*

SHOULDERS:

___ Level   ✓ Right high/Left low   ___ Left high/ Right low

___ Left rounded forward   ___ Right rounded forward   ___ Muscle development even

___ Other_____

CLAVICLES:

___ Level   ✓ Other *Right side higher*

ARMS:

___ Hang evenly   ___ Left rotated: ___ medial   ___ lateral   ✓ Right rotated: ___ medial   ___ lateral

___ Other _____

ELBOWS:

___ Even   ✓ Other *Right side higher*

WRISTS:

___ Even   ✓ Other *Right side higher*

FINGERTIPS:

___ Even   ✓ Other *Right side higher*

RIBS:

___ Even   ✓ Other *Right side does not move as freely as left*

___ Springy   ___ Other _____

WORKBOOK SECTION

box 10-7

COMPLETED PHYSICAL ASSESSMENT FORM—CONT'D

SCAPULA:

✓ Even   ___ Other _____

___ Move freely   ✓ Other *Right side limited mobility* _____

ABDOMEN:

___ Firm   ✓ Other *Weak muscles* _____

___ Hard areas: Describe _____

WAIST:

✓ Level   ___ Other _____

SPINE CURVES:

___ Normal   ✓ Other *Mild kyphotic curve* _____

GLUTEAL MUSCLE MASS:

✓ Even   ___ Other _____

ILAIC CREST:

✓ Even   ___ Other _____

KNEES:

✓ Even   ___ Other _____

PATELLA:

✓ Left movable   ___ rigid

✓ Right movable   ___ rigid

ANKLES:

✓ Even   ___ Other _____

FEET:

___ Relaxed   ✓ Other *Left foot more rigid than right* _____

ARCHES:

✓ Even   ___ High   ___ Flat   ___ Other _____

TOES:

✓ Straight   ___ Other _____

SKIN:

___ Moves freely   ___ Pulls   ___ Puffy   ✓ Other *Restricted between scapula and on upper chest*

SOFT TISSUE:

___ Normal   ✓ Tender   ✓ Restricted   ___ Flaccid   ✓ Hot   ___ Cold

___ Other _____

Location(s) of Tissue Change(s): *Base of neck and upper thorax* _____

Continued.

WORKBOOK SECTION

box 10-7

COMPLETED PHYSICAL ASSESSMENT FORM—CONT'D

FUNCTIONAL MOBILITY:

___ Normal ✔ Restricted ✔ Exaggerated ✔ Painful

___ Other _____

Location(s) of Mobility Change(s): *Left leg exaggerated, left ankle restricted and painful, shoulder movement exaggerated with breathing*

GAIT

HEAD:

___ Remains steady ✔ Other *More movement to right*

TRUNK:

✔ Remains vertical ___ Other _____

SHOULDERS:

___ Remain level ✔ Other *Right shoulder high*

ARMS:

✔ Motion is opposite leg swing ___ Motion is even left and right

___ Other _____

✔ Left swings freely ___ Right swings freely ✔ Other *Right overswings*

HIPS:

✔ Remain level ___ Twist during walking ___ Other _____

LEGS:

___ Swing freely at hip ✔ Other *Left leg does not swing as much as right*

KNEES:

✔ Flex and extend freely through stance and swing ___ Other _____

FEET:

✔ Heel strikes first at start of stance ✔ Plantar flexed at push-off ✔ Foot clears floor during swing phase

✔ Other *Walks on outside of left foot*

STEP:

___ Length is even ✔ Timing is even ✔ Other *Longer step with right leg*

OVERALL:

___ Rhythmic motion ✔ Other *Uneven stride*

WORKBOOK SECTION

box 10-8

COMPLETED TREATMENT PLAN FORM

Client Name: *Sue Williams*

Date: *00-00-00*

Choose One: ✓ Original plan   Reassessment (original dated _____)

Short-Term Client Goals:

To improve work and daily activity performance through (1) relaxation to support better sleep and (2) management of headache and arm tingling

Long-Term Client Goals:

Continuing stress management to manage headaches and disturbed sleep, maintain effectiveness at work, and support a healthy lifestyle

Therapist Objectives:

Normalize breathing function, reduce thoracic tension, and even stride in gait

Frequency, Length, and Duration of Visits:

Weekly massage 1 hour for 6 weeks, then reassessment

Progress Measurements To Be Used:

Frequency of headaches reduced by 50% and pain diminished from 8 to 4 on a scale of 1 to 10; decrease time to fall asleep by 30 minutes and increase sleep to 7 hours without interruption; reduce tingling in arms by 50%

Dates of Reassessment:

00-00-00

Massage Methods To Be Used:

General massage, connective tissue stretching, postisometric relaxation and lengthening, entrainment rocking

Additional Notes:

Client wears heels at work and spends most of the day in a seated position talking on the phone

Client Signature: *Sue Williams*

Date: *00-00-00*

Therapist Signature: *Robin Jones*

Date: *00-00-00*

WORKBOOK SECTION

box 10-9

COMPLETED SOAP CHART FORM

Client Name: _Sue Williams_

Date: _00-00-00_

S: SUBJECTIVE
Client States:

Tingling in arm, headache 8 on 1 to 10 scale, shortness of breath, disrupted sleep

O: OBJECTIVE
I Observed from Assessment Procedures:

Right side tension pattern, shortened chest muscles and connective tissue, weak abdominals, tight muscles in lower legs

What I Did This Session:

General massage, lengthened shoulders and lower leg muscles with muscle energy methods, mild connective tissue stretching on upper chest; taught lengthening for shoulders and lower legs

WORKBOOK SECTION

box 10-9

COMPLETED SOAP CHART FORM—CONT'D

A: ANALYSIS (ASSESSMENT OF EFFECTIVENESS)
The Results: What Worked/What Didn't:

Client reports decrease in headache (to 4 on 1 to 10 scale) and easier breathing. She feels sleepy and desires a nap. General massage with rocking entrainment seemed to be most effective. Client acknowledged the benefit of connective tissue stretching but did not enjoy the methods; will need to use the approach sparingly. Client willingly participated in muscle energy lengthening and found it effective.

P: PLAN
Plans for Next Session, What Client Will Work On:

Client will do lengthening exercises daily. Weekly sessions will continue using general massage with entrainment focus. Therapist will include small amounts of connective tissue stretching and continue to use muscle energy and lengthening on the thorax to help with breathing.

WORKBOOK SECTION

Problem-Solving Exercises

1. In general, excessive sympathetic activation would be balanced by a relaxing massage, and excessive parasympathetic activation would be balanced by a stimulation massage. If the client is functioning from sympathetic nervous system dominance and relaxation methods such as rocking and slow effleurage are used initially, the work often is irritating. By beginning with a more stimulating approach and using strokes such as rapid compression, proprioceptive neuromuscular facilitation, stretching, and tapotement, the design of the massage fits the client physiologically. After some of the nervous energy has been discharged, the client is ready for the more relaxing methods.

2. A finger pointing to a specific area may suggest an acupressure or motor point hyperactivity or a joint problem. What the pointing means depends on the area indicated. Because the client is drilling into a joint, it may be wise to refer him for joint dysfunction evaluation.

3. Damp areas on the skin show that the nervous system has been activated in that area. This small amount of perspiration is part of a sympathetic activation called a *facilitated segment.* Surface stroking, with pressure enough to drag, elicits a red response over hyperactive areas. Deeper palpation usually elicits a tender response. The small erector pili muscles attached to each hair also are under sympathetic autonomic nervous system control. Light fingertip stroking produces goosebumps over areas of hyperactivity.

4. Pulses should be compared by feeling for a strong, even, full pumping action on both sides of the body. If differences are perceived, the client should be referred to a physician. Sometimes the differences in the pulses can be attributed to soft tissue restriction of the artery, which is determined by the physician.

5. A major problem is very likely hypertonic muscles. If shortened postural muscles are found, they need to be lengthened. If shortened and weak phasic muscles are found, they first must be lengthened and stretched. Eventually, strengthening techniques and exercises will be needed. If the hypertonic phasic muscle pattern arises from repetitive use, the muscles must be fatigued with muscle energy/proprioceptive neuromuscular facilitation techniques and then lengthened.

Professional Application

It is important to be able both to understand the assessment procedures of chiropractic and provide the chiropractor with concise information for evaluation in the development of a total treatment plan. The ability to keep clear, concise client SOAP notes is valuable in comparing and coordinating the combined therapy.

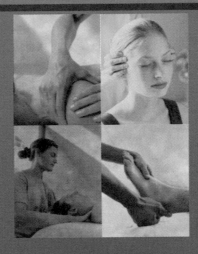

COMPLEMENTARY
BODYWORK SYSTEMS

objectives

*After completing this chapter, the student
will be able to perform the following:*

- Understand the physiologic mechanisms of complementary bodywork systems

- Identify overlap in the technical skills among the
various systems and integrate concepts of the styles
into the therapeutic massage system

- Consider a direction of interest for further study

THIS chapter introduces systems of structured touch other than therapeutic massage. Many different systems exist—far too many to be covered in this text. The individual systems cluster in the following categories:

1. Eastern and Oriental thought involving vital energy, chakras, meridians, and points
2. Reflex systems such as hydrotherapy and reflexology
3. Energetic systems such as polarity
4. Structural systems such as Rolfing, myofascial release, and craniosacral approaches

All the styles share in common with therapeutic massage the application of touch in a structured way to introduce various forms of sensory and mechanical information to the body to affect positive physiologic change. The language of each style is different and the theory base varies. The methods of assessment for each approach differentiate style variations more than any other part of the systems.

It is important to appreciate the similarities and differences of various bodywork approaches without becoming too concerned and overwhelmed with the language differences that tend to describe the same elements of anatomy and physiology.

COMPLEMENTARY BODYWORK SYSTEMS

section objectives

Using the information presented in this section, the student will be able to perform the following:

- **Identify similarities in bodywork methods**
- **Compare wellness massage with medical massage**

In the text *Zen Shiatsu—How to Harmonize Yin and Yang for Better Health*, Shitzuto Masunaga and Wataru Ohashi describe the interface of various bodywork methods as follows[9]:

Some professional therapists insist that a great difference exist among the three (anma [Chinese], Western massage, shiatsu [Japanese]) forms of treatment. I believe that a great difference cannot exist within a general field, in this case, manually applied stimulation to the human body. Of course, there are a variety of methods and schools, but basically they are similar . . . It is important to note that effectiveness of any treatment depends on both the practitioner and method working together. So the effectiveness of any treatment can vary greatly from one practitioner to another . . . All three methods of manipulation aim at stabilizing the functioning of the human body, the difference being whether they stimulate blood circulation and nerve interactions directly or indirectly. The effectiveness of manipulative therapy has been proven by modern scientific experiments involving cutaneous stimulation. From this point of view, no difference exists among the basic three techniques, though they were developed from different principles . . . The purpose of manipulative therapy is to work with a person's natural healing force to correct any internal malfunctioning particular to that person.

Many massage professionals continue their learning through the comprehensive study of one other bodywork approach. Others study many different bodywork modalities, some in considerable depth and others more superficially. Then they integrate the information into therapeutic massage variations, concepts, and an expanded look at the body.

This text does not attempt to describe the varied systems in depth; instead, this text is devoted to the professional practice of therapeutic massage. Providing only a brief description of these other systems would do an injustice to both the rich and complete massage system, as well as the rich and complete complementary bodywork systems, each of which are textbooks and lifetime studies of their own.

The author believes that expertise in any of the systems requires specific study. There is enough to learn about therapeutic massage without expecting also to develop expertise in the other various styles. Nor does it seem necessary to attempt to be proficient in multiple bodywork styles because the ultimate result of the application for all of them is essentially the same. In simple terms, pick one (maybe two) and learn it (them) well.

It is important to understand the basis of other methods because a client may respond better to a different manual system than therapeutic massage and informed referral is important. Methodology and technical skill among the systems overlap. It is helpful to be able to identify and use these overlapping areas.

What is presented in this text is a brief overview of these basic systems, suggestions for implementation of the basic concepts and techniques that overlap well with the massage therapy approach, and guidance for the development of an integrated system.

The information contained in this chapter is not sufficient training for the practitioner to be able to purposefully and intelligently understand and use these methods for anything other than a general enhancement of the skills already developed. However, with a commitment to further education, the methods mentioned can add efficiency, effectiveness, and enthusiasm for what therapeutic massage has to offer for wellness, prevention, rehabilitation, and client-directed healing. As you practice the various methods presented, pay attention to areas in which you display a particular interest and talent. This information can help direct you to specific avenues for continuing education.

The Basis of Bodywork

You can apply pressure, lift and stretch tissue, rock the body, stroke the skin, entrain the rhythms, move the joints, generate tissue repair by creating therapeutic inflammation, stimulate reflex responses, soothe the energy field, and provide interpersonal and professional support, compassion, and acceptance for the client. Regardless of the theoretical, historical, and cultural base, all the bodywork systems, including therapeutic massage, are built on this same foundation.

Expertise in any bodywork system consists of quality assessment to make effective decisions about the application of treatment to provide a service that benefits the client. Benefits range from pleasure and comfort care to ongoing management of chronic conditions and stress, as well as a therapeutic change processes. All these factors in some form are covered in this text.

Body, Mind, and Spirit

Bodywork—therapeutic massage as a complete system within the broader realm—serves the wholeness of the individual through a direct influence on the body and a respect for mind and spirit. The concept of the body/mind/spirit connection found in many complementary systems of bodywork leads to the acceptance of the unity and integrity of the individual. However, consideration must include different aspects of the person but never separate from the whole. As discussed at the beginning of this textbook, the skin is not separate from the emotions, nor the emotion separate from the organs, nor the organs separate from the muscles. No part is separate from the spirit or the larger context of our influence on others, society, culture, and the larger expanse of the universe.

In bodywork traditions, this interconnectedness is also apparent. For example, the ayurvedic medicine of India is similar to Oriental medicine. These practices are similar to the tribal medicine of Native Americans and other indigenous peoples. In Thailand, Tibet, Russia, and other parts of the world, the ancient traditions of medicine and folk health wisdom share a common difference with Western scientific thought. These systems identify body/mind/spirit lifestyle imbalance, termed in this text as *dysfunction* or "almost sick and not quite well." They introduce interventions to reverse this process before it cycles into body/mind/spirit disease.

Wellness Massage Versus Medical Massage

The main purpose of this textbook is to train the massage professional to use massage methods intelligently to promote health and well-being. Generally healthy people can benefit from the normalizing physiologic effects of hydrotherapy, connective tissue massage, lymphatic and blood circulation massage, trigger point work, acupressure, and reflexology. These methods, when integrated into the massage methods already used, can add another dimension to the effectiveness of the massage.

Sometimes the client may present the massage professional with minor problems that can be helped though the use of the techniques discussed in this chapter. These same methods can be used in various forms of health care and rehabilitative or athletic massage. For the massage

professional to use the methods in a more specific way, additional training is needed, especially in pathophysiology, pharmacology, and medical treatment protocols to understand the interface of massage therapy with these approaches. When dealing with medical conditions and working within the health care environment, the methods—massage manipulations and techniques as described in Chapter 9 or any of the various methods described in this chapter—do not change. Some methods are more appropriate for certain conditions, and others are chosen for different outcomes. What is different is the condition of the person receiving the massage. Additional education does not usually revolve around learning new methods, but instead learning how to choose and use methods with clients who present with various complex situations.

The massage professional servicing a client in the health care setting needs to increase his or her knowledge based on the function, dysfunction, or disease being addressed:

- Serving the athlete mandates understanding training protocols, common stress patterns, and injury rehabilitation of that particular sport.
- Working with stroke rehabilitation requires increased knowledge about stroke etiology, rehabilitation, and the use of massage as part of the overall rehabilitation and management process.
- Working with clients with depression is enhanced by understanding the manifestations of depression, mental health interventions, and psychotropic pharmacology.

The massage professional should confer with the medical team when dealing with clients who are undergoing medical intervention (e.g., medications, physical therapy, psychotherapy, chiropractic therapy). The massage should be integrated into the entire treatment protocol. Supervision by a licensed medical professional can help ensure that methods used for a client are monitored and evaluated for effectiveness in the treatment protocol.

Whether working in the wellness setting or in the health care environment, the attractiveness of therapeutic massage and complementary bodywork systems is their totality and the simple disciplines inherent in them that support healthy lifestyles. Chapter 13 explores this concept in further depth. This chapter provides an overview of complementary styles.

HYDROTHERAPY

section objectives

Using the information presented in this section, the student will be able to perform the following:

- **Explain the general effects of hot and cold water applications**
- **Incorporate simple hydrotherapy methods into the massage setting**

- **Suggest easy self-help techniques for clients using basic hydrotherapy**

Hydrotherapy is a separate and distinct form of therapy that combines well with massage. Water can be used in many different ways depending on the health needs and condition of the client and the facilities available for therapy.

Water therapy is as old as the human race. One of the first recorded mentions of the use of water as medicine involves the temples of the Greek god of medicine Aesculapius. At the temples, bathing and massage were part of the treatment for the sick. Hippocrates used water as a beverage for reducing fever and treating many diseases. He also stressed the value of using various types of baths, each with a different temperature, as a therapeutic tool to combat illness. Later, the ancient Roman physicians Galen and Celsus also recommended specific baths as an integral part of their remedies. Almost every warm-climate civilization has at some point in its history used baths for therapeutic reasons.[1]

Skillful use of hydrotherapy methods requires long-term study. The advanced-level massage therapist should be well trained in hydrotherapy. These methods have very powerful physiologic effects and have been used for centuries as part of the healing process. Before the development of antidepressant and stimulant medications, hot, warm, and cold applications were used to stimulate or sedate the autonomic nervous system. Cold shock was used instead of electric shock to treat depression. Warm baths of long duration were used to calm anxious persons. Herbal and mineral additives to water were also used for centuries to enhance the effects of hydrotherapy.

Water is a near-perfect natural body balancer and is necessary for life. It accounts for the largest percentage of our body weight. A universal solvent, it is a perfect detoxifier for our bodies. It is available in many forms, all of which are therapeutically beneficial. Water can relax or stimulate, anesthetize, and reduce or increase circulation. It works naturally and is nonallergenic, tissue-tolerant, inexpensive, and readily available.

Water's three forms (liquid, steam, and ice) allow for its use in a variety of temperatures. As a liquid, water can be pressurized and used as a relaxing massage shower or in a whirlpool for muscle and joint therapy. As steam, it provides relaxation and cleansing in a steam bath, humidity in a winter home, and a breathing aid to a congested child or older person. It can be used as an antiseptic as steam or when boiling. As heat, it can increase circulation, and as ice, it can reduce it. In this form, it is also an effective anesthetic and can minimize edema. When heated, water can increase body temperature and circulation; when cool, it can decrease it. As ice, it is an effective anesthetic and can minimize edema. In a flotation tank or soaking bath, water can reduce stress.

Water can be used internally by drinking it or by forcing streams of water into orifices, as in an enema, douche, bidet, or nose or ear bath. Water can be used externally in full or partial baths, showers, compresses, packs, hot water bottles, frozen ice bandages, and wrapped ice, and as steam in several different ways (Box 11-1).

Primary Physiologic Effects of Hydrotherapy

The effects of water are primarily reflexive and focused on the autonomic nervous system. The addition of heat energy or dissipation of heat energy from tissues can be classified as a mechanical effect. In general, cold stimulates sympathetic responses and warm activates parasympathetic responses. Short- and long-term applications of hot or cold differ. For the most part, short, cold applications stimulate and vasoconstrict with a secondary effect of increased circulation as blood is channeled to the area to warm it. Long, cold applications depress and decrease circulation. Short applications of heat vasodilate vessels and depress and deplete tone, whereas long, hot applications result in a combined depressant and stimulant reaction.

---

box 11-1

THERAPEUTIC USES OF WATER

Analgesic: pain relief—hot, warm and cold applications
Anesthetic: reduction in sensation—cold application
Antiedemic: reduces swelling—cold application
Antipyretic: reduces fever—cool to cold application
Antiseptic: kills pathogens—boiling water and high-pressure steam
Antispasmodic: reduces muscle spasm—hot, warm, and cold applications
Astringent: contraction of tissues—cold application
Burn treatment: first- and mild second-degree burns only—cool application
Diaphoretic: produces sweating—hot application
Diuretic: increases urine formation—drinking water
Emetic: produces vomiting—ingesting warm water
Expectorant: loosens mucus—hot and steam applications
Immunologic enhancement: increases white cell production—cold application
Laxative: promotes peristalsis of the bowel—ingestion of cold water or enema
Purifier: eliminates toxins—all forms of water
Sedative: reduces sympathetic arousal and encourages sleep—ingesting warm water
Stimulant: increases sympathetic arousal—short hot and cold applications
Tonic: increases muscle tone—cold and alternating hot and cold applications

Adapted from Nikola RJ: *Creatures of water-hydrotherapy textbook,* Salt Lake City, 1997, EUROPA/Healing Mountain School (1-800-407-3251).

Visceral Reflex-Cutaneous and Somatic Effects

Stimulation of certain nerve endings in organs results in both a muscle and skin response in a reflex loop. Usually the muscles spasm or increase in tension and the skin becomes more taut. This reflex is responsible for visceral referred pain patterns (Chapter 5, p. 202). Theoretically the reflex is a loop; therefore stimulation of muscle and skin can reflexively affect the corresponding organ. In general an organ is in a reflex pattern with the muscles and skin over it. Applications of hydrotherapy seem to have either sedation or stimulation effects to the specific organ.

Mechanical Effects

Different pressures of water can exert a powerful mechanical effect on the nerve and blood supply of the skin. Techniques that are used include a friction rub with a sponge or wet mitten, and pressurized streams of hot and cold water directed at various part of the body (Box 11-2).

Suggestions for Integration of Hydrotherapy with Therapeutic Massage

The basic techniques of hydrotherapy can be taught as self-help to clients. Although many massage therapy facilities do not have access to hydrotherapy equipment, simple hot and cold compresses can be used. A warm footbath is easy to incorporate into a massage and serves the double purpose of relaxing the client and freshening "stale" feet before the massage. A bag of frozen peas makes a great cold pack because it can mold to almost any area. Hot water bottles are safer to use than heating pads. They naturally cool down before they could burn someone. Water frozen in a paper cup with a stick in it makes an effective massage tool, especially when the practitioner is using ice as a counterstimulant to assist in lengthening and stretching procedures. Clean, pure drinking water should be available for both the client and therapist. Meticulous

---

box 11-2

EFFECTS OF HYDROTHERAPY USING HEAT, COLD, AND ICE APPLICATIONS

Effects of Heat
- Increased circulation
- Increased metabolism
- Increased inflammation
- Increased respiration
- Increased perspiration
- Decreased pain
- Decreased muscle spasm
- Decreased tissue stiffness
- Decreased white blood cell production

Applications of Hydrotherapy

As a *sedative,* water is a very efficient, nontoxic, calming substance. It soothes the body and promotes sleep.

Techniques: Use hot and warm baths to quiet and relax the entire body, salt baths, neutral showers to relax certain areas, or damp sheet packs.

For *elimination* the skin is the largest organ, and simple immersion in a long hot bath, sauna, or steam room can stimulate the excretion of toxins from the body through the skin. Inducing perspiration is useful in treating acute diseases and many chronic health problems.

Techniques: Use hot baths, Epsom salt or common salt baths, hot packs, dry blanket packs, and hot herbal drinks.

As an *antispasmodic,* water effectively reduces cramps and muscle spasm.

Techniques: Use hot compresses (depending on the problem), herbal teas, and abdominal compresses.

Effects of Cold and Ice
Cold
- Increased stimulation
- Decreased circulation—primary effect; increased circulation—secondary effect
- Decreased inflammation
- Decreased pain
- Decreased respiration
- Decreased digestive process
- Increased muscle tone
- Increased tissue stiffness
- Increased white blood cell production
- Increased red blood cell production

Ice
- Decreased circulation
- Decreased metabolism
- Decreased inflammation
- Decreased pain
- Decreased muscle spasm
- Increased stiffness

Application Type
- Ice packs
- Ice immersion (ice water)
- Ice massage
- Cold whirlpool
- Chemical cold packs
- Cold gel packs *(use with caution)*

attention to sanitation is necessary when using water applications.

Rules of Hydrotherapy

Hydrotherapy has a powerful effect on the body. The following rules, taken from the Ontario, Canada, curriculum guidelines for massage therapy, are suggested when using hydrotherapy in the massage setting:

1. Always take a thorough case history to check for possible contraindications. Contraindications include various circulatory and kidney problems, as well as skin conditions.
2. Always adapt the method to the individual and not vice versa. The procedures given for time, temperatures used, and other variables should be used as guidelines and not absolutes.
3. Have the client go to the bathroom before treatment begins.
4. Stay with the client during treatment, or have some way for the client to contact you, such as by using a bell.
5. Explain the complete treatment to the client beforehand so he or she knows what to expect and what is expected.
6. Make sure the room is draft-free, clean, and quiet. All equipment should be sanitary and in good working condition. Each client should have clean towels and sheets.
7. Keep the client from becoming chilled during or after the treatment.
8. When using cold temperatures, the water should be as cold as possible, within the tolerance of the client. A 10° difference is the minimum needed to create stimulation and change in the circulation.
9. Warm temperatures should be as warm as necessary and within the client's tolerance. Too hot a temperature can be debilitating.

---

box 11-2

EFFECTS OF HYDROTHERAPY USING HEAT, COLD, AND ICE APPLICATIONS—CONT'D

Contraindications for Ice
- Vasospastic disease (spasm of blood vessels)
- Cold hypersensitivity
  Skin: itching, sweating
  Respiratory: hoarseness, sneezing, chest pain
  Gastrointestinal: abdominal pain, diarrhea, vomiting
  Eyes: puffy eyelids
  General: headache, discomfort, uneasiness
- Cardiac disorder
- Compromised local circulation

Precautions for Ice
- Do not use frozen gel packs directly on skin.
- Do not use ice applications (cryotherapy) for longer than 30 minutes continuously.
- Do not do exercises that cause pain after cold applications.
- Do not use cryotherapy for treating persons with certain rheumatoid conditions, or for those who are paralyzed or have coronary artery disease.

Applications of Hydrotherapy

Ice is a primary therapy for strains, sprains, contusions, hematomas, and fractures. It has a numbing, anesthetic effect and helps control internal hemorrhage by reducing circulation to and metabolic processes within the area.

For *restoration and increasing muscle strength and increasing the body's resistance to disease,* cold water boosts vigor, adds energy and tone, and aids in digestion.

Techniques: Use cold water treading (standing or walking in cold water), whirlpool baths, cold sprays, alternate hot and cold contrast baths, showers and compresses, salt rubs, apple cider vinegar baths, and partial packs.

For *injuries,* the application of an ice pack controls the flow of blood and reduces tissue swelling.

Technique: Use an ice bag in addition to compression and elevation.

As an *anesthetic,* water can dull the sense of pain or sensation.

Technique: Use ice to chill the tissue.

For *minor burns,* water, particularly cold and ice water, has been rediscovered as a primary healing agent.

Technique: Use ice-water immersion or saline-water immersion.

To *reduce fever,* water is nature's best cooling agent. Unlike medications, which usually only diminish internal heat, water both lowers and removes heat by conduction.

Technique: Use of ice bags at base of neck, forehead, and feet, cold water sponge baths, and drinking cold water.

10. More is *not* better. It is not always more effective to use greater extremes in temperature or greater lengths of time. The aim is to achieve a positive change, and too much can overtax, damage, or set back the condition.

11. Ask pertinent questions during the treatment, including questions about comfort level and thirst, but keep talking to a minimum to allow the client to relax.

12. Check the client's respiratory rate and pulse before, during, and after treatments as required, especially with prolonged hot treatments. The pulse should stay fairly even.

13. Watch for discomfort and/or negative reactions to the treatment.

14. Stop the treatment if a negative reaction occurs.

15. Generally, short cold treatments are followed by active exercise. Prolonged cold and hot treatments are followed by bed rest and then exercise.

16. Apply cold compresses to the head with hot treatments and prolonged cold treatments.

17. Never give a cold treatment to a cold body. Always warm the body first. The easiest method for this is a warm foot bath.

Use Box 11-3 as a guide when classifying water temperatures for treatments.

Types of Water Application for Health Purposes

The types of water application used for health purposes include the following:

1. Local heat: Apply heat to a specific area of the body, such as a joint, the chest, throat, shoulders, or spine. Use a hot, moist compress or a hot water bottle.

2. Local cold: Apply cold to a specific area of the body. Use a cold compress, ice bag, ice pack, ice hat, or frozen bandage.

3. Sponging: Use alcohol, water, or witch hazel applied with a sponge to wash the body.

4. Tonic friction: Water sponging and washing combined with some form of friction, either from the hand or a rough wash cloth, produces a tonic effect in the body. Use cold friction massage or a cold sponge rub.

5. Baths: The body is immersed in cold, hot, or tepid water. Use foot, sitz, full, mineral, or herb baths. Any part of the body may be partially bathed, as in an arm, eye, or finger bath. A whirlpool is a bath in which the water is moving under pressure.

6. Compresses and packs: Compresses and packs are folded cotton, flannel, or gauze soaked in water or liquid medications or herbs. A pack covers a larger area than a compress.

7. Showers: Several kinds of water streams can be directed against the body. Alternate streams can also be directed against the body, or large quantities of water can be poured from a height.

8. Shampoo: When soap and water are used together on one or all parts of the body, it creates a shampoo. Use to cleanse hair or after sauna or steam room.

9. Steam: A vaporizer can cleanse the upper respiratory system, and a steam room or sauna increases body perspiration and releases many stored toxins. Cold steam, as from a humidifier, moistens dry rooms in winter and is important in preventing colds and sinus headaches.

10. Sauna (dry heat): An intense but tolerably heated room. Taking a tepid or cold shower after a sauna is recommended.

R.I.C.E. First Aid

Everyone should understand basic first aid. The **R.I.C.E. first aid** application of hydrotherapy is appropriate for most soft tissue injuries, especially sprains and strains. Always refer serious injuries to a medical doctor.

R.I.C.E. stands for

R—rest
I—ice
C—compression
E—elevation

R.I.C.E. decreases recovery time by decreasing the secondary injury to tissue caused by the inflammatory response. Less total damage results, decreasing the need for repair. Decreasing pain and muscle spasm results in a more normal range of motion and muscular strength. The

box 11-3
HOW TO CLASSIFY WATER TEMPERATURE

Very cold	32° to 56°—painful
Cold	56° to 65°—uncomfortable
Cool	65° to 92°—goose flesh
Neutral	92° to 98°—skin temperature
Warm to hot	98° to 104°—comfortable
Very hot	104° to 110°—red skin
Temperatures higher than 110° should not be used.	

11-1
PROFICIENCY EXERCISE

Visit a whirlpool, sauna, and steam room. Hotels may have this equipment available. Use the equipment and pay attention to how your body feels.

client can therefore return to activity much quicker, reducing other complications set up by the injury.

Rest allows the injured area(s) or the entire body to best use regenerative energy to heal.

Ice decreases metabolism, resulting in lessened secondary injury caused by swelling from the primary injury. Ice does not affect the original injury but keeps body processes from making the injury worse.

Compression increases pressure outside the vasculature. This helps control edema by promoting reabsorption of fluids.

Elevation reduces blood and fluid flow to injured areas.

A wrapped ice bag is the most effective initial therapy for many injuries, especially sports injuries. An ice bag held close to the injury site with an elastic bandage is ideal because the resulting compression reinforces the physiologic action of the application. An ice bath or ice massage is also effective.

To avoid frostbite, place a layer of fabric between the ice and the skin. Ice therapy varies with the injury and its severity. Most injuries respond within 24 to 48 hours. Ice bag compression should be used for 20 minutes, twice a day, or for shorter applications, four times a day. Apply ice periodically, not continuously. Between ice applications, rub the body part briskly with the hand. When heat is ineffective for muscle spasms, use ice. Often a sciatica attack that does not respond to moist heat will respond to one or two frozen bandages.

Be sure the injury has been evaluated by a physician. Apply ice to the injured area by immersion in ice water (ice bath) and massage with ice cubes or pops, an ice bag, or ice packs.

Ice application continues through four sensations (over a 10- to 15-minute time period): appreciation of cold (pain), warming, ache or throbbing, and skin anesthesia (numbness).

The effects of alternating hot and cold include constriction and dilation of vessels and decreased congestion. Techniques include hot and cold compresses, ice bags, warm or hot baths, hot packs, whirlpool baths, and alternating hot and warm or hot and cold showers. Do not use heat on a fresh injury; it increases the blood flow and inflammation and therefore produces tissue swelling (Proficiency Exercise 11-1).

LYMPH, BLOOD, AND CIRCULATION ENHANCEMENT

section objectives

Using the information presented in this section, the student will be able to perform the following:

- Explain the general effects of lymphatic and circulation enhancement massage

- Incorporate the principles of lymphatic and circulation massage into the general massage session

One of the most well-documented benefits of massage is stimulation of the lymphatic and circulatory systems. Many variations and styles of massage are used to stimulate lymph and blood circulation. When the massage is focused to stimulate the lymphatic or circulatory system specifically, a special type of massage is necessary. Because an entire body system is being stimulated, the approach is called **systemic massage.** In this section we discuss the important physiology and methods of focusing the massage to enhance lymph and blood circulation.

Lymphatic Drainage

Various styles are used for **lymphatic drainage.** One style is manual lymph drainage, which was developed by Emil Vodder. Another style, described by Eyal Lederman, an osteopathic physician, takes a somewhat different approach to lymphatic drainage than Vodder. Both methods provide the foundation for this section. Lymph drainage is a specific therapeutic method. As with all the methods presented in this chapter, specialized training is required to use it successfully.

All massage stimulates the circulation and lymph movement, but structuring a massage to focus on this system is a specific therapeutic intervention. When an individual body system is focused on and the effects of the massage are concentrated to a certain response, it is not uncommon for the client to feel the effects of the methods more than with general or local massage.

After undergoing massage involving the precise movement of lymph, the client may feel listless, fatigued, or achy for 48 hours. Some have described this feeling as a massage "hangover." The physiologic effects of toxin overload are similar to an alcohol hangover.

The Lymphatic System

The lymph system is a specialized component of the circulatory system, responsible for waste disposal and immune response. Lymph and blood are very similar, except lymph does not have red blood cells or platelets, has a slightly higher protein content, and carries bacteria and other debris. Lymph is the interstitial (around the cell) fluid.

The movement of lymph is along a pressure gradient from high to low pressure areas. Lymph moves from the interstitial space into the lymph capillaries through a pressure mechanism exerted by respiration, peristalsis of the large intestine, the compression of muscles, and the pull of the skin and fascia during movement.

This action is especially prominent at the plexuses in the hands and feet. Major lymph plexuses exist on the soles of the feet and palms of the hands. It is possible that the rhythmic pumping of walking and grasping facilitates lymphatic flow. As mentioned in Chapter 4, recent research indicates a possible primary intrinsic pumping mechanism inherent in the lymphatic system.

The lymphatic system permeates the entire tissue structure of the body in a one-way drainage network of vessels, ducts, nodes, lacteals, and lymphoid organs such as the spleen. It is helpful to visualize roots on a plant to get an idea of the extensive lymph network. Tiny lymph vessels, known as *lymph capillaries,* are distributed throughout the body, except in the eyes, brain, and spinal cord. The lymph is collected in the capillaries somewhat similar to the way water is drawn up into a plant's roots.

The lymphatic tubes merge into one another until major channels and vessels are formed. These vessels run from the distal parts of the body toward the neck, usually along veins and arteries. Valves within the vessels prevent the backflow of lymph.

Lymph nodes are enlarged portions of the lymph vessels that generally cluster at the joints. This arrangement assists movement of the lymph through the nodes by the pumping action when the joint moves. These nodes filter the fluid and produce lymphocytes.

All the body's lymph vessels converge into two main channels: the thoracic duct and the right lymphatic duct. Vessels from the entire left side of the body and from the right side of the body below the chest converge into the thoracic duct, which in turn empties into the left subclavian vein situated beneath the left clavicle. The right lymphatic duct collects lymph from the vessels on the right side of the head, neck, upper chest, and right arm. It empties into the subclavian vein beneath the right clavicle. Waste products are then carried by the bloodstream to the spleen, intestines, and kidneys for detoxification.

Massage Methods for the Lymphatic System

The pressure provided by massage mimics the compressive forces of movement and respiration. The pressure gradient from high pressure to low pressure is supported by creating low pressure areas in the vessels proximal to the area to be drained.

Simple muscle tension puts pressure on the lymph vessels and may block them and interfere with efficient drainage. Massage can normalize this muscle tension. As the muscles relax, the lymph vessels open and drainage is more efficient.

The methods of lymphatic massage are fairly simple, but lymphatic massage, when indicated, is a very powerful technique with bodywide responses. It stimulates the flow of lymph mechanically with pressure on the surface of the skin tracing the lymphatic routes. Disagreement exists about the intensity of the pressure used. Some schools of thought indicate the use of a very light pressure, and others, such as the technique described by Lederman, suggest a deeper pressure. Lederman indicates that the stronger the compression used, the larger the increase in the flow rate of lymph. Light pressure is used initially and then methodically increased as the area is drained.[8]

Although disagreement exists about methodology, all approaches have some validity. Therefore the method described in this text combines the various methods to support lymphatic movement in the body.

Rhythmic, gentle passive and active joint movement reproduces the body's normal means of pumping lymph. The client helps the process by deep, slow breathing, which stimulates lymph flow in the deeper vessels. When possible, position the area being massaged above the heart so that gravity can also assist the lymph flow.

The massage consists of a combination of short, light, pumping effleurage strokes beginning close to the torso and directed toward the torso; the strokes methodically move distally. This pattern is followed by long surface effleurage strokes. The direction is toward the drainage points (following the arrow on the diagram in Fig. 11-1). Pressure increases gradually as the entire pattern is repeated.

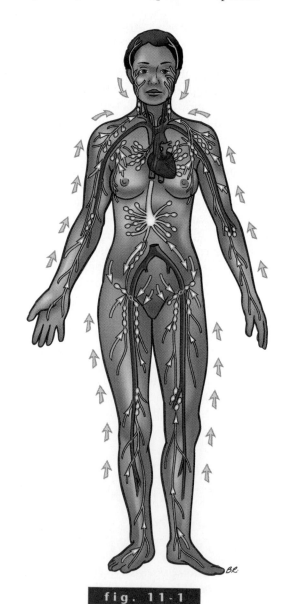

fig. 11-1

Direction of strokes for facilitating lymphatic flow.

The focus of the initial pressure is on the dermis, just below the surface layer of skin and the layer of tissue just beneath the skin and above the muscles. This is the superficial fascial layer. It does not take much pressure to contact the area. If too much pressure is applied, the capillaries are pressed closed. This nullifies any effect on the more surface vessels. With lymphatic massage, generally light pressure is indicated initially and increases to a moderate level during repeated application to the area.

This massage approach is appropriate for clients who are generally healthy. It is common to develop a somewhat sluggish lymphatic flow. The usual culprits are inactivity, consumption of junk food and beverages, and reduced water intake. All these factors stress the lymphatic system. Recovery from colds, influenza, and other common bacterial and viral infections can temporarily overload the lymphatic system. General massage with a focus as presented in this session, coupled with corrective action by the client of increased water intake, increased activity, and reduced junk food intake, can reverse the problem.

For professionals working with clients with lymphatic pathology, additional training is required, as is medical supervision (Proficiency Exercise 11-2).

Circulatory Massage

The purpose of circulatory massage is to stimulate the efficient flow of blood through the body. As with lymph massage, specific application for an impaired circulation disease process is out of the scope of practice for the massage professional, unless performed under appropriate supervision. In this situation, massage can be beneficial as part of the overall treatment plan.

Clients who are not sick can benefit greatly from increased efficiency in the circulatory system. This type of massage tends to normalize blood pressure, tone the cardiovascular system, and undo the negative effects of occasional stress. It is an excellent massage approach to use with athletes and anyone else after exercise. Circulatory massage also supports the inactive client by increasing the blood movement mechanically, but it in no way replaces exercise. Both circulatory and lymphatic massage are very beneficial for the client who is unable to walk or exercise aerobically.

The Circulatory System

The circulatory system is a closed system that is composed of a series of connected tubes and a pump. The heart pump provides pressure for the blood to move through the body via the arteries and eventually into the small capillaries, where the actual blood gas and nutrient exchange happens. The blood then returns to the heart by way of the veins. Venous blood flow is not under pressure from the heart. Instead it relies on the muscle compression against the veins to change the interior venous pressure. As in the lymphatic system, backflow of blood is prevented by a valve system.

Massage Methods for the Circulatory System

Massage to encourage blood flow to the tissues (arterial circulation) is different from massage to encourage blood flow from the tissues back to the heart (venous circulation). Because of the valve system of the veins and lymph vessels, any deep stroking over these vessels from proximal to distal (from the heart out) is contraindicated. A small chance exists of breaking down the valves if this is done. However, compression, which does not slide like effleurage or stripping, is appropriate for stimulating arterial circulation.

Compression is applied over the main arteries, beginning close to the heart (proximal), and systematically moves distally to the tips of the fingers or toes. The manipulations are applied over the arteries and with a pumping action at a rhythm of approximately 60 beats per minute or whatever the client's resting heart rate is. Compressive force changes the internal pressure in the arteries and encourages the movement of blood. Compression also begins to empty venous vessels and will form an arterial-venous pressure gradient encouraging arterial blood flow (Fig. 11-2).

Rhythmic, gentle contraction and relaxation of the muscles powerfully encourages arterial blood flow. Both active and passive joint movement support the transport of arterial blood.

The next step is to assist venous return flow. This process is similar to the lymphatic massage in that a combination of short and long effleurage strokes is used in combination with movement. The difference is that lymphatic massage is done over the entire body and the

---

11-2

PROFICIENCY EXERCISE

1. Fill a long balloon with water. Leave an air bubble in it. Use short effleurage strokes to move the bubble. Notice the level of pressure that moves the bubble most effectively.

2. Design a lymphatic self-massage. Incorporate deep breathing movement and compression action at the joints, palms, and soles of the feet.

movements are usually passive. With venous return flow, the effleurage strokes move distally to proximally (from the fingers and toes to the heart) over the major veins. The effleurage stroke is short, about 3 inches long. This enables the blood to move from valve to valve. Long effleurage strokes carry the blood through the entire vein. Both passive and active joint movements encourage venous circulation. Placing the limb or other area above the heart brings in the gravity assistance (Fig. 11-3) (Proficiency Exercise 11-3).

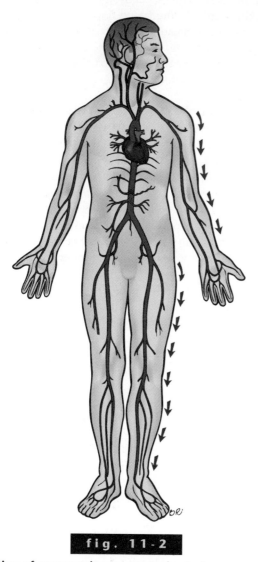

fig. 11-2

Direction of compression over arteries to increase arterial flow.

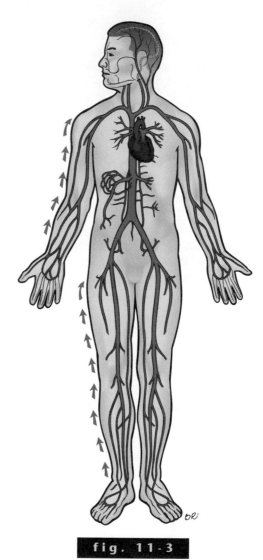

fig. 11-3

Direction of effleurage strokes to facilitate venous flow.

11-3
PROFICIENCY EXERCISE

1. Hook a hose up to a faucet and barely turn on the water. This simulates the heart pump. Use compression to facilitate the movement or "circulation" of the water in the hose.

2. Obtain a 3-foot piece of clear, soft plastic tubing. As if sucking on a straw, draw up a small amount of water into the tubing. Massage the water to the other end of the tube. This is similar to venous return massage.

REFLEXOLOGY

section objectives

Using the information presented in this section, the student will be able to perform the following:

- Explain the physiologic benefits of foot and hand massage
- Incorporate the principles of reflexology into the general massage session

In the bodywork community, **reflexology** means the stimulation of areas beneath the skin to improve the function of the whole body or of specific body areas away from the site of the stimulation. Eunice Ingham has been given credit for formalizing the system, which is based on the theory that certain points in the foot and hand affect other body organs and areas. Historically, the approach seems to have originated in China. Foot reflexology is the most popular type of reflexology.

Another approach to reflexology is referred to as *zone therapy.* It is postulated that there are ten zones running though the body. Reflex points for stimulation can be located within the zones.

Reflexology applies the stimulus/reflex principle to healing the body. The foot has been mapped to show the areas to contact to affect different parts of the body. Charts mapping these areas vary somewhat. Typically, the large toe represents the head, and the junction of the large toe to the foot represents the neck. The next toes represent the eyes, ears, and sinuses. The waist is about midway on the arch of the foot, with various organs above and below the line. The reflex points for the spine are along the medial longitudinal arch. It is thought that this stimulus/response reflex is conducted through neural pathways in the body that activate the body's electrical and biochemical activities (Fig. 11-4).

The medical definition of *reflexology* is "the study of reflexes." *Reflexotherapy* is treatment by manipulation applied to an area away from the disorder. In physiologic terms a reflex is an involuntary response to a stimulus.

This discussion of reflexology attempts to explain why foot and hand massage is beneficial through standard physiology and avoids the issue of whether actual corresponding points on the foot or hand exist that relate directly to other body areas. An explanation based on standard anatomy and physiology is better suited to the format of this textbook and may be better accepted by the public.

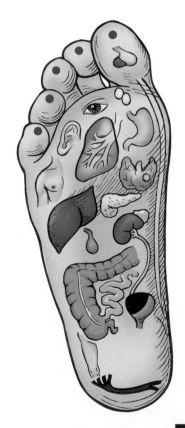 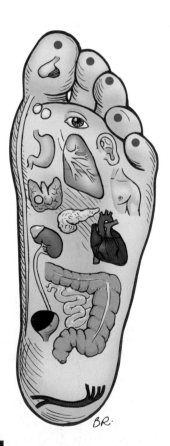

fig. 11-4

A generalized reflexology chart.

Physiologic Reflexes of the Foot

The foot is a very complex structure. The ankle and foot consist of 34 joints, with many joint and reflex patterns (Box 11-4). Extensive nerve distribution exists to the feet and hands. The position of the foot sends considerable postural information from the joint mechanoreceptors through the central nervous system. The sensory and motor centers of the brain devote a large area to the foot and hand.

It seems logical to assume that stimulation of the feet activates the responses of the gait control mechanism and hyperstimulation analgesia, with activation to the parasympathetic autonomic nervous system. Bodywide effects are the result. This fact alone is helpful in explaining the benefits of foot and hand massage.

Many nerve endings on the feet and hands correlate with acupressure points, which, when stimulated, trigger the release of endorphins and other endogenous chemicals. In addition, major plexuses for the lymph system are located in the hands and feet. Compressive forces in these areas stimulate lymphatic movement.

Reflex Phenomena

Reflex phenomena must be put into perspective. The whole body, including the hands, head, ears, and torso, has reflex points. If you consider all the reflexology points, acupuncture points, neurolymphatic points, motor points, and other reflex points, the body can be seen as a point. Because of the reflex nature of the body and the inherent ability for the body to self-regulate in response to stimulation, it is usually not necessary to become too overly focused on a particular system's name and use for a point.

More applicable is the ability to identify these various points during assessment procedures, analysis of the body context of the point, and effective treatment of the point. Assessment usually indicates an area tender to palpation if the point is hypersensitive or the reflex structure associated with the particular point is hyperreactive. The opposite is true if the point area feels empty, numb, or disconnected from the surrounding tissue.

Two basic treatment processes exist. If a reflexive point is tender and therefore likely to be overactive, relaxation and sedating methods are used. If the point is underactive, stimulation methods are applied. If you are not sure which application is appropriate, trust the innate balancing ability of the body. Alternately use both approaches, allowing the body to choose.

The professional can truly become overwhelmed with so many different names for the same phenomenon. The simplicity of the body response patterns is uniquely profound. It is not necessary for complicated methodology to confuse the issue of the generation of healing energy.

Methods of Massage for the Foot

An excellent way to massage the foot is to apply pressure and movement systematically to the entire foot and ankle complex. This pressure will stimulate the circulation, nerves, and reflexes. Moving all the joints stimulates large-diameter nerve fibers and joint mechanoreceptors, initiating hyperstimulation analgesia. The result is a shift in proprioceptive and postural reflexes. The sheer volume of sensory information flooding the central nervous system has significant effects within the body supporting parasympathetic dominance.

Foot massage is usually boundary-safe. Most people will accept foot or hand massage when the idea of removing the clothing is objectionable. Hand and foot massage is likely to be the most effective form of self-massage. The hand and foot have similar motor cortex distribution patterns. The stimulation of the hands during the massage does not override the sensations to the feet being massaged. The hands are massaged while they are massaging the feet (Proficiency Exercise 11-4).

---

box 11-4
REFLEXES ASSOCIATED WITH THE FOOT

Achilles tendon reflex—Plantar flexion/extension of the foot resulting from the contraction of calf muscles following a sharp blow to the Achilles tendon; similar to the knee jerk reflex

Extensor thrust—A quick and brief extension of a limb after application of pressure to the plantar surface

Flexor withdrawal—Flexion of the lower extremity when the foot receives a painful stimulus

Mendel-Bekhterev reflex—Plantar flexion of the toes in response to percussion of the dorsum of the foot

Postural reflex—Any reflex concerned with maintenance of posture

Proprioceptive reflex—Reflex initiated by movement of the body to maintain the position of the moved part; any reflex initiated by stimulation of a proprioceptor

Rossolimos reflex—Plantar flexion of the second to fifth toes in response to percussion of the plantar surface of the toes

---

11-4
PROFICIENCY EXERCISE

1. Exchange foot massages with another student or visit a professional reflexologist for a foot massage. Compare the effects with those of a full-body massage.
2. Using a skeletal model, move each of the joints of the foot. Then move each of the joints of your foot.
3. Massage your feet daily for 15 minutes for a period of 2 weeks and take notice of the effects.

CONNECTIVE TISSUE APPROACHES

section objectives

Using the information presented in this section, the student will be able to perform the following:

- Modify existing massage methods to address the connective tissue more specifically
- Explain the principles of deep transverse friction massage

Methods that affect the connective tissue of the body have been discussed throughout the text. Connective tissue systems range from the very subtle, light work of craniosacral and fascial release concepts, to the very mechanical **deep transverse frictioning** of Cyriax. This section provides specific introductory information about deep transverse friction and myofascial approaches. Refer to Chapter 4, Chapter 5, and Chapter 9, to review previously presented information on connective tissue methodology.

The basic connective tissue approach consists of mechanically softening the tissue through pressure, pulling, movement, and stretch on the tissues, which allows them to rehydrate and become more pliable. The process is similar to softening gelatin by warming it. If you want connective tissue to stay soft, water must be added. This is one reason why it is important for the client to drink water before and after the massage.

Connective Tissue Dysfunctions

People can develop several basic connective tissue dysfunctions. Connective tissue may shorten, lose fluidity, and adhere, causing binding, pulling, and restricted movement. Another common problem is overstretched connective tissue at the joint, resulting in laxity and destabilization of the joint. This sets the stage for protective muscle spasms, causing a reduction in joint space.

It is possible that the normalization of connective tissue will allow the joint to function properly; however, this process may become problematic. The purpose of the connective tissue is to stabilize; and stabilization may require that the joint remain out of optimal alignment. Dr. Gurevich, a Russian physician, explained the pattern of degeneration as usually beginning with dystonia or disruption of tone. (Sometimes a direct trauma to a joint may cause it to misalign, as opposed to increased or decreased muscle tension pulling joints out of alignment.)

Bones are designed to fit at the joint in a specific way. When this fit is disrupted, the next step is a protective muscle spasm, followed by connective tissue reorganization to stabilize the area. Areas of disruption in joint play or joint alignment eventually include a connective tissue component in the dysfunction.

Gurevich taught that the treatment sequence is first massage, including connective tissue approaches, then mobilization (movement of jointed areas within comfortable range of motion), and finally joint manipulation. Massage and mobilization are within the scope of bodywork practice, whereas joint manipulation is not. The services of a chiropractor, osteopath, or other professional trained in joint manipulation are desirable for problems that require direct manipulation of the joint.

Professional experience suggests that the longer the problem has existed, the more mechanical the techniques required initially. Mechanical techniques include all gliding, kneading, skin rolling, and compression styles of bodywork as long as the contact elongates and drags or pulls on the tissue for sustained periods. The connective tissue responds relatively slowly, sometimes taking 60 seconds or longer. Conversely, neuromuscular techniques usually elicit a response in 15 to 30 seconds.

The stretching, pulling, or pressure on the connective tissue is a little different from that of neuromuscular methods. Neuromuscular techniques usually flow in the direction of the fibers to affect the proprioceptive mechanism and create a quick response. Connective tissue approaches are slow and sustained, usually against or across the fibers. Connective tissue stretching is elongated or telescoped at the point of the barrier.[2,3] It is important to induce a small inflammatory process in the dysfunctional area. This process initiates the reorganization of tissue by stimulating tissue repair mechanisms.[5,8]

Another of the body's responses to inflammation is the generation of healing potentials from controlled injury. Injured tissue also yields a current known as the *current of injury*. First detected by Galvani in 1797, this current can encourage healing processes for days until the miniature wound heals.[5] In acupuncture the insertion of a needle into a muscle generates a burst of electrical discharges, which can cause a shortened or hypertonic muscle to relax instantly or within minutes.

Deep Transverse Friction

The most specific localized example of connective tissue work is Dr. James Cyriax's cross-fiber frictioning concept. This method is effective, especially around joints where the tendons and ligaments become bound. Deep transverse friction is always a specific rehabilitation intervention. It introduces therapeutic inflammation through the creation of a specific and controlled re-injury of the tissues. Cyriax asserts that the essential component of a transverse friction massage is that it applies concentrated therapeutic movement over only a very small area. The key element is that friction moves the tissue against its grain[4]:

During treatment by deep friction, great precision in sitting (positioning) of the patient and of the physiotherapist's hand is essential; throughout the session the physiotherapist keeps her mind on her fingertip. This type of work involves her in much more concentration and care than most of her other work. Nothing about it is routine; each patient and each lesion must be assessed and given expert and individual attention.

Although mastery of this type of deep transverse friction is beyond the scope of the technical development of this textbook, it is a valuable form of rehabilitative massage. Any massage practitioner working in a medical setting should be trained in the techniques. The additional skills required are not so much in the delivery of the methods, which are fairly straightforward, but in the assessment of where to friction and how to incorporate it into a comprehensive rehabilitation plan. Specific anatomic knowledge is required for the precision of which Dr. Cyriax speaks.

The frictioning can last as long as 15 minutes to create the controlled re-injury of the tissue, which introduces a small amount of inflammation and traumatic hyperemia to the area. The result is the restructuring of the connective tissue, increased circulation to the area, and temporary analgesia.[4]

Proper rehabilitation after the massage is essential for the friction technique to be effective and produce a mobile scar on re-healing of the tissue. The frictioned area needs to be contracted painlessly without putting any strain on the frictioned tissue. This is done by fixing the joint in a position in which the muscle is relaxed and then having the client contract the muscle as far as it will go. This is sometimes called a *broadening contraction* (Fig. 11-5).

Cyriax asserts the following[4]:

Thus, deep transverse frictions restore mobility to muscle in the same way as manipulation frees a joint. Indeed, the action of deep transverse friction may be summed up as affording a mobilization that passive stretching or active exercises cannot achieve. After the friction has restored a full range of painless broadening to the muscle belly, this added mobility must be maintained. To this end, the patient should perform a series of active contractions with the joint placed in a position that fully relaxes the affected muscle, i.e., the position that allows the greatest broaden-

ing. Strong resisted movement should be avoided until the scar has consolidated itself; otherwise, started too soon they tend to strain the healing breach again.

Methods of Deep Transverse Friction

Cyriax teaches that when massage is given to a muscle, tendon, ligament, or joint capsule, the following principles must be observed:

1. The right spot must be found.
2. The therapist's fingers and the client's skin must move as one. Care must be taken to not cause a blister. The client must understand that deep friction massage to a tender point can be painful.
3. The friction must be given across the fibers composing the affected structure.
4. The friction must be given with sufficient sweep. Pressure only accesses the tender area; it does not replace the friction. Circular friction is not recommended. Only a back-and-forth friction is effective.
5. The friction must reach deep enough. If it does not reach the lesion, it is of no value.
6. The client must be placed in a suitable position that ensures the appropriate degree of tension or relaxation of the tissues to be frictioned.
7. Muscles must be kept relaxed while being frictioned. Because the connective tissue of the muscle is affected, the massage must penetrate into the muscle and not stay on the surface.
8. Tendons with a sheath must be kept taut during friction massage.
9. Broadening contractions are used between sessions to promote circulation and mobile scar development during the healing process.

Using Cyriax's principles, this textbook introduces a modified version of these methods that can be incorporated into a general massage session for small areas of ad-

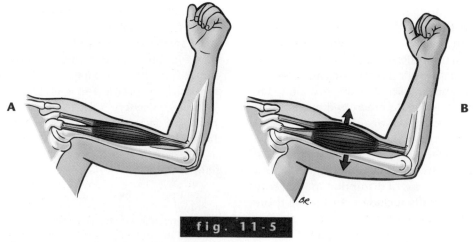

fig. 11-5

Broadening contraction. **A,** Beginning point. **B,** Contract muscle by flexing the joint.

hered tissue. The modified version of deep transverse friction will not have the same effects on an area of adhesion, but the ability to move the tissue in a transverse way may keep the development of adhesions in check when a person develops minor soft tissue tears from overstretching or minor muscle pulls.

To accommodate the lack of precise location about the anatomic structures, the friction suggested is done over a broader area for a shorter time, using the following procedure:

- Locate the area to be frictioned.
- Place the muscle in a relaxed position.
- Provide friction as described in Chapter 9.

Myofascial Approaches

Other forms of connective tissue massage exist. Bindege-webmassage, developed by Elizabeth Dickie, consists of light stokes without oil with a focus on the superficial fascial layer (between the skin and muscles). Rolfing, developed by Ida Rolf, and its various offshoots, such as Hellerwork, are methods of structural integration focused to bring the physical structure of the body into an efficient relationship with the perpendicular alignment of the body in gravity. The focus is normalization and redirection of the deeper fascial components of muscles and fascial sheaths. Osteopathy and physical therapy theory and practice contribute to the body of knowledge for **myofascial approaches.**

These styles of bodywork are often called *deep tissue massage, soft tissue manipulation,* or *myofascial release.* The procedures described in this textbook are only a portion of these systems, and additional training is required to learn these valuable methods in more detail. Craniosacral therapy, which is a subtle connective tissue approach reaching many structures deep within the body, is a valuable technique to perfect. John Barnes' Myofascial Release Seminars and the Upledger Institute's CranioSacral Therapy Seminars are reliable sources of additonal training.

The Nature of Fascia

The nature of connective tissue has been addressed in Chapters 4, 5, 9, and 10. Fascia, which is a form of connective tissue, is the specific focus of myofascial approaches.

Fascia in some form surrounds and separates almost every structure and cell in the body. It forms the interstitial spaces (space between individual cells). Fascia is involved in structural and visceral support, as well as separation and protection, and therefore influences respiration, elimination, metabolism, fluid flow, and the immune systems. Fascia is stress responsive, becoming thicker in response to real or perceived threats, as well as any other activation of the sympathetic autonomic nervous system. This emotional response of this fascial guarding system is sometimes called *body armoring.* It is an important factor in the relationship between body and emotional expression. This factor is often a component of body/mind approaches.

Anatomically, fascia can be classified as superficial or subcutaneous fascia and deep fascia. Superficial fascia lies between the skin and the muscles. Deep fascia surrounding the muscles weaves diagonally through the body, creating fascial sheaths (Chapter 10). Subserous fascia lies between the deep fascia and the membranes lining the body cavities. A deep level of fascia interconnects the cranium, spine, and sacrum, joining the connective tissue coverings of the central nervous system with the unity of the body. These classifications of fascia layering are artificial because fascia is one large, interconnected, three-dimensional microscopic dynamic grid structure that connects everything with everything. Through the fascial system, if you pull on the little toe you affect the nose and if the structure of the nose is dysfunctional it can pull anywhere in the body, including the little toe.

Fascia is loose irregular connective tissue with a loose and multidirectional network of collagen and elastin fibers. Fascia has a large percentage of ground substance. As indicated in Chapter 4, ground substance is thrixtropic and is a colloid substance; therefore fascia has many thrixtropic and colloid qualities.

Although fascia generally orients itself vertically in the body, it will orient in any directional stress pattern. For example, scar tissue may redirect fascial structures, as can trauma, repetitive strain patterns, and immobility. This redirection of structural forces occurs as a result of compensation patterns. During physical assessment the body will appear "pulled" out of symmetry or stuck. There are also three or four transverse fascial planes (depending on the resource you use). Transverse planes exist for joints as well. Adhesions result when fascia attempts to stabilize itself by attaching to surrounding tissue. Stabilizing formations can orient in any direction. Breakdown of the fascial system is a primary factor in the aging process.

Myofascial Dysfunction

Dysfunction in the fascial network compromises the efficiency of the body, requiring an increase in energy expenditure to achieve functioning ability. Fatigue and pain often result. Fascial shortening and thickening restrict movement, and the easy undulation of the expression of the body rhythms and entrainment mechanisms are disturbed. Twists and torsions of the fascia bind and restrict movement from the cellular level outward to joint mobility and easy gait function. This bind can be equated to ill-fitting clothing, or more graphically, "fascial wedgies." The dysfunctions are difficult to diagnose medically, are not apparent with standard medical testing, and are a factor in many elusive chronic pain and fatigue patterns.

Fascial dysfunction is seldom simple and almost always multidimensional, often encompassing body/emotional phenomena because body armoring is an effective coping strategy. Introducing corrective intervention is a therapeutic change process akin to remodeling a house as presented in Chapter 5. If the person is unable to respond effectively to a change process, management approaches can be offered, but effects are more involved in symptom management than structural change.

The methods themselves are deceivingly simple in relationship to the amount of changes that can be experienced. Therefore a solid respect for myofascial approaches is in order. Use them wisely after considering the broader picture of the client's state of being and ability to cope with active change.

Myofascial Methods

In most instances a lubricant is not used during myofascial approaches because the drag quality on the tissue is to be encouraged and lubricant reduces drag.

Methods that affect primarily the ground substance require a quality of slow sustained pressure and agitation. Most massage methods can soften the ground substance as long as the application is not abrupt. Tapotement and abrupt compression are less effective than slow effleurage or gliding methods that have a drag quality. Kneading, petrissage, and skin rolling that incorporates a slow pulling action are effective as well.

The fiber component is affected by stretching methods that elongate the fibers past the normal give of the fiber and enter the plastic range past the bind (see Chapter 9). This creates either a freeing and unraveling of fibers or a small therapeutic (beneficial and controlled) inflammatory response that signals for change in the fibers.

Tissue Movement Methods

The more subtle connective tissue approaches rely on the skilled development of following tissue movement. The process is as follows:

1. Firm but gentle contact is made with the skin.
2. Downward or vertical pressure is increased slowly until resistance is felt. This barrier is soft and subtle.
3. Downward pressure is maintained at this point, and horizontal pressure is added until the resistance barrier is felt again.
4. Sustain the pressure and wait.
5. The tissue will seem to creep, unravel, melt, slide, quiver, twist, or dip, or some other movement sensation will be noticed.
6. Follow the movement, gently maintaining the tension on the tissues, encouraging the pattern as it undulates though various levels of release.

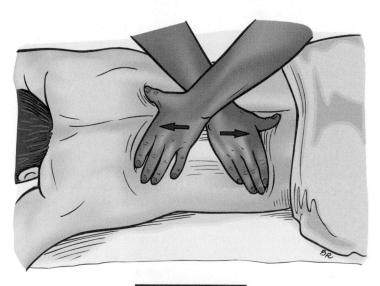

fig. 11-6

Light compressive force is applied, molding the hand to the skin. The hands are then separated without adding additional compressive force, providing for a fascial stretch.

11-5

PROFICIENCY EXERCISE

1. Make some gelatin using only half the required water. Let it set. Massage it into liquid form. Pay attention to the type of massage you use.
2. Get some plastic wrap, and twist and wad it into a ball. Smooth it out. What methods did you need to use?
3. Take the same plastic wrap and pull it. Take out all the slack, and telescope and elongate the tissue. What did you have to do to accomplish the stretch?

7. Close your eyes; do not interpret the process. Become fascinated with the journey. Eventually the tissue will become still.
8. Wait and sustain the stillness.
9. Slowly and gently release first the horizontal force and then the vertical force.

Following tissue movement is simple after the student stops thinking about the process and begins to experience it. A curious result of this type of work is the development of vasomotor responses on parts of the skin not directly addressed during the fascial tissue movement method. Theory suggests that these are areas with internal fascial connections that were pulled during the method. To continue the process, introduce vertical pressure over the vasomotor reddening and begin again.

Fascial Restriction Method

Fascial restriction involves an area larger than a small, localized spot. It is palpated as a barrier or an area of immobility within the tissue. It is worked initially using routine massage techniques. If the area does not release, the pressure must be more specific. The process is as follows:

1. Stabilize the tissue with one hand.
2. With the fingers of the other hand, pull the tissue in the direction of the restriction.
3. Use the heel of the hand or the arm to separate the tissue.
4. Maintain the pressure until a softening occurs.

Twist-and-release petrissage and compression applied in the direction of the restriction can also release these fascial barriers (Fig. 11-6).

The important consideration for all connective massage methods is that the pressure actually moves the tissue, puts tension into it, elongates it, and holds it long enough for energy to build in it and soften it. The development of connective tissue patterns is highly individualized and because of this, systems that follow a precise protocol and sequence are often less effective in dealing with these complex patterns (Proficiency Exercise 11-5).

TRIGGER POINT THERAPY

section objectives

Using the information presented in this section, the student will be able to perform the following:

■ **Describe a trigger point**
■ **Locate a trigger point**
■ **Use two methods to massage a trigger point**

Dr. Janet Travell did extensive research and is considered the foremost authority in myofascial pain involving trigger points.[11] Dr. Leon Chaitow has integrated additional information about trigger point therapy.[2,3] These two experts are the resources for the information in this section about trigger point therapy.

Some confusion exists about the synonymous use of the two terms *neuromuscular therapy* and *trigger point therapy. Neuromuscular therapy* is the umbrella encompassing a variety of treatment approaches, one of which is trigger point therapy. *Trigger point therapy* is one of many techniques useful in the treatment of myofascial problems. As with most of the methods discussed in this chapter, additional training is required by the therapist to become efficient and use trigger point methods more effectively. In general massage applications it is not uncommon to encounter a mild trigger point activity that can be dealt with effectively by using the methods discussed in this section.

Trigger Points

A **trigger point** is an area of local nerve facilitation of a muscle that is aggravated by stress of any sort affecting the body or mind of the individual. Trigger points are small areas of hyperirritability within muscles. If these areas are located near motor nerve points, the patient may experience referred pain caused by nerve stimulation. The area of the trigger point is often the motor point where nerve stimulation initiates a contraction in a small sensitive bundle of muscle fibers that, in turn, activates the entire muscle.[5,7,12]

A trigger point area is often located in a tight band of muscle fibers. Palpation across the band may elicit what is called a *twitch response*, which is a slight jump in the muscle fibers.

Any of the more than 400 muscles can develop trigger points. Accompanying the development of the trigger points is the characteristic referred pain pattern and restriction of motion associated with myofascial pain.

With classic trigger points the referred pain pattern can be traced to its site of origin. The distribution of the referred trigger point pain does not usually follow an entire distribution of a peripheral nerve or dermatomal segment.[8]

Perpetuating Factors

Perpetuating factors to the development of trigger points are reflexive, mechanical, and systemic. Reflexive perpetuating factors include the following:
- Skin sensitivity in the areas of the trigger point
- Joint dysfunction
- Visceral dysfunction in the viscerally referred pain pattern
- Vasoconstriction
- A facilitated nerve segment

Mechanical perpetuating factors include the following:
- Standing postural distortion
- Seated postural distortion
- Gait distortion
- Immobilization
- Vocational stress
- Restrictive or ill-fitting clothing and shoes
- Furniture

Systemic perpetuating factors include the following:
- Enzyme dysfunction
- Metabolic and endocrine dysfunction
- Chronic infection
- Dietary insufficiencies
- Psychologic stress

Assessment for Trigger Points

It is often difficult to decide whether the tender spot is really a trigger point, a point of fascial adhesion requiring friction, a motor point, or some other irritable reflex point, including any active acupuncture points. Because stretching of trigger point areas is essential to effective treatment, if doubt exists regarding the nature of the point, treat it as a trigger point.

The massage therapist usually finds trigger points during palpation or general massage using both light and deep palpation consisting of gliding strokes (Box 11-5). Dr. Chaitow recommends that gliding strokes should cover a region of 2 to 3 inches at a time.

Both Dr. Travell and Dr. Chaitow agree that some pain is elicited during assessment and treatment, but they both recognize that the *pain elicited during treatment should be*

---

box 11-5

PALPATING FOR TRIGGER POINTS

In performing light palpation, the therapist may notice trigger points from the following responses:

Skin changes: The skin may feel tense with resistance to gliding strokes. The skin may be slightly damp as a result of perspiration on the skin from sympathetic facilitation, and the hand will stick or drag on the skin.

Temperature changes: The temperature in a local area increases in acute dysfunction but decreases in ischemia, which indicates fibrotic changes within the tissues.

Edema: Edema is an impression of fullness and congestion within the tissues. In instances of chronic dysfunction, edema is replaced gradually with fibrotic (connective tissue) changes.

Deep palpation: During deep palpation, the therapist establishes contact with the deeper fibers of the soft tissues and explores them for any of the following:
- Immobility
- Tenderness
- Edema
- Deep muscle tension
- Fibrotic changes
- Interosseous changes

---

well within the client's comfort zone. The muscle must be relaxed to be examined effectively. If the pressure is too great, severe local pain may overwhelm the referred pain sensation, making accurate evaluation impossible. Trigger points that are so active that referred pain is already being produced have no need for exaggerated pressure.

Only muscles that can actually be treated at the same visit should be examined. Palpating for trigger points can irritate their referred pain activity, so only areas intended for treatment should be palpated (Fig. 11-7).

Methods for Treating Trigger Points

Trigger point therapy is not to be done for extended periods. Because of the nature of the syndrome and the irritation involved, 15 minutes is a sufficient amount of time to spend on trigger points. On some occasions 30 minutes of therapy can be tolerated, but this should not become a standard practice.

All the basic neuromuscular techniques, including the muscle energy techniques (Chapter 9), deal effectively with trigger points *if* the hyperirritable area within a muscle is hyperstimulated, then lengthened, and the connective tissue in the area softened and stretched. Direct pressure, dry needling (acupuncture), spray and stretch, or ice massage are suggested for trigger areas by Dr. Janet Travell and other professionals in the field. Direct manipulation of proprioceptors by pushing or pulling on a muscle belly or its attachments is also very effective. Positional release with the appropriate stretching is one of the most effective ways to treat trigger points.

After a trigger point has been identified, the massage therapist uses a pressure technique, muscle energy, or a direct manipulation and stretch method to eliminate the point. Positional release and lengthening and direct manipulation are the least invasive and gentlest methods (p. 383). The integrated muscle energy method is more aggressive than positional release or direct manipulation but less aggressive than pressure or pinching methods. These methods often are effective and are worth trying before the more intense pressure or pinching techniques.

As a reminder, positional release consists of identifying the painful point and positioning the body in the easiest position that reduces the pain at the point. Positional release is a first step to the integrated muscle energy method, which then introduces muscle contraction before lengthening (see Chapter 9).

Direct manipulation methods consist of pushing together at the belly of a muscle to affect spindle cells and pushing on tendons to affect tendon receptors. If the belly of the muscle is pressed together and the desired effect is not experienced, the next step should be to separate the tissue from the middle of the muscle belly toward the tendons. The local area must be lengthened. This lengthening is performed either directly on the tissues or through movement of a joint (Fig. 11-8).

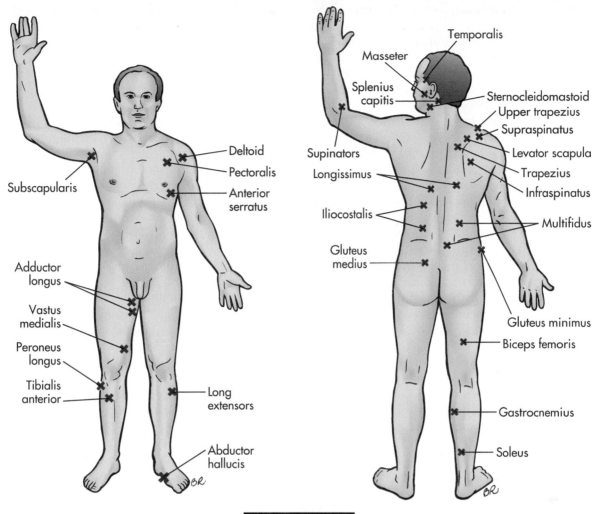

fig. 11-7

Common trigger points.

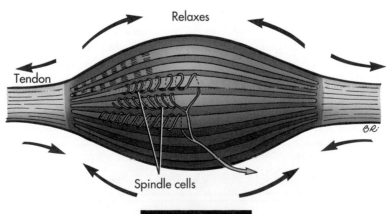

fig. 11-8

Direct manipulation of proprioceptors.

If the trigger point remains after the less invasive methods have been attempted, pressure techniques should be tried. The pressure may take the form of *direct pressure,* in which the trigger point is pressed by the therapist against an underlying hard structure (bone), or *pinching pressure,* when no bony tissue lies underneath, as in the "squeezing" of the sternocleidomastoid muscle.

This process can end the hyperirritability by mechanical disruption of the sensory nerve endings mediating the trigger point activity. When using the direct pressure technique, the therapist must hold the compression long enough to stimulate the spindle cells.[8]

The pressure technique must be done properly. Dr. Travell has pointed out that referred pain is usually sensed by the client within 10 seconds of applied pressure. It is therefore unnecessary to maintain pressure for longer than 10 seconds when trying to locate the trigger.

After the trigger has been located, the *time of applied pressure* will be different than the time used to locate the trigger. Dr. Chaitow recommends a procedure of gradually intensifying pressure, building up to 8 seconds, then repeating the process for up to 30 seconds or as long as 2 minutes. The procedure should end when the client reports the referred pain has stopped or the therapist feels a "release" in the trigger point tissue.

Sufficient duration is determined by the fiber construction of the muscle. Muscles are made up of red or white fibers, which can be slow or fast twitch. The type of fiber a muscle comprises is determined by whether the muscle functions as a postural endurance muscle or a phasic movement muscle and the demands exerted by the client's lifestyle. It is easier to fatigue phasic muscle fibers than endurance muscle fibers. After the muscle is fatigued, a period of recovery ensues in which the fibers will not contract and the muscle can be lengthened effectively and stretched if necessary.

Dr. Chaitow also recommends variable pressure rather than constantly held pressure from beginning to end to avoid further irritation to the trigger area. Students should not misinterpret this idea of variable pressure. It is not a "bouncing" in and out of the tissue but rather a carefully changing pressure for a specific purpose. The pressure used reflects the therapist's sensitivity to what is happening as the tissue responds; the therapist applies more pressure as the tissue shows it is relaxing and accepting more pressure. When the massage therapist senses that the tissues are becoming tense, pressure is decreased.

As an alternative, deep cross-fiber friction over the trigger point can be effective, followed by lengthening and stretching. This method is beneficial if the massage therapist suspects that the connective tissue around the trigger point has become immobile.

Dr. Travell recommends that after treating with pressure methods, the practitioner again stimulate circulation to the local area with circular friction, pétrissage, and/or vibratory massage techniques. Localized treatment of the muscle should always end with lengthening and stretching, whether passive or active, of the affected muscle. Dr. Travell and Dr. Chaitow agree that gradual, gentle lengthening to reset the normal resting length of the neuromuscular mechanism of a muscle and stretching to elongate shortened connective tissue of the treated (involved) muscle must follow any other interventions. Incomplete restoration of the full length of the muscle means incomplete relief of pain. Failure to lengthen and stretch the area results in the eventual return of original symptoms. Muscle energy approaches are more effective than passive stretching in achieving the proper response (see Chapter 9). They enable the muscle to "learn" that it can now return to a fuller resting length and more complete range of motion.

After treatment of a trigger point, the target (referred) area should be searched to uncover and deal with satellite or embryonic triggers. Immediately after treatment, moist heat (hot towel) over the region is soothing and useful. The area will require rest for a few days and avoidance of all stressful activity.[10]

As seen with the previous skills the actual application of trigger point methods is fairly basic. The learned professional's skill is required more in the assessment, decision making concerning appropriateness and intensity of treatment, and choice of methods. As with myofascial approach methods, the application of treatment protocols is deceivingly simple, especially when used with a client who has a multifaceted and complex situation. Often multiple methods are required in these situations. Trigger point release is a good example of an integration of multiple methods because effective intervention uses multiple techniques, massage manipulations, muscle energy methods, stretching methods, and hydrotherapy methods (Proficiency Exercise 11-6).

---

1 1 - 6
PROFICIENCY EXERCISE

1. Place a dried pea under a half-inch piece of foam. Locate the pea with light and deep palpation.
2. Working with a partner, use light palpation to locate an area of suspected trigger point activity. After an area is found, use deep palpation to find the exact area of the trigger point. Then use the methods described in this section to normalize the area.

ACUPUNCTURE

section objectives

Using the information presented in this section, the student will be able to perform the following:

- Explain the basic physiology of acupuncture points and the effects of acupuncture
- Locate an acupuncture point
- Use simple methods to stimulate acupuncture points

The richness of Oriental health theory and the unity of its body/mind/spirit connection is based on the energy of life. Life force called *Ch'i energy* flows through the body through interconnected pathways as water flows through the streams, rivers, lakes, and oceans of the earth. When Ch'i energy flows through the body like pure water, all of life's processes are balanced. However, if obstruction or stagnation in the life force develops, it becomes the basis for disease.

The Tao, or "Way," supports the balanced function of all the senses and teaches a lifestyle of moderation that avoids both depravation and excess. Ch'i energy is the vital force of life and Tao is the path or way to sustain the Ch'i energy.

Concern is expressed in the taking of pieces from the totality of being expressed in the Tao. Western science has lifted technique from this simultaneously simple but complex all-encompassing system. Very often, technique separated from its theoretical basis is less effective. Although technique can stimulate physiologic functions, it cannot support the human experience. The small section presented in this textbook is based on a very limited part of the total Oriental medicine system. As you begin to develop an understanding of these methods, be mindful and respectful concerning the larger structure of the body of knowledge from which they have been taken.

Many bodywork systems have evolved from this thought. Shiatsu (finger pressure) from Japan is the most familiar Oriental bodywork system. Shiatsu and acupressure are sometimes considered the same method. However, Shiatsu is much broader in its application of methods and diagnosis. Basically, Shiatsu is a form of Oriental massage in which the fingers are pressed on particular points of the body to ease aches, pain, tension, fatigue, and symptoms of disease.[9,10,12] The points are called *tsubo* or acupuncture points and are located along meridians described later in this section. One distinguishing method of Shiatsu diagnosis is through areas on the *Hara* (abdomen or center) and the back. Pressure in these areas or along the meridians identify energy (in Japan, *Ki*) flow as either *kyo* (under energy) and *jitsu* (over energy). Shiatsu restores balance by sedating the jitsu and strengthening or stimulating (toning) the kyo.

Acupuncture is becoming accepted by Western science.

It is one branch of Chinese medicine that has been proven effective in the treatment of many diseases and dysfunctions. The exact origin of acupuncture is unknown. Although it remains a mystery in some respects, Western science is close to validating its phenomena. Whatever physiologic factors underlie acupuncture, the beneficial changes that occur clearly are a sound basis for acupressure treatment.

Acupuncture can be defined as the stimulation of certain points with needles inserted along the meridians (channels) and "AhShi" (meaning ouch) points outside the meridians. AhShi and traditional acupuncture points have a high degree of correlation to trigger points. The purpose of acupuncture is to prevent and modify the perception of pain (analgesia) or normalize physiologic functions.

Acupressure is a modified version of acupuncture that substitutes pressure for needle insertion. The effects of acupressure are not as dramatic as those of acupuncture but are still effective, especially if repeated often with the pressure held long enough. There are hundreds of acupuncture points in the human body, with approximately 360 of the most used points located on 12 paired and 2 unpaired centrally located meridians.

Meridians

According to Chinese theory, the meridians are internally associated with organs and externally associated with the surface of the head, trunk, and extremities. Meridians seem to be energy flows from nerve tracts in the tissue and are located in the fascial grooves.[5]

Yin and Yang

The Oriental perspective considers body functions in terms of balance between complementary forces. These complements, which are often thought of as opposites, are actually a portion of a continuum. A circle is a good example: no matter where you stand on a circle you can look across and see the other side. In this idea of duality, we often forget that a circle is one concept; it is broken into sections only through the limitation of our perceptions.

Yin and yang are representations of the above concept. Yin and yang functions are complementary pieces of the whole (Fig. 11-9). When functioning equally and in harmony, the natural balance of health exists in all areas of

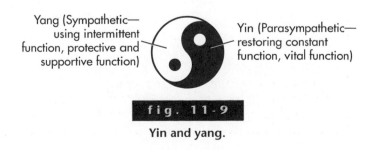

Yang (Sympathetic—using intermittent function, protective and supportive function)

Yin (Parasympathetic—restoring constant function, vital function)

fig. 11-9

Yin and yang.

the body, mind, and spirit. Conversely, if part of the continuum becomes out of sync with the rest, stress is put on the entire circle. Thus imbalances and symptoms might occur in many areas.

The body is physiologically a closed system. There cannot be areas of "too much" energy in the body without reciprocal areas of "not enough" energy. Just as muscles work in pairs and facilitate and inhibit each other, so do meridians. There are yin meridians or channels and yang meridians or channels.

Yin meridians are associated with parasympathetic autonomic nervous system responses and functions of the solid organs essential to life (e.g., the heart). The energy is considered "female" or of a negative charge. (Terminology

and metaphor tend to become confused with the terms *female* and *negative*. In this context the terms mean the functions draw energy of sustenance and nurturing in and restore or reproduce.) Yin meridians are located on the inside soft areas of the body and flow from the feet up (Chinese anatomic position with arms lifted into the air).

Yang meridians are associated with sympathetic autonomic nervous system responses and hollow organs whose functions are supportive to life, but not essential (e.g., the stomach). The energy is considered "male" and a "positive" charge. (Again, in metaphor these terms mean that the energy of transformation and transportation is expended in short bursts as necessary and moves out from the body). Oriental philosophy teaches that a balance

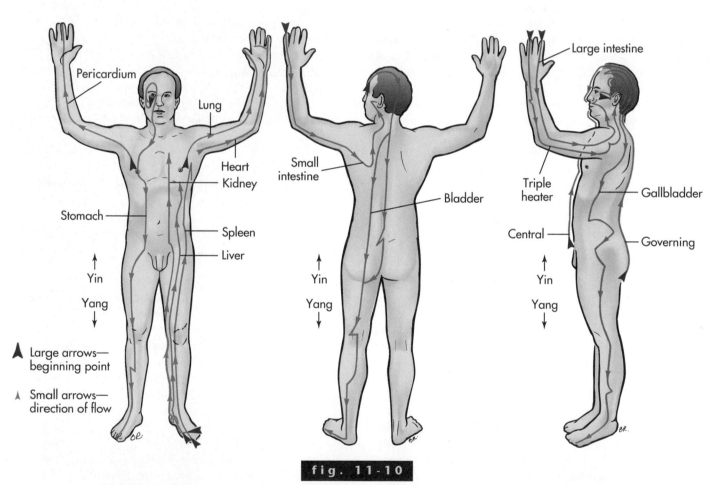

fig. 11-10

Typical location of meridians. Meridians tend to follow nerves. Yin and yang meridians are paired as follows:

Yin meridian	*Yang meridian*
Pericardium	Triple Heater
Liver	Gallbladder
Kidney	Bladder
Heart	Small intestine
Spleen	Stomach
Lung	Large intestine

must exist between the forces of yin and yang for health to exist. This balance changes according to the weather, seasons, and other rhythms of nature (Fig. 11-10).

The Five Elements

Chinese medical thinking is based on the relationship of the human being with nature. The five elements of nature become a basis for examination, diagnosis, and treatment to support health and relieve disease. The concepts of health parallel natural occurrences of life force energy as represented in the five elements. The five elements are wood, fire, earth, metal, and water. Each organ is represented by an element and each element has qualities of colors, sounds, smells, fluid secretion, anatomy, emotions, time, seasons, numbers, flavor, foods, planets, moon phases, dreams, and more (Fig. 11-11).

The human being is a reflection of the universe, and the five elements become a metaphor for the life processes of people. Qualities of the five elements become the basis for life. In Oriental medicine the five elements are the basis for diagnosis and treatment.

The vastness of this model and its elegance is far beyond the scope of this textbook. Therefore no attempt is made to present scaled-down versions of these systems. The student is referred to the reference list for further study. Students who are drawn to these concepts are en-

couraged to explore them in depth as they continue their path of knowledge.

During the natural course of therapeutic massage the physical aspects of these meridians and points are addressed. The next section investigates briefly methods to incorporate with therapeutic massage.

Location of Acupuncture Points

Acupuncture points usually lie in a fascial division between muscles and near origins and insertions. A point feels like a small hole, and pressure elicits a "nervy" feeling. Unlike a trigger point, which may only be found on one side of the body, acupuncture points are bilateral (i.e., located on both sides of the body) and located on the central or governing meridian. To confirm the location of an acupuncture point, locate the point in the same place on the other side of the body.

Methods of Treatment of Acupuncture Points

To stimulate a hypoactive (not enough energy) acupuncture point, use a short vibrating or tapping action. This method is used if the area is sluggish or a specific body function needs stimulation.

To sedate a hyperactive (too much energy) acupuncture

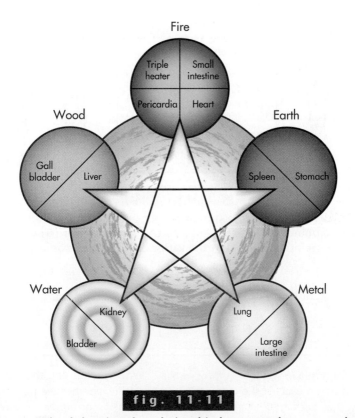

fig. 11-11

Five-element wheel showing the relationship between elements and organs.

point for pain reduction, elicit the pain response within the point itself. Use a sustained holding pressure until the painful over-energy dissipates and the body's own natural painkillers are released into the bloodstream. The pressure techniques are similar to those used for trigger points, but it is not necessary to lengthen and stretch an acupuncture point after treatment.

As with other reflex points, if you are unsure as to the nature of the hypoactive or hyperactive state of the acupuncture point, alternately apply both techniques and allow the body to adjust to the intervention.

It is often difficult to determine whether you are dealing with a trigger point or an acupressure point because the two often overlap. It may be wise to lengthen and

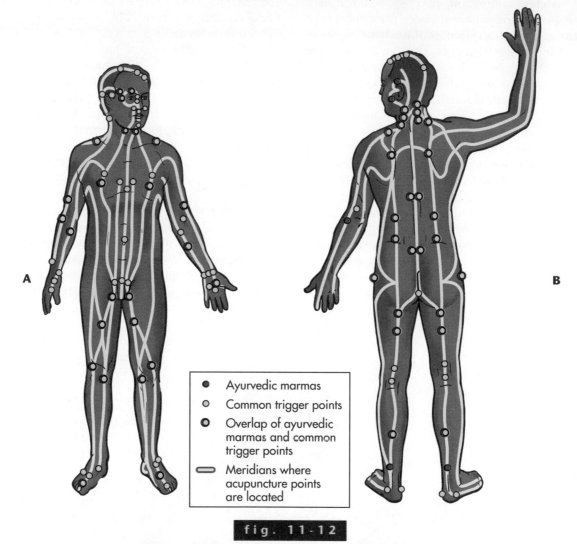

- ● Ayurvedic marmas
- ○ Common trigger points
- ◉ Overlap of ayurvedic marmas and common trigger points
- ⬭ Meridians where acupuncture points are located

fig. 11-12

Comparison of Ayurvedic marmas, common trigger points, and traditional meridians where acupuncture points are located. Anterior **(A)** and posterior **(B)** view of overlapping locations of various points suggest that the various points share common anatomy and physiology.

11-7
PROFICIENCY EXERCISE

1. Working with a partner, perform a massage that incorporates running the hand down each of the meridian grooves in the body. Stop at each hole or point you feel.

2. When performing this massage and locating a point, decide whether the point needs to be stimulated with vibration or tapping or sedated with sustained direct pressure. How did you decide?

stretch the area gently after the use of direct pressure methods. The process does not interfere with the effect on the acupressure point, but without it a trigger point cannot be treated effectively (Proficiency Exercise 11-7).

AYURVEDA

section objective

Using the information presented in this section, the student will be able to perform the following:

■ Identify and understand introductory Ayurvedic terminology

Ayurveda is a system of health and medicine that was developed in India. The foundation of its theory base is similar to Oriental systems. As with all the complementary systems presented in this chapter, Ayurveda is a distinct and rich body of knowledge on its own. The language of Ayurveda is being used more often in Western society, and students should be familiar with some of the terms used to describe Ayurvedic principles of thought.

Ayurveda means life knowledge or right living. Ayurveda is grounded as a body/mind/spirit system in the Vedic scriptures. The tridosha theory is unique to this system. A dosha is a body chemical pattern. When the doshas combine, they constitute the nature of every living organism. The three doshas are Vata (wind), Pitta (bile), and Kapha (mucus). These three combine to form five elements (similar to Oriental theory) of ether, air, fire, water, and earth.

Bones, flesh, skin, and nerves belong to the *earth element*. Semen, blood, fat, urine, mucus, saliva, and lymph belong to the *water element*. Hunger, thirst, temperature, sleep, intelligence, anger, hate, jealously, and radiance belong to the *fire element*. All movement, breathing, natural urges, sensory and motor functions, secretions, excretions, and transformation of tissues belong to the *air element*. Love, shyness, fear, and attachment belong to the *ether element*.

People display temperament based on the degree of influence or dominance of a particular dosha. This is considered an inherited genetic quality and influences a person through his or her entire life. The balance of function within the dosha system equates to health.

The points connected with this system are called *Marmas*. About 100 of these points exist, and they are concentrated at the junctions of muscles, vessels, ligaments, bones, and joints. These junctions form the seat of vital life force (in India, *Prana*). Marmas have a strong correlation to common trigger points and the location of the traditional meridians (Fig. 11-12).

In Ayurveda, Chakras are considered the seven centers of the Prana located along the spinal column, interrelated with the nervous system and endocrine glands. These are subtle centers of consciousness that are the link between the universal source of intelligence and the human body. The massage methods of Ayurveda are tapping, kneading, rubbing, and squeezing. The use of specialized oil preparations is integral to the systems.[6]

POLARITY THERAPY

section objectives

Using the information presented in this section, the student will be able to perform the following:

■ Explain the basic theory of polarity therapy
■ Incorporate the principles of polarity therapy into the massage session

Polarity is a holistic health practice that encompasses some of the theory base of Oriental medicine and Ayurveda. Polarity therapy was developed by Dr. Randolph Stone in the middle 1900s. It is an eclectic, multi-faceted system.

Life force energy (Ch'i, Ki, Prana) has not been a popular subject of Western scientific research. The abstract quality and esoteric nature of the concept is still primarily held in the knowledge base of "spiritual truth." Many spiritual disciplines practice the "laying on of hands." Polarity therapy is also a respectful, compassionate, and intentional laying of the hands on the body.

A physiologic explanation can be postulated as to the result of this therapeutic "laying on of hands" process. Entrainment is one of the most plausible of the physiologic responses. Some polarity techniques involve rocking motions; therefore all physiologic benefits of rocking as discussed in Chapter 9 apply. Gentle stimulation by polarity methods to the joint receptors generate reflex responses to the associated muscles.

As with all methods of healing touch, something exists beyond the physiologic explanation for the benefit. This "something" is intangible but very real in the experience of it. Therein remains the mystery.

The bodywork principles of polarity blend easily with massage and will be briefly explored. The intention of the touch is the same as that of therapeutic massage, explained in Chapters 1 and 2 and as a theme throughout this text. Nothing is ever forced. The experience belongs to the client. The practitioner offers the methods not by protocol but through a practiced development of decision making, guided by intuition. When there is no attachment to the outcome on the part of the professional for his or her own individual sense of achievement, the methods become "free" to influence the experience of the client.

As discussed in previous sections of this chapter, the application of polarity methods are simple. However, the ability to deliver the methods in a purposeful and individualized way, detached from expectation, but fascinated with the outcome, is a goal of advanced learning. Eventually one learns that the more complex the client situation, the simpler the methods used. Because of its simplicity, polarity is one of the gifts to bodywork.

Principles and Applications of Polarity Therapy

The purpose of polarity therapy is to locate blocked energy and, by using the principles outlined here, release it. When blocked energy is released, body systems and organs can function normally and healing can take place naturally.

Polarity therapy does not treat illness or disease; it affects the body (life) energy, which flows in invisible electromagnetic currents through the body's organs and tissues. Instead, it stimulates the energy that is inactive in a diseased body part. The following principles apply:

1. The head and spinal column form the central neutral (0) energy axis of the body.
2. Long vertical currents of energy travel from head to foot on the right side of the body flowing down the front and up the back. Positive (+) outward energy is expressed through the right side.

   The right side represents the following:
   Warmth
   Heat
   Sun
   Yang
   Positive, expanding energy
3. On the left side of the body, the vertical currents flow up the front and down the back. Negative (−) inward energy is expressed through the left side.

   The left side represents the following:
   Cooling
   Contracting
   Moon
   Yin
   Negative, receptive energy
4. There are five electromagnetic currents on each side

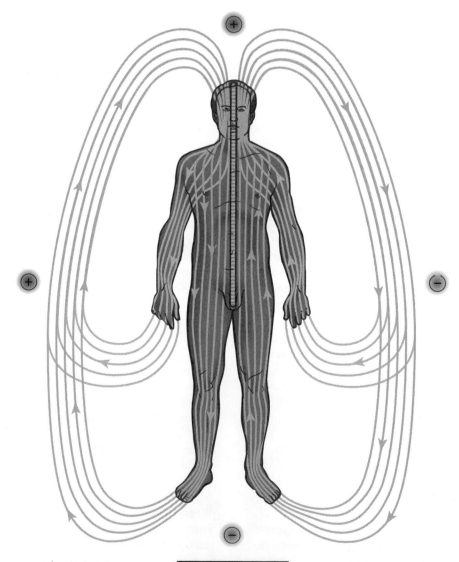

fig. 11-13

Electromagnetic currents travelling vertically on the body.

of the body. Each current is related to an element. The elements are ether, air, fire, water, and earth. The currents relate to the organs and functions of its area (Fig. 11-13).

The Five Major Body Currents

The five major body currents are ether, air, fire, water, and earth.

Ether is associated with hearing, the voice, the throat, and the quality of nothingness.

The core current of the torso flows from north to south (head to pelvis to back). The ether element represents pure vibration and responds to gentleness and love.

Color: sky blue
Sense: hearing
Food: pure air

Air is associated with respiration, circulation, and the heart, lungs, and speed. It flows from east to west (from front to back in a circular pattern). With a balanced air element, we are calm and relaxed.

Color: emerald green
Sense: touch
Food: fruits and nuts

Fire is associated with digestion, the stomach, the bowels, warmth, and the heat of the body. A diagonal current found on both sides of the body, it starts at the shoulders and goes to the opposite hip. It is part of the figure-eight energy and is activated by touch, food, and exercise.

Color: yellow
Sense: sight
Food: grains

Water is associated with generative power, creativity, the pelvic organs, sexuality, glandular secretions, emotional drive, equilibrium, and balance. A long current that splits the body in half, it extends from the head to foot, including the arms and legs. The right side moves clockwise, the left side counterclockwise.

Color: orange
Sense: taste
Food: leafy green vegetables, seaweed, watery foods

Earth is associated with the elimination of solids and liquids, the bladder, the rectum, the formation of bone, structure, and support. A zigzag current is solid straight lines from one side to the other.

Color: red
Sense: smell
Food: tubers, meat, dairy

Each electromagnetic current—ether, air, fire, water, and earth—passes through a corresponding finger and toe, giving its name to the finger and toe; e.g., the middle finger, or the fire finger (Fig. 11-14).

The polarity (positive [+] or negative [−]) of these electromagnetic currents is shown in Fig. 11-14. Positive and negative are opposites. The use of positive and negative labels is only relative; it is a way of showing relationships.

The right side of the body is positive (+), whereas the left side of the body is negative (−). The head is positive, whereas the feet are negative. The front of the body is positive, whereas the back is negative. The top is positive, whereas the bottom is negative. Each joint is neutral and is a crossover for energy currents, which change polarity at the crossover. The neutrality of the joints allows them to be flexible. Each finger and toe has an individual polarity (see Fig. 11-14).

Blocked energy usually registers as soreness, tenderness, or pain. A simple way to bring energy to an area where it is blocked is to place your left hand on the pain and your right hand opposite that area—on the back, front, or side of the body. This principle is used in many techniques such as pelvic release or in the treatment of back pain.

Reflexes

Reflexes are points along an energy current that connect with other points along that current. When stimulated, a reflex point can affect the other reflexes on the same energy path. Manipulations that stimulate the foot and hand poles use the reflex principles located there (Fig. 11-15).

Positive and Negative Contacts

Because all polarity contacts are bipolar, it is necessary to have both hands in contact with the body so that energy can move from one hand to the other through the blockage. If the energy block is on the front of the body, place the left hand over the painful, blocked area and the right hand on the back of the body directly opposite the left hand. This double contact will draw energy through the body from front to back, side to side, and top to bottom contacts.

In practice a positive contact (e.g., the right hand, or fire finger) activates and gives energy. The opposite is also

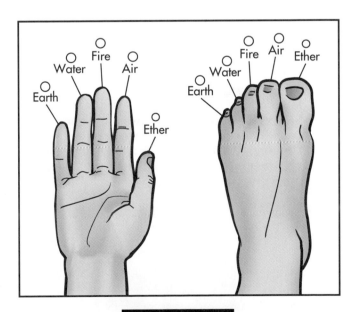

fig. 11-14

The finger and toe chart.

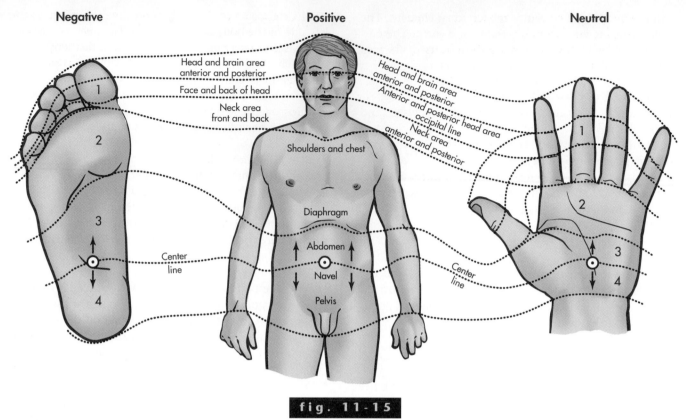

Negative

Positive

Neutral

Head and brain area anterior and posterior

Face and back of head

Neck area front and back

Shoulders and chest

Diaphragm

Abdomen

Navel

Pelvis

Center line

Head and brain area anterior and posterior

Anterior and posterior head area

occipital line

Neck area anterior and posterior

Center line

fig. 11-15

Reflex relationships among hand, foot, and body.

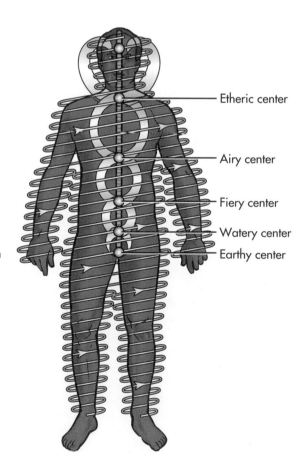

Etheric center

Airy center

Fiery center

Watery center

Earthy center

fig. 11-16

Brain wave currents criss-crossing the spine from the brain to the coccyx. These currents resemble the Caduceus, the ancient Greek symbol for medicine. Each crossover point is known as a *chakra*, or *energy center*.

true—a negative contact (e.g., the left hand, or air finger) is relaxing and receives energy.

Fig. 11-15 illustrates the foot reflexes as they relate to the rest of the body. In addition to those in the feet, there are reflexes in the hands, arms, legs, and head. Alternately stimulating a reflex and its corresponding body part can free blocked energy and allow normal functioning.

The negative poles of the body are most frequently obstructed. The negative pole is stimulated first, then the positive pole, to send currents over the entire body.

Using diagonal contacts on the body activates the serpentine brain wave currents illustrated in Fig. 11-16.

How to Apply a Polarity Method

- With most procedures, stimulate the area (rub briskly) for a few minutes, then hold and feel the energy. Hold for 30 to 60 seconds. If after stimulating for 2 minutes you feel no energy, hold for 1 minute longer and then move on.
- When possible, keep the client's body centered between your hands.
- Be careful not to cross your hands on your client's body.
- When stimulating points, use the fleshy pads of your fingers.
- Be gentle; never force. Forcing creates tension, which blocks energy. A light, gentle touch moves energy.
- When you feel the energy, the blocked energy is released. Life energy has intelligence. After it is moving, it knows what to do and where to go.
- People heal at different rates; therefore don't expect a physical result after completion of a procedure. Be neutral when working with a client. Don't let your expectations be a part of the energy.
- If the manipulations are ineffective, place your hand on your client's body and send love. Visualize energy flowing through your hands to your client (Proficiency Exercise 11-8).

11-8
PROFICIENCY EXERCISE

1. Design three original massage sessions that incorporate a principle from each topic covered in this chapter.
2. Exchange massage with three students using one of the massage sessions developed in this chapter.
3. While giving 10 general massages to "practice clients," mentally note each time you use one of the methods in this chapter.
4. Using professional journals and massage school catalogs, find a continuing education opportunity for each method discussed in this chapter.

SUMMARY

The addition of these methods to the massage professional's skills can provide a more specific focus during the massage. For example, a client could enjoy a relaxing foot bath and sip a cup of hot tea while waiting for the appointment. The client and the massage therapist may drink a glass of pure water together. A cold compress could be placed on the back of the neck, forehead, or other area of the body during the massage.

Use of effleurage could be focused to move lymph and blood in the veins, whereas compression could move down the arteries to stimulate arterial blood flow.

Effleurage, specifically applied into the grooves of the body, may stimulate the meridians. Compression, vibration, and tapping of the acupuncture points may normalize body function.

Petrissage, stretching, and friction methods applied slowly and deliberately to drag, pull, and elongate might soften and normalize the connective tissue.

The occasional trigger point might be treated with direct pressure or friction, with a hot compress applied afterward. An ice pack may sometimes be a better choice after friction to control the amount of inflammation.

Every joint in the hands and feet may be moved and attention given to compression on the bottoms of the hands and feet to stimulate lymphatic flow. The client can be instructed in deep breathing to further encourage lymph movement.

Awareness of the energy patterns of the body and the compassionate "laying on of hands" becomes part of every technique.

As a result of the massage interaction, the client should experience a pleasant, relaxed, and alert state in response to the physiologic shifts in the body.

Each bodywork system is complete within itself; however, extensive overlap exists in both the application of techniques and physiologic effects. Although further study of the methods presented will benefit the massage professional, the ability to become proficient in the application of any of the systems, including therapeutic massage, is a life-long study. Just as studying a foreign language tends to improve proficiency in a person's primary language, the study of bodywork systems complementary to therapeutic massage improves the understanding and technical application of massage modalities. All bodywork systems are forms of structured professional touch complementing, not replacing, each other.

REFERENCES

1. Buchman DD: *The complete book of water therapy: 500 ways to use our oldest natural medicine,* New York, 1979, E.P. Dutton.
2. Chaitow L: *Soft-tissue manipulation,* Rochester, Vt., 1988, Healing Arts Press.

3. Chaitow L: Workshop notes, Lapeer, Mich. 1988, 1991, 1992, 1993.

4. Cyriax J, Coldham M: *The textbook of orthopaedic medicine treatment by manipulation massage and injection,* vol 2, ed 11, East Sussex, England, 1984, Bailliere Tindall.

5. Gunn C: *Reprints on pain, acupuncture and related subjects,* Seattle, 1992, University of Washington.

6. Johari H: *Ayurvedic massage: traditional Indian techniques for balancing body and mind,* Rochester, Vt., 1996, Healing Arts Press.

7. Kreighbaum E, Barthels KM: *Biomechanics: A qualitative approach for studying human movement,* ed 2, New York, 1985, Macmillan.

8. Lederman E: *Fundamentals of manual therapy: physiology, neurology, and psychology,* New York, 1997, Churchill Livingstone.

9. Masunaga S, Ohashi W: *Zen shiatsu: how to harmonize yin and yang for better health,* New York, 1997, Japan Publications.

10. Ohashi W: *Do-it-yourself shiatsu: how to perform the ancient Japanese art of acupuncture without needles,* New York, 1976, Penguin Books.

11. Travell JG, Simons DG: *Myofascial pain and dysfunction: the trigger point manual,* Baltimore, 1983, Williams and Wilkins.

12. Yao JH: *Acutherapy,* 1984, Acutherapy Postgraduate Seminars, 808 Paddock Lane Libertyville, Il. 60048.

WORKBOOK SECTION

Short Answer

1. Why is continuing education required to use the methods presented in this chapter effectively?

   _____

   _____

   _____

   _____

2. What are the primary effects of hydrotherapy?

   _____

   _____

   _____

   _____

3. What are some simple hydrotherapy methods that the massage practitioner can use that do not require special hydrotherapy equipment?

   _____

   _____

   _____

   _____

4. What are some important contraindications and precautions for the use of ice?

   _____

   _____

   _____

   _____

5. What is systemic massage and what results can be expected from this type of massage?

   _____

   _____

   _____

   _____

6. What are the basic procedures for lymphatic massage?

   _____

   _____

   _____

   _____

7. What are the basic procedures for circulation massage?

   _____

   _____

   _____

   _____

8. What are the physiologic mechanisms that make reflexology a valuable massage approach?

   _____

   _____

   _____

   _____

9. What are the recommended methods for foot massage?

   _____

   _____

   _____

   _____

10. Why is hand and foot self-massage beneficial?

   _____

   _____

   _____

   _____

11. What are connective tissue approaches?

   _____

   _____

   _____

   _____

WORKBOOK SECTION

12. What is the intent of connective tissue massage?

_____

_____

_____

13. Why is additional education so important before using connective tissue approaches?

_____

_____

_____

14. What is a trigger point?

_____

_____

_____

15. How are trigger points located?

_____

_____

_____

_____

16. What methods are used to normalize trigger points?

_____

_____

_____

17. After the treatment of a trigger point, what types of therapy follow?

_____

_____

_____

_____

18. What is the Western terminology for acupuncture points, meridians, and yin and yang?

_____

_____

_____

19. What wisdom do the Eastern approaches offer for the massage practitioner?

_____

_____

_____

20. Where are acupuncture points located?

_____

_____

_____

21. How are acupuncture points treated?

_____

_____

_____

22. How does polarity therapy combine the knowledge base of both Oriental and Ayurvedic systems?

_____

_____

_____

23. How can the principles of the therapeutic methods presented in this chapter be integrated into a massage?

_____

_____

_____

_____

WORKBOOK SECTION

Matching

Match the term to the best definition.

1. Acupressure _____

2. Ayurveda _____

3. Cryotherapy _____

4. Hydrotherapy _____

5. Myofascial release _____

6. Polarity therapy _____

7. Reflexology _____

8. Shiatsu _____

9. Systemic massage _____

10. Trigger point _____

11. Yang _____

12. Yin _____

a. the portion of the whole realm of function of the body, mind, and spirit of Eastern thought that corresponds with parasympathetic autonomic nervous system functions.

b. the portion of the whole realm of function of the body, mind, and spirit of Eastern thought that corresponds with sympathetic autonomic nervous system functions.

c. an area of local nerve facilitation resulting in hypertonicity of a muscle bundle and referred pain patterns.

d. therapeutic use of various types and temperatures of water applications.

e. methods used to tone or sedate acupuncture points without the use of needles.

f. a system of health case that uniquely developed the tri-dosha system.

g. the therapeutic use of ice.

h. massage primarily structured to affect one body system. This approach is usually used for lymphatic and circulation enhancement massage.

i. a system of bodywork that affects the connective tissue of the body through various methods that elongate and alter the plastic component and ground matrix of the connective tissue.

j. an eclectic system that combines principles of Oriental theory and Ayurveda.

k. a massage system directed primarily to the feet and hands.

l. an acupressure- and meridian-focused bodywork system.

WORKBOOK SECTION

Various reflexes are associated with the feet. Match the reflex with the description.

1. Achilles tendon reflex _____

2. Extensor thrust _____

3. Flexor withdrawal _____

4. Mendel-Bekhterev _____

5. Postural reflex _____

6. Rossolimos reflex _____

7. Proprioceptive _____

a. plantar flexion/extension of the foot resulting from contraction of calf muscles following a sharp blow to the Achilles tendon. Similar to the knee-jerk reflex.

b. flexion of the lower extremity when the foot receives a painful stimulus.

c. plantar flexion of the toes in response to percussion of the dorsum of the foot.

d. a quick and brief extension of a limb on application of pressure to the plantar surface.

e. reflex initiated by movement of the body to maintain the position of the moved part. Any reflex initiated by stimulation of a proprioceptor.

f. any reflex that is concerned with maintenance of posture.

g. plantar flexion of second to fifth toes in response to percussion of the plantar surface of the toes.

WORKBOOK SECTION

Labeling

Label the correct muscle names to show the locations of common trigger points in Fig. 11-17.

A. Abductor hallucis

B. Adductor longus

C. Anterior serratus

D. Biceps femoris

E. Deltoid

F. Gastrocnemius

G. Gluteus medius

H. Gluteus minimus

I. Iliocostalis

J. Infraspinatus

K. Levator

L. Long extensors

M. Longissiums

N. Masseter

O. Multifidus

P. Pectoralis

Q. Peroneus longus

R. Soleus

S. Splenius capitis

T. Sternocleidomastoid

U. Subscapularis

V. Supinators

W. Supraspinatus

X. Temporalis

Y. Tibialis anterior

Z. Trapezius

AA. Upper trapezius

BB. Vastus medialis

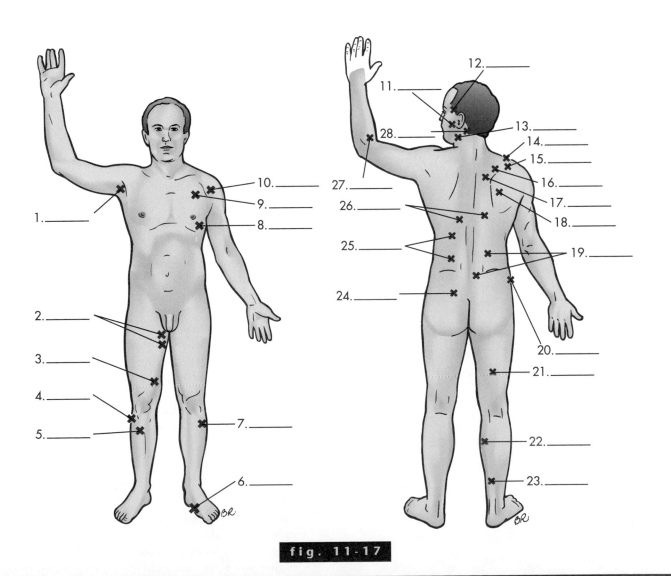

fig. 11-17

WORKBOOK SECTION

Additional Exercise

When using hydrotherapy, the effects of the various forms and temperatures must be known so that the desired results can be achieved. Read the results on the left side, then place an X in the correct columns to match with proper form and temperature. Some of the effects will show up in more than one answer.

	Effects of heat	Effects of cold	Effects of ice
1. Increased circulation			
2. Decreased circulation			
3. Increased metabolism			
4. Decreased metabolism			
5. Increased stimulation			
6. Increased inflammation			
7. Decreased inflammation			
8. Decreased pain			
9. Decreased muscle spasm			
10. Decreased tissue stiffness			
11. Increased tissue stiffness			
12. Increased muscle tone			

Problem-Solving Exercises

1. How can you tell the difference between a trigger point and an acupuncture point?

   _____

   _____

   _____

   _____

2. A client wants a general relaxation massage but has some mild circulatory sluggishness. What style of massage would you use to best serve the client?

   _____

   _____

   _____

   _____

Professional Application

1. You are a massage therapist who has been in practice for about 3 years. An increasing number of your clients seem to have connective tissue problems. What types of continuing education would help you to work most efficiently with these clients?

   _____

   _____

   _____

   _____

2. You find yourself with a job opportunity working in a pain management clinic with a team of health care professionals that consists of an osteopathic physician, nurse practitioner, psychologist, physical therapist, acupuncturist, and nutritionist. Based on the information in this chapter, develop a presentation concerning the integration of complementary bodywork modalities with massage therapy. (Use a separate piece of paper.) Include recommendations for additional education for yourself. Justify or explain the benefit of continuing education in one of the modalities in this chapter. Explain why you think this modality would offer the most benefit combined with therapeutic massage. Also consider what other modalities the other bodywork professionals may be using in the clinic. Use the clinical reasoning model as you prepare your presentation.

ANSWER KEY
Short Answer

1. Each method has so much to offer, it is impossible to provide a thorough study in the few pages devoted here, when a book could be written on each topic. A higher skill level is attained with concentrated study.

WORKBOOK SECTION

This chapter provides only a sample so that students can try the methods and more purposefully choose the focus of future study. An entry-level course of approximately 500 class hours is not enough class time to adequately cover these methods.

2. The effects are mainly reflexive and focus on the autonomic nervous system. The addition of heat energy or dissipation of heat from the tissue may be classified as mechanical in effect. In general cold stimulates sympathetic responses and heat activates parasympathetic responses. Short and long applications of hot or cold produce different results. Most short, cold applications stimulate and increase circulation. Long, cold applications depress and decrease circulation. A short application of heat depresses and depletes tone, whereas a long, hot application results in a combined depressant and stimulant reaction.

3. Hot and cold compresses can be used. A foot bath is easy to incorporate. A bag of frozen peas makes a great ice pack. Hot water bottles are safer to use than heating pads. Water frozen in a paper cup with a stick in it makes an effective ice massage tool. Pure drinking water for clients and yourself is also an excellent hydrotherapy method.

4. The following conditions contraindicate the use of ice: vasospastic disease, cold hypersensitivity, cardiac disorder, compromised local circulation, rheumatoid conditions, an area of paralysis, and coronary artery disease. When using ice, it is important to consider the following precautions:
   - Do not use frozen gel packs directly on skin.
   - Do not use cryotherapy applications for extended time periods. 15-minute therapy sessions are recommended.
   - Do not do exercises that cause pain following cold applications.

5. Systemic massage entails focusing massage on a specific body system; two forms of systemic massage are lymphatic and circulation massage. When a massage is concentrated on a particular body system, the effects of the massage are more dramatic.

6. The massage consists of a combination of short, pumping, and active effleurage strokes, followed by long surface effleurage strokes, deep breathing, and passive range of motion. The direction of action is toward the drainage points. The focus of the pressure is on the dermis just below the surface layer of skin and the layer of tissue just beneath the skin and above the muscles and then may gradually increase.

7. Compression is applied over the main arteries, beginning near the heart or proximally to it, and systematically moving distally, ending at the tips of the fingers or toes. The strokes are applied over the arteries and pump at a rhythm of approximately 60 beats per minute, or with the client's resting heart rate. The next step is to assist venous return flow. A combination of short effleurage strokes, long effleurage strokes, and joint movement is used. With venous return flow, the effleurage strokes move distal to proximal, or from the finger and toes to the heart, over the major veins. The short effleurage stroke is about 3 inches long and moves the blood from valve to valve. Long effleurage strokes carry the blood through the entire vein. Passive and active joint movements help venous circulation. Placing the limb or area above the heart allows for gravity assistance.

8. The foot has many joint and reflex patterns. Sensory information about position and posture from the joint kinesthetic receptors is extensive. Sensory and motor centers of the brain devote a large area to the feet and hands. There is extensive nerve distribution to the feet and hands. The position of the foot sends a great deal of postural information through the central nervous system. Stimulation of the feet seems to activate the responses of the gait control mechanism hyperstimulation analgesia (parasympathetic dominance). Bodywide effects are achieved by this technique. Many nerve endings in the feet and hands correlate with acupressure points, which, in turn, release endorphins and other endogenous chemicals when stimulated. In addition, major plexuses for the lymph system are located in the hands and feet. Compressive forces in this area stimulate lymphatic movement.

9. An excellent way to massage a foot is to apply pressure and movement systematically to the entire foot and ankle complex. The pressure stimulates the circulation, nerves, and reflexes. Moving the joints stimulates large-diameter nerve fibers, initiating hyperstimulation analgesia and joint kinesthetic receptors. The result is a shift in proprioceptive and postural reflexes. This same approach can be used to massage the hands.

10. Hand and foot massage is likely to be the most effective form of self-massage. The hands and feet have similar motor cortex distribution patterns. The stimulation of the hands during the massage does not override the sensations to the area being massaged. The hands are massaged while massaging the feet.

WORKBOOK SECTION

11. Techniques that specifically alter the configuration of the connective tissue are classified as connective tissue approaches. The methods can vary from mechanical methods, such as Cyriax's deep transverse friction, to the very subtle approaches of craniosacral therapy. Connective tissue methods stretch, pull, drag, elongate, and move the tissue.

12. The intent of connective tissue massage is to either soften the ground matrix, or plastic component, of connective tissue, or introduce small amounts of inflammation, which triggers connective tissue restructuring.

13. To use frictioning, extensive anatomic knowledge is required. Frictioning must be done very specifically, and because it introduces an inflammatory response the effect is a controlled injury of tissue. Without the anatomic knowledge and assessment required, the precise location of an adhesion will not be known and healthy tissue may be damaged. Additional training is required to skillfully follow tissue movement to work effectively with the craniosacral system.

14. A trigger point is an area of local nerve facilitation of a muscle that can be aggravated by stress of any sort affecting the body or mind of the individual. Trigger points are small areas of hypertonicity within muscles. If these tight areas of muscle fibers are located near motor nerve points, referred pain may result from nerve stimulation. Often the area of the trigger point is the point where nerve stimulation initiates a contraction in a small sensitive bundle of muscle fibers (motor point) that in turn activates the entire muscle.

15. Using light palpation, the massage practitioner needs to notice whether the skin feels tense and whether there is resistance to gliding strokes. The skin may be slightly damp with perspiration on the skin from sympathetic facilitation. The temperature in a local area increases in acute trigger points, but decreases in chronic trigger points, as a result of ischemia, which is an indication of fibrotic changes within the tissues around the trigger point. Edema produces an impression of fullness and congestion within the tissues. In instances of chronic dysfunction, edema is replaced gradually with fibrotic (connective tissue) changes and the tissue texture feels cemented. During deep palpation the massage therapist establishes contact with the deeper fibers of the soft tissues and explores them for immobility, tenderness, edema, muscle tension, and fibrotic changes. With both light and deep palpation, gliding strokes cover a region of 2 to 3 inches at a time. The trigger point is painful to pressure and refers pain to other areas.

16. The trigger point is hyperstimulated by using various methods such as compression, pushing together or apart on the spindle cells, or active contraction of the muscle. Hyperstimulation is followed by stretching of the muscle fibers containing the trigger point.

17. After treatment of a trigger point, the target (referred) area should be searched to uncover satellite or embryonic trigger points that need to be treated. Immediately afterward, the area needs to be massaged to increase local circulation. Placing a damp warm or hot towel over the region is soothing and useful. The area requires rest for a few days, avoiding all stressful activity.

18. Most acupuncture points correspond with motor points or nerve endings; meridians lie over or close to main nerve tracts; yin is parasympathetic, and yang is sympathetic.

19. A person is body, mind, and spirit. These are not separate pieces but a part of a whole. Health is achieved when harmony exists in all areas.

20. Acupuncture points usually lie in fascial division between muscles, near the origin and insertion. The point feels like a small hole and pressure elicits a "nervy" feeling. Unlike a trigger point, which may only be on one side of the body, acupuncture points are bilateral (located on both sides of the body). To confirm the location of an acupuncture point, locate the point in the same place on the other side of the body.

21. To stimulate a hypoactive or "not active enough" acupuncture point, use a short vibrating or tapping action. This method is used if the area is sluggish or a specific body function needs stimulation. To sedate a hyperactive or "too active" point for pain reduction, elicit the pain response within the point itself. Use a sustained holding pressure until the painful overenergy dissipates and the body's own painkillers are released into the bloodstream. The pressure techniques are similar to those used for trigger points, although it is not necessary to lengthen an acupuncture point after treatment.

22. Dr. Stone trained in both systems and incorporated the methods with a Western knowledge base to create an eclectic multifaceted system.

23. Using massage manipulations and techniques in a deliberate way during the general massage session adds to the effectiveness of the massage. Thought and intuition are used to allow the client's body to influence the approach used during the massage.

WORKBOOK SECTION

Matching

1. e   7. k
2. f   8. l
3. g   9. h
4. d   10. c
5. i   11. b
6. j   12. a

1. a
2. d
3. b
4. c
5. f
6. g
7. e

Labeling

1. U	8. C	15. W	22. F
2. B	9. P	16. K	23. R
3. BB	10. E	17. Z	24. G
4. Q	11. N	18. J	25. I
5. Y	12. X	19. O	26. M
6. A	13. T	20. H	27. V
7. L	14. AA	21. D	28. S

Additional Exercise

Heat 1, 3, 6, 8, 9, 10
Cold 1, 5, 7, 8, 11, 12
Ice 2, 4, 7, 8, 9, 11

Problem-Solving Exercises

1. Acupuncture points are bilateral. You should be able to find the same spot on the other side of the body. Trigger points usually are only on one side of the body.
2. Focus compression methods initially over the main arteries and then switch to effleurage strokes and joint movement for the major portion of the remainder of the massage.

Professional Application

1. Classes in trigger point therapy, deep transverse friction, myofascial release, and craniosacral therapy.
2. Answers not provided. There are a variety of solutions.

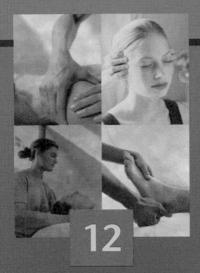

12

SERVING SPECIAL POPULATIONS

objectives

After completing this chapter, the student will be able to perform the following:

- Develop a massage environment to best serve individuals with special needs

- Demonstrate the communication skills that are important for working with a client with special needs

- Gather information on additional training to help the practitioner better serve clients with special needs

- Integrate therapeutic massage into the health care environment

IN this chapter we examine ways massage professionals can show respect for and help those who need special consideration. The intent is to help massage professionals focus the benefits of therapeutic massage for clients with specific needs. Integration of therapeutic massage into the health care environment also is presented because many clients who have special needs also require the support of a number of different health care professionals. Clients actively undergoing health care intervention can be considered a special population as well. Each section offers a general description of the special situation, the application for massage, and directions for obtaining further training and information.

The following special populations or circumstances are considered:

Abuse
Athletes
Breast massage
Children
Chronically ill individuals
The elderly
Infants
Medical intervention and support
Physically challenged individuals
  • Amputation
  • Burns
  • Hearing impairment
  • Mobility impairment
  • Size (height and weight)
  • Speech impairment
  • Visual impairment
Pregnant women
Psychologically challenged individuals
  • Addictions
  • Chemical imbalances in the brain
  • Developmental disabilities
  • Learning disabilities
  • Mood disorders
  • Posttraumatic stress disorder
The terminally ill

In exploring each situation it is important always to see the individual as a person first, with the special need as only a secondary consideration. There are no visually impaired, hearing impaired, sick, or abused people, but there are people who have visual or hearing impairments, who deal with various illnesses, or who have been abused. Basic massage skills are sufficient to serve all people because they facilitate general health enhancement and increase well-being. Specific rehabilitative massage requires additional education, but the most common application of therapeutic massage in conjunction with medical treatment is general, nonspecific support that is within the training levels presented in this text.

The basic skills presented in this textbook seldom change when applied in special situations. Effleurage for a person with special needs is still effleurage. The difference is in the recipient of the treatment and the way the treatment is done. Working with special populations requires additional knowledge about the specific situations or conditions addressed. The practitioner also must keep in mind the effects of or need for any training protocols, counseling, developmental stages, medical treatments, or accommodations (e.g., barrier-free access) in conjunction with the therapeutic massage.

It is the massage professional's responsibility to learn as much as possible about the situation with which the client is dealing. If the work is with tennis players, the therapist should learn about tennis; if the work is with survivors of abuse, the therapist should learn about abuse; if the work is in pain management, the therapist needs to understand pain and treatment protocols; if the work is with children with attention deficient disorder (ADD), the massage therapist must understand ADD and its treatment protocols.

The scope of these individual studies is beyond the context of this textbook but not beyond the massage professional's scope of further study. By using the clinical reasoning model, the massage professional can develop intervention plans and justification for the benefits of therapeutic massage as part of a comprehensive treatment program. The best way to obtain information about special needs is to ask the client directly. Various research avenues are available, and the Internet is an especially wonderful source of information. After the practitioner understands the client's particular situation, the physiologic effects of massage that provide the most benefit can be identified and intervention plans can be developed (Box 12-1).

We all need help at times. For most of us, however, the condition with which we require assistance is limited or short-lived. Those with disabilities or special needs live with their challenge *every day.* Life may be harder, and the person may be experiencing more stress. Massage can be a wonderful way to reduce stress, promote well-being, and provide a respite from the daily challenges faced by those with special needs.

ABUSE

section objectives

Using the information presented in this section, the student will be able to perform the following:

■ **Define** *abuse*

■ **Explain state-dependent memory**

■ **Recognize dissociation**

■ **List the elements needed in additional training to work specifically with abuse issues**

■ **Respond resourcefully if a client reacts emotionally during a massage**

---

box 12-1

USE OF THE CLINICAL REASONING MODEL TO DETERMINE SELF-STUDY NEEDS, DEVELOP A TREATMENT PLAN, AND JUSTIFY THE EFFICACY OF MASSAGE THERAPY

Example
Therapeutic massage for children with attention deficit disorder

1. Gather facts to identify and define the situation.

Key questions:
What is the problem?
What are the facts?

Attention deficit disorder (ADD) is primarily an organic condition that tends to have a genetic manifestation. It is characterized by the inability to sustain focused attention, a condition called **distractibility** or **inattention**. Often one or more of the following also are present: free association to many thoughts, impulsivity, moodiness, anxiety, withdrawn or spaced-out behavior (more prevalent in females), propensity to high-stimulation activities and behavior, bad temper, impatience, poor impulse control, and hyperactivity (in attention deficit/hyperactivity disorder [ADHD]).

ADD tends to be a biochemical disorder of dopamine, norepinephrine, and serotonin imbalance.

Stimulant medication is used to normalize the neurochemical imbalance. Stimulant medication increases sympathetic arousal, which can lead to side effects of appetite suppression, digestive upset, headache, and sleep difficulties.

Massage affects the neurochemicals involved in ADD by increasing dopamine and serotonin levels and increasing the norepinephrine level during the first 15 minutes. Massage inhibits sympathetic arousal if it lasts approximately 30 minutes or longer and acts as a form of sensory stimulation.

Research and Information Available
1. Corydon V, Clark G: *ADHD throughout the life span,* Las Vegas, 1997, Random Clark Publications [2253-A Renaissance Drive, Las Vegas NV 89119, (800) 613-6867].
2. American Psychiatric Association: *Diagnostic and statistical manual of mental disorders: DSM-IV,* 1994, The Association.
3. Castro M: *Homeopathic guide to stress,* New York, 1997, St. Martin's Griffin.

4. Field TM: Touch Research Institute, University of Miami Medical School, Department of Pediatrics (D-820), P.O. Box 016820, Miami, Florida 33101.
5. Fritz S: *Mosby's visual guide to massage essentials,* St Louis, 1996, Mosby.
6. Horacek HJ Jr: *Brainstorms: understanding and treating the emotional storms of attention deficit/hyperactivity disorder from childhood through adulthood,* New Jersey, 1998, Aronson Inc. [http://www.aronson.com].
7. Michigan Department of Social Services: *What you should know about stress and your child,* 1995, Channing L. Bele.
8. Muir M: Body-based therapies for childhood disorders. In *Alternative complementary therapies,* vol 3, no 6, 1997 [2 Madison Ave., Larchmont, NY 10538-1962, (914) 834-3100)].
9. Stress can trigger ADHD: http://gehur.ir.maim:edu.
10. Child health talk: childhood stress, http://www.kidshealth.org/ai/chtl.
11. Youngs BB: *Stress in children,* New York, 1995, Arbor House.

2. Brainstorm possible solutions.

Key question
What might I do?
What if . . . ?

If massage stimulates the same neurochemicals as the medications, it might be possible to lower the dosage of medication. Because it stimulates sympathetic arousal, massage may support effective use of medication at a lower dosage. Mild cases of ADD might be controlled with massage and similar methods.

Because massage can also inhibit sympathetic arousal, it may alleviate some of the side effects of the medication, allowing the use of a higher dosage if necessary. It may also reduce generalized stress in both child and parent.

Possible interventions include the following:

• Self-help methods
 A simple hand massage routine
 Complicated finger tapping exercises to provide sensory stimulation
 Progressive relaxation

Words synonymous with *abuse* include *exploit, misuse, prostitute, batter, mishandle, mistreat, molest, ravish, violate, harass, condemn, persecute, torment, belittle, ridicule, insult, offend, neglect, ignore, berate, criticize, defile, desecrate, dishonor, attack, reject,* and *pervert.* Words that have the opposite meaning are *honor, respect, consider, regard, protect, defend, preserve, praise, value, safeguard, shelter, sustain, support, tolerate, appreciate, approve, recognize, understand,* and *accept.*

When people are abused, whatever the form of abuse, they must learn to survive as best they can at the time of the abuse. These survival mechanisms take many forms, such as dissociation, hypervigilance, aggressive behavior, learning to "disappear," low self-esteem, and withdrawal. Posttraumatic stress disorder is common. These patterns may generalize into many life situations.

If the abuse happens to a young child, the victim's cop-

box 12-1

USE OF THE CLINICAL REASONING MODEL TO DETERMINE SELF-STUDY NEEDS, DEVELOP A TREATMENT PLAN, AND JUSTIFY THE EFFICACY OF MASSAGE THERAPY—CONT'D

A breathing pattern consisting of a short inhale through the nose and long exhale through the mouth

Training methods such as blowing up a balloon, blowing through a flute, and blowing bubbles

Stimulation of acupressure points

Entrainment mechanisms (e.g., rhythmic rocking)

- Professional massage

  Full-body, broad-based compression for 30 to 45 minutes

  Shiatsu technique

  Chair massage for 15 to 30 minutes

- Massage methods taught to parents

  Compression

  Slow-stroke massage

  Assisted progressive relaxation

  Rocking

3. Evaluate possible interventions logically and objectively; look at both sides and pros and cons.

Key question

What would happen . . . ?

Headaches and stomachache could be helped the most by massage interventions. The interventions could help reduce stress symptoms and off-task behavior, although not every child would respond to the same type of intervention.

Medication could be used effectively, although dosage would need to be monitored.

Parental involvement is necessary because the physiologic benefits of the methods are most effective if reinforced daily. However, parental participation could be minimal and inconsistent.

The child would usually relax with a very firm pressure. Light pressure would usually stimulate and agitate. Disrobing would be problematic.

Drawbacks to this program include cost, parental consistency, and time factors. Also, children under age 10 may not be old enough to learn self-help methods.

4. Evaluate the effect on the people involved.

Key question

How would each person involved feel?

The child would enjoy the interventions, although a great deal of energy would be needed to keep such children focused.

Appreciation of these children is necessary to work effectively.

These children become bored and inattentive when required to do repetitive tasks.

5. Develop intervention plan and justification statements.

Bodywork methods clearly have much to offer in the management of behavioral difficulties and stress faced by children with ADD/ADHD. Many interventions could be used such as teaching self-help methods, clinical sessions, and parental teaching and coaching.

Massage methods provided over the clothing would be emphasized to avoid the need for lubricant and disrobing. The longer 30- to 45-minute session for stress management and relaxation would be recommended for the clinical sessions. The shorter 15-minute massage would be helpful in focusing attention for task concentration such as doing homework. This 15-minute session could be taught to the parent.

Self-help methods could be taught to older children. A simplified version of the soothing massage could be taught to parents to encourage effective sleep and provide a calming effect. Parents could benefit from the same massage methods for stress management.

Consistent self-massage by the child and massage by the parent to provide various forms of sensory stimulation are necessary to achieve benefits. Continuing education and encouragement for the parents, who are also stressed, is important. A supportive coaching role can be provided to complement the bodywork interventions.

---

ing mechanisms develop around a twisted reality. The younger the child, the more difficult effective survival will be, and possibly the more magnified the inappropriate survival mechanisms that develop.

People most often think of **abuse** as physical or sexual torture. It is safer to consider the acts of the "monster" or sociopath than to recognize the subtler abuses we all have experienced. Most abusers are members of the family (in-

cluding siblings) or friends. Mixed signals can be very devastating; those who have experienced both abuse and support from the same person have difficulty with trust and esteem. Guilt is common and secrecy the norm.

Subtler forms of mistreatment, especially emotional abuse, also are common. The effects of the abuse should not be judged by their intensity. Children or adults who have been deceived have had their trust violated and their personal power taken away, just as the person who has been raped has. Abuse removes a person's self-empowerment, no matter what the means. The severity of the results depends on the frequency of the abuse, whether someone was able to validate the victim's self-worth, whether the victim received help in coping at the time, and inner resources. The older we are, the more inner resources we have to support effective coping.

State-Dependent Memory and Dissociative Behavior

Sexual and physical abuse attack the very form of a person, and the body remembers in some way. The technical term for this is **state-dependent memory.** This type of memory is encoded in the brain in a manner that includes the position, emotion, and chemicals, as well as the nervous system activation and all other combined physiologic effects that influence the internal functions, at the time the experience occurred. Later, when the physical and emotional states change, the memory may be vague or forgotten.

State-dependent memory functions in all life experiences. When a person gets ready to hit a baseball or drive a car, the individual assumes the appropriate position, and the body remembers what is required. In a traumatic experience, this mechanism locks in all the factors that coincide with the experience. In the future, this repressed memory may be triggered by any one of the sensations and physiologic factors involved in the state-dependent memory. For example, the sense of smell often triggers a memory. When working with massage, the pressure, location of the touch, and position or movement of the client may trigger the client's memory.

The myelinization of nerves and the development of the nervous system continue from birth to about 3 years of age. During this period memories are transient and spotty and may be stored in the memory centers in scattered ways. During the first year of life, the senses of touch, sound, smell, taste, and vision are functioning and in some ways are more keen than in the adult. However, the processing, storage, and retrieval of all this information are not keenly developed. Abuse is particularly devastating when it occurs during this crucial time of learning about the world and of dependence on a caregiver to meet not only basic needs (e.g., food, clothes) but also the need for connection, bonding, and love. Physical, sexual, or emotional abuse at this time is recorded by the body but is not always understood, coped with, or remembered in detail.

A person who experiences abuse during the formative years may have difficulty sorting it all out in adulthood. The memories may be spotty or piecemeal, or only one of the sensations (e.g., smell, touch, position) may be encoded in the memory. It is important not to discount this memory pattern simply because all the pieces do not fit together to form a whole picture. It may be affirming to know that all the pieces do not have to fit together for the

person to have enough information to resolve and integrate past experiences and develop more resourceful behavior for the present and future.

Sexual abuse in an older child often is laden with mixed signals, role confusion, and secrecy. Role confusion occurs when the child takes on the duties or family function of one of the parents. Because the child is older, memories may be clear, or, because of state-dependent memory patterns, they may be clouded or shut off and separated. The perpetrator may develop a relationship with the child and then use the child to meet the adult's or older adolescent's sexual needs. Again, feelings, emotions, roles, coping styles, and behavior all shift somehow to put the abuse into a form that can be survived.

Physical abuse (e.g., beatings, neglect) and emotional abuse (e.g., criticism, unrealistic expectations) demand survival as well. How many times have we been expected to do something that we did not have the skill, physical ability, or knowledge to accomplish and were belittled after trying our very best? This type of abuse riddles the self-esteem with holes.

Some life experiences that may affect a person in a manner similar to abuse are illness, medical procedures, hospitalization, accidents, or other trauma. The success of the individual's coping skills depend on the type of support received during and soon after the traumatic event, as well as the dynamics surrounding the situation. A child who attempts to hide the pain during a medical procedure so as not to upset the parents is being denied full emotional and physical expression in the situation. If the medical staff does not explain the procedure so that the child comprehends, or if the child is too young to understand, this too may become a difficult situation to integrate into a person's life experiences. If a parent or support person is physically separated from or emotionally unavailable for a child or adult during a crucial time, this can have a lasting effect.

Abuse of an adult, such as occurs with rape, violent crime, stalking, spouse beating, and abuse of the elderly, also must be considered. Typically, adults feel powerless in the situation and may feel as though the abuse is deserved or that they somehow did something to cause it. If elderly persons are also mentally impaired, such as with Alzheimer's disease, they may become childlike in their reasoning and survival mechanisms.

The touch of the massage therapist may remind the body of the abuse. It is possible that as the body remembers, it can somehow resolve and integrate the experience. Often the client does not remember the details or recall who, what, where, when, or how. Instead, a vague uneasiness or **dissociation** develops (i.e., detachment, discontentedness, separation, isolation). One mechanism for surviving physical, sexual, and emotional abuse is to "leave the body" and therefore not feel the abuse or to believe that the abuse is happening to someone else.

Many types of dissociative coping mechanisms are valuable in times of emergency and survival. However, if the pattern of dissociation becomes repetitive and generalized, one result is that the person becomes unable to feel. One way to relearn feelings and appropriate touch is through giving and receiving massage.

The massage professional should be aware of a client's dissociating during a massage. It is not our job to change the dissociative pattern by reminding the client to remain aware of her body unless the client specifically requests it. More specialized training is required to deal effectively with all the ramifications of a client's shift in coping style. This frequently involves professional counseling.

The massage practitioner should never remove a coping mechanism for a client or imply guilt for using it when it still serves a purpose. It takes time to learn to cope differently. Most of the time people dissociate in order to avoid feeling pain. The timing and situation must be just right to be able to focus the energy necessary to "feel" again. The process must happen gently, at the client's pace, and must never be hurried. The client leads, and the therapist follows that lead. As this happens, the practitioner can begin to recognize the pattern of the dissociation and the massage techniques or positions that seem to trigger the pattern. With this information the therapist can alter the approach to the massage, providing the client the opportunity to stay with the body more easily.

For example, if the therapist notices that every time the left knee is bent, a client's body becomes unresponsive, the eyes distance, or breathing shifts, then it is best to work with the knee in a different position. Also, the practitioner can have the client move into the position rather than being moved, which is more empowering for the individual. Over time, it becomes easier to notice these little steps, which will reacquaint the client with his body.

Some people who have been abused use self-abuse, which can take many forms, including a destructive lifestyle, addictive processes, and self-inflicted trauma. It may seem hard to understand, but self-abuse may be calming for the person. Endorphins and other chemicals are released during self-abuse. The mechanisms of counterirritation and hyperstimulation analgesia come into play. The massage professional may notice bruises, cuts, burns, or other injuries on the client's body. In a professional manner, the professional should bring these areas to the client's attention and note them in the client's record. Acknowledging an injured area to a person who abuses herself may cause the person to feel guilty or ashamed, tell a cover story, or ignore the question.

Occasionally a client demands or requests very deep massage when the soft tissue condition does not indicate the need for this type of invasive work. Self-abuse mechanisms may be involved in this situation. It is important not to become involved in a situation that perpetuates an abuse pattern. The therapist needs to trust her intuition and should not force the person to face the situation by confronting him with the possibility of self-abuse mechanisms. If the therapist is uncomfortable, the client must be told of the discomfort.

The decision to deal actively with an abusive history requires commitment and time from the client. Professional help and support groups often are needed. Also, some individuals do not want to recover their memories of abuse; this is a valid response for these clients. The practitioner must not suggest that a client was abused or that the client needs to deal with her situation. Our job is to honor, respect, consider, regard, protect, defend, preserve, praise, value, safeguard, shelter, sustain, support, tolerate, appreciate, approve, recognize, understand, accept, and never to harm.

Boundaries are very important. Review the importance of respect for personal boundaries (see Chapter 2).

Listening and believing what the body and the client say are significant. The client may personalize (transference) the nurturing touch of the therapist and may want to involve the therapist in the experience. Referral is important. When a person is actively exploring personal abuse and its results, it is important that the massage therapist not take on the client's problems (countertransference).

Reenactment and Integration

The reenactment of abuse is different from an integration process that may result from the physical triggers produced by massage. **Reenactment** involves reliving the event as though it were happening again right now. **Integration** involves remembering the event, yet being able to remain in the present moment, with an awareness of the difference between then and now, to bring some sort of resolution to the event.

Reenactment does not necessarily provide the awareness and understanding necessary to integrate the physical response and emotional feelings into the client's experience in an empowering way. Instead, with reenactment the client repeats an abusive pattern and feels disempowered and lost. The massage professional must be aware of the potential for harm to a client by deliberately triggering a reenactment response. Without the additional and necessary support of qualified counselors and other support personnel to provide for an integration process, a reenactment is undesirable.

If a client should respond during the massage by crying, shaking, panicking, becoming agitated or fearful, or demonstrating another emotional pattern, it is important for the massage professional to be quiet and let the person experience the emotion. In some instances it is best to continue to massage the area in the same way as that which triggered the response, slow down, and allow the body to integrate the information. The client should be asked no questions other than "Do you want me to continue?" The practitioner should be calm and accepting of the response and should never try to encourage or stop the response.

It is important not to interfere with the person's experience by interjecting suggestions. At other times it is appropriate to stop the massage and wait for the response to dissipate. If needed, tissues should be provided in an unobtrusive way. It is important for the therapist to stay connected with the client, but distanced from the client's experience. The emotional experience belongs to the client, not to the practitioner, who works as a support in a quiet, simple way. When the emotional response dissipates, the massage can be continued. If the client asks what happened, a simple explanation based on state-dependent memory is sufficient. Similar explanations, as previous mentioned, help the client understand what happened. A client who seems unsettled and needs additional help coping should be referred to a qualified counselor.

Confidence, respect, and trust are necessary to provide the type of massage that enhances the well-being of those who have been or are being abused. Always remember that confidentiality is a sacred trust; the therapist does not talk about clients or any experience with clients to anyone else.

Working with those who have been physically or sexually abused is rewarding work, but it can be very difficult. Additional training is needed to serve clients who have a history of abuse. The actual techniques of massage are no different, but an understanding of coping mechanisms and somatic (body) memories requires additional study. Bodywork in some form may be a valuable tool for some individuals who want to resolve these issues, whereas for others it is not the best choice. Effective decision-making

---

12-1

PROFICIENCY EXERCISE

1. Find and read three books that deal with abuse.
2. Visit a safe house or shelter for abused women and talk with the volunteers who work there.
3. Contact the child protection agency in your community and obtain information on recognizing child abuse and reporting suspected cases.
4. In the space provided, describe an incident in which you felt abused. Also describe an incident in which you feel you abused someone.

I felt abused when:

I abused someone when:

---

skills and support and supervision by qualified professionals determine the appropriateness of massage interventions for this population (Proficiency Exercise 12-1).

ATHLETES

section objectives

Using the information presented in this section, the student will be able to perform the following:

- List the experts in the care and training of athletes
- Explain the three types of restorative massage
- Explain the concept of event sport massage
- List the necessary components of additional sports massage training

An **athlete** is a person who participates in sports either as an amateur or a professional. Athletes require precise use of their bodies. The athlete trains the nervous system and muscles to perform in a specific way. Often the activity involves repetitive use of one group of muscles more than others, which may result in hypertrophy, changes in strength patterns, changes in connective tissue formation, and compensation patterns in the rest of the body. These factors contribute to the soft tissue difficulties that often develop in athletes.

Massage can be very beneficial for athletes if the professional performing the massage understands the biomechanics required by the sport. If not, massage can impair optimal function in the athletic performance. Because of the intense physical activity involved in sports, an athlete may be more prone to injury. All injuries must be referred for evaluation.

The experts for athletes are sports medicine physicians, physical therapists, athletic trainers, exercise physiologists, and sports psychologists. It is especially important for competing athletes to work under the direction of these professionals. With athletes the psychologic state is crucial to performance; often the competition is won in the mind.

Athletes depend on the effects of training and the resulting neurologic response for quick, precise functioning. It is easy for massage therapists to disorganize the neurologic responses if they do not understand the patterns required for efficient functioning in the sport. The effect is temporary, and unless the athlete is going to compete within 24 hours, it is not significant. However, if the massage is given just before competition, the results could be devastating. Any type of massage before a competition must be given carefully.

Restorative Massage

According to Patricia Benjamin and Scott Lamp, authors of the textbook *Understanding Sports Massage*, there are three forms of restorative massage: recovery massage, remedial massage, and rehabilitation massage.[1]

Recovery Massage

Recovery massage focuses primarily on athletes who want to recover from a strenuous workout or competition when no injury is present.

The method used to help an athlete recover from a workout or competition is similar to a generally focused, full-body massage using any and all methods from Chapter 9 to support a return to homeostasis. Massage focused on circulation enhancement (as presented in Chapter 11, p. 475) also is appropriate, as are the other methods presented in Chapter 10, except for deep transverse friction, specific myofascial release, and extensive trigger point work.

Remedial Massage

Remedial massage is used for minor to moderate injuries. Methods used in remedial massage include all methods presented in Chapters 9 and 11, as well as selective use of deep transverse friction and myofascial and trigger point work.

Rehabilitation Massage

Rehabilitation massage is used for severe injury or as part of the postsurgical intervention plan. Methods of massage used in rehabilitation massage vary. Immediately after injury or surgery, more nonspecific, general stress reduction, and healing promotion massage techniques are developed. Attention is given to the entire body while the area

of injury or surgery heals. Any immobility, use of crutches, or changes in posture or gait during recovery probably will set up compensation patterns. Massage can manage these compensation patterns while the physician, physical therapist, and trainer focus on the injured area. During active rehabilitation, massage can become part of the recovery process, supervised by an appropriately qualified professional, as part of a total treatment plan.

If a massage professional plans to work with an athlete on a continuing basis, it is important that the practitioner come to know the athlete and become part of the entire training experience. The therapist should learn about the sport, what is required of the athlete's body and mind, how best to use massage to enhance performance, and how to support the body in compensating patterns.

Promotional or Event Massage

Promotional massages usually are given at events for amateur athletes. The massages are offered as a public service to provide educational information about massage. It is important to receive written documentation of informed consent from each person receiving a massage at these events (Box 12-2). One way to do this is to develop an informed consent statement on the top of a sign-in sheet and have each participant read it and sign before receiving

---

box 12-2

SAMPLE INFORMED CONSENT FORM FOR USE AT SPORTING EVENTS

Name: _____

Sporting event: _____

Date: _____

I have received, read, and understood informational literature concerning the general benefits of massage and the contraindications for massage. I have disclosed to the massage practitioner any condition I have that would be contraindicated for massage. Other than to determine contraindications, I understand that no specific needs assessment will be performed. The qualifications of the massage practitioner and reporting measures for misconduct have been disclosed to me.

I understand that the massage given here is for the purpose of stress reduction. I understand that massage practitioners do not diagnose illness or disease, perform any spinal manipulations, or prescribe any medical treatments. I acknowledge that massage is not a substitute for medical examination or diagnosis, and it is recommended that I see a health care provider for those services.

I understand that an event sports massage is limited to providing a general, nonspecific massage approach using standard massage methods but does not include any methods to address specifically soft tissue structure or function.

Participant's Signature: _____ Date: _____

Participant's Signature: _____ Date: _____

Participant's Signature: _____ Date: _____

the massage. A short brochure or pamphlet explaining the benefits, contraindications, and cautions of sports massage is given to each participant.

The sports event massage lasts about 15 minutes and is quick paced. This type of public, promotional environment is one area where following a sports massage routine is important.

The use of lubricants is optional, and the massage practitioner may choose not to use them because of the risk of allergic reaction, staining an athlete's uniform, or other unforeseen factors.

It is important to watch for any swelling that may indicate a sprain, strain, or compression fracture and refer the athlete to the medical tent for immediate evaluation. It also is important to watch for thermoregulatory disruption, hypothermia, or hyperthermia and refer the individual immediately if these are noted.

If a massage professional is doing promotional work at sports massage events and is working with many unfamiliar athletes, it is best to do postevent massage. With this technique, the effects of any neurologic disorganization caused by the massage are not significant.

No connective tissue work, intense stretching, trigger point work, or other invasive work should be done with an athlete at a sporting event. The massage should be superficial, supportive, and focused more on circulation enhancement.

The Sports Massage Team

Often a group of massage professionals and supervised students work an event as a team. A team leader who is familiar with the sport usually is in charge at the sporting event. All the massage practitioners participating follow a similar routine. If this "team spirit" also is adopted by the massage professionals, each person does essentially the same routine consistently throughout the event. Remember, each member of a sports massage team represents the entire profession. The attitude should be one of helpfulness and concern, and therapeutic opinions must be avoided.

Pre-Event Massage

Pre-event, warm-up massage is a stimulating, superficial, fast-paced, rhythmic massage that lasts 10 to 15 minutes. The emphasis is on the muscles used in the sporting event, and the goal is for the athlete to feel that her body is "perfect" physically. Avoid uncomfortable techniques. The warm-up massage is given in addition to the physical warm-up; it is not a substitute. This style of massage can be used from 3 days before the event until just before the event. Massage techniques that require recovery time or are painful are strictly contraindicated. Focus on circulation enhancement and be very careful of overworking any area. Sports pre-event massage should be general, nonspecific, light, and warming. Avoid friction or deep, heavy strokes. Massage should be pain free! It is suggested that only massage therapists who work on an ongoing basis with a particular athlete give the athlete a pre-event massage.

Intercompetition Massage

Intercompetition massage, given during breaks in the event, concentrates on the muscles being used or those about to be used. The techniques are short, light, and relaxing. It is suggested that only massage therapists familiar with a particular athlete give him an intercompetition massage.

Postevent Massage

Postevent, warm-down massage can reduce muscle tension, minimize swelling and soreness, encourage relaxation, and reduce recuperation time. The massage techniques can spread muscle fibers to minimize fascial adhesions and encourage circulation. Be aware of possible sprains, strains, and blisters. Use ice for inflammation and areas of microtrauma.

12-2

PROFICIENCY EXERCISE

1. Look through professional journals and send for information about three advanced sports massage training sessions.
2. Contact a university with a sports team and speak with the athletic trainer to discover ways in which massage might be used to enhance athletic performance.
3. Contact a local exercise club or physical therapy department and talk with the exercise physiologist about how massage could enhance the work being done.
4. Volunteer to work at a sponsored sports massage event held by your school or local professional massage organization.
5. With your classmates, organize a sports massage event for a local sporting function.
6. Obtain a catalog from a university that offers degrees in athletic training or exercise physiology. List the classes required to earn these degrees.

In athletes, regular massage allows the body to function with less restriction and accelerates recovery time. Many specialized training programs for sports massage are available. If the massage professional intends to work with athletes, additional training must be pursued. Such training should include the physiologic and psychologic functions of an athlete; overuse and repetitive use syndromes; the biomechanics of specific sports; the use of cryotherapy, ice massage, and other hydrotherapy methods; injury repair and rehabilitation; education in training regimens; and education by exercise physiologists, athletic trainers, and sports psychologists (Proficiency Exercise 12-2).

BREAST MASSAGE

section objectives

Using the information presented in this section, the student will be able to perform the following:

- Determine when breast massage is appropriate
- Consider ethical principles in deciding when breast massage is performed

Massage of the female breast is a controversial issue. A conservative approach is taken in this textbook.

Breast massage can be appropriate for certain conditions such as fibrosis and the development of scar tissue after surgery (surgery for breast cancer is the most common cause of such scar tissue). Surgery for breast cancer may involve either removal of only the cancerous tissue or a mastectomy. Often reconstructive surgery is performed. The massage practitioner must attend to contraindications and cautions in connection with treatments given after surgery. For example, radiation over the area can weaken the bones, predisposing them to fracture.

Breast implants are another consideration. Care must be taken to apply gentle pressure over the implants.

Breast reduction surgery is performed for both cosmetic and health reasons. The same attention to scar tissue development and healing is taken as with other surgical procedures.

As for any surgery or area of healing, specific massage to the area is not provided during the acute phase. After the initial healing is complete and the attending physician approves the treatment, gentle massage that mobilizes the tissue around the surgical area can be performed. After 4 weeks, if healing is progressing well, the scar itself can be gently massaged. The most common method used is a very gentle form of skin rolling. After 3 months myofascial methods can be used.

When working with existing scar tissue, the work progresses slowly and deliberately. Most scar tissue tends to be less pliable than the surrounding tissue. It also tends to shorten and pull. Breast surgery can result in a pulling forward of the shoulder and tension in the midback.

Myofascial methods (as presented in Chapter 11) are effective for managing scar tissue. More generalized massage manipulation such as effleurage and pétrissage prepares the tissue for more specific work.

If breast massage for a specific condition is deemed appropriate by a health care professional and the client is referred to the massage professional, the following measures are recommended:

- Work with specific informed consent for breast massage.
- Work with another professional in the room, much as a male gynecologist has a female nurse present during examinations. If this is not possible, male therapists should refer a female client to a female therapist.
- Use careful draping. Do not expose the entire breast unless absolutely necessary. Do not expose both breasts.
- Work gently, professionally, and confidently.
- Avoid the nipple area.

Ethical Considerations in Breast Massage

Breast massage as part of a general massage serves no specific physiologic purpose that cannot be achieved in ways other than breast massage; therefore the concerns may outweigh the benefit. The ethical principles discussed in Chapter 2 serve as the basis for decision making regarding the appropriateness of breast massage for either men or women. The massage professional should particularly consider the following:

- *Proportionality:* The benefit must outweigh the burden of treatment.
- *Nonmaleficence:* The practitioner must do no harm and must prevent harm from occurring.
- *Beneficence:* The treatment must contribute to the client's well-being.

Anatomically the breast is part of the integumentary system. It becomes a functional part of the female reproductive system only during lactation. In both men and women, the breast is considered an erogenous zone. An erogenous zone is an area of the body where sexual tension concentrates and can be relieved through stimulation. Other erogenous zones are the mouth, genitals, and anus. These areas usually have some sort of erectile tissue that engorges with blood when stimulated. The nipple consists of this erectile tissue. The controversy over the appropriateness of massage of the female breast centers on the breast as an erogenous area.

Soft tissue under the breast tissue can be accessed effectively by placing the client in the side-lying position, in which the breast tissue falls away from the chest wall toward the table. In the supine position the breast tissue usually falls to the side, allowing massage over the sternum and intercostal area. These two positions provide adequate access to the soft tissue of the chest wall. For this reason, there is no reason to massage through the breast tissue proper to reach these areas.

Breast examination and teaching breast self-examination

1 2 - 3
PROFICIENCY EXERCISE

Investigate the surgical procedure for breast cancer, breast augmentation with implants, or breast reduction. Write an intervention plan and justification statement for the use of therapeutic massage. Use the model in Box 12-1 as an example.

Therapeutic massage for _____

1. Gather facts to identify and define the situation.

Key questions
What is the problem?
What are the facts?

2. Brainstorm possible solutions.

Key question
What might I do? or What if . . . ?

3. Evaluate possible interventions logically and objectively; look at both sides and pros and cons.

Key question
What would happen if . . . ?

4. Evaluate the effect on the people involved.

Key question
How would each person involved feel?

5. Develop intervention plan and justification statements.

are adequately undertaken by other health care professionals. It is not necessary for the massage professional to provide such services.

General massage of the breast is not recommended for either male or female clients. To avoid discrimination it is suggested that both male and female clients be draped effectively with a chest drape and that the breast area proper be excluded from the massage (Proficiency Exercise 12-3).

CHILDREN

Using the information presented in this section, the student will be able to perform the following:

- Apply general massage methods to ease growing pains
- Train family members in massage techniques for use at home

Providing massage services for children is not much different from providing massage for adults. For the purposes of this textbook, children are people ranging in age from 3 to 18 years of age. Children love physical contact. It is interesting that the horsing around and wrestling that children do looks a lot like massage. Because children and adolescents may have shorter attention spans than adults, a 30-minute massage usually is sufficient.

From age 3 to puberty the physical growth is mostly in height. At adolescence, growth in height accelerates under the influence of increased hormonal levels, and sexual maturation ensues as well. Both physical and emotional growing pains are common. Physical growing pains occur because the long bones grow more rapidly than the muscle tissue, resulting in a pull on the periosteum or connective tissue bone covering, which is a very pain-sensitive structure. Massage can help by gently lengthening the muscles and stretching the connective tissue, providing symptomatic relief of pain through the effects of counterirritation, hyperstimulation analgesia, gait control, and release of endorphins.

Adolescents live in bodies that are changing every second. Hormonal levels fluctuate constantly, and moods swing in response to this. Growth is accelerated, and natural sleep-wake patterns often are disrupted. It is not uncommon for a teenager to be up all night and want to sleep all day. Massage may help an adolescent become more comfortable with this ever-changing body. It certainly helps with growing pains. Use special caution when working with adolescent boys. The reflexive sexual erection response is sensitive, and almost anything can trigger an erection. The therapist should be sensitive to this by not using a smooth sheet over the groin area when working with male adolescents. Instead, keep the sheet bunched in this area to disguise any physical response to the massage.

It also is important that the practitioner never work with children or adolescents unless a parent or guardian is present. Part of the massage time can be used to teach the parent or guardian some massage methods to help the child and to teach the child some massage methods for use on the parent. Massage provides a structured approach to safe touch. It may help families stay connected during both good and difficult times (Fig. 12-1) (Proficiency Exercise 12-4).

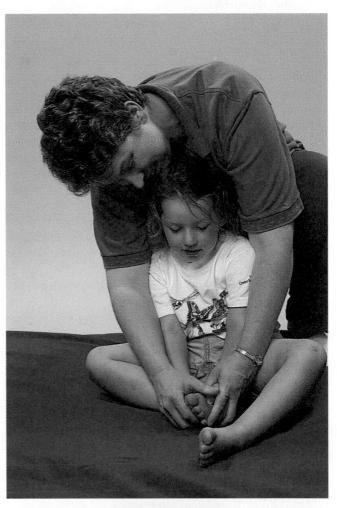

fig. 12-1

Parent massaging her child. (From Fritz S: *Mosby's visual guide to massage essentials,* St Louis, 1997, Mosby.)

12-4

PROFICIENCY EXERCISE

1. Give massages to three children or adolescents of various ages. Make sure the parent or guardian is present.
2. On separate sheets of paper, develop a one-page handout with five massage techniques that families can share.

CHRONIC ILLNESS

section objectives

Using the information presented in this section, the student will be able to perform the following:

- Explain the basic etiology of chronic illness
- Explain the difference between acute illness and chronic illness
- Develop realistic expectations for working with people who have a chronic illness

Chronic illness is defined as a disease, injury, or syndrome that shows either little change or slow progression. Dealing with chronic illness is difficult for the person who has it, for the physician and the health care team, and for the massage therapist. In many situations not much can be done except to make day-to-day living with the illness more tolerable. Healing is an option in some situations, but even then healing is a long process that requires work, commitment, and support. **Acute illness** or injury is a short-term condition that resolves through normal healing processes and, if necessary, supportive medical care. Compared with chronic illness acute conditions are dealt with relatively easily because healing produces measurable results.

The dynamics of family relationships, work situations, emotions, and coping skills play an important role in the etiology of a chronic illness. Chronic illness affects every aspect of a person's life and the lives of those around him. An entire family's dynamic functioning pattern may be set up around a chronically ill family member. Shifting illness patterns may be difficult. Entire relationship dynamics may change if the chronically ill individual improves. Personal and professional responsibilities that the client has been able to avoid because of the illness must be addressed if chronic conditions improve. Benefit gained by chronic illness is called *secondary gain*. This process may be subconscious and therefore difficult for the client to recognize or change.

The dynamics required to support chronic illness patterns reach far beyond the physiology of the disease, and professional counseling may be required. Working with chronic illness does not often produce measurable results. More often a slow deterioration is seen, or at best a stabilization. For this reason, working with chronic illness does not fit easily into the current medical system, which is geared mostly toward acute and traumatic care.

Long-term debilitating diseases such as Parkinson's disease, multiple sclerosis, systemic lupus erythematosus, rheumatoid arthritis, fibromyalgia, chronic fatigue syndrome, asymptomatic human immunodeficiency virus (HIV) infection, acquired immunodeficiency syndrome (AIDS), and disk problems that cause back pain respond well to the short-term relief of symptoms massage pro-

vides. Massage also can reduce general stress by helping the individual to cope better with the condition.

Chronic illness follows an uneven cycle, with good and bad periods. On good days the person may overexert herself and deplete an already weakened energy source. The immune system may be compromised, making the person with a chronic illness more susceptible to infections such as colds and influenza. Because most chronic illness patterns have good days and bad days, the intensity of massage sessions must be geared to the daily condition. It may be better to give massages more often for shorter periods when the symptoms are more active.

One approach to rehabilitating chronically ill individuals is a hardening or toughening program. **Hardiness** is the physical and mental ability to withstand external stressors. Individuals with chronic illnesses often reduce their activity levels, isolate themselves, and become less hardy. Massage, hydrotherapy, specially designed hardening programs, and exercise can increase a person's hardiness.

People with chronic illnesses usually are under a physician's care and may be taking medications. The massage practitioner must work closely with the medical professionals involved in order to understand the effects of the various treatments and medications. Because massage affects the physiology, its effects influence the effects of the medications. Appendix C presents some guidelines for determining the interplay of massage with various medications.

Mind/body approaches, behavior modification, relaxation techniques, spiritual healing, and other types of interventions and alternatives are helpful to those with chronic illnesses. All these approaches tend to empower the client, rallying the powerful internal resources that human beings have. It is important not to discount a method that a person may use for self-help. The only caution about alternative interventions is that some of those offering such services do not have the client's greatest good as their top priority. Instead, they prey on the misery of the chronically ill. These people usually offer cures, charge high fees for treatment sessions and require frequent sessions, and try to convince the client that their way is the only way, making the client dependent on them. This type of behavior is unethical.

The massage professional who wants to work with the chronically ill must have realistic expectations. Instead of developing a massage approach to bring about a cure for the illness, which is out of the scope of massage practice, the focus should be on helping the client feel better for a little while. Although this can get very frustrating for the practitioner, we can see that our work has value if we remember that we may be the only ones who provide this type of care, that not getting worse is an improvement, that some people need their illness to survive, and that massage eases their suffering in the illness pattern.

A clinical reasoning process is necessary to make appropriate decisions as to the type of care most beneficial for a client with a chronic illness (see Chapter 5). Treatment plans revolve around therapeutic change, condition management, or palliative care. Because of the nature of chronic illness, the emotional factors involved, and possible secondary gain, the treatment most often chosen is condition management, with palliative care provided during acute episodes of the illness. This recommendation does not mean that an actual therapeutic change plan is not possible; it simply is not as common.

The massage therapist's expectations must be realistic and professionally detached from the outcome of the client with a chronic illness. *Often the client's present situation is the best that can be achieved under the existing circumstances.* If each pattern presented by a client is seen as a solution, it is easier to understand why approaches that relieve the symptoms and support healing often are met with resistance.

For example, caffeine is known to disturb sleep. A client with a chronic fatigue syndrome pattern consumes four or five cups of coffee after noon and finds that she cannot sleep at night. Massage has been ineffective in supporting sleep. The client will not stop drinking coffee in the afternoon because she cannot function at work if she doesn't. So what do you do? There is no easy answer, and survival mechanisms reinforce short-term solutions even if the behaviors create long-term problems.

Often additional training is required just to understand chronic illness patterns, the effects of the medication involved, and the skill necessary to work in conjunction with other health care professionals. As with athletes, if work is to be done with someone who has a chronic illness, the massage therapist should understand as much as possible about the illness. By using this information and consulting with the physician and other health professionals involved in the client's care, the massage practitioner can integrate the effects of massage into the comprehensive treatment plan, helping the client to achieve the highest quality of life possible.

A resourceful goal for working with people with

chronic illness is helping a client rediscover the fact that each person is in charge of her own life, and the illness is not. The illness may have been allowed to take over the person's life and personal power. "Healing" may be the act of reasserting control of one's life, not getting rid of the disease. The benefits of massage may provide enough relief to enable the client to find the necessary inner resources for dealing constructively with the effects of chronic illness, enhancing the client's quality of life and the lives of those around him or her (Proficiency Exercise 12-5). *(Author's note: I speak from personal experience and continue to learn from an endocrine condition and a compressed disk in my lower back.)*

THE ELDERLY

section objectives

Using the information presented in this section, the student will be able to perform the following:

- **Provide a rationale for the benefits of massage for the elderly**
- **Understand the need for fee and time adjustments when working with the elderly**

The age range for the elderly is considered to be 70 years or older. However, some 60-year-olds have the problems of the aged, and some 85-year-olds have a physiologic condition better than that of some 60-year-olds. Because of this, it may be well to consider the physiologic condition rather than the chronologic age in individuals over age 60.

In the industrialized societies, the fastest growing segments of the population are those over age 80. People in their advanced years can benefit greatly from massage. Although the massage methods are no different, elderly persons do present specific difficulties. Muscle tissue has diminished and been replaced by fat and connective tissue. Connective tissue in general is affected during the aging process. It becomes less pliable, is slower to reproduce, and more easily forms fibrotic tissue. Bones are not as flexible and are more prone to breaking. Joints are worn, and osteoarthritis is common. Skin is thinner, and circulation is not as efficient. Medications may be prescribed to control blood pressure and other conditions. People who are elderly are not sick because of these conditions because the aging process is normal.

The body tends to collapse a bit during aging. The spaces provided for the nerves are reduced, and bones and soft tissue structures can put pressure on the nerves, resulting in sciatica and thoracic outlet syndrome. Feet hurt because the intricate joint structure of the foot has broken down. Circulation to the extremities is diminished, often resulting in a burning pain. These conditions are not life-threatening, but they surely can cause a person to feel mis-

---

12-5
PROFICIENCY EXERCISE

1. Choose one chronic illness and investigate it thoroughly.
2. Develop an educational brochure explaining the benefits of massage as part of a plan for coping with the chronic illness you have investigated. Share the brochures with fellow students.

erable. If only temporarily, massage can help ease the discomfort of these conditions.

Many of the elderly take several medications. The elderly also are more sensitive to the dosage level of medication and less able to self-regulate homeostatic processes. The massage professional must be attentive to the physiologic interactions between the effects of massage and the medications. Regular massage may allow reduction of the dosages of some medications.

Elderly persons often are depressed. This frequently is a chemical depression as well as a situational condition. Massage stimulates neurochemicals that can lift mild depression temporarily. Dementia conditions such as Alzheimer's disease have shown temporary improvement after massage. Wandering behavior has diminished, and an increased awareness of the current environment has been observed.

Lack of appetite and weight loss can be problems with advanced age, but the parasympathetic stimulation caused by massage can increase appetite and improve digestion for elderly clients. Sleep also can be improved. Many elderly people have periods of insomnia or disrupted sleep patterns. Improved sleep supports restorative mechanisms and increases vitality.

Many elderly people are alone. Their spouses have passed away, and their families are busy with their own lives. We all need to be touched. If a person is not physically and emotionally stimulated, neurologic function begins to deteriorate. The interaction with a massage therapist can provide both physical and emotional stimulation for the elderly. If nothing else, the physical contact with another human being provides sensory stimulation, with beneficial results.

Because the elderly often are alone or isolated in extended care facilities and have a limited income, the massage therapist should take into consideration not only the fees charged but also the amount of time spent with the elderly client. Many elderly persons want to talk. This social interaction may be just as important as the physical interaction of the massage. If the massage professional listens attentively, much can be learned from the elderly, who have many years of experience to share. The time should be given willingly. However, professional boundaries need to be maintained. When the massage practitioner tells an elderly person how much time can be spent, most respect the time boundary.

If a person does not have adequate cognitive functioning skills, as in cases of dementia caused either by the aging process or by medications taken for other conditions, she will be unable to give informed consent for the massage. The guardian, physician, or other health care professional must intervene to give the necessary permission.

As in the previous discussions, if work is to be done with elderly persons, the massage practitioner may need more training to learn about their special needs. In most cases a general massage session using the skills presented in this text and an attentive, caring attitude are sufficient for interacting professionally with the elderly (Fig. 12-2) (Proficiency Exercise 12-6).

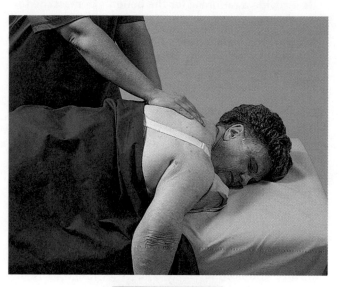

fig. 12-2

An elderly client receiving a massage. Note the placement of a foam support needed because of kyphosis.

12-6

PROFICIENCY EXERCISE

1. Volunteer to give massages at a local senior citizens' center for at least 4 weeks or a total of 32 hours.
2. Contact a local nursing home and ask if there is a resident who has few visitors and would appreciate receiving a massage. Commit to a minimum of two massages per month for 6 months.

INFANTS

section objectives

Using the information presented in this section, the student will be able to perform the following:

- **Explain the importance of the first year of life for an infant**
- **Explain the importance of organized sensory stimulation for infants**
- **Teach parents to massage their babies**
- **Understand the importance of a confident touch when working with infants**

Most authorities designate babies from birth to 18 months of age as infants. For the purposes of this textbook, the classification is expanded to 3 years of age because infants are still developing neurologically until that time. One or both parents must provide informed consent for the massage and must be present during any professional interaction with the infant.

Compared with other mammals, human infants are born about halfway through the gestation period, while the head is still small enough to pass through the birth canal. Otherwise, babies would stay in the womb at least another year. The womb is a much safer place to be unless the pregnant mother uses tobacco, drugs, alcohol, or other chemicals that cross the placental barrier, or if she does not provide adequate nutrition and care for herself and thus her baby.

Protection, nutrition, connection, bonding, stimulation, and soothing acceptance are crucial for human infants. Infants are born with a need for sociability, along with the more basic needs for food, shelter, and so forth. The people of most cultures massage their infants. Although this practice has been almost lost in the Westernized world, it is being revived. Research by Dr. Tiffany Field and her associates shows that premature infants who have been massaged fare much better than those who have not. Massage provides an organized, logical approach to sensory stimulation, which is important for infants because part of their growth is learning to sort and organize sensory stimulation.

Physiologically, the infant's growth pattern is not complete until 3 years of age. By 12 months of age (when, if our heads were not so big, a child would just have been born), the infant can move independently from place to place but still is utterly dependent on the protection of a parental person or family group. Two-year-olds are still babies. Three-year-olds are quite different in both function and body form. By the time a child can control bladder and bowel functions reliably (about age 3), cognitive functions are better able to be organized. Now is the time to work on learning the meaning of "no," picking up toys, and sharing. This infant is ready to pass into childhood.

Understanding the limitations of these walking infants is important. How many 2-year-olds have been spanked for not sharing toys or putting toys away, when physically and developmentally they are incapable of understanding the concept? Touch then becomes negative in connotation. Lots of hurts happen at this age. The parents' expectations often are too high, resulting in frustration on the part of both parents and child. These "wonderful and challenging" twos are a great time to take time out and give a massage. If the child is approached appropriately, this experience can be calming for both the parent and the child, and touch then becomes a very positive experience.

When working with any person, the massage professional needs to "meet" the person where he or she is at that moment. This is most important when working with infants. A fussy baby or a 2-year-old in a tantrum are caught up in the physiologic process. It takes time for both the nervous and endocrine systems to calm down. When verbal skills are not sufficient to express the problem, crying may be a way to burn off internal agitation that has built up through the day. A parent or massage practitioner who expects the infant to settle into the massage immediately may be disappointed. Relaxing takes time. Repetitive long strokes and rhythmic movement of the limbs can initiate a calming response in an infant. Even bilateral (on the side) pressure is calming. Swaddling provides this type of consistent, even pressure that reduces neural activity. If the baby stiffens with the massage, the tactile stimulation most likely is too intense, too light and uneven, or painful. The infant nervous system is very sensitive. Confining the massage to the feet or rhythmic rocking may be preferable to stroking for infants who seem highly tactile sensitive. When just the right combination of methods is found, the infant will respond to the touch calmly.

It is appropriate to teach parents to massage their own babies. Massage may be especially helpful for parents who have trouble bonding with their infants. Bonding is the attachment process that occurs between parent and child. Although bonding is considered primarily an emotional response, it is theorized that some biochemical and hormonal interaction may support the process. The hormone oxytocin is present in both the mother and the father and may be a factor in the bonding process. Massage through skin stimulation increases the oxytocin level.

Other than in a hospital-type setting, the massage practitioner is unlikely to develop a clientele of infants. But teaching infant massage can be an exciting career addition. Classes are available to massage therapists on teaching infant massage. The skills a beginner has usually are sufficient to work in well-baby care. Consideration must be given to a shorter massage time (15 to 30 minutes), to the smaller, still developing anatomy, and to the needs of the parents as they learn to communicate with their babies through touch. A confident touch is important; babies can detect nervousness immediately. To them this is not a "safe" touch, and they will not respond and may even try to withdraw. The parents may then feel rejected by the infant. Learning massage is an excellent way for parents to become confident with their touch (Fig. 12-3).

Infants born to mothers addicted to drugs and alcohol have a nervous system that is especially challenged. Research is underway to determine if the gentle, organized, tactile approaches of massage can help these special babies. The initial findings are promising. Babies, especially babies of drug-addicted mothers, sometimes are abandoned, and hospitals place these infants in what is called a *boarder nursery*. A hospital may be open to the volunteer efforts of a massage therapist, which could provide a great learning experience for both the massage professional and the hospital staff.

Remember, each baby is different. "Listen" to these little bodies, structure the massage to best meet their needs, and the baby will respond with a purity that fills your heart (Proficiency Exercise 12-7).

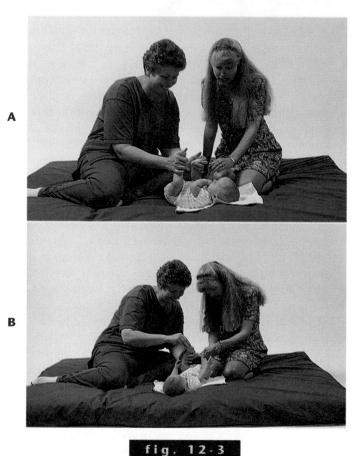

A

B

fig. 12-3

A and B, A parent being taught infant massage by a massage therapist.

12-7
PROFICIENCY EXERCISE

1. Using professional journals, investigate resources for learning more about infant massage.
2. Find a litter of puppies or kittens and massage these "babies."

MEDICAL INTERVENTION AND SUPPORT

section objectives

Using the information presented in this section, the student will be able to perform the following:

- Explain the importance of supervision in the health care setting
- Describe the written and verbal communication necessary for working in the health care environment
- List special considerations for working with clients undergoing medical treatment either in the health care environment or home health care setting

Working with clients in a health care environment (e.g., hospital, rehabilitation center, extended care facility, mental health facility) involves special considerations. Also, more and more people are being cared for in their homes by visiting nurses and home health workers. In both these situations the massage professional functions as part of a health care team, following the objectives of a comprehensively designed treatment plan.

The entire plan is supervised, usually by a physician. In the health care environment the massage therapist often is supervised directly by a nurse, a physical therapist, an occupational therapist, or some other qualified health care professional. When working with a client undergoing medical intervention outside the organized health care environment, attention must be given to the total health care program, and an effective interaction must be maintained between the supervising personnel and massage professional. Often in these situations the client is the main interface, but it may be necessary occasionally to speak directly with the physician or psychologist.

The interaction with other health care professionals is very important. A balance must exist between professional exchange of information, with each member of the team carrying out her part of the treatment plan, and the expectation of extensive face-to-face communication. These professionals are very busy, and it is unlikely that they will be able to speak at length with the massage professional about a particular client. Although this may be unfortunate, it is the reality, and brevity, along with precise information, becomes important.

Most communication is done in written form through treatment orders and charting. The massage professional's charting and record-keeping skills must be very effective to work in the health care environment.

When working outside the medical setting, exchange of information between the massage therapist and other members of the health care team is possible only with the client's consent. This is obtained by having the client complete a release of information form (see Chapter 2, p. 54). Cooperative interaction is necessary to coordinate various home care situations. Independent action must be tempered by awareness of the total health care picture for the client and by respect for the other health care professionals involved.

The health care environment presents special considerations. Universal precautions and other sanitation procedures must be followed precisely. Working around various types of equipment and devices (e.g., intravenous lines) must be considered. The massage often must be modified because the client is unable to assume the classic position of lying on a massage table. Many such clients are confined to a bed or wheelchair. Privacy often is compromised, and interruptions are common. The environment may be noisy and busy with other activity.

Various medications and their interaction with the effects of the massage must be considered. The effects of medical tests or preparation for tests can affect massage intervention. For example, many testing procedures require fasting before the test. This stresses the body, and the intensity of massage would need to be modified.

Therapeutic massage has much to offer in the health care environment. Clients are stressed, and the relaxation approaches of massage support the other medical interventions and the healing process in general. Massage before surgery can help with presurgery anxiety. Comfort or palliative care for support while a person undergoes invasive medical procedures can ease the discomfort somewhat. Massage provided during drug rehabilitation programs supports the recovery process. Massage for the medical staff promotes their ability to serve effectively, because the health care staff can be stressed and overworked. The possibilities for massage in the health care environment are numerous.

The massage provided in the situations just described usually is very basic and primarily focused on palliative care. The challenge of working in the health care environment is not how to work with the specific client, but rather how to work effectively with the health care professionals serving the client. The skill levels presented in this text are sufficient for this type of care, provided the professional is qualified to work in the complex health care environment. To function in the health care environment, the massage professional must be skilled and knowledgeable in the following areas:

- Clinical reasoning
- Problem solving
- Preparing justifications for treatment
- Setting qualifiable and quantifiable goals
- Medical terminology
- Pathology
- Medical tests and procedures
- Medications
- Assessment
- Developing treatment plans
- Analyzing the effectiveness of methods used
- Charting
- Communicating information effectively

These skills can be developed through continuing education of the massage professional, or through comprehensive massage training of individuals who already have these skills, such as nurses and physical therapy assistants. For those who already have health care training, it is unrealistic to expect that simple exposure to massage is sufficient to enable them to work effectively with the vast knowledge base of massage. It is just as unrealistic to believe that a massage professional with an entry level education can function effectively in the health care environment. Because therapeutic massage falls within the paraprofessional realm, it seems most logical to extend the education of massage professionals who want to work in a health care setting and provide supervision of the massage professional by qualified health care personnel.

This text, in combination with anatomy and physiology studies (the recommended text for such studies is *Mosby's Basic Science for Soft Tissue and Movement Therapies* by Sandy Fritz, 1999, St Louis, Mosby), covers the information needed to work in a supervised health care setting *if* sufficient time is available in classes to truly digest and integrate the full content of the text. Five hundred contact hours of education (15 to 20 credits) is not enough time for full integration and professional application of the skills needed to work in the health care setting. Programs of 1000 to 2000 contact hours (30 to 45 credits) would more realistically provide the time for development of these special skills (Proficiency Exercise 12-8).

12-8

PROFICIENCY EXERCISE

1. Obtain a course catalog from a college and compare your current massage education with the curriculum required for a nurse, a physical therapy assistant, an occupational therapist, a respiratory therapist, or other similar health care professional.

2. Discuss with a physician, chiropractor, physical therapist, or psychologist the skills she would want to see in a massage professional who would work with her in the professional setting.

PHYSICALLY CHALLENGED INDIVIDUALS

Using the information presented in this section, the student will be able to perform the following:

- Communicate more effectively with people who have a physical disability
- Adjust the massage environment to better support those with physical disabilities
- Become aware of subtle discrimination

According to the guidelines of the Americans with Disabilities Act, a **physical disability** or impairment is any physiologic disorder, condition, cosmetic disfigurement, or anatomic loss that affects one or more of the following body systems: neurologic, musculoskeletal, special sense organ, respiratory (including speech organs), cardiovascular, reproductive, digestive, genitourinary, hemic and lymphatic, skin, and endocrine. Extremes in size and extensive burns also may be considered physical impairments.[2]

People with physical impairments can benefit from massage for all the same reasons that any other individual can. The client's body may develop a compensation pattern for the disability. For instance, a person in a wheelchair could have increased neck and shoulder tension from moving the chair. In addition, dealing with a physical impairment daily can make routine functions more stressful. The following are some guidelines that may help the therapist provide services for these clients. A person with a disability should be treated the same as anyone else. The right of individuals to choose the kind of help they need must be respected.

A therapist must never presume to know, understand, or anticipate a client's need. *It is important to ask!* A concerned therapist does not try to pretend that the disability does not exist, but rather responds professionally. The disability affects only a small part of the whole person. After the client has provided the necessary information about the disability, the therapist should accept the impairment as part of how the person functions.

Personal Awareness

People who are not physically challenged may be uncomfortable around those who are. This discomfort comes from not knowing what to do or say, from being afraid of the person's disability, or from various other causes.

It is common to put the disability first rather than the person. If the disability is first in the therapist's mind, the person is not. Lack of knowledge is a huge contributing factor to this form of subtle discrimination. Overcompensation and patronization by the nondisabled person makes normal communication difficult. The massage professional is responsible for acting professionally and communicating effectively with all clients, including those who have disabilities. Not understanding how to interact effectively is not an excuse because the best source of information is the person with the impairment. Ask your client to explain his or her limitations; what assistance, if any, might be needed; and how that assistance should be given if requested.

The practitioner should use good judgment when deciding whether to ask if assistance is needed and then should wait until the person accepts the offer before providing assistance. The client can give the best directions on how to proceed.

For example, in offering assistance it may be best to say, "If you need any assistance, I am glad to help. Tell me what you need." If the offer is declined, no offense should be taken. If the person is abrupt, it may be that this question has been asked many times already but not in such a pleasant or respectful manner.

If another person is present, all remarks should be directed to the client and not to the companion. Talking to the companion rather than the client is very degrading; it occurs when the therapist is more comfortable with the able-bodied companion and therefore finds it easier to address that person.

Sometimes we are uncomfortable and cannot move beyond these feelings. The client will sense our discomfort. Simple disclosure allows communication and understanding. For example, when working with a severely burned client, I found that the texture of the skin was difficult for me to massage. It unsettled me. The client also was very disfigured. He could sense my discomfort but did not understand the source and assumed it was from his appearance, which was not a factor. Because he was familiar with people's reaction to his appearance, the client asked me about the cause of my discomfort. Simple disclosure and the understanding that resulted helped me to deal more effectively with the tactile difficulties I was having and helped the client to understand the source of my feelings. This was a valuable lesson in the importance of simply, professionally, and honestly using disclosure as described in Chapter 2. It often is difficult to communicate these types feelings and difficult for professionals to accept their personal limitations. Sometimes referral to a practitioner who is not affected by a particular situation is the best choice for both the massage professional and the client.

Supporting Clients with a Visual Impairment

Many people with a visual impairment have some type of sight. Comparatively few people have no vision at all. When assisting a client with a visual impairment, the therapist should never push or pull on the person. Instead, if guiding is necessary, the therapist should stand just in front and a bit to the left of the client, who can then touch the therapist's right elbow when following.

Useful directions should also be given to a person with a visual impairment. If asked where something is, the therapist should not point and say "over there." Instead, terms such as *left, right, about 10 steps,* and so on are much easier to follow. It is not necessary to speak more loudly to individuals with a visual impairment; they usually can hear just fine.

The conversation should begin with the therapist addressing the client by name so that she is aware of being spoken to. The therapist then should state his name but should not touch the client until the person is aware of his presence in the room.

If a person with a visual impairment places anything anywhere, it should not be moved. If a door is opened, the direction of the opening (toward or away from the person) and the location of the hinges (left or right) should be explained. It is best to let the client open the door in order to be better oriented to its position.

If a service dog is harnessed and working, be it a guide dog for someone with a visual impairment or any other support service, the therapist must not pet, feed, or in any other way interact with the dog. This distracts the dog and makes its job difficult. It must become very tiresome for a person with a service dog to be stopped repeatedly and asked if someone can pet the dog (Fig. 12-4).

Supporting Clients with a Speech Impairment

It may be difficult to understand a person with a speech problem. The therapist should ask the person to repeat anything that was unclear until it is understood and then should repeat what was said so that the person can clarify if necessary. If the therapist cannot understand what is being said, the client should be informed of this. If necessary, a notepad can be used to put communication in writing.

Supporting Clients with a Hearing Impairment

To gain the attention of a client with a hearing impairment, the therapist should lightly tap him once on the shoulder or discreetly wave a hand. If no interpreter is present, all talking should be done in a normal tone and rhythm of speech.

If a client can lip read, it is important that the therapist always face the person and not cover her own mouth when talking. A normal voice tone and speed should be used. If the therapist normally speaks quickly, the speed should be slowed a bit. If necessary, a notepad can be used to put communication in writing.

Hearing aids amplify sound; they do not make sound clearer. Reducing background noise helps the hearing impaired to hear better. With this in mind, it may be wise to

ask before using any music during the massage session. Getting too close to a hearing aid can make it squeal, therefore care must be taken when massaging the ears.

Supporting Clients with a Mobility Impairment

There are many types of mobility impairment and many reasons for it. Just because a person is paralyzed does not mean that a particular area has no feeling. Furthermore, just because a person uses a wheelchair does not mean that the person is paralyzed.

When speaking to a client in a wheelchair, it is best to do so from eye level. Looking up strains the neck. The process obviously requires the massage therapist to sit down.

A wheelchair must never be pushed unless the person in the chair gives permission. The individual also will give directions for pushing the wheelchair over barriers.

When transferring a client from a wheelchair to the massage table (Fig. 12-5, *A*), the client can give the best di-

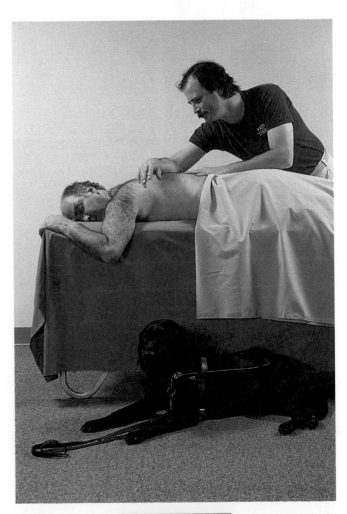

fig. 12-4

The guide dog is trained to lie quietly by the massage table.

rections on how to proceed. A transfer to a mat on the floor may be easier to accomplish, in which case the massage should be given there. The most efficient transfer is a lateral transfer to a table that is the same height as the wheelchair. This entails a shift in body mechanics by the massage therapist to a lower table (Fig. 12-5, *B*).

Special care must be taken in giving a massage to a person with paralysis because normal feedback mechanisms are not functioning. Clients with catheters or other equipment must instruct the therapist in the handling of the devices. In most cases the catheter can be ignored.

If the client has undergone amputation and uses a prosthesis, she may or may not want the device removed during the massage. Permission must be granted to massage the amputated area. If the client is comfortable with this, massage can be especially beneficial if a prosthesis is used. Although no scientific validation is available, professional experience has shown that massage strokes carried the full length of the amputated limb seem to feel good to the client.

Supporting Clients with a Size Impairment

If the client is short, a stool may be needed to help reach the massage table, clothing hangers, or restroom fixtures. The massage professional should casually sit down to establish eye contact with the client so that the person does not have to look up, which strains the neck.

A very large person may not trust the massage table and may be more comfortable on a floor mat. Getting up and down from the floor may be difficult. Sometimes seated massage is the better option. Ask the client what is preferable. If the practitioner is nervous about doing the massage on the massage table, the client must be told (disclosure) because the therapist's anxiety will affect the quality of the massage.

Supporting Clients with Burns and Disfigurements

People who have been burned may face an assortment of challenges ranging from impaired mobility to disfigurement. As burns heal, scar tissue replaces functional epithelial tissue. All the functions of the skin are compromised, including excretion, sensation, and protection. Scar tissue tends to contract and pull, which can make the area of the healed burn feel shortened or tight. Severe contractures sometimes develop and must be treated medically. Myofascial release, craniosacral therapy, and other connective tissue techniques can soften and gently stretch connective tissue. Massage of this type may reduce the effect of this shrinkage somewhat. Professionals who want to serve clients who have been burned need additional training in these methods.

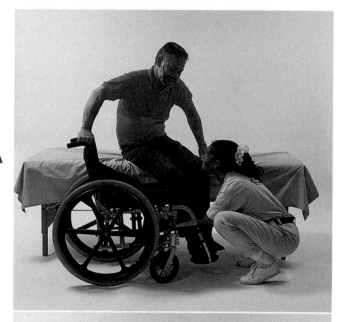

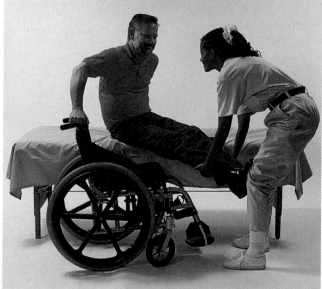

fig. 12-5

A, A transfer from a wheelchair to the massage table.
B, A low table that allows a lateral transfer is best.

12-9

PROFICIENCY EXERCISE

Contact your local building department and speak with the person in charge of the barrier-free code requirements. Find out the requirements and the reason for each.

Many disfigurements tend to draw our attention because the mind is designed to notice differences. Although many disfigurements do not limit function in any way, they can create social difficulties. Attempting not to notice a disfigurement usually fails. The client recognizes the situation exists and has various levels of comfort with the condition. Honest communication is effective in redirecting the attention from the disfigurement to the person over time. The practitioner might offer a simple statement such as, "I can't help but notice (the particular disfigurement). I'm not uncomfortable, but the difference naturally draws my attention. Please be patient with me until I become more familiar with you."

Barrier-Free Access

All massage facilities must be barrier free. Commercial buildings usually are required by law to have barrier-free access and elevators, as well as restroom facilities accessible to individuals with a handicap (Proficiency Exercise 12-9).

PSYCHOLOGICALLY CHALLENGED INDIVIDUALS

section objectives

Using the information presented in this section, the student will be able to perform the following:

- ■ **Understand the importance of verifying informed consent when working with individuals who have a psychologic disability**
- ■ **Structure a massage to support other psychologic interventions**

The Americans with Disabilities Act defines **mental impairment** as any mental or psychologic disorder such as mental retardation (developmental disabilities), organic brain syndrome, emotional or mental illness, and specific learning disabilities.[2]

We will consider the following:

- Addictions
- Chemical imbalances in the brain
- Developmental disabilities
- Learning disabilities
- Mood disorders
- Posttraumatic stress disorder

Again, the actual massage approach is no different when working with psychologically challenged individuals. The important factor is the person receiving the massage. Practitioners who want to work with clients with psychologic challenges need additional training to be able to understand the physiology and psychology of the various disorders and the challenges these clients face. An understanding of psychotropic pharmacology is important because massage and these medications affect the body in similar ways. This type of work should be supervised closely by a psychologist or psychiatrist.

At times we are all challenged psychologically. It is important to understand how our minds work and the interaction of the mind/body connection. Results of current research are becoming available that show the link between the mind, the body, and health. A dedicated student of massage will seriously consider taking some psychology courses at a community college or other educational center and keeping up to date on the new findings. Massage will continue to have a very important place in mind/body medicine and treatments, along with other forms of mental health services.

The Importance of Informed Consent

Informed consent is an important concern when working with clients influenced by drugs (both prescribed and not), internal chemical imbalances, and developmental disabilities. Special care must be taken to ensure that the client is able to provide informed consent. When doubt exists, the massage should not be given.

Addictions

Individuals withdrawing from chemical and alcohol addictions may find that massage helps reduce stress levels. The type of chemical to which the person is addicted determines the types of stressful experiences incurred. The therapist listens to the client and helps decide whether the massage could calm an anxious client or give a boost to a depressed client. Heavy connective tissue massage should be avoided during withdrawal phases. Toxins released from this type of massage may overtax a system already burdened with withdrawal detoxification.

Chemical Imbalances in the Brain

Certain types of mental disability arise from an imbalance of brain chemicals. Hyperactivity, ADD, bipolar (manic-depressive) disorder, schizophrenia, seasonal affective disorder, obsessive-compulsive disorder, and clinical depression are just a few brain chemical disorders.

Medication is important in helping these individuals. The massage professional should never make the client feel guilty for taking medication or suggest that medication is not necessary. Medication must be monitored carefully by a physician, with the smallest effective dosage given to avoid side effects. Massage cannot replace medication, but the client who receives regular massage may be able to reduce the dosage and duration in some situations. In other situations the side effects of certain medications can be managed with massage. It is very important to work with the client's physician and chart the client's response to the massage carefully.

Developmental Disabilities

Massage for those with developmental disabilities has the same effect as for everyone else. Care must be taken to communicate at the client's level of understanding but not below functioning level. Adults with developmental disabilities are not children and should not be treated as such. Developmentally disabled people may become frustrated and anxious during a day of challenges. Life is more difficult for them to manage. If accepted by these clients, massage is soothing, calming, and beneficial, but remember, not everyone likes to be touched, and the individual's needs must be respected.

Autism is believed to be a developmental disorder characterized by impaired social interaction and communication and a restricted repertoire of interests. Contrary to popular belief, most children and adults with autism do want to be touched. A very reliable, structured touch with firm, consistent pressure usually is preferred. Massage applied in a very deliberate way within the client's comfort level has been shown to increase social interaction somewhat and reduce anxiety.

Learning Disorders

Difficulties with processing sensory input, which occurs in some learning disorders, may be helped by the organized, systematic, sensory stimulation of massage. Having a learning difficulty is stressful. *(Author's note: I have dyslexia, as well as an inner ear dysfunction that makes hand-eye coordination difficult. Thank goodness for computers, spell checkers, and editors.)* Life is more difficult when one is dealing with any special situation. Stress from dealing with the environment aggravates the learning difficulty. Self-esteem is hard to maintain when a person has been made to feel stupid in school because he or she could not write, spell, or read. People with learning disabilities are not stupid, they just need to learn differently. Massage helps reduce their stress, thereby facilitating learning and enabling them to feel more positive about themselves.

Psychiatric Disorders

Psychiatric disorders such as anxiety, panic, depression, and eating disorders interplay in a combination of autonomic nervous system functions and hormone neurotransmitters, neuropeptides, and other brain chemicals. **Anxiety** is an uneasy feeling usually connected with increased sympathetic arousal responses. **Panic** is an intense, sudden, and overwhelming fear or feeling of anxiety that produces terror and immediate physiologic change that results in paralyzed immobility or senseless, hysteric behavior. A panic attack is an episode of acute anxiety that occurs at unpredictable times with feelings of intense apprehension or terror. It may be accompanied by a feeling of shortness of breath that leads to hyperventilation, dizziness, sweating, trembling, and chest pain or heart palpitations. Most symptoms can be directly related to overactivation of the sympathetic autonomic nervous system.

Depression is characterized by a decrease in vital functional activity, mood disturbances of exaggerated emptiness, hopelessness, and melancholy, or unbridled periods of high energy with no purpose or outcome.

It is common to see anxiety and depressive disorders in conjunction with fatigue and pain syndromes. **Pain and fatigue syndromes** are multicausal and often chronic, nonproductive patterns that interfere with well-being, activities of living, and productivity. Some such syndromes are fibromyalgia, chronic fatigue syndrome, infection with the Epstein-Barr virus, sympathetic reflex dystrophy, headache, arthritis, chronic cancer pain, neuropathy, low back syndrome, idiopathic pain, somatization disorder, and intractable pain syndrome.

Acute pain, as well as acute "episodes" of chronic conditions, can be factors in these syndromes. Panic behavior, phobias, and the sense of impending doom, along with the sense of being overwhelmed and of hopelessness, are common with these conditions. Mood swings, hyperventilation, sleep disturbance, concentration difficulties, memory disturbances, outbursts of anger, fatigue, and changes in habits of daily living, appetite, and activity levels are symptoms of these conditions and syndromes.

Eating disorders involve mood disorders, physiologic responses to food, and control issues. They are complicated situations that usually require professional intervention. The job of the massage therapist is to be aware of a possibility of an eating disorder and to refer the client. Any substantial weight loss must be referred to a physician. Individuals who have anorexia nervosa (a starving disorder) lose a great deal of weight. It is more difficult to recognize bulimia, which involves binge eating and purging by vomiting and laxatives. The teeth and gums are affected by the stomach acids, and the massage professional may notice this. Referral should be made because of symptoms, not because the therapist is attempting to diagnose the disorder.

Hyperventilation syndrome often is a significant underlying factor with anxiety and panic. Massage can normalize the breathing muscles, which must be done to correct a dysfunctional breathing pattern.

Because acute and chronic pain are managed somewhat differently it is important to make the distinction between the two. Intervention for acute pain is less invasive and focused on supporting a current healing process. Chronic pain is managed with either symptom relief or a more aggressive rehabilitation approach that incorporates a therapeutic change process.

When working with clients who have psychiatric disorders, the most common approach is general stress reduction massage. This type of massage may take the edge off the mood through the influence of massage on the autonomic nervous system. The type of massage given can be adjusted to be a little more stimulating or a little more relaxing. The key is to begin where the person is at the time of the massage. Someone who is anxious initially may resist long, slow strokes and instead may do better with a strategy that begins with active joint movement, postisometric relaxation, lengthening and stretching, and rapid compression and gradually shifts into a calming, rocking massage with long, slow strokes. The person who is a little depressed may not initially want to join in with an active participation massage. Instead, the work might begin with rocking and long, slow strokes and end with stimulating active joint movement, rapid compression, and *tapotement.*

Massage affects the brain chemicals by encouraging the release of serotonin, dopamine, and the endorphins, which alter mood. It also affects the release of various hormones that influence mood. Massage has a strong normalizing effect on the autonomic nervous system and can support other interventions for psychiatric disorders.

Posttraumatic Stress Disorder

Posttraumatic stress disorder involves the reexperiencing of flashback memory, as well as state-dependent memory,

somatization, anxiety, irritability, sleep disturbance, concentration difficulties, times of melancholy or depression, grief, fear, worry, anger, and avoidance behavior. Excessive stress can manifest as a number of disorders, such as cardiovascular problems, including hypertension; digestive difficulties, including heartburn, ulcer, and bowel syndromes; respiratory illness; susceptibility to bacterial and viral illnesses; endocrine dysfunction, particularly adrenal or thyroid dysfunction; delayed or diminished cellular repair; sleep disorder; and hyperventilation syndrome, to mention just a few. Posttraumatic stress disorder can have long-term effects.

Trauma occurs as a result of physical injury by violent or disruptive action or by a toxic substance or as a result of psychic injury caused by a short- or long-term severe emotional shock.

Because therapeutic massage is effective in normalizing the effects or physiologic manifestations of stress on the body, it can be an effective tool in the management of or recovery from posttraumatic stress disorder (Proficiency Exercise 12-10).

12-10

PROFICIENCY EXERCISE

Based on the information presented in this section, choose one psychologic challenge and write an intervention plan and justification statement for the use of therapeutic massage. Use the model in Box 12-1 as an example.

Therapeutic massage for _____

1. Gather facts to identify and define the situation.

Key questions
What is the problem?
What are the facts?

2. Brainstorm possible solutions.

Key question
What might I do?
What if . . . ?

3. Evaluate possible interventions logically and objectively; look at both sides and pros and cons.

Key question
What would happen if . . . ?

Continued.

PREGNANCY

Using the information presented in this section, the student will be able to perform the following:

- Explain the importance of prenatal care
- Describe the three basic stages of pregnancy
- Design a general massage session to meet the needs of a pregnant woman
- Teach a support person basic massage methods to use during labor

Early prenatal care provided by qualified health care professionals is very important for pregnant women. Pregnancy is not an illness; it is a natural event. Prenatal care is needed to ensure that proper nutrition is provided for the mother and that the pregnancy is progressing normally and to identify any potential problems early. If a woman is planning to become pregnant, it is useful for her to build and maintain her health for about 6 months beforehand. This means eliminating all alcohol, drugs, and nicotine, normalizing her weight, developing a moderate exercise program, and eating a nutritious diet. These activities help prepare the best environment for the baby's growth. Smoking, alcohol, and drug use are very dangerous to the unborn child. Excessive stress also is dangerous to the developing infant and can be the cause of miscarriage and inability to conceive.

Pregnancy is divided into three distinct segments: the first, second, and third trimesters. A pregnant woman un-dergoes extensive physical and emotional changes during each of these stages.

The First Trimester

During the first 3 months (the first trimester), the woman's body must adjust to tremendous hormonal changes, which are likely to cause mood swings. The most common complaint is morning sickness or nausea, which results from the physical adjustment to the growing baby. This is also a very vulnerable time for the developing baby. Massage given at this time is general wellness massage, which may help balance the mother's physiologic responses. Positioning is not a concern, unless the breasts are tender, because the abdomen has not yet started to expand. Deep work on the abdomen is avoided so as not to disrupt the attachment of the baby to the uterine wall. Surface stroking can be pleasurable to the client.

The Second Trimester

The second trimester usually brings a leveling of the hormones, and the woman feels better. During this time she may start to show and feel the first movements of the baby. If the pregnancy was planned, this is a joyful time. If not, the physical evidence of the growing baby may cause additional stress for the mother. Toward the end of the second trimester, the connective tissue begins to soften to allow the pelvis to spread. The joints seem to become sloppy. The muscles of the legs, gluteals, and hip flexors must provide joint stabilization. Overstretching must be

---

12-10

PROFICIENCY EXERCISE—CONT'D

4. Evaluate the effect on the people involved.

   Key question
   How would each person involved feel . . . ?

5. Develop an intervention plan and justification statements.

avoided. Carpal tunnel syndrome is common among pregnant women and may be perpetuated even after the birth as a result of caring for the infant. Support for the abdomen is important (Fig. 12-6).

Be attentive for strain in the back muscles during positioning. Keep the head in alignment with the spine. Using a support so that the shoulder lies comfortably and does not fall forward or toward the ear is helpful. Support between the knees helps keep the hips in the neutral position and relieves stress in this area. A support under the top arm may also be comfortable (see Fig. 12-6). As in the first trimester, deep work on the abdomen must be avoided.

The Third Trimester

During the last (third) trimester, the weight of the growing baby, the postural shifts, and the movement of the internal organs may cause discomfort for the pregnant woman. Because many of the internal organs are pushed up and back the diaphragm does not work as efficiently. The mother uses her neck and shoulder muscles to breathe, possibly causing discomfort or thoracic outlet symptoms. Hyperventilation syndrome may develop. Massage offers temporary relief of these symptoms.

About 2 weeks before birth (in the first pregnancy), the baby turns head down and drops into the birth canal. This provides more space for the diaphragm to work and breathing becomes easier, but pressure on the bladder causes frequent urination. Impingement on lymph vessels may cause the legs and feet to swell. Edema or fluid accumulation may be a symptom of more serious complications, and the client should be referred to a physician immediately if these are noted. The low back may ache from the postural shift. The breasts have enlarged in preparation for lactation. A woman may not feel very attractive at this point and most likely is not very comfortable physically. Fatigue and sleep disturbances may result. Massage is gentle, supports comfort, and assists circulation. If a comfortable position cannot be found, allow the client to change position often and use the restroom as needed. General massage may help the woman feel better for a little while and support comfortable sleep.

Labor

Labor occurs as the baby moves down the birth canal prior to birth. Education and birthing classes are important, especially for first pregnancies. It may be appropriate to teach the woman's support person some massage techniques before the onset of labor. Massage given by the support person helps that person to feel useful and involved with the pregnancy and birthing process. Massage of the lower back and stroking of the abdomen may provide comfort and a point of focus during labor. Massaging the feet often is helpful. Massage can relax the body and divert the attention of the nervous system, thereby providing distraction

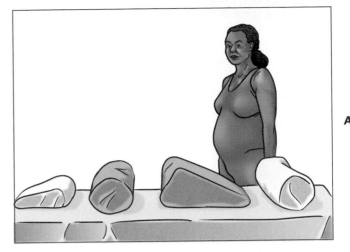
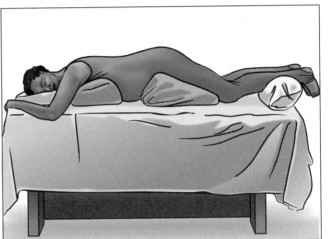
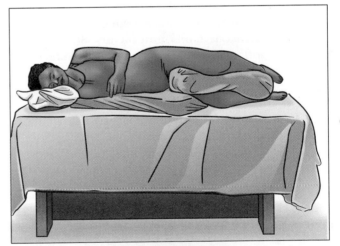

fig. 12-6

A, Placement of supports when massaging a pregnant woman. **B,** Supports for the prone position. **C,** Supports for the side-lying position.

during early labor. Labor proceeds easier and faster if the woman is relaxed and works with her body.

During a phase of labor called *transition,* it is not uncommon for the woman not to want to be touched. Transition occurs just before the second stage of labor, with the actual movement of the baby down the birth canal. The contractions at this time are very hard and have not yet been replaced by the urge to push. After delivery, massage may help the woman's body return to normal, it may reduce the stress of taking care of a new baby, and it may give the client some time to take care of herself.

Recommendations for Massage during Pregnancy

Unless specific circumstances or complications are involved, massage for pregnant women should be a general massage. Do not massage vigorously or extremely deeply, do not overstretch, and do not massage the abdomen other than with superficial stroking. Avoid massage on the inside of the ankle because there is a reflex point in that area that stimulates uterine contractions (this area is located on the spleen meridian). Watch for fever, edema, varicose veins, and severe mood swings. After birth, postpartum depression can become a serious problem for some women. Refer a client with these conditions to her physician immediately.

There are times when pregnancy is not a joyous event, as in an unwanted pregnancy. The practitioner must not try to convince the woman that she really does want the baby or try to change her mood. She must be supported with caring, quiet touch and listening.

Interrupted pregnancies also are difficult. Whether the cause is spontaneous abortion in the first 3 months, induced abortion, or miscarriage, an interrupted pregnancy is a strain on a woman's body and emotional well-being. If a client has had an interrupted pregnancy, watch for emotional changes at what would have been the projected time of birth. Extra caring and support are helpful then.

The massage professional must have permission from the physician or licensed midwife to work with a woman during pregnancy. Giving a general massage to a pregnant

woman can be a very rewarding experience, one that allows the massage professional to watch the miracle of life develop (Proficiency Exercise 12-11).

TERMINAL ILLNESS

section objectives

Using the information presented in this section, the student will be able to perform the following:

- **Obtain additional information about the process of dying**
- **Explain the importance of comfort measures**

When nothing further can be done to prolong life, care focuses more on comfort measures. The experts in terminal illness are the dedicated hospice nurses and staff members who treat death with dignity. It has been said that the staff members of hospices are midwives to the dying.

In order for the massage practitioner to work successfully with those dealing with a terminal illness, the practitioner must be aware of his or her personal feelings about death. It is strongly encouraged that every massage professional who wants to work with clients during this very important, challenging, and special time of life become hospice volunteers and take the training that hospices offer.

No one knows when a person is going to die. However, two very powerful psychologic forces influence living and dying: hope and the will to live. Attitudes about death vary. Adults usually have more fears about death than children do. They fear pain, suffering, dying alone, the invasion of privacy, loneliness, and separation from family and loved ones. They worry about who will care for and support those left behind. Elderly people usually have fewer of these fears than younger adults. They may be more accepting that death will occur and have had more experience with dying and death. Many have lost family members and friends. Some welcome death as freedom from pain, suffering, and disability.

Dr. Elizabeth Kubler-Ross has written about death, and her works have much to offer. Bernie Siegal's books also are excellent. Massage professionals interested in working with the terminally ill would benefit from reading their works.

Massage has much to offer in comfort measures for the terminally ill. Being bedridden and immobile is painful. Massage can distract the sensory perception and provide temporary comfort measures. It provides continued human contact and can give caregivers something useful, rewarding, and positive to do for their loved one who is dying.

Massage can become an important stress reduction method and a means of support for family members and caregivers. Caring for someone who is terminally ill can be very stressful. This support person may need to receive

---

12-11

PROFICIENCY EXERCISE

1. Contact your local hospital or other agency offering childbirth classes. See if it would be possible to attend as an observer.
2. Locate a pregnant dog, cat, or horse. While giving the animal a massage, gently palpate the abdomen.

massage simply to have someone take care of him or her for an hour. Teaching simple massage methods to the caregivers provides them with a means of meaningful and structured interaction with their loved one, as well as a means of connecting with and supporting each other.

The massage professional should be an integral part of the team that works to make this time of passage as gentle as possible. This means that once the decision to work with someone who is terminally ill has been made, it is important to stay with the process until the client dies (if possible). The therapist probably will grow to care for the person, will cry when death comes, and will mourn and grieve.

As always, it remains the client's choice as to what is wanted, and he or she must give informed consent. The client who is dying needs to retain as much personal empowerment as possible. It should not be discouraging if all that is done during a massage session is to stroke a client's hands. At this time, especially, it is crucial to "listen" and "allow" (Proficiency Exercise 12-12).

12-12

PROFICIENCY EXERCISE

1. Plan your funeral. List all plans and details regarding final arrangements.
2. Talk with an attorney about living wills.
3. Volunteer to provide massage for hospice staff members. Spend a minimum of 32 hours.
4. In the space provided, write about how you wish to be taken care of when it is your time to die. How much intervention do you want? Do you want to die in a hospital or at home? When do you want hospice services?

SUMMARY

Respect is important in any interaction with another person. In all situations, remember to see and address the person first, and then to accommodate the individual's special needs by offering assistance and following the directions provided by the client. Massage therapists who want to focus their professional skills to best meet the specific needs of a person will seek out training and information pertinent to the therapeutic needs of each client. Often the knowledge base required to provide massage to many populations becomes too extensive, and it becomes necessary to specialize. When this is the situation, such as when a massage professional obtains additional training for sports massage, the information is built on the fundamentals of massage and the additional training is focused on the application of the massage fundamentals for the special situation.

The wise professional recognizes when less intervention is more appropriate. It requires much learning, great skill, and patiently developed empathy to therapeutically hold someone's hand.

REFERENCES

1. Benjamin PJ, Lamp SP: *Understanding sports massage,* Champaign, Ill., 1996, Human Kinetics.
2. McGladrey, Pullen: *The Americans With Disabilities Act (rev.),* New York, 1994, Panel Publishers.

WORKBOOK SECTION

Short Answer

1. What is the single most important factor for effective communication with those who have special needs?

   _____

   _____

   _____

   _____

2. What special massage skills are needed to work with those with special needs?

   _____

   _____

   _____

3. What is the best source of information about any special situation?

   _____

   _____

   _____

   _____

4. What is a general definition of abuse?

   _____

   _____

   _____

   _____

5. What importance does state-dependent memory have in working with those who may have a history of abuse?

   _____

   _____

   _____

   _____

6. What responses might the massage practitioner receive when pointing out an area of injury to a client who self-abuses?

   _____

   _____

   _____

   _____

7. How should a massage practitioner respond if a client experiences an emotional response during the massage?

   _____

   _____

   _____

   _____

8. Why is massage beneficial for athletes?

   _____

   _____

   _____

   _____

9. What is restorative massage for athletes?

   _____

   _____

   _____

   _____

10. What type of massage is provided at sports events?

    _____

    _____

    _____

WORKBOOK SECTION

11. What adjustment to a massage session may need to be made when working with children?

_____

_____

_____

_____

12. Why do children like massage?

_____

_____

_____

_____

13. What is a major benefit of massage for children and adolescents?

_____

_____

_____

_____

14. Why is it important to teach parents and children some basic massage methods to share with each other?

_____

_____

_____

_____

15. Who gives informed consent for massage for those under 18 years of age?

_____

_____

_____

_____

16. What is a realistic goal for the massage professional when working with those who have a chronic illness?

_____

_____

_____

_____

17. What is the importance of hardiness, and how does massage encourage it?

_____

_____

_____

_____

18. Why is close supervision by the physician or other health professional important when working with those who have a chronic illness?

_____

_____

_____

_____

19. What can the massage therapist learn from working with the elderly?

_____

_____

_____

_____

20. What special physical conditions are common among the elderly?

_____

_____

_____

_____

21. Are special skills required for working with the elderly?

_____

_____

_____

_____

22. Why is massage beneficial for infants?

_____

_____

_____

_____

23. Who is the best person to massage a baby?

_____

_____

_____

_____

24. What key elements are important when massaging an infant?

_____

_____

_____

_____

25. What are the unique concerns of working in the medical environment or with those receiving home health care?

_____

_____

_____

_____

26. What are important things to remember when working with clients who have a physical disability?

_____

_____

_____

_____

27. When working with those who have an emotional or developmental disability, what important factor must the massage therapist consider?

_____

_____

_____

_____

28. How can massage be beneficial in withdrawal from addiction, in learning disabilities, and in developmental disabilities?

_____

_____

_____

_____

29. Are special massage skills required when working with pregnant women? Explain.

_____

_____

_____

_____

30. What part can teaching massage to the expectant father or other support person play?

_____

_____

_____

_____

31. What can providing massage for someone who is dying teach us?

_____

_____

_____

_____

WORKBOOK SECTION

32. What is the best source of information about working with the dying?

_____

_____

_____

_____

33. What can massage offer to someone who is dying?

_____

_____

_____

_____

Problem-Solving Exercises

1. You are working at an organized sporting event as a volunteer for the local sports massage team. You notice that one of the other team members is doing deep invasive work on one of the clients. What should you do?

_____

_____

_____

_____

2. A client begins to shake and to breathe very deeply during the massage. What do you do?

_____

_____

_____

_____

3. An elderly client wants you to stay after the massage and have a cup of coffee. What do you do?

_____

_____

_____

_____

4. A young father is having trouble holding his newborn baby. What can you do?

_____

_____

_____

_____

5. A client with a speech difficulty needs to provide informed consent. How could this be accomplished?

_____

_____

_____

_____

_____

6. A client is near death. She does not want a full massage but needs to be touched. What can you do?

_____

_____

_____

_____

Professional Application

You are asked to give a presentation to a group of nurses at a local hospital. They are looking for ways to use massage in various outpatient situations. They need a general explanation of ways massage would be beneficial in many different conditions. What major points would you make during the talk?

_____

_____

_____

_____

_____

_____

WORKBOOK SECTION

Research for Further Study

A major approach for massage is generalized, nonspecific, body supportive care. It does not seek to intervene but rather tries to provide support and nurture health. Brainstorm the various applications for massage in special needs situations and then find research to support some of the concepts.

_____

_____

_____

_____

ANSWER KEY

Short Answer

1. Always remember to interact with the person who has a special need. Do not allow yourself to become focused on the special situation. Consider the person first.

2. In providing wellness personal service massage, as opposed to rehabilitative massage, the skills are no different than those presented in this text. What is different is the situation presented by a client. An athlete has certain needs based on the sport, the pregnant woman based on the pregnancy, and those with a chronic illness based on the illness pattern. The massage practitioner needs additional training in the various situations and conditions to use the fundamental massage skills purposefully.

3. The client is the best source. Even if the client lacks technical knowledge about a particular illness, sport, pregnancy, disability, or emotional pattern, he or she is still the only one who really understands the effects of any situation.

4. Abuse is the deliberate taking away of a person's self-empowerment.

5. The touch of the massage professional may trigger a memory pattern. Each memory, including all the sensory information, nervous system functions, and endocrine functions in play at the time of the experience, is stored in a multidimensional way. When the body state changes, the memory becomes vague and less clear. Because massage produces changes in the nervous and endocrine systems and is a source of sensory stimulation, a state that holds a memory pattern for a client could be re-created. This may help a person resolve and integrate a past experience, provided appropriate professional support is available. Often only pieces of a memory are retrieved. This is common with body memories. The massage may trigger a physiologic response, yet no visual or sequential memory is retrievable. Just because a person does not remember who, what, when, why, or how does not mean that the memory is not valid.

6. The client may discount the injury, provide a cover story, feel guilty or ashamed, or be surprised that the injury is there. It is important for the massage therapist not to press the issue and to realize that self-abuse is a coping mechanism that may calm the person. The massage therapist must not perpetuate an abuse pattern by providing invasive massage.

7. Stay connected with the client but distanced from the experience, which belongs to the client. Continue the massage methods that triggered the response if the client agrees. Ask the client if he or she would like you to continue. Slow the methods and allow the body time to integrate and resolve the body memory. Refer the client if additional coping and counseling skills are indicated.

8. Compensating patterns that may develop from any sport respond well to maintenance massage methods. In addition, recovery occurs quicker and performance is enhanced by regular massage.

9. There are three forms of restorative massage: Recovery massage primarily focuses on the athlete who wants to recover from a strenuous workout or competition when no injury is present. Remedial massage is used for minor to moderate injuries. Rehabilitation massage is used for severe injury or as part of intervention after surgery.

10. Organizing a sports massage team to provide general circulation enhancement massage is a great public education and promotional concept. It is important to develop a simple 15-minute routine that all massage practitioners can use. A similar concept can be used for seated neck and shoulder massage in a corporate office.

11. Children's attention spans are shorter, therefore the massage may need to take less than an hour; 15 to 30 minutes is typical.

12. Touch is important during the growing years. Massage is an organized approach to touch, and the nervous system likes to learn from it. Wrestling and horsing around, both activities that many children do, may provide massagelike responses.

WORKBOOK SECTION

13. Massage provides temporary relief from growing pains.

14. Massage is a great, organized, and safe way to touch. This may help families stay in touch during both difficult and good times.

15. The parent or guardian provides informed consent and must supervise the massage session.

16. It is important for the massage professional to focus on helping the client feel better for a while rather than trying to eliminate the chronic illness. Chronic illness presents a variety of problems in living. For many, "healing" is the act of taking back self-control; not getting rid of the illness but learning to live with it in a resourceful manner. Massage can help the process by providing temporary symptomatic relief in a chronic illness.

17. Hardiness, or toughening, is the ability to physically and mentally withstand external stressors. Because of a decrease in physical activity and isolation, those with a chronic illness becomes less hardy. Massage is a gentle, organized, and controlled way to provide both physical and mental stress. It provides the client the opportunity to begin to assimilate and adjust to the sensory input in a way that increases hardiness.

18. Many people with a chronic illness are taking medication or undergoing other medical interventions. It is important for the medical professional to be able to monitor the effects of different therapies. Because massage interacts with both the nervous and endocrine systems, it is important that massage effects be monitored as part of the entire therapeutic outcome. Medication and the resulting side effects may be able to be reduced through a multidisciplinary approach to dealing with chronic illness.

19. The elderly have years of experiences to share. Patience, respect for time, and the importance of listening can be learned from the elderly.

20. Because of reduced joint space and changes in soft tissue, it is common to find nerve compression and resulting pain.

21. It is important to understand the physiology of aging and the physical changes that take place. The elderly client may take medication to control various physiologic processes, but in general, basic massage skills and an attentive, caring spirit are all that is required.

22. Massage provides an organized sensory stimulation that helps the nervous system to grow and begin to integrate information. It also provides a bonding method for parent and infant.

23. Primary caregivers gain the most from massaging the baby. The massage professional serves both the infant and the caregivers by teaching infant massage.

24. Infants instinctively know when a touch is not safe. They will not respond well to a nervous touch but depend instead on a confident touch. It is important to honor an infant's physiologic state and give him or her time to respond to the touch.

25. Supervision as part of a health care team requires tempering of independent treatment and clearing of all interventions to make sure that they coordinate with the total treatment plan. Charting is essential, as is attention to effective communication. The environment may be noisy and have interruptions and lack of privacy. The client may be taking medications or using special equipment such as intravenous lines.

26. Ask the client to explain the disability to you, as well as any limitations and the type of assistance needed. Then pay attention to the person, not the disability.

27. Special care must be taken to ensure that the client is able to provide informed consent.

28. Any form of disability makes daily life more stressful. Massage is a great way to reduce general stress levels.

29. Fundamental massage skills are sufficient for working with pregnant women. As in the aging process, pregnancy is a normal event, not a sickness. General wellness personal service massage is indicated. Consideration must be given to positioning, and emotional swings linked to hormonal changes need to be taken into account. The abdomen is never massaged deeply, and changes such as swelling should be referred to the physician or midwife. Oriental approaches sometimes indicate avoidance of the spleen meridian.

30. Massage gives that person something to do that is beneficial both as the pregnancy progresses and during labor.

31. Those who are dying are doing meaningful and serious work in going through this process. Being privileged to share in the process can teach us how to die with dignity.

32. A hospice is one of the best sources, and the massage practitioner is encouraged to support and learn from the dedicated individuals who work in hospices.

33. Massage supports other comfort measures. Physical touch can be an important link to this world. Just listening as the person puts his or her life in order and staying with the person throughout the process is important. Gentle touch and a spirit willing to connect and to mourn an inevitable loss are all that is necessary.

WORKBOOK SECTION

Problem-Solving Exercises

1. This is inappropriate behavior and could injure the client. Either speak with the sports massage team leader or quietly ask to speak with the team member and remind him or her that invasive work is inappropriate and could cause harm.
2. Gently ask the client if she is comfortable and would like to continue with the massage. If she wants to end the session, do so gently and with a sense of closure. If she chooses to continue, stay general with the approach and be quietly supportive.
3. This is a judgment call. Acknowledge that the social aspect of the massage is very important, and if you choose to stay for a bit more conversation, realize that you are establishing a pattern that may need to be continued.
4. Teach him massage to provide a way to organize the touch and meet the needs of the infant.
5. The client can write the message or use other technologic means such as a voice synthesizer to communicate.
6. Gently stroke her hands and feet and listen to her.

Professional Application

- Massage is a good support for comfort care.
- Massage is good for symptomatic relief of pain.
- Massage evens the mood.
- Massage reduces general stress levels.

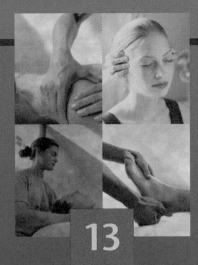

13

WELLNESS EDUCATION

objectives

*After completing this chapter, the student
will be able to perform the following:*

- Identify the basic components of a wellness program
- Locate resources to develop a wellness program
- Develop a personal wellness program
- Provide general wellness guidelines to clients

THIS chapter educates the massage professional about the general concepts of wellness. Massage is an important part of any wellness program because it restores body balance and provides a connection with other human beings. As such it is necessary for the massage professional to understand the components of "wellness." With this information the professional can explain to clients how massage fits into the overall wellness picture. It is not possible to define a step-by-step process that provides for wellness because each person is an individual and needs to develop a personal plan according to the general concepts of wellness. It is important to read this chapter with your heart and soul as well as with your mind.

Wellness programs can be built around the following factors:

Body
- Nutrition
- Light and dark exposure
- Sleep
- Breathing
- Movement
- Sensory stimulation

Mind
- Relationships with self and others
- Communications
- Beliefs
- Intellectual stimulation

Spirit
- Purpose
- Connection
- Faith
- Hope
- Love

We are considered *well* when body, mind, and spirit are in ideal balance.

We are not well when imbalance exists and balance cannot be restored.

In the words of renowned nutrition scientist Professor Jeffrey Bland, many people are "vertically ill." Such people are not sick enough to lie down, but they are certainly not well.[1] It seems to be more than the type of stress involved; it is the amount of stress that accumulates until the breakdown begins. It will be only a matter of time before physical health, the mind, or the quality of life simply falls apart under the accumulation of multiple stressors.

Each individual would benefit from the development of a personal wellness plan. Just as in designing a massage, no right or wrong way exists to formulate this plan. By following a few basic guidelines, whatever works is what is best for each person. Massage practitioners need to remember that as wonderful as massage is, it addresses only a part of the person. Wellness is about the whole person. The sensitive massage professional realizes that during a client's search for wellness, the time spent with the massage practitioner provides focused attention, acceptance, and effective listening, which are as important as the massage methods used.

This chapter examines the basic guidelines necessary for building a wellness program. It provides enough information to give some direction in the development and implementation of a wellness plan. As with massage, often the simpler the program the better it is. We are supposed to be well. Our bodies will recognize the best process.

Wellness has a domino effect. Simple alterations in lifestyle create a chain reaction throughout one's entire life. Consequently, it is necessary to commit only to a few carefully planned lifestyle alterations and then allow the rest of the "pieces" of our lives to fall into place.

Resistance usually occurs when an adjustment is necessary. We may initially resist change, which can come either from our own bodies or coping patterns, or from family and friends who interact with us. Remember, if our behavior changes, the people around us will have to change as well. Go slowly and allow the "pieces" (your own body, family, or friends) to comment, complain, support, and resist but do not give in and quit. Persist with the wellness program and give your body and your family and friends time to get used to your new lifestyle.

Making a change to wellness takes determination. Letting go of behavioral patterns is difficult. It is very hard to do this alone, so relationships with those who are supportive and believe in us (e.g., support groups, professional therapy) are helpful. The massage professional can be an important support person for the client making wellness changes in his or her life.

STRESS

Stress is our response to any demand on the body or mind to respond, adapt, or alter. It is a state of readiness to survive, requiring hypervigilance from the body and mind. It is our emotional reaction to stress that may be the difference between positive action and/or destructive breakdown, especially if many of the stressors seem beyond our control.[1]

An expert on stress, Hans Selye, said the following[4]:

The ancient Greek philosophers clearly recognized that, with regard to human conduct, the most important, but perhaps also the most difficult thing was 'to know thyself.' It takes great courage even just to attempt this honestly . . . Yet it is well worth the effort and humiliation, because most of our tensions and frustrations stem from compulsive needs to act the role of someone we are not.

Before any wellness program can be developed, a person needs to at least "explore thyself." The next step is to analyze and explore the stressors that we all encounter in our daily lives. The three major elements of stress are the stressor itself, the defensive measures, and the mechanisms for surrender.

Stressors are any internal perceptions or external stimuli that demand a change in the body. The **defensive mea-**

sures are the ways our bodies defend against the stressor, such as the production of antibodies and white blood cells or behavioral and emotional defenses. Sometimes defending is not the best way to deal with stress. It is important and resourceful to know when to quit or surrender. Hormonal and nervous stimuli encourage the body to retreat and ignore stressors. On an emotional level this is sometimes called **denial,** which can be an important method of coping with stress.[4]

It has long been known that mental excitement and physical stressors cause an initial exhilaration, followed by a secondary phase of depression. A law of physics states that for every action there is an opposite and equal reaction. Certain identifiable chemical compounds, such as the hormones produced during the acute alarm reaction phase of the general adaptation syndrome (discussed in Chapter 4), possess the property of first keying up for action and then causing a depression. Both effects may provide great protective value to the body. It is necessary to be keyed up for peak accomplishments, but it is equally important to relax in the secondary phase of depression. This prevents us from carrying on too long at top speed (Box 13-1). Selye says the following[4]:

The fact is that a person can be intoxicated with his own stress hormones. I venture to say that this sort of drunkenness has caused much more harm to society than the alcoholic kind. We are on our guard against external toxicants, but hormones are parts of our bodies; it takes more wisdom to recognize and overcome the foe which fights from within. In all our actions throughout the day, we must consciously look for signs of being keyed up too much, and we must learn to stop in time. To watch our critical stress level is just as important as to watch our critical

quota of cocktails. More so. Intoxication by stress is sometimes unavoidable and usually insidious. You can quit alcohol and, even if you do take some, at least you can count the glasses; but it is impossible to avoid stress as long as you live, and your conscious thoughts often cannot gauge its alarm signals accurately. Curiously the pituitary is a much better judge of stress than the intellect. Yet, you can learn to recognize the danger signals fairly well if you know what to look for.

Depending on our conditioning and genetic makeup, we all respond differently to general stress. As a whole, each person tends to respond consistently, with one set of signs, in individualized patterns caused by the malfunctioning of whatever happens to be the most vulnerable part in his or her physiology. When warning signs appear, it is time to stop, change the activity, and divert the body's attention to something else.

If proportionately too much stress occurs in any physical or emotional area of the body, the energy needs to be diverted to a different area. If a person is thinking too much, then he or she should use the larger muscles of the body (e.g., gardening, taking a brisk walk). If too much exercise is causing stress, balance can be restored by reading a novel, watching a movie, or listening to soft music. If too much stress occurs in the body as a whole, rest is required. If we do not rest of our own accord, the body may become ill so that we will rest for awhile.

WELLNESS COMPONENTS

Wellness training requires an extensive amount of information about diet, exercise, lifestyle, and behavior patterns. It is important to seek out those with experience to provide that information. Do not depend on only one information source. Talk with two, three, or four "experts" and read three or four books on each topic before making decisions about what could be done to benefit or improve

---

box 13-1

COMMON STRESS RESPONSES

- General irritability, hyperexcitation, or depression
- Pounding of the heart
- Dryness of the throat and mouth
- Impulsive behavior and emotional instability
- Overpowering urge to cry, run, or hide
- Inability to concentrate
- Weakness or dizziness
- Fatigue
- Tension and extreme alertness
- Trembling and nervous tics
- Intermittent anxiety
- Tendency to be easily startled
- High-pitched, nervous laughter
- Stuttering and other speech difficulties
- Grinding teeth
- Insomnia
- Inability to sit still or physically relax

- Sweating
- Frequent need to urinate
- Diarrhea, indigestion, queasiness, and vomiting
- Migraine and other tension headaches
- Premenstrual tension or missed menstrual cycles
- Pain in the neck or lower back
- Loss of or excessive appetite
- Increased use of chemicals, including tobacco, caffeine, and alcohol
- Nightmares
- Neurotic behavior
- Psychosis
- Proneness to accidents

The massage professional recognizes that these signs of stress result from fluctuations in the autonomic nervous system and resulting endogenous chemical shifts.

your wellness. Remember, only a few symptoms combine to create a huge array of illness and disease patterns. Fortunately, a combination of only a few lifestyle changes is required to redirect a disease pattern toward a more resourceful and healing pattern.

When developing a wellness program, consider your mental and physical history. Our sense of self in relation to others is also important. If this connection with others is not respected and nurtured, the wholeness of our life is strained. This strain may interfere with our spiritual, emotional, and physical health.

Many of us have been sick, or at the very least "vertically ill." It may take extraordinary effort to reverse these situations. That is when we realize maybe we should have taken better care of ourselves in the first place. Taking care of ourselves is what wellness and massage are all about.

Communication

People are not designed to be alone; therefore we must be able to communicate effectively with each other. If we do not communicate effectively with others and with ourselves, our energy is confused and our responses scattered. Communication is one of the biggest problems for humans because it is so subjective. It is very difficult to be truly objective; knowing this is an important part of wellness. Wellness requires assuming responsibility for our communication. Chapter 2 provides guidelines for communication in the professional world, but these same skills enhance communication in all personal interactions.

Demands

Today, many of the demands placed on us are outside the design of the body: too much to know, too much to do, too many responsibilities, and too many places to be. Our lives have become hurried, and a constant battle for time exists. Too many options exist with too many choices, and it all costs too much.

Wellness often revolves around simplification of lifestyle. Simplification requires choices, boundaries, discipline, and "letting go" in many dimensions.

Loss

Sometimes an event in life removes some part of us. It could be a body part, a body function, a relationship, a member of our family, or a job. Loss heals though grieving. Grief is a physiologic response that includes stimulation of the sympathetic autonomic nervous system. The emotional response is first alarm, then disbelief and denial, progressing to anger and guilt. This process progresses to finding a source of comfort and finally adjustment to the loss. To heal, we need to reconstruct that part or learn to live resourcefully without it.

Seeking Help

Many professionals can help us with specific therapeutic interventions as the wellness program is developed. Doctors, counselors, other health care providers, educators, and religious and spiritual advisors all play an important part in helping us become well again or maintain our wellness. Ultimately, each of us must do the work and take responsibility for who, what, and where we are, but it is important to use what help is available. For example, if a person has a large tumor growth and a surgeon can safely remove it, then the doctor's help will give the body a head start on healing.

Intuition

A balance exists between intuition and research in wellness. In developing a wellness program, it is important to consider these two very important sources of information. Hippocrates advised "do no harm." A wellness program relies on adherence to this advice, in addition to a balance between what science knows and *what we know we need*. A wellness program needs to change as we change. When a good wellness program is carried out, a person looks forward to getting back to living life to the fullest and, at the appropriate time, dying with dignity (Proficiency Exercise 13-1).

Body

Our bodies are our dwelling places in this life. They are the most concrete aspects of our being. The care of our bodies is an important part of any wellness program. Areas that require attention in a wellness program to support the body are the following: nutrition, breathing, exercise and stretching, relaxation, sleep, and feelings.

Nutrition

Proper nutrition is easy to explain, but people do not always follow recommendations. This is because nutrition involves more than just eating. Eating affects the mood; mood influences feelings; and behavior supports feelings. The issue of food therefore becomes an emotional topic.

The basics of balanced nutrition are explained in the Department of Agriculture's new guide to good eating. The original four food group recommendations have been

---

13-1

PROFICIENCY EXERCISE

Begin to build a library about wellness. Take an inventory of books and magazines you already have. Categorize them and commit to adding one new book at least every 3 months. Explore your public library and become familiar with what wellness resources it has to offer.

changed to a pyramidal shape, which suggests a diet high in vegetables, grains, legumes, and fruit. The protein requirement from animal sources has been decreased. Dairy needs are moderate to small. When purchasing any animal products, you may want to locate naturally raised and hormone-free products.

Although fat and sugar requirements in the diet are minimal, human beings have a strong urge for sweets and fats. It is this instinctive craving for fat and sugar that contributes to most dietary problems. In early days of human existence these two substances were difficult to find. Human beings had to have a deep instinctual desire to fight the bees for their honey, and the animals for their fat or to gather fatty seeds. Today these substances are in abundance, but our primitive nature still acts as though we need to store up for a future famine.

An ideal diet is low in fats and sugars and moderately low in protein and dairy, with the bulk of the calories coming from complex carbohydrates.

Cycles of high and low blood sugar are produced by unbalanced diets, aggravated by improper spacing between meals, and supported by substances such as coffee, tea, alcohol, and cola drinks. These fluids stimulate adrenaline production, which forces sugar to be released into the blood. The body then pushes sugar levels down again with insulin.

Drinking enough pure water is very important to a wellness program. Because our bodies are more than 70% water, most diets recommend at least 64 ounces of water per day for efficient body function.

Adequate fiber and water in the diet support bladder and bowel habits that support wellness. Eating on a regular schedule is important to support body rhythms that in turn support wellness.

Nutritional supplements. Many people take nutritional supplements. Experts disagree on the value of these. The food source is compromised by depleted soil and artificial fertilizers and tainted by pesticides and other chemicals. In addition, nutritional value is compromised by long-term storage and preservation. It is difficult to obtain optimal nutritional value from the food we eat without extraordinary attention to our diet, which requires time, dedication, and discipline.

Supplementation is a plausible answer to this problem. The only recommendation offered is that the closer a supplement is to a "real food," the better the body will be able to use it. It is usually best to take supplements with food to enhance absorption.

Herbs, which are very powerful substances, should not be used as nutritional supplements or medicines without knowledge of their effects (Proficiency Exercise 13-2).

Breathing

Breathing provides us with air—a very essential nutrient. Breathing patterns are a direct link to altering autonomic nervous system patterns, which in turn affect mood, feelings, and behavior. Almost every meditation or relaxation system uses breathing patterns. Other ways to modulate breathing are through singing and chanting.

Proper breathing is important, but most of us do not breathe efficiently. For many the air quality is not very good. The rest of us may be in too big of a hurry to breathe deeply. Slow, deep breathing takes time. The simple bellows breathing mechanism is a body-wide coordination of muscle contraction and relaxation. A good way to recognize the full-body effect of breathing is to do the following activity:

Tighten your feet by gripping the floor with your toes. Take a deep breath and feel what happens. Relax your feet and again notice what happens. Tighten the gluteal muscles and take a deep breath. Then relax the muscles and take another deep breath, again noting what happens. These exercises should demonstrate that breathing involves more muscles than the diaphragm and intercostals.

The shoulders do not move during normal relaxed breathing. The accessory muscles of respiration located in the neck area should be activated only when increased oxygen is required for the fight-or-flight response. This is the pattern for sympathetic dominance breathing. If the person does not balance the oxygen/carbon dioxide levels through increased activity levels, hyperventilation can occur. Patterns of hyperventilation can perpetuate anxiety states. (See Box 4-3, p. 167.)

The accessory muscles of respiration (such as the scalenes, sternocleidomastoid, serratus posterior superior, levator scapulae, rhomboids, abdominals, and quadratus lumborum) may be constantly activated for breathing when forced inhalation and expiration are not needed. This will result in dysfunctional muscle patterns. Often tightness in the quadratus lumborum or shoulder pain is not identified as an inefficient breathing pattern during assessment by the massage professional.

Phases of breathing. Breathing includes three phases of inspiration (bringing air into the body) and two phases of expiration (moving air out of the body). **Quiet inspiration** takes place when an individual is resting or sitting quietly. The diaphragm and external intercostals are the prime movers. As **deep inspiration** occurs, the actions of quiet inspiration are intensified. When people need more

---

13-2

PROFICIENCY EXERCISE

Keep a food diary for 2 days. If your diet is not well balanced, decide what it would take to develop a plan that cuts fat and sugar intake and increases water intake to recommended levels.

oxygen, they breathe harder. Any muscles that can pull the ribs up are called into action. **Forced inspiration** occurs when an individual is working very hard and needs a great deal of oxygen. Not only are the muscles of quiet and deep inspiration working, but also the muscles that stabilize and/or elevate the shoulder girdle to elevate the ribs directly or indirectly.

Expiration is divided into two phases. **Quiet expiration** is mostly a passive action. It occurs through relaxation of the external intercostals and the elastic recoil of the thoracic wall and tissue of the lungs and bronchi, with gravity pulling the ribcage down from its elevated position. Essentially no muscle action is occurring. **Forced expiration** brings in muscles that can pull down the ribs and muscles to compress the abdomen, forcing the diaphragm upward.

Normal breathing consists of a shorter inhale in relation to a longer exhale. The ratio of inhale time to exhale is one count inhale and four counts exhale. The ideal pattern ranges between two to four counts for the inhale to 8 to 16 counts for the exhale. A reverse of this pattern is the basis for hyperventilation syndrome. Bodywork and breathing retraining methods seek to restore normal breathing.

Some people may wonder why tightening the feet interferes with breathing. It seems to be a chain reaction between prime mover and antagonist muscle patterns. For the abdominals to contract to compress the abdominal cavity, their antagonist patterns have to relax all the way up and down the body.[2]

Consider breathing mechanisms during assessment. By placing your hands on the shoulders of a client while she breathes, you can determine whether she is using her accessory muscles for relaxed breathing. The shoulders should not move up and down. Observation indicates whether the client is using accessory muscles to breathe because the chest movement is concentrated in the upper chest instead of the lower ribs and abdomen. The accessory muscles show increased tension and a tendency toward the development of trigger points if the breathing pattern is dysfunctional. These situations can be identified with palpation. Connective tissue changes are common because breathing dysfunction is often chronic.

Therapeutic massage can normalize many of these conditions and support more effective breathing. It is very difficult to breathe well if the mechanical mechanisms are not working efficiently. Many who have attempted breathing retraining have become frustrated by their inability to accomplish the pattern. They may find more success after the body and mechanism of breathing are more normal. The breathing retraining program presented in Box 13-2 can be taught to clients. The box can be photocopied and used as a handout. Three common activities can help normalize a breathing pattern: yelling, crying, and laughing because all three support an extended exhale. Each of these activities is sustained for 3 to 5 minutes and can be valuable in any breathing retraining program (Proficiency Exercise 13-3).

Exercise and Stretching

Our bodies are designed for purposeful movement toward a goal such as gathering food for the day or running for safety. Our bodies still function as though this were the reality, but we do not need to work as hard to gather our food in the grocery store and seldom do we really have to run or fight for our lives.

Exercise and stretching programs are important parts of any wellness program because they provide the activity our body was designed to have. Now we run in place and ride stationary bikes. Exercise has become an essential purpose unto itself. Fitness programs need to be appropriate; it is important to modify exercise systems and stretching programs to fit the individual. There are many resources available to study exercise and stretching programs.

General recommendations include 30 minutes daily of moderate aerobic activity, which increases the heart and breathing rates. A variety of activities can keep the exercise program from becoming boring. Running, dancing, mowing the yard, and giving massage are examples of aerobic activity. The required activity level varies for each person. Some of us need vigorous activity such as racquetball, whereas others fare better with swimming, walking, or gardening.

Muscles and bones need to work against a load or weight to remain healthy, so resistance or weight training of some sort is also needed. Fifteen to 30 minutes of resistance weight training three or four times a week is adequate for most people. Carrying groceries is an example of weight lifting that can be worked into daily activity. The easiest weight training programs build weight-bearing exercise into daily motions in addition to the formal workout.

Slow stretching can replace the bending and reaching for which our bodies are designed. Static positions are very hard on the body because muscles and connective tissue shorten to mold the body to this static position (e.g., talking on the phone and holding the receiver to the ear with the shoulder). Many types of stretching programs exist. Yoga-type approaches are usually excellent stretching systems. It is important that the stretching be slow, gentle, and sustained.

Frequent 5-minute stretches and breathing breaks should be built into everyone's day, especially for those who maintain static positions. If this is done, productivity may increase and there may be less fatigue at the end of a busy day.

Any exercise and stretching program must begin slowly. Activity levels can be increased gradually each week. It takes about 6 weeks for those who are new to movement to reach a level of comfort with the new moves; additional activities may be added more slowly at that point (Proficiency Exercise 13-4).

Relaxation

Relaxation methods initiate a parasympathetic response. Because muscle tension patterns are habitual, most suc-

box 13-2

BREATHING RETRAINING SEQUENCE

The following breathing retraining sequence should be taught to those who lift their shoulders during quiet and deep inspiration.

Phase I (Fig. 13-1)
1. Have clients sit in a relaxed position.
2. The clients place their hands in their laps and interlace the fingers.
3. The fingers and thumbs are pressed firmly into the top on the body of the hand.
4. This position is held as long as possible without discomfort while the client breathes normally.

Phase II (Fig. 13-2)
1. Clients sit in a relaxed upright position in chairs with arms.
2. The clients' arms are placed on the arms of the chairs.
3. Clients firmly press the forearm closest to the elbow into the arm of the chair.
4. Clients remain in this position as long as comfortably possible and breathe normally.

These exercises accomplish an inhibition of the accessory muscles. Essentially, in these positions the client cannot use these muscles to breathe, and the intercostal muscles and diaphragm are supported.

The client does these exercises as often as possible throughout the day. An attempt should be made to accumulate 30 minutes of time per 24-hour period.

Phase III—Stretching to Open the Chest Wall (Fig. 13-3)
1. The clients stand in a corner with their arms in line with the shoulders spread out on the walls facing the corner.
2. The clients firmly press their arms into the wall for a count of five.
3. The clients relax the arms while allowing the body to fall gently into the corner to stretch the soft tissue of the chest. They hold this position 10 to 30 seconds.
4. The clients move fingers up the wall until resistance is felt and repeat the sequence.

Phase IV
The clients exhale in the following manner:
1. Clients tighten toes, buttocks, and abdominals to prepare to compress the abdomen.
2. They lift the chin into the air and relax the shoulders.

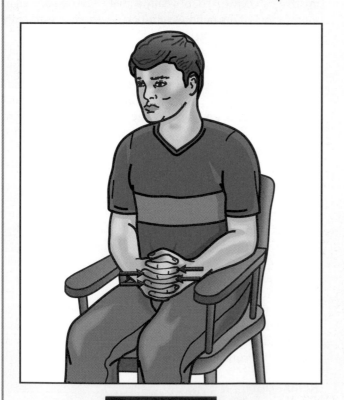

fig. 13-1

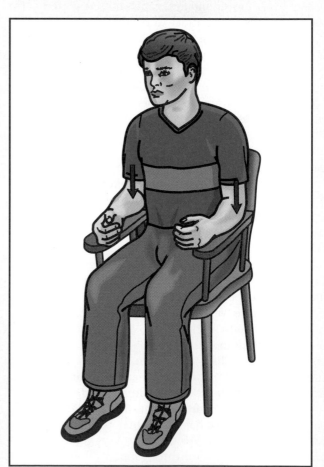

fig. 13-2

box 13-2

BREATHING RETRAINING SEQUENCE—CONT'D

3. They slowly exhale through the mouth in a manner similar to blowing out a candle while tightening the muscles listed previously even tighter. Clients exhale until as much air as possible is expelled without straining.

4. At the bottom of the breath, which is when no further air can be exhaled without strain, the clients stop breathing. (This is different from holding the breath, which requires effort.) It is a resting phase of 3 to 5 seconds.

5. Before the clients begin to inhale, they relax all muscles, drop their chins to their chests, and keep the shoulders relaxed.

6. Clients inhale slowly through the nose until the lungs are comfortably full. This is the top of the breath.

7. They then stop breathing for 3 to 5 seconds and repeat the sequence beginning with Step 1.

The exhalation should take two to four times as long as the inhalation.

Many additional resources exist for retraining breathing patterns. Find one that is comfortable and use it regularly.

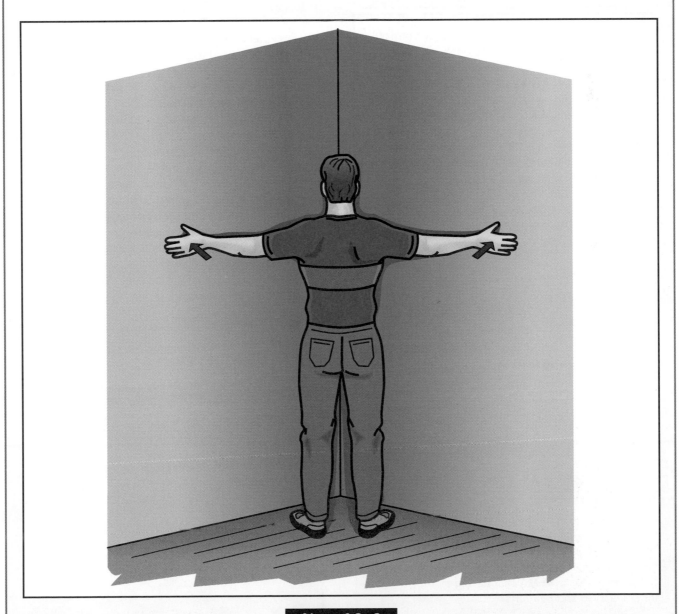

fig. 13-3

cessful relaxation methods combine movement, stretching, tensing, and then releasing muscles (progressive relaxation). The heart rate and breathing rate are synchronized (entrainment) while the individual focuses on a quiet or neutral topic, event, or picture. This is called *visualization*. Slow, rhythmic music can be a beneficial component to add to a relaxation program. Most meditation and deliberate relaxation processes are built around this pattern. The focus of relaxation is to quiet the physical body, not to create a spiritual experience; however, many prayer systems use similar patterns, which are beneficial for relaxation as well.

Almost any type of pleasurable, simple, repetitive activity that requires focused attention induces the relaxation response. Gardening, needlepoint, playing music, watching fish in an aquarium or birds at a bird feeder are all forms of relaxation if there is no need to achieve, compete, or produce results in a specific period. Knitting a sweater for pleasure and having to finish one in a week are two different activities. Relaxation takes time, and when something is urgent, it usually interferes with the ability to relax.

Mindfulness is a concept of relaxation. Being mindful is similar to the centering or focusing methods presented in Chapter 8. Mindfulness is being attentive to the moment, secure that we have learned from and then have let go of the past, and that we are planning for the future without worry. A human "doing" is not mindful. Mindfulness is about a human "being."

Just as tension patterns are habitual, relaxation can become a habit. Typically, it takes 8 to 10 weeks of consistent reinforcement to build a habit pattern. Unlike exercise, which can be varied to prevent boredom, a relaxation sequence needs to be the same each time to reinforce the conditioned response to the habit structure. It is important to use the same location, music, time of day, smells, colors, position, and breathing pattern in the sequence. Any of the components of the relaxation program can soon become triggers to relaxation.

A person should experiment with relaxation methods until the right program is found, then consistently use it every day for at least 15 minutes. (It takes this long for the physiology to make a shift from an aroused state to a relaxed one.) Many audiocassette programs provide progressive relaxation and self-hypnosis. These cassettes pull together all the components of a relaxation program. This type of resource can be very useful (Proficiency Exercise 13-5).

Sleep

Restorative sleep is necessary for wellness. Lack of quality sleep is becoming a major health concern. Many people

---

13-3

PROFICIENCY EXERCISE

1. This exercise helps you understand how normalizing breathing affects the entire body. Begin by doing a simple physical assessment by moving yourself into forward trunk flexion, side-bending lateral trunk flexion, trunk extension, neck flexion, extension, and lateral flexion. Identify the areas of your body that seem most restricted. Now yell or howl as loud as you can for 1 minute. Next pretend to cry and sob for 1 minute. Finally belly laugh as hard and as long as you can.

   Now perform the simple physical assessment again. In the space provided describe the results.

2. Develop a "how to breathe" handout to give to clients. Include at least three different breathing patterns.

13-4

PROFICIENCY EXERCISE

Locate an exercise and stretching program taught by a qualified instructor at your local community center, community education center, or health club, or purchase an exercise and stretching video. Participate in the program for 6 weeks, monitoring all movements for correctness and comfort.

13-5

PROFICIENCY EXERCISE

In the space provided, design a daily 15-minute relaxation program especially for you.

do not get enough sleep. An absolute minimum of 6 hours of uninterrupted sleep are required, with 8 to 9 hours necessary for most people.

Interruptions to sleep are many. These interruptions include pain that repeatedly wakes the person, external random noise (such as traffic noise), tending infants and children, varied work schedules, a restless or snoring bed partner, sinus or other respiratory difficulties such as coughing, and urinary frequency. The list of possible interruptions is endless. Regardless of the perpetuating factors, sleep is compromised and deep sleep stage is seldom achieved.

Others have disrupted sleep patterns because of insomnia, snoring, sleep apnea, hormone fluctuations, high cortisol (stress hormone) levels, medications, and stimulant intake such as caffeine. Again, quality sleep is sacrificed.

Light/dark cycles regulate sleep patterns. For effective sleep we need adequate exposure to daylight, which stimulates scrotonin. We also need adequate exposure to darkness. With the advent of artificial lighting we spend less and less time in the dark, which disturbs sleep. Absence of light supports release of melanin, a pituitary hormone that is involved with the sleep pattern.

During sleep the body renews, repairs, and generally restores itself. Growth hormone is an important factor in this process, with more than half of its daily secretions taking place during sleep. If the deeper stages of sleep are not sustained, the body's restorative mechanisms are compromised. Sleep disturbances are a major factor in many chronic fatigue and pain syndromes.

Sleep, especially during dreaming, is when we seem to repair, sort, and restore emotionally (Proficiency Exercise 13-6). Dreaming is still a mystery but research indicates that it is essential for emotional well being. Methods to support effective sleep are presented in Box 13-3.

Feelings

Feelings are the body's interpretation of emotions. They occur as a response to the effect of hormones, neurotransmitters, and other endogenous chemicals. People use chemical substances such as food, nicotine, alcohol, and drugs to create feelings. Behaviors such as the need to create crises, eating disorders, accident proneness, hypervigilance, panic, illness, and codependent relationships generate feelings.

Often if a person's physiology can be changed, his or her feelings can also be changed. The easiest way to change the physiology is to move, as in exercising or breathing.

A massage will also change the physiology. This is perhaps why massage "feels" so good. Being touched in a resourceful way supports wellness. Sensory stimulation is essential for the body to thrive. Many people are deprived of touch, and many adults exchange touch only in the context of a sexual relationship. Touch is essential for wellness. Touching generates and expresses feelings. The power of touch was explored in the very beginning of this text.

When feelings are unresourceful, an opposing response must be activated to restore a balance. For example, if you are weighed down with too much thinking, moving around and pulling some weeds in the garden creates a balance. If feeling angry, find a way to laugh. If feeling down, help someone. If feeling anxious and alone, get a hug or a massage (Proficiency Exercise 13-7).

Mind

The mind is the part of us that reasons, understands, remembers, thinks, and adapts. It coordinates the conscious and subconscious part of us that influences and directs

---

13-6

PROFICIENCY EXERCISE

In the space provided, analyze your personal sleep pattern using the information in this section. Identify three activities that support restorative sleep and three activities that can be improved.

My current sleep pattern is as follows:

Three current activities that support sleep are the following:

1.

2.

3.

Three activities that could improve sleep are the following:

1.

2.

3.

box 13-3

SUPPORTING RESTORATIVE SLEEP

Therapeutic massage supports restorative sleep in the following ways:

- It reduces sympathetic autonomic nervous system activity and cortisol levels.
- It promotes parasympathetic autonomic nervous system dominance.
- It relieves or reduces pain and discomfort that may interrupt sleep.

Self-help measures for supporting restorative sleep include the following:

- Maintain a regular sleep/wake cycle. Get up and go to bed at the same time every day, including days off.
- Get at least 30 minutes of daylight exposure by being outside or placing yourself in front of an open window.
- Exercise moderately on a regular basis but do not exercise aerobically 4 hours before sleeping.
- Reduce stimulant intake substantially and ingest no stimulants 10 hours before sleeping. If you go to bed at 11:00 PM, do not drink colas or coffee after 1:00 PM.
- Concentrate protein food intake 6 hours before going to sleep. Eat carbohydrates after this time. Do not eat a heavy meal before going to bed. Do not go to bed hungry. Eat a *small* snack of complex carbohydrates without sugar with some dairy product such as yogurt 30 minutes before bed if hungry. Although a protein, turkey is high in tryptophan, which encourages sleep. A small turkey sandwich is a possible bedtime snack.
- Stretch gently 1 hour before retiring. A slow, rhythmic pattern is best.
- Get into the dark or soft lighting (only enough light for

safe movement) 1 hour before bedtime. Stretching in the dim light is an excellent way to begin the wind-down process to prepare for sleep.
- Develop a bedtime ritual that you follow consistently. The ritual should begin 30 minutes before going to bed. Make sure to stay in dim lighting. This ritual should be 15 minutes long. It can include hygiene such as washing and brushing teeth but should not consist of full body application of water, because both hot and cold application can stimulate the body. (A warm bath 1 hour before sleep is relaxing.) Meditating or reading something that is gentle and can be finished in 5 or 10 minutes may be helpful. Listening to soft and gentle music is soothing. Various aromas are considered relaxing and are available in such forms as scented candles, incense, and essential oil diffusers. Drinking a cup of relaxing herbal tea is soothing. Meditate, pray, and review your day in a thankful way. After you develop this ritual it needs to be reinforced. Do it the same way every night. Eventually the ritual will signal the body into a sleep pattern.
- When drowsiness occurs, immediately relax into sleep. The drowsy pattern lasts only about 15 minutes and then a new body rhythm cycle begins, which lasts about 90 minutes.
- If you miss the sleep window, continue with calm activities until the sense of drowsiness again occurs. Then go to bed.
- Sleep in the dark. Especially do not sleep with the television on.
- Get up at the same time in the morning regardless of when you went to bed.
- Avoid long naps. A short 15- to 30-minute nap is usually all right during midday fatigue.

PROFICIENCY EXERCISE

Honestly identify two personal behaviors that have a repetitive pattern, one resourceful and one unresourceful. What feelings are generated by these behaviors? For the unresourceful behavior identify one alternative resourceful behavior to generate similar feelings.

Example
Resourceful behavior: Watching uplifting human interest movies
Feelings: Empowerment, security, connectedness
Unresourceful behavior: Overeating at night
Feelings: Being connected, fulfilled, cared for
Replacement behavior: Playing with my dog

Your Turn
1. Resourceful behavior:

   Feelings:

   Unresourceful behavior:

   Feelings:

   Replacement behavior:

2. Resourceful behavior:

   Feelings:

   Unresourceful behavior:

   Feelings:

   Replacement behavior:

mental and physical behavior. The mind processes what we believe. We can change our mind (beliefs) fairly quickly, although habitual belief patterns are difficult to overcome. Belief changes need to be supported over time to be reflected in lifestyle and wellness programs. The body responds to mind changes, but more time may be required for the effects of that response to manifest in the organic form of the body's anatomy and physiology. Patience is required to objectively identify body changes in response to mind changes. This interaction between mind and body is the basis for current approaches to mind/body medicine. The mind involves emotions, behavior, self-concept, and coping.

Emotions

Emotions are feelings driven by thoughts. They lead to actions that represent the consequences of how we think and what we do. What we think and feel and how we live are all inextricably linked.

The immune system is controlled directly by the mind. The science of psychoneuroimmunology has clearly established that unresolved emotions and thought patterns of hate, fear, anger, and jealousy reduce the efficiency of the body's defenses.[1]

In 1975, Dr. Robert Adder conditioned rats to dislike sweetened water by injecting them with a chemical to make them feel ill whenever they drank it. After the injections stopped for some time, some rats began dying. On investigation, Adder found that the chemical he had used was a suppressor of immune function. The rats had not only become conditioned to feeling ill whenever they drank sweet water but also were also mimicking its other effects and depressing their immune systems. This ability to depress the immune function was proof of nervous system control over the immune system. Many subsequent tests have confirmed this finding in human beings.[1]

As human beings, we *learn* to be helpless, addictive, and have low self-esteem. We learn to hate. The important point to remember is that if we learned the maladaptive behavior in the first place, we can also learn a more resourceful behavior to use instead.

Emotions can be very powerful. If used resourcefully, they can provide us with the empowerment to reach our goals. Many good things have come from an emotion turned into resourceful behavior.

Wellness encompasses a full range of emotion. Some of us pride ourselves on not feeling certain emotions, but if we can experience an emotion in a resourceful way, it is not healthy to deny its expression. For example, if something as powerful as anger is turned inward, it does not lead to positive outcomes. But if expressed resourcefully, to the person or situations involved, then a sense of resolution takes place and we can get on with our lives, free of the anger.

Wellness comes from using the emotion instead of the emotion using us. Used resourcefully, emotions can pro-

vide the motivation to achieve wellness; used unresourcefully, they can make us ill and be destructive to those who share our lives.

Sometimes we need someone, such as a daughter, who loves us in spite of ourselves to put our emotions and resulting behavior into perspective (Proficiency Exercise 13-8).

Behavior

Behavior is what we do in response to feelings, to trigger thoughts and feelings, and occasionally to avoid feelings. Resourceful behavior results in feeling good about what has happened. Unresourceful behavior still results in a good feeling (or we would not do it), but often we feel bad about what happened, and/or others feel bad.

Addictive behavior can take many forms. A person who is addicted to food, drugs, alcohol, exercise, pain, crisis, or loss will develop a lifestyle that both protects and supports the substance or behavior of choice. Addictions require a great deal of time and energy. Addictive behavior throws the balance of wellness off course. It takes hard work and lots of support to change an addictive behavior. Sometimes a less damaging addiction is replaced by a more damaging one, and vice versa.[1] A person may alter a food habit by creating an exercise dependency. Whichever is the more damaging addiction needs to be evaluated. Behavior changes that are at least steps in the resourceful direction should not be discouraged. To truly alter behavior, a person must evaluate his or her sense of self (Proficiency Exercise 13-9).

Self-Concept

What we think about ourselves and how we talk to ourselves are very important contributors to wellness. Some people do not have a positive self-concept.

Most of us want a purpose and a sense of achievement, success, and self-confidence. This is achievable when we stop comparing ourselves with one another. Instead, wellness involves reaching out to others for support and information.

Rather then basing their personal value on an external standard, healthy people develop internal standards of

---

13-8
PROFICIENCY EXERCISE

List any emotions that gave you the drive to complete this therapeutic massage educational program.

self-worth. We need to own both our successes and our mistakes and attempt to correct the mistakes. It is healthy to "clean up our own messes." Putting relationships and mistakes back in order can resolve issues and allow energy to be used in more beneficial ways.

It is also healthy to clean up a mess that someone else may have left. Often the person or situation that made the mess does not, or will not, assume responsibility for it. If we wait for it to be cleaned up, we may have to live with the mess for a long time.

Part of wellness is eliminating physical, mental, and spiritual messes and clutter that we no longer need, regardless of who is responsible. As adults, it is also our responsibility to disallow preventable messes. Sometimes we have to be very strong with other people about what we will and will not allow in our space.

Some messes are not created by anyone such as natural disasters. When people unite in communities to clean up these messes, wellness is supported.

Another threat to wellness is misjudging our worth. Everyone is good at something; no one is good at everything. Measure success and self-worth by how good you feel about your accomplishments, instead of by money or fame. Especially with massage, an inner sense of accomplishment is important. Massage is a quiet, unpretentious profession. It does not usually receive a lot of public glory. Massage is an important and needed service and its benefits often cannot be objectively measured. As with any type of prevention activity, it is difficult to know what did not happen because someone took preventive measures.

When we have developed a healthy relationship with ourselves, we can also develop and sustain healthy relationships with others. Supportive relationships are important to wellness. If a relationship continues to generate messes in your life, maybe it is not a resourceful relationship. This does not mean that effort and concern are not required for family and friends or even concern for a population more globally. What is important is that we are empowered in a relationship and free to give and receive with a balance of energy exchanged. Sometimes one gives more and other times one receives more, but the total outcome is mutual support for one another's highest good that supports wellness (Proficiency Exercise 13-10).

Coping

Wellness is the ability to live each day and be able to say we did our jobs well, as we enter sleep with a thankful heart. How we lived that day is the coping part, and sometimes the simplest things can make a difference.

One day, when things were going particularly poorly in an office, a 5-year-old boy walked through. He stopped and said, "Good morning everybody. Have you noticed that the sun is shining today?" It was a better day for all after that.

Resourceful coping consists of commitment, control, and challenge. **Commitment** is the ability and willingness to be involved in what is happening around us to have a purpose for being. This purpose is more than what we do, it is how we serve. It is possible to serve in many ways. A career in massage can be a path of service or just a job. Purpose and service have nothing to do with the task. Picking up garbage is as much a service as is being a doctor. Cleaning house, cutting hair, building houses, and packing cartons are all paths of service. The commitment is to make a difference and serve well, including performing a task well to support wellness.

Control is characterized by the belief that we can influ-

13-9
PROFICIENCY EXERCISE

List three addictive behaviors. For each, list three alternative behaviors that are less damaging, yet may generate similar feelings.

Addictive behavior: _____

Alternative behavior:

1.

2.

3.

Addictive behavior: _____

Alternative behavior:

1.

2.

3.

Addictive behavior: _____

Alternative behavior:

1.

2.

3.

13-10
PROFICIENCY EXERCISE

Clean up two "messes," one you made in someone else's life and one someone made in your life. Notice how your self-concept blossoms.

ence events by the way we feel, think, and act. This is internal control, not external control. *Internal control* involves adjusting ourselves to the situation and looking for ways to respond resourcefully. Those who exert *external control* attempt to control circumstances and people. It is impossible to control the weather, most circumstances, and most people. Relying on external control is a poor coping mechanism.

The eternal wisdom expressed in the saying "grant me the serenity to accept the things I cannot change, the courage to change the things I can, and the wisdom to know the difference" speaks to self-concept and internal versus external control.

Living each day as a **challenge,** filled with things to learn, skills to practice, tasks to be accomplished, and obstacles to overcome supports wellness. Beginning each day with the affirmations of "I greet the day and all that it holds" may generate an attitude of challenge. Those who see change as a challenge cope much better than those who do not. Using available resourceful coping mechanisms to cope with change in life allows the individual to welcome changes as leading to personal development.

Poor stress-coping skills in the form of attempted external control and unproductive emotions such as unresolved anger suppress our immune systems and predispose us to infection and poor health. It is the individual's response to the stress that determines the effect on immunity, and not the stress itself.[1] Wellness includes learning more efficient ways to cope with life (through counseling and behavior modification programs if needed).

To improve coping skills, pay attention to people who cope well and ask them to share how they cope. Attending seminars and reading books on effective coping, assertiveness, and development of internal control provide additional resources. Professional counseling can be helpful. Remember, we learned the coping mechanisms we currently have and we can learn even better ways to cope (Proficiency Exercise 13-11).

Spirit

Our spirit is the part of us that transcends. Our spiritual selves "know." Spiritual wellness consists of faith, hope, and love.

Faith

Faith is the ability to believe, trust, and know certain things that science cannot prove. Faith is the strength of wellness and involves the expression of that connecting strength each day through faith in ourselves, our partners, our families, and humanity as a whole. Faith is essential to wellness (Proficiency Exercise 13-12).

Hope

Hope is the belief, assurance, conviction, and confidence that our future will somehow be okay. It is the belief that the choices we make now will be the most resourceful choices as we create our future (Proficiency Exercise 13-13). Without hope, no sense of continuity exists. To quote Temple Grandin, an admirable woman with autism, "I like to *hope* that even if there is no personal afterlife, some energy impression (of me) is left in the universe . . . I do not want my thoughts to die with me."[3]

Love

Love has no concrete explanation. Love is a prerequisite for wholeness, and wholeness is necessary for wellness.

13-11

PROFICIENCY EXERCISE

In the space provided, take an inventory of yourself to see what coping mechanisms you possess. List three effective coping mechanisms and three that are not as effective. Choose one of these ineffective coping mechanisms and develop a plan to change it.

Effective coping mechanisms:

1.

2.

3.

Ineffective coping mechanisms:

1.

2.

3.

Plan for change of one ineffective coping mechanism:

13-12

PROFICIENCY EXERCISE

On a separate sheet of paper, write a poem, story, or song or draw a picture about your source of faith. This piece of art is just for you, so do not be concerned that anyone else will see it.

This is not romantic love; it is bigger, stronger, more empowering, and mightier. It is quiet, gentle, forgiving, and nonjudgmental.

A teenage boy was struggling to put these most important issues into perspective. He came to his mother and said, "I have figured out the meaning of life." Wondering this herself, she asked her son what he had discovered. The son replied, "When I play my music and I feel great and those who listen to me feel great, then I have shared my love, and my power gets bigger and so does theirs. But if I play my music, and only I feel great and those who listen feel bad and weak, then I have taken their power and this is evil. This is the meaning of life." This love celebrates the irrepressible process of life. This is the love of wellness (Proficiency Exercise 13-14).

13-13

PROFICIENCY EXERCISE

Complete the following sentence ten different ways.

I hope

I hope

I hope

I hope

I hope

I hope

I hope

I hope

I hope

I hope

13-14

PROFICIENCY EXERCISE

During a learning experience, one or two people may emerge who teach us more than we expected to learn. Often the learning has nothing to do with the courses we are studying. This is a love sharing. Go to those who have shared their love with you and say "Thank you."

SUMMARY

Wellness is more than the components discussed in this chapter. Wellness is living life in a simple, gentle, respectful way—for ourselves and with others. Wellness is the result of the healing that takes place on multiple levels when we take care of ourselves, which then extends to caring for others and the planet in general.

Someone once said, "When half the world is receiving a massage and the other half is giving a massage, we shall have peace." Wellness is peace within and sharing that peace in simple ways. Sharing this peace consistently with respect and compassion can support the wellness of us all and provide peace for our world.

REFERENCES

1. Chaitow L: *The body/mind purification program,* New York, 1991, Fireside.
2. Lippert L: *Clinical kinesiology for physical therapist assistants,* Portland, 1991, Author.
3. Sacks O: An anthropologist on Mars, *The New Yorker,* p 106, Dec 27, 1993, Author.
4. Selye H: *The stress of life,* ed 2, New York, 1978, McGraw-Hill.

NOTE: This chapter has no questions or workbook exercises other than requesting that the readers read this chapter with their hearts and souls as well as their minds.

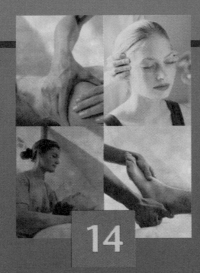

14

BUSINESS CONSIDERATIONS FOR A CAREER IN THERAPEUTIC MASSAGE

o b j e c t i v e s

After completing this chapter, the student will be able to perform the following:

- Determine his or her personal motivation for developing a therapeutic massage career
- List the pros and cons for independent and employee status
- Develop a 5-year business plan
- Design a marketing strategy and advertising materials for a massage business
- Negotiate rental and employment contracts
- Develop a business management and record-keeping system

WHAT is a career? A common dictionary definition of **career** is a chosen pursuit, a life work. What is a job? Dictionaries define a **job** as a regular activity performed for payment.

Therapeutic massage can be either a job or a career. Which do you want? The answer to that question will determine in large part how you proceed with professional development. This text in general and this chapter in particular view therapeutic massage from the perspective of a career path.

This chapter presents specific information for those who want to develop a massage business, but it does not attempt to be a course in small business management. The information presented here is unique to therapeutic massage. It is sufficient to guide the student toward additional learning opportunities and to generate classroom discussion. This chapter takes the position that the nuts and bolts of business are no different for massage than for any other professional service business. Detailed information on topics such as marketing methods, financial record keeping, and tax requirements can be found in business textbooks. Resource books on the business aspects of massage therapy also are available (see Appendix D), and professional organizations often provide business information.

This chapter does what generic business texts cannot do—it shares the experience of being a massage professional and of walking this career path or holding a job in therapeutic massage. Throughout the text, the student has been encouraged to pose questions, to use clinical reasoning as a problem-solving method, and to challenge information. It has been suggested that you seek your authorities carefully and compare information from many different experts. It is no different in the business world.*

This chapter is built on the author's experiential base, which has been expanded by the experiences of many other massage professionals. The experiential base is supported by solid, standardized business information.

---

*To substantiate the validity of the business information in this chapter, a brief business profile of the author is presented:

- Certificate in bookkeeping
- 21 years as a massage practitioner
- 12 years in full-time private practice (30 to 40 clients a week)
- 3 years in part-time practice (10 to 20 clients a week)
- Professional practice locations: health club, on-site (private homes, small businesses, and corporations), chiropractor's office, full-service beauty salon, private country club, home office
- 6 years of professional practice with a psychologist in private practice
- Owner of a massage therapy school (director and instructor for 13 years)
- Employer of 39 associates
- Owner and manager of two commercial properties for 7 years

Businesswise, for this author "been there, done that" fits, and the experience gained over these many years has provided a realistic knowledge of a career in therapeutic massage.

SELF-EMPLOYMENT OR EMPLOYEE STATUS

section objectives

Using the information presented in this section, the student will be able to perform the following:

- **Compare and contrast the pros and cons of self-employment and employee status**
- **Understand the commitment required to develop a massage therapy business**

Currently many massage practitioners are **self-employed.** Successful self-employment requires an entrepreneurial spirit. An entrepreneur is one who organizes, operates, and assumes the risk of a business venture. Much of this chapter focuses on the self-employed massage professional.

However, not everyone is cut out for self-employment. The hours are long, and 100% commitment is required. Self-employed people must be self-starters with a broad range of professional and business skills. Some people think that self-employed individuals get to be their own boss—not so; instead of one or two bosses, every client becomes the boss. Self-employment requires an entrepreneurial spirit and a deep internal commitment. During the latter part of this century therapeutic massage has been provided primarily by self-employed massage professionals. The entrepreneurial spirit runs high in the massage/bodywork profession, but times are changing.

The profession has seen a steady increase in available jobs and career opportunities in the more traditional **employee** market, in which the massage practitioner goes to work for an individual or a company at an hourly wage or salary.

More employment opportunities are opening up for massage professionals in the personal service industry and the medical establishment. The most rapid expansion of employment opportunities is occurring in the health care system. Massage professionals are working as technicians for physicians, physical therapists, mental health professionals, and other health care professionals.

The service industry is growing as well. The concept of the "day spa," a place where people can "get away" in their local area for a day of pampering, including massage, is catching on. Full-service cosmetology businesses offer employment opportunities as well.

The fitness industry is another source of employment. Many health clubs offer the services of a massage professional. The recreational industry (e.g., hotels, cruise ships, retreats, resort centers) also is an active employer of massage practitioners.

More and more independent massage therapy clinics are opening as well, which is an exciting trend. The owner or manager of these clinics handles all business responsibilities and hires massage practitioners to do the work (Fig. 14-1).

Career Resource Directory

The variety of career opportunities available to a trained massage or bodywork practitioner is almost unlimited. Massage and bodywork practitioners work in a variety of atmospheres. Below is a list outlining some of the opportunities.

Airports
Athletic clubs

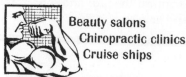

Beauty salons
Chiropractic clinics
Cruise ships

Corporate wellness programs
Dance studios
Dance touring companies

Golf & country clubs
Hospitals
Hotels
Medical clinics
Orthopedic clinics
Mall locations
Physical therapy clinics
Physicians offices
Plastic surgery rehabilitation clinics
Private establishments

Private employment by celebrities
Private out-call practice
Professional athletic teams
Resorts
Ski resorts
Spas
Sports medicine clinics
Truck stops

Hotels & Resorts

Most four- and five-star hotels and resorts include at least minimal spa facilities on their properties. The following chains are known for employing massage and bodywork practitioners. You should also contact privately-owned hotels and resorts in your area.

Clarion
Embassy Suites
Four Seasons Hotels
Hilton Hotels

Hyatt Regency Resorts
Intercontinental Resorts
Radisson Hotels
Registry Resorts

Sheraton
Ritz Carlton
Stouffer
Westin Resorts

Cruise Lines

Cruise lines offer an exciting opportunity for both travel and employment. Hiring for several cruise lines is handled through the concessionaire, Coiffure Trans Ocean Inc. They hire for Princess, Crystal, Crown, Royal, Norwegian, Cunard, Commodore, Seaborne, Admiral, American Hawaii, and other cruise lines. *Coiffure Trans Ocean Job Line: 305/358-8739.*

Day & Destination Spas

Day and destination spas are very popular places to be hired as a massage or bodywork practitioner. Some destination spas such as the Golden Door, Canyon Ranch, and La Costa employ as many as sixty massage and bodywork practitioners. There is also an opportunity to be hired overseas as there are a tremendous number of spas in Europe, the Caribbean, and other exotic destinations. In these situations, practitioners will often be required to learn a variety of spa therapies, such as herbal wraps and paraffin baths, which can add to your skills and allow you more variety in your practice. For more information on approximately 250 spas in the United States, Canada, the Caribbean, the Bahamas, and Bermuda, get the book *Fodors Healthy Escapes,* available from any bookstore or your local library. Consult your local telephone book for information on day spas in your area.

fig. 14-1

Career resource directory. (From Associated Bodywork & Massage Professionals [ABMP], 28677 Buffalo Park Road, Evergreen CO 80439-7347. Phone: [800] 458-ABMP or [303] 674-8478. Fax: [303] 674-0859. http://www.abmp.com/.)

You can be either self-employed or an employee, and you can either have a career or hold a job in massage. However, don't think that you must be self-employed to have a career. Each option has its advantages and disadvantages, and only you can decide what is an advantage and what is a disadvantage. For example, one person may feel that the independent decision making involved in self-employment is an advantage, whereas a person who has difficulty coming up with independent ideas would categorize this as a disadvantage.

The key is, "Know thyself." If you have the commitment, drive, skill, and discipline necessary for self-employment and are willing to make the 100% commitment it takes to build and maintain a massage therapy practice, this is the best option for you.

Questions a professional must ask himself or herself are: "How disciplined am I? Do I wait until the last minute to do a job? Am I on time, or do I usually run late? Do I keep myself organized?"

The very skills that make a wonderful massage therapist—intuition, sensitivity, an ability to respond to the moment—can be a source of difficulty in meeting the business requirements of planning ahead, keeping bills paid on time, carefully planning business strategy, and staying in one place long enough to carry out the business plan. If you do not have either the self-discipline or the skills necessary for self-employment, employee status may be the better choice.

Experience supports this observation: Many excellent massage professionals are inherently poor at business management. The intuition, spontaneous feelings, and people orientation of those entering the profession do not necessarily work in harmony with the logical, impersonal, structured nature of business. Individuals who want to develop a career in massage frequently are gentle, intuitive people who may find the concepts of developing and enforcing policy statements and determining fee structures difficult. Many people have difficulty with the discipline and organization required to manage a small business. It is difficult to watch excellent massage professionals fail in their effort to serve the public because they did not recognize that they would do far better in an employee situation. It is equally disturbing to see those with the entrepreneurial spirit constrained in the structure of someone else's business dream.

Technical business information often seems alien to the student of therapeutic massage. This chapter shares information about business issues. It is important that the student understand the steps involved in setting up and managing a small business. These issues are not contrary to the service orientation and the gentle, caring attitude necessary for a practitioner of therapeutic massage. Rather, careful attention to these concerns is part of the responsibility of the massage professional.

Whether you are self-employed or an employee, an understanding of business practices related to the massage profession is important. Therapeutic massage is the same as any other business. It is important to market the product—your skills as a massage practitioner—and attend to the record keeping and financial commitments required to run a business (Box 14-1).

---

box 14-1

BUILDING A BUSINESS: APPLYING THE PREGNANCY AND CHILD-REARING METAPHOR

Consider your education in therapeutic massage as a pregnancy. It takes time for the baby to grow until it has developed enough to survive in an unprotected environment. It is the same with going to school to learn therapeutic massage. The time will come for the baby (the professional practice) to be born. This is a natural process but not without its struggles and hard work. Graduation, the birth from school, comes for the student as well. Everyone is excited about the baby, but soon the parents (the massage practitioner) realize that for about 2 years, this new little life will require constant care, hard work, attention to detail, and very long, focused hours. The 2-year-old child seeks independence, but constant supervision is necessary until the child is about 5 years old. At age 5 the child has learned many lessons and can begin some self-care as the parents supervise from a little farther away. Each year after that, the child becomes more independent, although attention from the parents is still necessary, just as it is with a new business.

A professional should plan to give a new business 2 years of constant attention to enable it to develop strong roots from which to grow. It will take about 5 years before attention to the business can be eased and small portions of it entrusted to another supervising person for short periods. Yet, careful attention and participation will always be required if a business is to remain successful. Building a business is hard work that in time reaps rewards.

MOTIVATION

section objectives

Using the information presented in this section, the student will be able to perform the following:

- Understand the importance of motivation in successfully developing a business
- Determine a suitable market for an individual massage therapist

- Explore personal strengths and weaknesses that would aid or impede the development of a successful business
- Develop a personal application of methods to prevent burnout

To succeed at anything, a person must be motivated. Some sort of internal drive must provide the energy to do what is needed to accomplish a goal. One of the primary reasons that businesses fail is lack of drive and **motivation**. Without the motivation to stay with the commitment, people give up during difficult times. This is especially true of small businesses with single owners, a category that includes most massage businesses.

Motivation begins with knowing what one wants. Plans must be developed, but the massage professional must be willing to change if a strategy is not working. If success is the goal, then quitting cannot be an option. The following are some important points:

- *Know thyself.* No one should persist with something that goes against his or her core values, no matter how successful the process may be for someone else.
- *Follow your dream.* Success flows from desire and motivation. Desire and motivation are the driving forces for the dreams that come from deep within us to bring us joy and healing. Hard times and hard work are part of the process of building a new business. If we follow our dreams and live our purpose, the hard work provides a rewarding, intrinsic sense of satisfaction.
- *Accept that experience is the best teacher.* We learn from our mistakes as well as from our successes. Implementing plans is the only way to find out whether they work. It may become obvious over time that another approach is more advantageous, but being afraid to make mistakes will limit you as a professional.
- *Ask "What's in it for me?"* To succeed in any endeavor, we need to recognize the benefits to be gained from the process. This is an important consideration in any decision. It is not a selfish attitude; rather, it is a smart approach. People will not put energy into something that does not give them satisfaction. This concept applies to money as well. Business is business, and earning money is part of any successful business operation. However, money itself is a poor source of motivation. Motivation is a deeper-felt sense that comes from the heart and soul.
- *Recognize that self-concept matters.* People have ideas about who they should be, and these often conflict with what we have been told and believe that we are. Self-esteem is very important to success in business practices. Trying to live up to others' expectations is a bad business practice. A successful business is built on who we are, not on what others want us to be. Develop your ability to use all aspects of yourself to the best advantage.

- *Believe in your product.* Understand and be able to explain the benefits of therapeutic massage. It is most acceptable to explain the benefits of massage in terms of physiologic responses that all people share. Explanations of this type are easy for most people to understand.
- *Provide a quality product.* The massage practitioner must be a skilled technician. Clients pay for the benefits they experience from massage. Repeat business is based on your ability to continue to produce those benefits. To be truly successful the practitioner must put the person, not his or her condition, first. People seek caring, nurturing, and nonjudgmental touch as much as technical skill.

It is not only one's massage skills that are brought to the therapeutic massage business. Each professional also brings personal strengths and weaknesses, successes and failures, and experiences and learning. It is important to use all our strengths. It is even more important to recognize the areas in which we are not as strong because these limitations influence our business activities in a negative way.

It is wise to hire help to support areas in which weakness is noticed. Each business person needs a diverse group of support people to use as consultants, such as a lawyer, an accountant, a skilled bookkeeper, an advertising/marketing consultant, and an adviser for business planning. Consulting with these resource people need not be expensive. Local Chamber of Commerce and Small Business Administration (SBA) offices offer free services. The SBA supports an organization of retired business people known as the *Service Corps of Retired Executives* (SCORE). The members of this organization want to help others succeed.

It is essential that the massage professional talk to many people and listen to their experiences about successes and mistakes. This information can be extremely helpful with regard to inherent problems in business. This core information, along with the fundamentals of therapeutic massage, lays the foundation for a successful practice.

Although experts, authorities, and mentors are helpful, no single individual has all the answers or knows the whole truth. Each of us must find his or her own answers. Truth is personal, empowering, and freeing. Many motivational tapes, books, and speakers are available that can be used for inspiration. The following overlapping themes, which can be found in most of these sources, are the kernels of truth:

- Whatever we believe—with emotion and feeling—becomes our reality.
- What we do with confidence can become our self-fulfilling prophecy.
- We attract into our lives that which harmonizes with our dominant thoughts.

Burnout

When a person is burned out, motivation is lost. **Burnout** occurs when you use up your energy faster than you can replenish it. For massage therapists this means taking better care of others than we take of ourselves. Burnout can be a problem in most service professions. Taking care of others is a big job. If we do not take care of ourselves also, we soon have nothing to give others or ourselves. Each of us must take care of our physical needs. You must rest, eat well, and have regular massages. Pay attention to emotional needs. Surround yourself with people who believe in you. Take care of your spiritual needs, which connect the value of what you want to accomplish with a much higher purpose. Follow the wellness guidelines presented in Chapter 13.

The actual practice of massage is simple, repetitious touch, which sometimes can get boring. It is important to keep yourself excited about the benefits of such simple applications of touch. One of the best ways to do this is to continue your education. Classes make you think and bring you together with other massage professionals.

These are good opportunities to share and learn together. State-licensed massage schools and professional organizations are the best sources for massage education. Many classes on business practices and motivation are available from these sources.

It also is important to get away from massage for a bit. The massage professional occasionally should take classes or vacations that have nothing to do with massage or muscles. If you commit to saving your earnings from one massage a week, you will have $1000 to $2000 a year to spend on continuing education and vacations. You deserve it. Take care of yourself, and let others take care of you. Take a vacation, and burnout will be less of a problem.

After a person begins to live life—including business life—*on purpose*, the energy to develop the business concept will be available. Living on purpose is the key to motivation. It means drawing strength from knowing that what we have to offer is valuable. When the massage practitioner truly believes this, he or she can begin developing a business concept or seeking rewarding employment (Proficiency Exercise 14-1).

---

1 4 - 1
PROFICIENCY EXERCISE

In the space below, explore your beliefs in order to find motivation for developing your career in therapeutic massage.

1. Answer the following questions:

   What do I believe—
   about therapeutic massage as a professional service . . .

   about my abilities as a massage professional . . .

   about myself as a person . . .

   about my future clients . . .

2. Complete the following statement five times:

   I feel confident about

   I feel confident about

   I feel confident about

   I feel confident about

   I feel confident about

3. Complete the following statement five times:

   A dominant thought that influences my life is

   A dominant thought that influences my life is

   A dominant thought that influences my life is

   A dominant thought that influences my life is

   A dominant thought that influences my life is

DEVELOPMENT OF THE BUSINESS

section objectives

Using the information presented in this section, the student will be able to perform the following:

- Locate the resources needed to write a resume
- Develop a mission statement to use as the basis for a business plan
- Develop business goals
- Develop a personal start-up cost worksheet

The Resume

A resume is a compilation of professional and personal data about a person. Before we can develop a business plan and set goals, it is important to find out who we are. A good resume becomes part of the promotional materials we use when self-employed, and it must be used to apply for a job in the massage field. The resume should list not only massage experience, but also other work experience as well. This is very important. We are the sum total of all our experiences, and we bring that knowledge base into all work and business situations. Many professional resources are available to help you develop your resume. Contact the local Chamber of Commerce or a nearby library branch to locate such assistance (Proficiency Exercise 14-2).

The Business Plan

It is important to have a plan when setting up a business. To make the plan workable, the professional needs to know where she is in the present, what her path has been, and what she has learned from her accumulated experiences. After this information is available, future plans can be made.

One business plan option is to move gradually into a new massage business by working at it part time while letting the business grow slowly (keeping your full-time job). Another option is to commit to the new massage business full time. If the practitioner chooses to do this, he will need to have enough money saved up to support his basic needs for about a year.

Either path is acceptable. You will need to decide what fits for you. This is the type of information that becomes formalized when developing a business plan.

In all business planning it is important to find and fill a need. What is the massage need that you, as a practitioner, are willing to fill? The answer to this question becomes the basis of your mission statement.

A *mission statement* expresses the intent of the business plan. In order to develop a mission statement, it is important to answer this question: What will be the main focus of my business?

An example of a mission statement follows:

My business mission is to serve the blue-collar labor population in my area by providing therapeutic massage and self-help education at a reasonable cost, with flexible appointment hours, and at an easily accessible location.

The development of the formal business plan begins while the student is still in school. Education in the skills needed to carry out the mission statement is the first step of the business plan. Also part of a business plan is the development of a financial plan to support the educational process and the first year of business, a time when income may be low. While in school, students should use the expertise of teachers and other students to explore career options (Proficiency Exercise 14-3).

The Goal-Setting Plan

After the "big picture" concepts of the business plan are in place, smaller steps to implement the plans are identified. These are goals. Goals are important because they provide direction and landmarks for achievement (Box 14-2).

Goals may change over time. Goal setting can be compared to taking a trip. To stay fresh and alert during a trip, it is important to stop and rest. If these stops are planned ahead of time, the journey seems shorter. The journey to a successful business is similar when attainable goals are placed along the way.

In planning for a trip, it is important to identify any

14-2

PROFICIENCY EXERCISE

1. Draft your resume.
2. Contact your local community college, library, or public service organization and attend a class in resume writing.

14-3

PROFICIENCY EXERCISE

Pretend that you are a successful massage practitioner 5 years from now. You have been asked to return to your massage school and speak to the business class about how you succeeded in your business. Talk into a tape recorder for 30 minutes as though you were addressing the class. Play back the tape, and write down the steps you took that led to a successful business. Use these steps to develop an outline for a business plan. Then meet in groups of four students and share your outlines with one another.

obstacles that may be encountered. What are your financial and personal resources? It is the same with a business. Review the support available from others. Be willing to learn along the way.

Basic survival skills promote self-sufficiency in business as well as in life. A good question to ask is, "What is the worst possible thing that could happen as a result of this decision?" Think ahead to possible solutions should the worst happen, and try to determine whether the business could survive that experience. What would be gained? It is important to take calculated risks. If these risks are small and entered into slowly, you can change strategies if need be (Proficiency Exercise 14-4).

The clinical reasoning model used throughout this text is an invaluable tool for setting attainable goals (Box 14-3).

Start-Up Costs

Start-up costs are the initial expenses required to begin a business. When giving a massage, the student is taught to keep it simple and to go slowly. The same ideas apply to business. When beginning a massage business, it is not necessary to have a suite of offices. The least expensive way to do business is to develop an on-site massage business for private homes or offices and have the business office in your home.

Beginning small with the bare essentials keeps start-up costs under $3000. A basic portable table should not cost more than $400. Business cards and a simple brochure are needed, as well as client/practitioner statements, policy and procedure booklets, receipt books, and client information forms. The total cost for these is about $300. It is a good idea to have a separate telephone line and answering machine, which together cost about $200. Membership in one of the professional organizations also provides liability insurance; the membership and insurance usually cost less than $300. Linens and supplies should cost about $300, and opening a bank account, plus miscellaneous expenses, takes about $500. An expenditure of $1000 for initial advertising is reasonable.

With the use of a small office, the start-up cost jumps to about $5000. This includes the expenses detailed above plus office costs, such as rent (about $1000 because renting office space often requires payment of the first and last months' rent up front) and office furniture and utility hook-ups (another $1000).

As previously mentioned, in addition to these start-up costs, you should have a minimum cash reserve equal to

---

box 14-2

GUIDELINES FOR SETTING GOALS

1. State goals in the present tense. Act as though your goal has already been achieved. Make sure you are the main character. Use the pronouns *I, me,* and *my.*
2. Make sure your goals are realistic and attainable. Can you achieve these goals from your own resources with little help from others? If the activity of a specific person is necessary to achieve your goal, rethink it. What other people may be able to be part of the goal? Avoid depending on only one other person.
3. Speak positively. Avoid words such as *should, would, could, try,* and *never.*
4. Set target deadlines for yourself; they will give you something to work toward.
5. Make sure your goals are small steps toward your ultimate plan. For example, graduating from school is too big to be a goal; it is more like a mission statement. Completing all the exercises in this chapter within 4 weeks is an attainable goal.

14-4

PROFICIENCY EXERCISE

Picture yourself 5 years from now enjoying a successful massage therapy business. A new student comes to you and asks you how you achieved your success. You begin to tell the story of the past 5 years and all the steps it took to get where you are now. All the steps you list are possible goals. When you begin by visualizing the end result, all you have to do is identify the probable steps that you got there. *In the space provided, write down two professional goals that you identified.*

Goal 1

Goal 2

box 14-3

USING THE CLINICAL REASONING MODEL FOR GOAL SETTING

1. Gather facts to identify and define the situation. (This can be the mission statement.)

Key questions

What is the desired outcome?
What are the facts?
My business mission is to serve the blue-collar labor population in my area by providing therapeutic massage and self-help education at a reasonable cost, with flexible appointment hours, and at an easily accessible location.
I will need a group of people for a client base.

2. Brainstorm possible goals.

Key questions

What might I do?
What if . . . ?
What are the possibilities?
What does my intuition suggest?
What if I contact the XYZ manufacturing plant as a potential population?
What if I contact the ABC packing company as a potential population?

3. Evaluate each possible goal identified in Step 2 logically and objectively; look at both pros and cons.

Key Questions

What would happen if . . . (insert each brainstormed idea from Step 2)?
What are the costs, resources needed, and time involved?
What are the logical cause and effect of each possibility identified?
What are the pros and cons of each goal suggested?
What are the consequences of not acting?
What are the consequences of acting?
What would happen if I contacted the XYZ manufacturing plant?
- *I would need a massage room on site.*
- *Travel time to work would be 45 minutes.*
- Pro: *This plant has 300 employees, a large potential client base.*
- Con: *This plant has a history of striking.*
What would happen if I contacted the ABC packing company?

- *I could work at my existing office site.*
- *I am 15 minutes from work on foot.*
- Pro: *This company is in a growth phase*
- Con: *This company has only 50 employees.*

4. Evaluate the effect of each possible goal on the people involved.

Key question

How would each person involved feel if . . . (insert each brainstormed idea from Step 2)?
For each goal, what would be the impact on the people involved: client, practitioner, and other professionals working with the client?
How does each person involved feel about the possible goals?
Does a feeling of cooperation and agreement exist among all parties involved?
How might people feel if I contact the XYZ manufacturing plant?
- *This company is quite traditional. The president is sometimes resistant to change. I am socially acquainted with the plant manager, and he might like the idea.*
How might people feel if I contact the ABC packing company?
- *This company is very progressive in terms of human resources. I have a personality conflict with one of the vice presidents but have a good rapport with the other members of the human resources board.*

5. Choose a goal and develop an implementation plan after carefully processing Steps 1 through 4.

Based on this process, I believe the most attainable goal is to contact ABC packing company.

6. Implement the plan and set a date for reevaluation

Implementation plans are step-by-step procedures that detail what must be done to achieve the goals; these procedures can be considered subgoals.
Steps for implementing the goal of contacting the ABC packing company:
- *Develop a presentation packet (1 week)*
- *Send a letter of inquiry (tomorrow)*
- *Make an appointment for an interview (2 weeks)*

PROFICIENCY EXERCISE

1. Talk with three massage practitioners and ask them what it cost to start their massage businesses.

2. Use professional massage publications and other resources to complete a sample start-up cost worksheet.

the amount of money needed to cover basic business and personal living expenses for 6 months to 1 year. Many people begin a business without these cash reserves and do fine. Others give up the business venture because they don't have enough money to pay bills. This situation forces them to find other jobs. Keeping a cash reserve allows you to focus on developing your business with less financial worry (Proficiency Exercise 14-5).

THE TARGET MARKET

s e c t i o n   o b j e c t i v e s

Using the information presented in this section, the student will be able to perform the following:

- Develop a word-of-mouth marketing plan
- Develop an informational brochure, business card, and media story
- Design a fee structure for therapeutic massage services
- Determine whether third-party insurance reimbursement is available or appropriate for the practice of therapeutic massage

When developing a business, it is important to know the market. Many opportunities are open for the massage business, ranging from the service approaches of stress reduction massage to the allied health opportunities of working in clinical settings. The future for massage is bright. Research has provided the long-awaited verification of the benefits of massage. Educational standards continue to improve, and the profession is becoming standardized and formalized. These developments should achieve a broader acceptance of therapeutic massage and bodywork methods. As a result, more people will consider using massage as part of a health maintenance program.

Massage probably will assume a larger role in corporate stress reduction programs. Athletes will use the services of a massage practitioner more often. Pain control clinics will see its value. Both elderly and young persons can benefit from the nurturing touch of the massage therapist. Opportunities for the development of the massage business will be even greater after people understand the benefits of massage. The need for consistently well-trained practitioners will increase.

There is no typical massage business. Successful massage professionals can be found practicing in many different formats. Massage professionals may be full-time employees of a chiropractor or may work part-time out of their homes. A business could be developed entirely at one location or in three or four locations. A massage therapist may do massage one day at a local manufacturing business for the employees and the next day may do home (on-site) visits for local business people. The third day could be spent teaching a self-help massage class for the local community education program. On the fourth day, the therapist may see clients at a full-service cosmetology establishment in the morning and, that evening, provide on-site massage for a local support group dealing with stress.

With all the possibilities available to the massage practitioner, it is necessary eventually to narrow the focus to one, two, or three specific markets so that advertising and promotional activities are manageable.

Answering the following questions begins the process of narrowing and developing a target market for a therapeutic massage business:

- Where do you plan to work?
- What potential client groups or populations are available within a half-hour drive of the location?
- What type of massage or bodywork do you enjoy giving?
- What group or type of people do you want to help most?
- How are you going to reach those potential clients?
- When do you want to be available to do massage?

By the fifth year of business, a solid focus, narrow target market, and consistent clientele usually have been established (Proficiency Exercise 14-6).

Marketing

Marketing encompasses the advertising and other promotional activities required to sell a product or service. Advertising is a must when starting a new business, and many forms of advertising are very costly. For massage, some types of advertising work better than others.

Word of mouth is the best advertising. Meeting people and talking with them is far more effective than placing an ad in a newspaper. Having satisfied clients who tell other potential clients about you is even better. In the beginning, the massage practitioner must talk with many people to develop a client base. It takes time to build a business. It is important not to become discouraged because if you want to succeed quitting is not an option.

The massage practitioner should persist in handing out business cards and brochures and giving demonstrations until the clients are found. Placing an ad and then sitting in an office waiting for clients to call does not work. Suc-

---

14 - 6

PROFICIENCY EXERCISE

Locate the phone numbers of all the service clubs (e.g., Rotary International) in your community (the local phone book often lists these organizations). Send a short letter of introduction to three of the organizations, offering to do a 30-minute presentation about therapeutic massage for the group. Follow up with phone calls. Arrange to do a presentation (as a student) for the group.

cess comes by arranging to speak at service clubs and churches in the area or by volunteering to work at races and local events. Businesses may want to offer a stress management class. Local school districts often have adult education classes, and short classes teaching simple massage routines are popular. Charitable organizations often have auctions, which are wonderful opportunities to give away gift certificates for massage (Fig. 14-2).

Being visible in the community helps to generate business. Not everyone supports massage, however; do not take negative responses personally.

A regular base clientele numbering about 100 is sufficient to support a thriving therapeutic massage business. Some clients will have weekly standing appointments, others biweekly appointments, and the rest will visit monthly or occasionally. It may be necessary to talk to 2000 people to find 100 clients.

The main marketing obstacle to personal service wellness massage is convincing the public that regular massage is beneficial to a total lifestyle program focused on managing stress and striving for wellness. A wellness massage business is built on those who obtain therapeutic massage regularly. Clients who get a massage on a weekly, bimonthly, or monthly basis are the mainstay of a personal service massage business. A successful business of this type depends on quality, consistent, personal attention to the client. Clients who are happy with the work are the best source of word-of-mouth advertising.

The Brochure

The brochure is the primary tool for educating the public and potential clients about the services offered. It should give specific information about the following (Proficiency Exercise 14-7):

1. *The nature of the services offered.* The brochure should explain clearly that therapeutic massage is a general health service. It should state that no specific treatment of any kind is given for preexisting physical or mental problems. All specific problems of a medical, structural, psychologic, or dietary nature will be referred to the appropriate licensed professional. Written permission and supervision by the medical professional or other licensed health professional will be required in order for the massage practitioner to work with any conditions that fall within that specific scope of practice.
2. *A description of the services offered.* The brochure should give a simple explanation of the process of a massage. It should include a full description of the types of services offered and the procedures followed in rendering those services. It should explain that the client may remain dressed and will always be properly draped. It should be clearly stated that the client may stop the session at any time and may choose not to have any area of the body touched or to have any particular technique used.
3. *The qualifications of the practitioner.* Verifiable credentials documenting education, training, and experience should be outlined in a manner that allows potential clients to verify the competence of the practitioner. A valid organization that issues the credentials, such as a school or continuing education provider, must have a record of the practitioner having completed the course.
4. *The client's financial and time investment.* Include a realistic statement of costs and fees in the brochure. Emphasize that the effects of massage are temporary and that massage is best used as a maintenance system. State that the massage practitioner will teach self-help

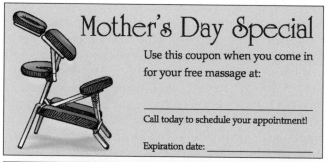

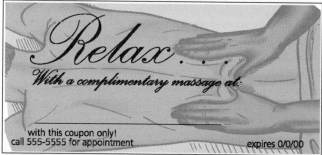

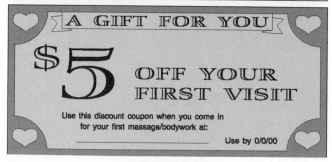

fig. 14-2

Sample coupons and gift certificates.

14-7

PROFICIENCY EXERCISE

1. Locate three different professional brochures. Evaluate them against the criteria listed in this section.
2. Develop a sample professional brochure for your future business.

to the client if requested. The best results from massage are maintained when treatment is given on a weekly or biweekly basis. Therapeutic massage, when used occasionally, provides only temporary effects.

5. *The client's role in health care.* Include the importance of the client's responsibility in his or her personal health care. It is important that the client realize that the massage practitioner is a facilitator in the wellness process.

The Media

Local newspapers often run stories about new and unusual businesses. A word of caution about newspapers: the massage professional should write the story in order to eliminate embarrassing mistakes. Including a black and white photo of the professional giving a massage is a great idea. It is also beneficial to provide the writer copies of other good news stories about therapeutic massage.

Media advertising (newspaper, radio, and television) is very expensive and not the best idea initially. The clientele developed most likely will be located within a 30-mile radius of the business location. A direct mailing to a specific area is more effective than newspaper advertising.

Before advertising in the Yellow Pages of the phone book, which also is very expensive, the massage professional must be sure that the business location will not change for at least a year. The advertisement will be locked in for a year after the phone book has been distributed, and the contract must be paid even if the business moves.

It is much more cost effective to use media advertising the way automotive companies do: A group of massage professionals in the area can advertise together. By splitting the cost, newspaper, radio, and television advertising (which is expensive for one person) becomes affordable. Whenever a cooperative venture such as group advertising is formed, the professionals involved *must get the agreement in writing with the help of an attorney.* Never make oral contracts or agreements. Fig. 14-3 presents some sample advertisements.

When developing any written material or advertising, potential clients need to know the answers to these basic questions:

- Who? (You)
- What? (Therapeutic massage)
- Where? (Address and phone number)
- When? (Appointment times)
- How? (They can reach you by phone)

This information should be on a business card. The card should be simple and direct and should not list all the therapist's credentials. It is convenient to put the information about the next appointment date on the back of the card (Proficiency Exercise 14-8).

Reimbursement
Setting Fees

Another concern for the client is how much the massage will cost. Setting fees and using incentives are great marketing tools. When trying to decide how much to charge

for massage services, it is helpful to investigate what others located within a 1-hour radius of the business location are charging. Consider setting your fees in the midrange of current fees in the area.

It is possible to offer incentives and coupons to generate business interest (see Fig. 14-2), but it usually is unwise to attempt to undercut the competition by charging very low fees. There is much to be gained when massage therapists work together to educate the public about the advantages of massage. The range for massage fees usually is as follows: 30 minutes, $20 to $30; a full hour, $35 to $60. For sessions under 30 minutes it is common to charge $1 per minute (Box 14-4).

Plan on spending half the gross income of the business (all income generated by business activities) on overhead expenses and setting aside one third of the net income (gross income minus business expenses) to pay income taxes.

Always remember that each hour spent doing massage requires at least 1 hour of business management time. Giving 20 1-hour massage sessions is at least 40 hours of work.

The half-hour massage is the most expensive per minute for the client because of the linen usage and necessary paper costs. It costs the massage professional as much to do a half-hour massage as it does an hour massage. The hour massage and the hour-and-a-half massage are more cost effective.

For an on-site massage session the practitioner travels to the client's home or business, and travel and set-up time must be figured into the cost. Because the therapist is already organized to do massage, other sessions at the same location can be provided at the regular rate. If a person is housebound for health reasons, the massage therapist commonly takes this into consideration when setting fees. The massage professional who has only an on-site business saves on rental and utility costs, which may influence the on-site fee structure. Remember that time is money, and it takes longer to do an on-site massage than one in the office.

Another way to determine the fees appropriate for your area or target market is to calculate the average hourly wage of the people in your target market and multiply that by three (up to a maximal hourly fee, which usually is $75). For example, if the employees of ABC packing company make $8 per hour, then the fee for a 1-hour massage would be $24. If the target market is business professionals with an average hourly wage of $25, the fee could be $75. The justification for this structure is that people may understand the value of working 3 hours a week to provide self-care.

If the practitioner sets a fee of $40 an hour for the packing company population, it is unlikely that these clients will be able to afford weekly massage sessions, but regular every-other-week appointments are possible. If the $40 fee is set for the business professional population, weekly appointments are more likely.

Many therapeutic massage professionals give a discount to clients who schedule regular visits. This can be

Ad Samples

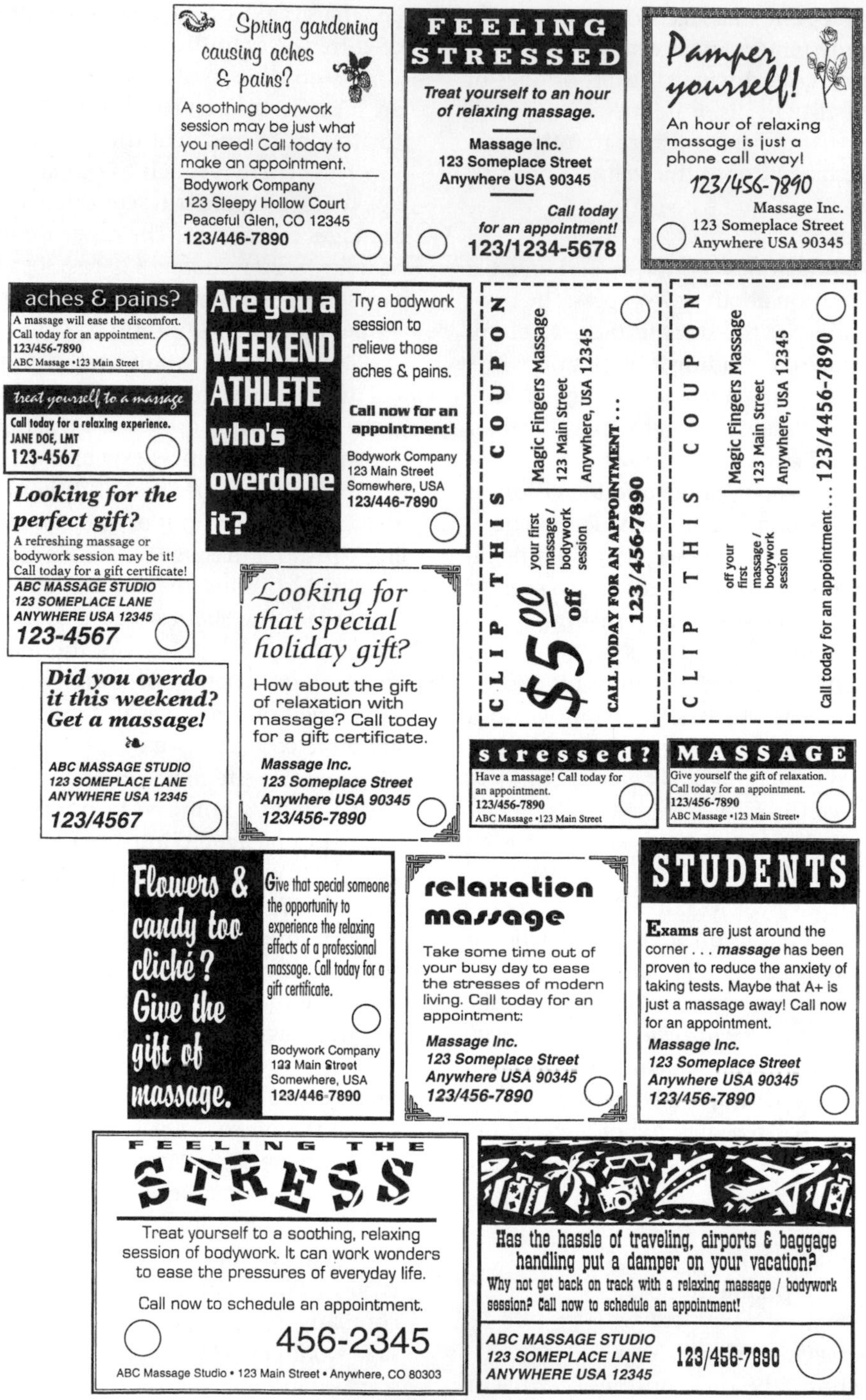

fig. 14-3

Sample advertisements. (From Associated Bodywork & Massage Professionals [ABMP], 28677 Buffalo Park Road, Evergreen, CO 80439-7347. Phone: [800] 458-ABMP or [303] 674-8478. Fax: [303] 674-0859. http://www.abmp.com/.)

done in a variety of ways. One possibility is a package of massages that the client pays for in advance. For example, a client pays for 10 massage sessions in advance with a $5 discount for each massage. The package deal for the $40 session would be 10 massages for $350 rather than $400.

Another option is to give a $5 discount to anyone who books a weekly appointment.

Many massage professionals underestimate the value of their service, whereas others overestimate themselves. When considering money and how much to charge for a

---

box 14-4

TYPICAL MASSAGE FEES

½ hour	$25
1 hour	$40
1½ hours	$55

On-site 1-hour massage: $80 (special circumstances may reduce this fee)

The pricing structure for rural areas is somewhat lower than for urban areas.

It is essential to consider "real time" when planning the business. There is always time between massage sessions:

45 minutes to do a half-hour massage
1 hour and 15 minutes to do an hour massage

1 hour and 45 minutes to do an hour-and-a-half massage
3 hours to do an hour on-site massage
Now consider the actual amount of money generated per hour:
Two half-hour massages can be done in 1½ hours: income generated, $50 ($33 per hour).
It takes 3 hours to do two 1-hour massages: income generated, $80 (about $27 per hour).
It takes 3½ hours to do two 1½-hour massage sessions: income generated, $110 ($33 per hour).
It takes 3 hours to do an on-site 1-hour massage: income generated, $80 ($27 per hour).

14-8

PROFICIENCY EXERCISE

1. Cut out three newspaper stories about new businesses in your area.
2. Write a newspaper story about yourself. Include a picture of yourself.
3. Cut out three current, positive magazine or newspaper articles about therapeutic massage.
4. Design a small ad for your future massage business that is suitable for the Yellow Pages. Call an ad representative from your local telephone company and find out how much it would cost to run the ad.
5. Design a piece of direct mail advertising for your future massage business. Locate a direct mail advertising source and find out how much the ad would cost and the expected rate of return on this type of advertising investment.
6. Contact your local newspaper and ask an ad representative to help you design a display ad for your future massage business. Find out how much it would cost to run the ad.
7. In the space provided below, design the front and back of a business card.

service, it is important to realize that people usually live according to an equal exchange for services rendered or for goods received. This is called the *equity hypothesis*. It is important to charge what a massage is worth in time value. If the fee is too high, the professional does not support those stable weekly and biweekly clients who are the mainstays of a massage practitioner's business. However, if fees are too low, the clients may begin to feel as though they are taking advantage of the massage professional, and the therapist may begin to resent the time spent with the clients. This situation does not foster a gentle, caring, nonjudgmental touch.

It is important to review fees yearly. A good time is at the end of the year when taxes are filed (this usually happens in April, so May is a good time to raise rates). Clients should be notified at least 30 days in advance of any price changes. Also, a full schedule of clients for 3 months is an indicator that a rate increase might be considered (Proficiency Exercise 14-9).

Insurance or Third-Party Reimbursement

Insurance companies do not usually pay for wellness-oriented, personal service therapeutic massage. The paperwork requirements for collecting insurance are extensive. Most massage professionals are unable to bill the insurance company directly for reimbursement. The managed care system is affecting the ability to bill insurance directly and is reducing the number of health care providers who can bill directly.

If the massage therapist is an employee of a licensed medical professional or of a managed care corporation with access to insurance billing codes and is working under direct supervision, the massage services may be available for billing. In this situation the massage therapist receives an hourly wage or salary. The burden of collecting from the insurance company falls on the physician, chiropractor, physical therapist, dentist, psychiatrist, or corporate entity, not on the massage practitioner.

Occasionally a client can collect from the insurance company by providing a prescription for massage from the physician and a receipt showing payment, the diagnostic code from the physician, and a description of the procedure. It is important to have the insurance company preapprove payment for therapeutic massage. This is done by having the client contact the insurance company before any massage begins. Documentation on the benefits of massage, the physician's prescription, and any other information required by the insurance company are presented for review. This usually is the client's responsibility. Based on this information, the insurance company determines whether the client will be reimbursed for the massage services and notifies the client in writing of the decision. The client pays the massage professional directly, and the massage professional provides the receipt with the physician's diagnostic code, the procedure used, and the duration of the session. Responsibility for collecting insurance reimbursement falls to the client.

A good deal of controversy exists about the advisability of dealing with insurance companies. Some massage professionals seem to do well with insurance reimbursement. Workers' compensation and smaller insurance companies are more apt to pay. Therapists who choose to deal with insurance companies, however, must be very careful. Many massage practitioners have been unable to collect insurance payments due and have lost a considerable amount of money. It remains to be seen what effect the managed health care system will have on independent health care professionals, including massage practitioners.

Personal service massage is not likely to fall under the accepted coverage of current or future health care plans. However, the possibility exists that future insurance coverage will be available for preventive heath care. Some managed care systems currently are investigating various options for extending some limited coverage in this area.

Massage is a wonderful addition to any wellness program. If insurance coverage becomes available in this realm,

---

14-9
PROFICIENCY EXERCISE

1. Investigate the fee structure for massage therapy in your area.
2. After you have determined the average fee in your area, decide how many massage sessions per month *you* could afford. What could you afford to pay for a massage session twice a month?
3. On a piece of paper, develop a sample incentive plan. Explain how you would track the discounts.

14-10
PROFICIENCY EXERCISE

1. Contact a local chiropractor, physical therapist, mental health professional, or physician's office, and talk with the billing clerk about the paperwork involved in insurance reimbursement. Ask how much the insurance company covers for various treatments.
2. Call your personal health insurance company and ask whether massage therapy is covered, what the requirements are for receiving coverage, and how much is reimbursed for a massage session.

it probably still will fall under the medical umbrella and will not be accessible to the independent massage practitioner.

The current widespread lack of health insurance coverage for therapeutic massage services should not discourage the new massage professional from starting a business. Many health care professionals are discouraged and frustrated with the health insurance system and the limits it places on their attempts to provide their patients with quality care. Some professionals are even beginning to refuse to participate in health insurance programs; they have begun to adjust their fee schedule and are returning to a cash-for-services system.

Jobs will become available for those who wish to work in the medical system, those who wish to have access to health insurance reimbursement, and also for those who want to be independent business people providing massage services outside the medical establishment on a cash-for-services basis. It is beneficial for both the client and the therapist to have options. As the future unfolds, both business opportunities will continue to develop.

Remember, payment by the client for services rendered is the most dependable income base (Proficiency Exercise 14-10).

THE BUSINESS STRUCTURE

section objectives

Using the information presented in this section, the student will be able to perform the following:

- Negotiate lease agreements based on a flat fee or on a percentage of gross receipts
- Determine average overhead expenses and yearly income

Self-Employment

A common business structure in the massage profession is the self-employed massage professional. Typically the professional becomes affiliated with an established business such as a health club, chiropractor, or full-service cosmetology business by renting a room in that business establishment. It is important to make sure that any agreement of this type is written in contractual form and reviewed by an attorney (Box 14-5).

One pitfall of this type of arrangement is created when the owner or manager of the business wants the massage practitioner to function as an employee but, for payment and tax purposes, to be classified as self-employed. With this arrangement, the business owner does not have to pay matching payroll taxes or benefits.

With true self-employment status, it is important to realize that the professional essentially is renting space from the owner. The massage business is completely independent in the way business is conducted. The business owner cannot direct the massage practitioner regarding what hours to work, what kind of work to do, or what to wear.

Facility Rental

There are two basic ways to pay the owner of the existing business. One is to give the owner a percentage of every massage performed. The rate varies from 10% to 50% (the average is 30%). With this arrangement, the business owner profits from every massage done and may be more likely to support your business with word-of-mouth advertising and referrals. It also is common to advertise together.

Under the other type of agreement, the practitioner pays the owner a monthly rent. Rental fees vary depending on the business location and the area of the country. It is difficult to give a range, but most rooms in established businesses can be rented for $100 to $500 per month. One formula for figuring rent involves calculating the percentage of the total square footage of the space. For example, let's say that the room you want to rent is 12 feet by 12 feet, or 144 square feet. The business occupies 2000 square feet. The 12 × 12 room is about 7% of the total available space. The owner pays $2800 per month for rent ($14 per square foot); 7% of $2800 is $196. The business owner needs to make some money to apply the business principle of making a reasonable profit. A 50% return is normal; 50% of $196 is $98. The rent for the space would be $196 plus $98, or $294.

It may be a better choice at first to pay a percentage for each massage. If there is a slow week or very few massages are given, the professional is not obligated to pay a monthly bill. As the business builds, it is common to end up paying more per month with a percentage agreement than with a flat fee. If a mutually beneficial relationship is desired, a compromise can be negotiated, such as an upper limit cap on monthly rent. This is the type of information that must be included in a written legal agreement, or contract.

Hourly Wage Employment

It is becoming more common to hire massage technicians at an hourly wage. A beginning wage is $7 to $10 per hour. The average yearly net income for a full-time technician is approximately $20,000 to $25,000. This is about $10 per hour based on a 40-hour workweek. Remember that income taxes must be paid on this amount. When working for an hourly wage, the practitioner usually is paid for the time spent at the job location, regardless of whether massage is given. Sometimes an agreed salary is offered instead of an hourly wage. Those who work for a salary often are paid on the basis of completion of certain tasks rather than the number of hours worked. A salary structure for therapeutic massage might be $400 per week based on completion of 20 massage sessions per pay period. An hourly wage may seem like less than a self-employed practitioner earns, but overall the actual amount in the therapist's pocket is about the same.

box 14-5

SAMPLE FACILITIES AND SERVICES AGREEMENT WRITTEN IN CONTRACT FORM

Agreement, made this _____ day of _____, 20__, by and between _____, Therapist,

DBA, Cantonville, Maryland, and _____.

Whereas, _____ Massage Therapist, DBA, is a massage therapist and an independent contrac-

tor wishing to use the facilities and services of _____ at _____ for the express

purpose of the rendition of therapeutic massage services or activities related to massage therapy.

TERMS OF AGREEMENT

1. Fee for a 1-hour therapeutic massage is $40. Massage Therapist receives 75% of massage fees and _____ receives 25%. The same percentage applies regardless of the cost of the massage.
2. Fees may be adjusted only on agreement by both parties.
3. This contract is in effect through March 31. At that time either party may cancel or modify the agreement. A new contract will be issued from April 1.

The following facilities and services will be provided by the chiropractor for massage therapist:

A. Storage for all massage supplies
B. Use of the facility and its services, i.e., telephone, bathroom, microwave, refrigerator
C. Booking and confirmation of all massage therapy appointments
D. All collection of money, whether cash or insurance
E. A room for massage therapist use in the rendition of therapeutic massage services or activities related to massage therapy, and _____ also furnishes electricity, heat, and cleaning for this room
F. Promotion of therapeutic massage as an enhancement to chiropractic care

The massage therapist will abide by the following conditions:

A. Bring all necessary supplies associated with therapy
B. Launder all sheets
C. Pay any and all own costs associated with being an independent contractor, i.e., liability insurance and professional membership
D. Control own hours and schedule
E. Not be held accountable for any expenses incurred by facilities or services not included in this agreement
F. Keep all tips
G. Keep all client information confidential
H. Work at facility by appointment only
I. Reconcile all accounts and pay proper percentage to chiropractor at the end of each month

Cancellation of use of facilities and services is to be in writing, giving at least 30 days' notice, thereafter releasing each party from all financial and legal obligations with the other.

Having read the terms of this agreement, _____ does hereby agree to terms and by signing does

agree to use _____ facilities and services to begin on _____.

_____   _____

Date: _____   Date: _____

Comparing Self-Employment and Employee Earnings

To earn $20,000 of net income, a self-employed massage therapist has to generate about $40,000 gross income. Based on 50 weeks of work per year, and 20 massage clients per week at $40 per client, the gross receipts are $40,000 per year. Fifty percent will be spent on overhead costs, including rent, advertising, linens, supplies, phone, mailings, and postage. It also is important to remember that the self-employed massage therapist must consider "real time," which is the amount actually put into the business. At a minimum, for every hour spent giving a massage, at least 1 hour will be spent on business work such as records, clean up, advertising, and marketing. Remember—self-employed people never really leave their business.

When all factors are considered, the earnings end up being about the same whether the practitioner is an hourly wage employee or the owner of his or her business.

Advantages and Disadvantages of Self-Employment

The advantages of self-employment should be considered. For example, the business income could be increased by subletting the space (make sure any rental agreement allows for this). Likewise, after the first few years the advertising and marketing expenses decline because you have established a repeat business with clients who return regularly for massage, and net income increases. Some feel that self-employment offers more freedom to self-direct the business structure, as well as flexibility in scheduling work hours and long-term financial security. Disadvantages include numerous responsibilities both for business concerns and for client services, isolation and lack of peer support and supervision if working alone, and an inability to leave the business for any length of time. Income can vary, and no group benefits are available, such as insurance packages or paid vacations. Membership in professional associations can offset the benefit issue because group insurance programs are available through them.

Advantages and Disadvantages of Employee Status

Employees who have established long-term relationships with their employers often get pay increases. Over a 5-year period the massage practitioner could start at the lowest end ($7 per hour) and work up to $15 per hour. When choosing a career option, consider that as a therapeutic massage employee, you are not responsible for any of the business concerns and can focus most of your professional energy on client services. Employee status usually involves working with other professionals in some way, creating an environment of support and supervision. Some businesses may offer benefits and paid vacations. Income usually is stable.

The disadvantages of being an employee might include adherence to business rules and regulations, less flexibility in work scheduling, and a shared work space.

Requirements of an Employee

In applying for a therapeutic massage position, you must submit a resume and a personal list of career expectations for the job. It is important to understand the job description, the hours that will be spent on the job, and obligations to the employer—and it is vital to get all this in writing, along with any special arrangement that may be made. This document should be signed and dated by all parties involved so that everyone has an original copy. The job interview may include performing a massage session as a skills test.

Many employers complain about the quality and commitment of their employees. The massage/bodywork industry is no different. If you choose to be an employee, the information in this text should help you understand the commitment and responsibility required of an employer to create an environment that allows to you pursue your career as a massage professional free of business responsibilities (Proficiency Exercise 14-11). As an employee, keep in mind the "Do's" and "Don'ts" listed in Box 14-6.

14-11

PROFICIENCY EXERCISE

Develop your personal pro and con lists for self-employment and employee status.

Self-employment

Pros	Cons

Employee status

Pros	Cons

---

box 14-6

EMPLOYEE "DO'S" AND "DON'TS"

Don't

- Gossip
- Complain without providing a viable solution
- Be dishonest
- Behave unethically
- Behave irresponsibly

Do

- Be on time for work
- Look and act like a professional
- Be consistent and accurate with recording requirements of the business
- Be courteous and supportive
- Be assertive and communicate openly with your employer
- Develop a sense of commitment and loyalty to your employer
- Take your responsibilities seriously
- Improve your skills
- Own your mistakes and correct them
- Be willing to extend yourself in the short term for everyone's long-term gain
- Be a team player
- Be flexible and creative
- Use problem-solving skills to resolve potential conflict
- Commit to the job

MANAGEMENT

section objectives

Using the information presented in this section, the student will be able to perform the following:

- **Use a step-by-step procedure to set up business management practices**
- **Set up business files**
- **Develop the paper trail required for business records**

Management consists of all the activities required to maintain a business, particularly record-keeping and financial disbursement. The KISS principle (*keep it simple and specific*) is an excellent concept to help organize the details of business practices. Of course, there are many ways to set up a business operation. A business consultant and an attorney usually are the best advisers. The simplest business arrangement, the sole proprietorship, is detailed in this textbook. The steps in setting up this arrangement are as follows:

1. Obtain all necessary licenses
2. Choose a business location
3. Determine the legal structure of the business
4. Register the name of the business
5. Register for tax purposes
6. Arrange for insurance
7. Open business banking accounts
8. Set up investments
9. Keep records
10. Develop a client-practitioner agreement and policy statement

Obtaining Licenses

Massage professionals usually deal with two distinct types of licenses: professional and business. Professional licensing shows that you have achieved the skills to practice your profession; such a license may be issued by the state or by a local government body (see Chapter 2). With massage, difficulties occasionally arise with local licensing in the form of massage parlor ordinances. If this problem is encountered, it is important to organize a group of massage professionals and other supporters in the local community and work to change the ordinances.

If a state licenses massage, the massage professional usually must show proof of a certain level of education and pass some sort of licensing test. To find out about licensing in any state, it is best to contact the Department of Licensing and Regulation at your state capital. Usually the licensing department for massage is in the occupational license department. This agency can provide the necessary information.

A business license, which is obtained from the local government, allows that governmental body to regulate the type and location of business operations. If a profession is licensed, the professional may need to show a copy of the license to obtain a business license. Any required forms should be filled out carefully.

Choosing a Business Location

When deciding where to locate your business, remember that each community has specific zoning regulations. These regulations protect the investment of those who own property. Without zoning, someone could put a junkyard next to a home. Usually the zoning that a massage business requires is general office or commercial zoning. Because of difficulties with local ordinance control of massage establishments, there may be restrictions on locations for a massage business. To obtain this information, the practitioner should visit local government offices and ask to see the zoning ordinances.

A permit or business license may be needed. It is important that the business owner develop a good working relationship with government officials. These officials usually have a sincere concern for their communities, and the massage professional must respect this. Often these officials need to be educated about therapeutic massage. As with a massage, go slowly and be gentle and understanding.

Difficulty with massage parlor ordinances have diminished substantiality over the past 5 years, but the problem still exists. Hopefully, growing public awareness about therapeutic massage eventually will resolve this problem.

Determining the Legal Structure of the Business

A *sole proprietorship* (one-owner business) is the simplest way to set up a business. Partnerships and corporations are complicated business structures, and the need for them should be discussed with an attorney. This chapter is structured around the sole proprietorship.

Registering the Name of the Business

Registering the name of your business is known *as obtaining a DBA* (i.e., *doing business as* _____). When choosing a business name, the public's interpretation must be considered. One person chose *BODY-WORKS* and received calls about automotive body repair. The fee to register the name of your business is about $20, and it usually is done at the county clerk's office. The clerk will check to see whether anyone else in the county is using the name and then issue the DBA. This document may be needed to open a business checking account.

Registering for Tax Purposes

Federal, state, and local taxes must be paid. A sales tax identification number may also be needed. Information about federal taxes can be provided by the Internal Revenue Service (IRS) at 1-800-829-1040. State tax information can be obtained from the Department of the Treasury in any state. Information about local taxes can be obtained from both the county and local government offices. The IRS has many publications and counseling services that help explain payment of business taxes. The business owner is strongly urged to seek the advice of a business attorney or certified public accountant regarding legal tax requirements.

One third of a gross business income usually is needed to cover various taxes. This money must be set aside every month and left untouched. One of the biggest problems new business owners have is nonpayment of taxes because the tax money was spent on overhead expenses. The best protection is to pay the government first, because the penalties are high and tax laws are difficult. A professional tax preparer can help a great deal with management of your taxes.

Arranging for Insurance

The massage practitioner needs professional liability insurance, often called *malpractice insurance*. The term *malpractice* refers to professional negligence or maleficence. Negligence is an unintentional wrong. A negligent person fails to act in a reasonable and careful manner and consequently causes harm. Maleficence is causing deliberate harm. Clients expect a certain level of professional education, standards of practice, and responsibility for conduct. Unfortunately, in the highly litigious climate of today's world, the best protection against a lawsuit is insurance. Insurance reduces the risk of having a liability claim filed against you personally. To advertise this, however, only invites a lawsuit. Accurate and comprehensive records are the next best protection; anything that seems even slightly important must be documented.

The best place to obtain liability insurance is through the professional organizations. Those that have been in existence for 5 years or longer are the Associated Bodywork and Massage Professionals (ABMP), the American Massage Therapy Association (AMTA), and the International Myomassetics Federation (IMF). (The addresses and phone numbers of these organizations can be found in Appendix D.) There are other professional organizations for massage and bodywork professionals, and careful investigation into their insurance plans is recommended. The insurance costs usually are part of the dues structure of these organizations and thus available at a reasonable cost. It is very expensive to obtain insurance from private companies.

Premise liability insurance also is needed. This is often called "trip and fall" insurance. It can be obtained through professional organizations or from a local insurance agent. Because home business offices are not covered under a homeowner's policy, additional coverage in the form of a business rider is needed. The insurance agent also can discuss fire and damage insurance on equipment.

The more complicated a business, the more comprehensive the insurance coverage must be. Sale of products requires *product liability insurance*. *Independent contractor liability insurance* protects the contractor against third-party claims from hired independent contractors, and so on. The insurance agent and the insurance representative of the professional organization can provide additional information.

Opening Business Banking Accounts

A business checking account can be opened at a local bank. The DBA usually is required to use a business name. Self-carbon checks make record keeping easier. All income from the business is deposited in the checking account, which serves as a record of gross income. Payments for all expenses are written out of this checking account, which provides a record of business deductions. What is left over is called the *net income.*

If the massage professional is disciplined enough to pay off a charge card every month, then a business credit card is a good idea. The monthly statement is a good record of business expenses.

Taxes are paid quarterly on the net income. It is wise for the professional to contact a good bookkeeper or accountant to help set up the payment schedule for taxes.

After all business expenses and taxes have been covered, the massage professional may write himself or herself a paycheck (called a *draw check*). This check should be deposited in a personal checking account, and personal expenses can be paid from this account. *Personal and business money must not be mixed.*

Setting Up Investments

It is a good idea for self-employed massage professionals to set up an individual retirement plan. After paying taxes, 10% of income could be invested in a long-term growth investment. A local bank or insurance company may have access to stable mutual funds. Individual retirement accounts (IRAs) are also available. Money can be invested in compound interest-bearing accounts in many ways. This takes discipline, but we inevitably get older, and it is important to plan for that time now.

Another investment to consider is giving away one massage per week to someone who really needs it. What is given out truly does come back tenfold. Remember the equity hypothesis. This person always has something to return to the massage professional. Maybe it is only a smile of appreciation, which can be worth more than gold.

Keeping Records: the Paper Trail

All business receipts must be saved and filed. Copies of all important documents should be stored in a location other than that of the originals. Everything must be dated, and no oral contracts should be made. Information should be organized monthly on a spreadsheet so that when it is time for the tax preparer to do the business and personal taxes, everything can be verified. This so-called paper trail is very important for a properly run business, and it must be established.

Comprehensive client files must be kept in order, as presented in Chapter 3. Payment records also are kept in the client files. Note whether payment was made by cash, credit card, or check. If given a check, note the check number. If cash, note the receipt number. If a monthly billing system is used, post the date the bill was sent and the date the check was received along with the check number. Any credit card information should be taken and recorded. Records must be kept current. If it is necessary to use professional liability insurance or if you are billed by a client's insurance company, the first thing the company will request is the client's records.

Anyone who wants to manage his or her own business is advised to take some classes in small business management at a community college or attend workshops offered by the local Chamber of Commerce. **For the self-employed, there is no avoiding the necessity of keeping accurate records.** Many commercial record-keeping systems are available. It is helpful to chose one and use it consistently. All massage professionals, whether they are employees or self-employed, must keep accurate, comprehensive client files. The success of your professional life depends on it.

Developing a Client-Practitioner Agreement and Policy Statement

It is essential to have the client read a *client-practitioner agreement and policy statement,* as presented in Chapter 2 (p. 50). The client-practitioner agreement and policy statement is the document in which you set the professional rules for the client. People usually do quite well with information presented to them in a clear, concise, up-front way. The potential for conflict increases if the rules are not understood and agreed or if they are changed too often in midstream. The client-practitioner agreement and policy statement prevents conflicts by clearly stating all policies. This agreement is more comprehensive than the brochure and becomes part of the informed consent process, but it is not protection against a lawsuit. It does have value in that it can do the following:

- Clarify for the client the nature of the service rendered
- Help protect against unwarranted and unrealistic expectations on the part of the client
- Serve the practitioner as a constant reinforcement of the scope and limits of his or her practice within acceptable legal parameters
- Serve as a valuable factual tool if required in court action

The agreement or policy statement should be presented in simple, easily understood language. It gives the practitioner an opportunity to define his or her practice. The practitioner-client agreement is of little value if it does not accurately describe the type of service offered to the public (Proficiency Exercise 14-12).

SUMMARY

This chapter is full of details, regulations, requirements, obligations, paperwork, and responsibility. Someone once said that the job is not complete until the paperwork is

PROFICIENCY EXERCISE

Using the information in this section and the outline provided below, develop a check list for your personal business management plan. The first one is done as an example to get you started

1. Obtain licenses
   - Check with the state about license requirements
   - Obtain a copy of licensing forms
   - Complete forms and return
   - Check with local government about license requirements for:
     Business license
        Obtain copy of licensing forms
        Complete forms and return
     Professional practice license or ordinance
        Obtain copy of licensing forms
        Complete forms and return

2. Choose a business location

3. Establish the legal structure of the business

4. Register the name of the business

5. Register for tax purposes

6. Arrange for insurance

7. Open business banking accounts

8. Set up investments

9. Keep records: the paper trail

10. Develop a client-practitioner agreement and policy statement

done. Be sure to do the paperwork, and use professional help in business where necessary. Success takes time and does not usually happen overnight. Persistence, flexibility, and determination are your keys to a successful business practice. Keep goals realistic and your professional dreams before you if you are to fuel the motivation to strive for success. Define success not only by money made but also by the value obtained from providing professional therapeutic massage services. Take care of yourself to avoid professional burnout so that you can continue to serve your clients in this wonderful and needed profession.

WORKBOOK SECTION

Short Answer

1. Why is motivation so important in building a massage business?

   _____

   _____

   _____

2. Why is it important for a massage professional to explore individual strengths and weaknesses when developing a business?

   _____

   _____

   _____

3. What is burnout, and how can it be prevented?

   _____

   _____

   _____

4. Why is it important to develop a good resume?

   _____

   _____

   _____

5. What is a business plan?

   _____

   _____

   _____

6. What are start-up costs?

   _____

   _____

   _____

7. What are the most effective marketing and advertising strategies?

   _____

   _____

   _____

8. What is the importance of a brochure?

   _____

   _____

   _____

9. How do you set fees?

   _____

   _____

   _____

10. What is real time?

    _____

    _____

    _____

11. What are the prospects of obtaining medical insurance reimbursement for personal service massage?

    _____

    _____

    _____

12. What are the three main types of business opportunities available for the massage professional?

    _____

    _____

    _____

13. What is the KISS principle, and why is it important?

    _____

    _____

    _____

14. What types of insurance does the massage professional need?

    _____

    _____

    _____

WORKBOOK SECTION

15. What is the importance of the paper trail?

_____

_____

_____

16. Why is the client-practitioner agreement and policy statement so important?

_____

_____

_____

17. Why does everyone, including employees, need to understand business operations?

_____

_____

_____

Additional Activity

In developing a client-practitioner agreement and policy statement, you need to be specific about certain areas of information. For each of the sections presented, put in the information that a client needs to know. When you are done, you will have a comprehensive outline to use in creating the booklet.

Use Box 2-6 (p. 50) in the text as a guideline for the information needed. For example, the text says to explain what type of work you provide. You are to list either therapeutic massage, reflexology, or whatever it is that you do.

Some of the answers for this section are samples you can use to compare your responses; others are a reiteration of the information that you will need to detail.

Client-Practitioner Agreement and Policy Statement
All entries should be specific as to the following items:

1. The nature of the service offered:

    a. _____

    b. _____

    c. _____

d. _____

_____

e. _____

_____

2. Description of the service offered:

    a. _____

    b. _____

    c. _____

    d. _____

    e. _____

3. Qualifications of the practitioner:

    a. _____

    b. _____

4. Client financial and time investment:

    a. _____

    b. _____

    c. _____

    d. _____

    e. _____

WORKBOOK SECTION

5. Role of the client in health care:

   a. _____

   _____

   b. _____

   _____

6. Type of service:

   a. _____

   _____

   b. _____

   _____

   c. _____

   _____

   d. _____

   _____

   e. _____

   _____

7. Training and experience:

   a. _____

   _____

   b. _____

   _____

   c. _____

   _____

   d. _____

   _____

   e. _____

   _____

8. Appointment policies:

   a. _____

   _____

   b. _____

   _____

c. _____

   _____

d. _____

   _____

e. _____

   _____

9. Client/practitioner expectations and informed consent:

   a. _____

   _____

   b. _____

   _____

   c. _____

   _____

   d. _____

   _____

   e. _____

   _____

   f. _____

   _____

   g. _____

   _____

   h. _____

   _____

   i. _____

   _____

10. Fees:

   a. _____

   _____

   b. _____

   _____

   c. _____

   _____

WORKBOOK SECTION

d. _____
_____

e. _____
_____

f. _____
_____

g. _____
_____

h. _____
_____

i. _____
_____

11. Sexual appropriateness:

a. _____
_____

b. _____
_____

12. Recourse policy:

a. _____
_____

b. _____
_____

Problem-Solving Exercises

1. Tom is notified that a client is unhappy with his massage fees and is considering finding another massage professional with lower fees. What steps can Tom take to support his fee structure?

_____
_____
_____
_____

2. Marilyn is having a meeting with a client who she feels may have difficulty understanding the scope of practice of massage. How can she use the client-practitioner agreement and policy statement booklet to help establish professional boundaries and obtain informed consent?

_____
_____
_____
_____

3. Calculate real time required to learn massage.

_____
_____
_____
_____

4. After graduation Terry begins a private massage practice. Business begins to build slowly but then levels off. Word-of-mouth advertising is not working as well as expected. What steps can Terry take to boost business?

_____
_____
_____
_____

Professional Application

1. A client calls about receiving a massage. You speak with her on the phone and offer to send her your client policies and procedures booklet. Two weeks later you still have not heard from the prospective client. You make a follow-up telephone call, and the client has specific questions about certain aspects of the policy booklet. This client tells you that a previous massage therapist did not have all these rules. What would you do?

_____
_____
_____
_____

WORKBOOK SECTION

2. Motivation Statement
   In the space below, list three things that have motivated you to become a massage practitioner.

   _____

   _____

   _____

   _____

3. Define the following items as they relate directly to you.

   Know thyself _____

   Follow your dream _____

   Whatever we believe with emotion and feeling becomes our reality

   _____

   Believe in your product _____

   Provide a quality product _____

4. Develop a personal application of methods to prevent burnout. Call it *The Burnout Plan* or give it some other clever name. List one idea for each of these areas:

   _____

   _____

   Care of physical needs _____

   Support person _____

   Care of spiritual needs _____

   Continuing education _____

   Get-away time _____

5. The business structure of therapeutic massage takes many forms. There is a difference between the massage employee and the self-employed massage professional. Choose which approach you plan to pursue, and list those areas of the chapter that most pertain to your professional development plan.

   _____

   _____

   _____

   _____

6. List five business goals. Use the five recommendations for goal setting presented in Box 14-2 as a guide (Box 14-2 is condensed for your convenience below):

   Hints for setting goals:
   1. State goals in the present tense.
   2. Make sure your goals are realistic and attainable.
   3. Speak in the positive.
   4. Set target deadlines for yourself.
   5. Make sure your goals are small steps toward your ultimate plan.

   In each goal, circle any portion that meets the first recommendation.
   Underline any portion that meets the second recommendation.
   Put a box around any portion that meets the third recommendation.
   Double underline any portion that meets the fourth recommendation.
   Double circle any portion that meets the fifth recommendation.

   Sample:

   I will (1,3) complete this exercise (2,5) within the next thirty minutes (4).

   _____

   _____

   _____

   _____

   _____

Research for Further Study

1. Compare the business procedures outlined in the text to another business operation, and identify both similarities and differences in those procedures.

   _____

   _____

   _____

   _____

   _____

WORKBOOK SECTION

2. The statement "business is business" applies to massage. List resources in your area for further business education such as community college courses, the Chamber of Commerce, and so forth.

_____

_____

_____

_____

ANSWER KEY
Short Answer

1. It takes time and commitment to build any business. The person must believe in the product or service. The massage professional must not quit when times get hard, especially during the first 2 years of the business. Motivation provides the inner strength to stay with a project long enough to succeed.

2. If we understand all aspects of ourselves, then it is easier to determine where difficulties may arise, where we will need help from others, or what other skills we may need to learn to support our weak areas. A successful business depends on maximal utilization of strengths and compensation for and understanding of weaknesses.

3. Burnout occurs when we expend more energy than we restore. It could also be described as taking care of others more than we take of ourselves. Burnout can be prevented by keeping our lives balanced. This can be achieved by getting a regular massage, taking classes, and taking a vacation.

4. A resume helps us present the professional experience, qualifications, and attributes that we bring to a business relationship.

5. A business plan is a map of a business's future. It provides direction, clarity of purpose, and a mechanism that sets smaller goals to achieve along the way.

6. Start-up costs are the amount of money it takes to begin a business. One start-up cost that often is forgotten is a reserve of money for subsidizing living expenses during the first year of business.

7. Depend most on word-of-mouth advertising and spread the word initially by making yourself visible in the community through public speaking and volunteer work. Encourage the local media (e.g., newspaper, radio) to do a story about your business. Direct mail is good. Yellow Page advertising is important after the business has been established in a location for 1 year. Form a group of massage and bodywork professionals in your community, and advertise as a group in the newspaper, on the radio, or even on television and share the advertising costs.

8. The brochure educates the public about your massage business in a comprehensive and concise manner.

9. Investigate the fees charged within a 1-hour drive of your location and set your fees midrange. To get the word out, you may have special introductory offers. It is always best to work with your fellow massage practitioners. Massage is a business of low competition because so much depends on the client-practitioner relationship. Clients continue to see you because they like you. By working together in a community, it is easier for massage professionals to educate the public about the importance of therapeutic massage.

10. Real time includes the time it takes to do a massage, as well as the time between massages and the time needed to complete the client's records. In addition, the massage professional must realize that the time spent on business record keeping and paperwork requirements will equal approximately the time spent performing actual massage.

11. Insurance companies are not focused on prevention at this time, therefore it is unlikely that wellness personal service massage will be reimbursed by insurance in the near future. However, the medical insurance programs are changing, and prevention may become a more important consideration. Until that time, cash for services rendered is a more dependable income base. Any proposed insurance coverage must be preapproved by the insurance company before a massage is given.

12. The main types of businesses developed by massage professionals are (1) self-employment, using leased or purchased space, (2) self-employment, paying a percentage of the income from each massage instead of rent for space, and (3) employee status, earning an hourly wage or salary.

13. KISS means *keep it simple and specific*. If a business management system is too complicated, most people will not consistently follow through with the record keeping.

14. Professional liability or malpractice insurance and premise liability insurance ("trip and fall" insurance) are crucial, and the massage professional needs this protection. Other types of insurance are available depending on the complexity of the business.

WORKBOOK SECTION

15. Without an adequate record-keeping system, we are unable to verify information, accurately report business income, keep track of clients' progress, or look back to learn from successes and mistakes in order to achieve a better business operation in the future.

16. This booklet, presented in a format the client can easily understand, enables the client and the therapist to set realistic expectations about what is required in the professional relationship. Thinking the details out in advance prevents many problems. The client-practitioner agreement and policy statement determines the boundaries of the professional relationship.

17. Understanding how a business works helps us appreciate the responsibilities and commitment of business owners and helps people to be better employees. We are all dealing with business concepts when we manage our personal lives. Business management is just one of those things we all need to understand.

Additional Activity

1. The nature of the service offered:
   a. Clearly explain that therapeutic massage is a general health service.
   b. State that no specific treatment of any kind is given for pre-existing physical or mental problems.
   c. Referrals will be made to the appropriate licensed professional for specific medical, structural, psychologic, or dietary problems.
   d. Written permission and supervision by a medical professional or other licensed health professional will be required to work with any conditions that fall within their scope of practice.

2. Description of the service offered:
   a. (Give a full description of the types of services offered and the procedures followed in rendering those services.)
   b. Clients may remain dressed and will always be properly draped.
   c. The client may stop the session at any time and may choose not to have any area of the body touched or any particular techniques used.
   d. (Simply explain the process of a massage.)

3. Qualifications of the practitioner:
   a. (List verifiable credentials documenting education, training, licensing, certifications, and experience to allow potential clients to verify for themselves the practitioner's competency.)
   b. (List the organization issuing the credentials, such as a school or continuing education provider.)

4. Client financial and time investment:
   a. Include a realistic statement of costs and fees in the brochure.
   b. Emphasize that the effects of massage are temporary, and massage is best used as a maintenance system.
   c. Indicate that the effects of the massage session can be increased with simple exercises. The massage practitioner will teach self-help to the client if requested.
   d. The best results from massage are maintained when massage is implemented on a weekly or biweekly basis.
   e. Therapeutic massage, when used occasionally, provides only temporary effects.

5. Role of the client in health care:
   a. Include the importance of the client's responsibility in personal health care.
   b. It is important for the client to realize that the massage therapist's role is as a facilitator in the wellness process.

6. Types of service:
   a. Our clinic offers relaxation, prenatal, and sports massages.
   b. Explain what this particular style of bodywork is good for and what its limitations are.
   c. Specify if you specialize in working with any particular group (e.g., the elderly, athletes) or with specific problems, such as headaches and back pain.
   d. State whether you do not care to work with certain situations, such as pregnant women or people with certain medical conditions.
   e. Have a referral network of related professionals that you use.

7. Training and experience:
   a. Licensing information. Does your state require licensing? If so, have the facts confirming that you are licensed available.
   b. State how long you have been in practice, what school you attended, if the school was approved by any professional organization, and how many classroom hours were required for graduation.
   c. Provide information about continuing education.
   d. Provide information about additional education if pertinent (e.g., that you are also an athletic trainer).
   e. Include the names of any professional organizations in which you are an active member.

8. Appointment policies:
   a. Define the length of an average session.

WORKBOOK SECTION

b. Inform clients which days you work, your hours, and whether you do on-site work, either residential or business.

c. Tell the client to expect that the first appointment will be longer than subsequent appointments, whether you take emergency appointments, and how often you suggest clients come for a massage session.

d. Be clear about the cancellation policy and your policy for late appointments.

e. Tell the client whether he or she can eat before an appointment or if physical activity should be altered or restricted before or after the session.

9. Client/practitioner expectations and informed consent:

a. Explain in detail what happens at the first bodywork session (i.e., paperwork, medical history, and so on).

b. Clients should know that they can get partly undressed or undressed down to their shorts or panties, and that clients are covered and draped during the session.

c. Explain the order in which you massage (face up or face down to begin), what parts of the body you work on and in what order, if you use oils, if a shower is available before or after the massage, or if bathing at home before the massage appointment is expected.

d. Make sure the client understands whether talking is appropriate during the session and that you should be informed if anything feels uncomfortable.

e. If you have low lighting and music is provided, the client should be comfortable with that aspect of the massage.

f. Make clear to the client the possibility of any reactions that may be expected.

g. Indicate that the goals for the massage session and proposed styles and massage methods will be discussed with the client before the massage and that consent must be provided for all massage procedures.

h. Inform the client that your profession has a code of ethics and indicate your policy on confidentiality.

i. If the client is in any way uncomfortable, it is permissible to be accompanied by a friend or relative.

10. Fees:

a. Fees are reviewed annually, and any increase will begin in April.

b. A sliding fee is available for retirees, those on disability, and other such individuals.

c. Cash, checks, and major credit cards are acceptable for payment.

d. Payment is expected at time of service; any arrangements for billing must be made in advance.

e. Clients are responsible for collecting from insurance companies.

f. Insurance covers our services only when the client is referred by a physician and has written preapproval from the insurance company.

g. Our fees are based on hourly rates.

h. A 20% discount is offered to all clients who purchase a series of five sessions.

i. To thank you for referring new clients to our office, we offer you a $5 discount on your next session.

11. Sexual appropriateness:

a. Sexual behavior by the therapist toward the client and the client toward the therapist is always unethical and inappropriate.

b. It is always the responsibility of the therapist or health professional to see that sexual misconduct does not occur.

12. Recourse policy:

a. If a client is unhappy or dissatisfied, a portion of the fees will be refunded.

b. If the matter is not handled in a satisfactory manner, clients can contact the Organization of Bodyworkers of Tylerville [insert your own local professional association here] to register any complaints.

Problem-Solving Exercises

1. Determine fees charged by other therapists in the surrounding area. Locate information about education levels and costs comparable to his that may validate higher fees.

2. Send a booklet to clients to read before the first massage. Use the booklets as a guide for carefully thought-out policies when interviewing the client.

3. Take into account the following and then total:
Time in school
Time spent commuting to school
Time spent completing homework
Time spent doing research
Time devoted to practice

4.

a. Talk with current clients about their satisfaction with his service and ask whether they are referring new clients.

WORKBOOK SECTION

b. Consider offering incentives for referrals.

c. Take continuing education and advertise about his new skills.

d. Do a direct mail with a special offer to current clients.

e. Volunteer to work at some special events.

Professional Application

1. Offer to have the client come in and talk with you.

Identify the areas of concern for the client, and expand on the information in the booklet.

Explain the professional aspects of informed consent.

Explain that knowledge and clarity on these aspects supports the professional relationship.

FINAL WORDS

ALTHOUGH this is the end of the textbook, it is just the beginning of your massage career. It has been quite a journey; it began with touch and continues with the ongoing evolution of you as a massage professional.

It will take some time to learn all the information presented in this book. In a year, after some massage experience, reread this textbook. You will be surprised what you can still learn from it, and you will be duly impressed with what you now understand. Most likely you will discover that the ability to think purposefully and use the reasoning process is your most valuable skill. When you can do this, you truly become your own best teacher.

Finishing this textbook and your course of study in therapeutic massage is an achievement. Be proud of yourself and all those who helped you in the learning process.

Your success now depends on your belief in your own ability. Nothing can stop you if you desire to achieve. Every obstacle is an opportunity to exercise your "achievement muscle." The origin of this muscle is in your faith and the insertion is in your hope. Its function is love and compassion for those you serve.

Success is the maximal use of the abilities you have. If a better way exists to do something, challenge yourself to find it, then share it with others. When in doubt, effleurage!

You never fail when you have done your best. Measure success by what really matters.

All great achievements require time, perseverance, and purpose. Go slowly, evaluate, and adapt to each change, seeing it as an opportunity for growth.

Massage creates space and substitutes one set of signals for another. Hopefully, a more resourceful set of signals frees the energy to reach for our highest potential without restriction. Massage brings an awareness of body, mind, and spirit. Pay attention to the subtleties and quiet messages of life. Let these things teach you.

Most importantly, massage touches people, and in turn, we are touched by them.

Thank you for letting me serve you through this textbook.

WORKS CONSULTED

T HE following works have been used by the author in the development of this text. They are listed by chapter in alphabetical order.

*Recommended reading for further study
**Recommended companion textbook and/or reference

CHAPTER 1

Arvedson J: *Medical gymnastics and massage in general practice*, London, 1930, JA Churchill.

Arvedson J: *The techniques, effects, and uses of Swedish medical gymnastics and Massage*, London, 1931, JA Churchill.

Basmajian JV, Nyberg R: *Rational manual therapies*, Baltimore, 1993, Williams and Wilkins.

Baumgartner AJ: *Massage in athletics*, Minneapolis, 1947, Brugess.

Beard G: A history of massage technic, *Phy Ther Rev* 32:613, 1952.

Beck M: *Theory and practice of therapeutic massage*, ed 2, Albany, NY, 1994, Milady.

Benjamin P: Massage therapy in the 1940s and the college of Swedish massage in Chicago, *Massage Therapy Journal* 32(4):56, 1993.

Cantu RI, Grodin AJ: *Myofascial manipulation theory and clinical application*, Gaithersburg, Md., 1992, Aspen.

Chaitow L: Massage moves mainstream into a UK university *International Journal of Alternative and Complementary Medicine*, 1993.

*Chaitow L: *Palpation skills, assessment and diagnosis through touch*, New York, 1997, Churchill Livingstone.

Chaitow L: *Soft tissue manipulation*, Rochester, Vt., 1988, Healing Arts Press.

Colton H: *Touch therapy*, New York, 1983, Kensington.

Despard LL: Textbook of massage and remedial gymnastics, ed 3, New York, 1932, Oxford University Press.

Garofano JS: *Therapeutic massage & bodywork*, Stamford, Conn., 1997, Appleton & Lange.

Graham D: The history of massage, *The Medical Record* (approximately) 1874.

Graham D: Massage, *Med Surg Rep* XXXL (10), 1874.

Graham D: *A treatise on massage its history, mode of application and effects*, ed 3, Philadelphia, 1902, Lippincott.

Greenman PE: *Principles of manual medicine*, Baltimore, 1989, Williams and Wilkins.

Greenman PE: *Principles of manual medicine*, ed 2, Baltimore, 1996, Williams & Wilkins.

Gurevich D: *Historical perspective*, unpublished article, 1992.

Johnson W: *The anatriptic art and medical rubbing*, London, 1866, Simpkin, Marshall and Co.

Kellogg JH: *The art of massage*, Battle Creek, Mich., 1929, Modern Medicine Publishing.

Kleen E: *Massage and medical gymnastics*, ed 2, New York, 1921, William Wood.

Knott M, Voss DE: *Proprioceptive neuromuscular facilitation: patterns and techniques*, ed 2, New York, 1968, Harper and Row.

Kruger L, editor: *Pain and touch*, ed 2, San Diego, 1996, Academic Press.

Lederman E: *Fundamentals of manual therapy physiology, neurology, and psychology*, New York, 1997, Churchill Livingstone.

Lewit K: *Manipulative therapy in rehabilitation of the locomotor system*, ed 2, Oxford, 1991, Butterworth-Heinemann.

McMillian M: *Massage and therapeutic exercise*, ed 3, Philadelphia, 1932, WB Saunders.

Millenson JR: *Mind matters, psychological medicine in holistic practice*, Seattle, 1995, Eastland Press.

*Montague A: *Touching the human significance of the skin*, ed 3, New York, 1986, Harper and Row.

Norstrom G: *Handbook of massage*, New York, 1896, The Faculty of Stockholm.

Northrup C: *Women's bodies, women's wisdom*, New York, 1994, Bantam Books.

Ornstein R, Sobel D: *The healing brain*, New York, 1987, Simon and Schuster.

Post SE: *Massage: a primer for nurses*, New York, 1891, Nightingale Publishing.

Roth M: *Handbook of the movement cure*, London, 1856, Groombridge and Sons.

Smith EWL, Clance PR, Imes S: *Touch in psychotherapy theory, research, and practice*, New York, 1998, Guilford Press.

Tappan FM: *Healing massage techniques, holistic, classic, and emerging methods*, ed 2, Norwalk, Conn., 1988, Appleton and Lange.

Tappan FM: *Massage techniques: a case method approach*, New York, 1961, Macmillan.

Tappan FM, Benjamin PJ: *Tappan's handbook of healing massage techniques, holistic, classic, and emerging methods*, ed 3, Norwalk, Conn., 1998, Appleton and Lange.

Taylor CF: *Theory and practice of the movement cure by the Swedish system*, Philadelphia, 1861, Lindsay and Blakiston.

Thomas Z: *Healing touch: the church's forgotten language*, Louisville, Ky., 1994, Westminster/John Knox Press.

van Why R: *History of massage and its relevance to today's practitioner*, 1992, The Bodywork Knowledgebase.

van Why R: *Lecture on the history of massage in four parts*, 1992, The Bodywork Knowledgebase.

van Why R: *Notes toward a history of massage*, ed 2, 1992, The Bodywork Knowledgebase.

CHAPTER 2

Administrative Rules of Michigan Occupational Regulations Department of Licensing and Regulation, Lansing, Mich., 1994, Michigan Department of Commerce.

American Massage Therapy Association: *American Massage Therapy Association code of ethics,* Chicago, Ill., The Association.

*Anderson KN, Anderson L, Glanze WD, editors: *Mosby's Medical, nursing, and allied health dictionary,* ed 4, St Louis, 1994, Mosby.

*Ashley M: *Massage: a career at your fingertips,* New York, 1992, Station Hill Press.

Bass E, Davis L: *The courage to heal: a guide for women survivors of child sexual abuse,* New York, 1988, Harper and Row.

Blanchard K, Peale NV: *The power of ethical management,* New York, 1988, William Morrow.

Carlson K, Barbara RA, Schatz A: Is state regulation of massage illegal? *Massage and Bodywork Quarterly* Fall:42, 1993.

Clouser KD, Hufford DJ, O'Conner BB: Informed Consent and Alternative Medicine, *Alternative Therapies* 2(2):76, 1996.

*Corey G, Corey MS, Callanan P: *Issues and ethics in the helping professions,* ed 4, Pacific Grove, Calif., 1993, Brooks/Cole Publishing.

Davis CM: *Patient practitioner interaction and experiential manual for developing the art of health care,* Thorofare N.J., 1994, Clack Incorporated.

Denny NW, Quadagno D: *Human sexuality,* ed 2, St Louis, 1992, Mosby.

Dubler N, Nimmons D: *Ethics on call,* New York, 1994, Harmony.

Guidelines for Core Curriculum for Massage Therapy School, Board of Directors of Masseurs—Province of Ontario: *Regulated Health Professions Act and the Massage Therapy Act,* Toronto, Ontario, Canada, June 1992.

Guidelines for Core Curriculum For Massage Therapy School, Board of Directors of Masseurs—Province of Ontario: *Therapeutic Massage Curriculum Guidelines,* Toronto, Ontario, Canada, June 1992.

Hands On 14(3), 1998, American Massage Therapy Association.

International Myomassethics Federation, Inc: *Code of ethics,* Huntington Beach, Calif., 1993, The Federation.

In touch with the future massage therapy in the 90s: issues of professional development, Chicago, 1990, American Massage Therapy Association.

Keirsey D, Bates M: *Please understand me, temperament in leading,* Del Mar, Calif., 1996, Prometheus Nemesis.

Keirsey D, Marilyn B: *Please understand me, character and temperament types,* ed 2, Del Mar, Calif., 1984, Prometheus Nemesis.

Kohn A: Shattered innocence, *Psychology Today,* p 54, February 1987.

Leflet D: *Hemme approach to ethics,* Bonifay, Fla., 1995, Hemme Approach Publications.

Legislative updates, *Touch Therapy Times* October 1993.

Lyons DJB: *Planning your career in alternative medicine: a guide to degree and certificate programs in alternative health care,* New York, 1997, Avery Publishing Group.

Massage laws nationwide, *Massage Magazine* p 128, July/August 1998.

McPartland JM, the Census Subcommittee on the Alternative Medicine Research Institute and Teacher's Academy: Census of bodyworkers and movement therapists in Vermont, USA, *Journal of Bodywork and Movement Therapies* 2(2):125, 1998.

Millenson JR: *Mind matters, psychological medicine in holistic practice,* Seattle, 1995, Eastland Press.

Mitchell BB: *Acupuncture and Oriental medicine laws,* Washington, D.C., 1997, National Acupuncture Foundation.

National Certification Examination for Therapeutic Massage and Bodywork: candidate handbook, Lansing, Mich., 1993, The Psychological Corporation.

Occupational Regulation Section of the Michigan Public Health Code, Articles 1, 7, 15, and 19 of Act 368 of 1978, Michigan Department of Licensing and Regulation, Lansing, Mich., 1978.

Oregon administrative rules, Board of Massage Technicians Chapter 334 Division 10 Massage Licensing, Portland, Ore., July 1991, Oregon Board of Massage Technicians.

Palmer D: Defining our profession: strategies for inventing the future of massage, *Massage and Bodywork Quarterly* p 28, Summer 1993.

Pearson JC, Spitzberg BH: *Interpersonal communication: concept, components, and contexts,* ed 2, Dubuque, Iowa, 1987, Wm. C Brown.

Sohnen-Moe C: Business ethics, *Massage* 44, 1994.

Sorrentino SA: *Mosby's textbook for nursing assistants,* ed 3, St Louis, 1992, Mosby.

State Medical Board of Ohio: *4731-1-05 Scope of Practice of Massage,* January 1992.

State of Florida: *Massage Practice Act,* Chapter 480. No. 1993.

Successful business handbook, Evergreen, Col., 1997, Associated Bodywork and Massage Professionals.

Texas Public Health Act. 4512K, Title 71: *Regulation of massage therapists and massage establishments,* Chapter 141, January 1990.

**Thibodeau GA, Patton K: *The human body in health and disease,* St Louis, 1992, Mosby.

Thomas C: *Bodywork: what type of massage to get and how to make the most of it,* New York, 1995, Williams Morrow.

Thomas J: Legislative updates, *Massage Magazine* p 121, July/August 1998.

Touch training directory, Evergreen, Col., 1993, Associated Bodywork and Massage Professionals.

Waites E: *Trauma and survival: post-traumatic and dissociative disorder in women,* New York, 1993, WW Norton.

Warren DM: An analysis of existing law governing licensed and unlicensed health practices, *American Holistic Medicine* 1, 1979.

Washington State: *The Law Relating to Massage Therapy,* 18.108 RCW, 1991.

Webster's new universal unabridged dictionary deluxe, ed 2, New York, 1983, Simon & Schuster.

Williams KM: Taking the "parlor" out of massage, *Zoning and Planning News* 7:6, 1989.

**Yates J: *A physician's guide to therapeutic massage: its physiological effects and their application to treatment,* Vancouver, B.C., Canada, 1990, Massage Therapists Association of British Columbia.

CHAPTER 3

*Anderson KN, Anderson LE, Glanze WD, editors: *Mosby's medical, nursing, and allied health dictionary,* ed 4, St Louis, 1994, Mosby.

**Birmingham JJ: *Medical terminology: a self-learning text,* ed 2, St Louis, 1990, Mosby.

**Brooks ML: *Exploring medical language, a student-directed approach,* ed 3, St Louis, 1994, Mosby Lifeline.

**Fritz S, Paholsky K, Grosenbach M: *Mosby's basic science for soft tissue and movement therapies,* St Louis, 1999, Mosby.

Gunn C: *Bones and joints,* ed 3, New York, 1996, Churchill Livingstone.

*Hinkle CZ: *Fundamentals of anatomy and movement, a workbook and guide,* St Louis, 1997, Mosby.

Lillis CA: *A concise introduction to medical terminology,* ed 4, Stamford, Conn., 1997, Appleton & Lange.

Lindsay DT: *Functional human anatomy,* St Louis, 1996, Mosby.

Seeley RR, Stephens TD, Tate P: *Essentials of anatomy and physiology,* ed 2, St Louis, 1996, Mosby.

Sorrentino SA: *Mosby's textbook for nursing assistants,* ed 3, St Louis, 1992, Mosby.

Stewart J: *Clinical anatomy and pathophysiology for the health professional,* Miami, 1994, MedMaster.

**Thibodeau GA, Patton K: *The human body in health and disease,* St Louis, 1992, Mosby.

Thibodeau GA, Patton KT: *Anatomy and physiology,* ed 3, St Louis, 1996, Mosby.

Thomas CL: *Taber's cyclopedic medical dictionary,* ed 16, Philadelphia, 1985, FA Davis.

Thompson DL: Goal-oriented SOAP charting: the search for functional outcomes, *Massage Magazine* p 82, May/June 1998.

*Thompson DL: *Hands heal: documentation for massage therapy,* Seattle, Wash., 1993, Thompson.

CHAPTER 4

Alcock J: *Animal behavior: an evaluatory approach,* Sunderland, Mass., 1989, Sinawer.

**Anderson LE, Glanze WD, editors: *Mosby's medical, nursing, and allied health dictionary,* ed 4, St Louis, 1994, Mosby.

Baldry PE: *Acupuncture, trigger points and musculoskeletal pain,* New York, 1989, Churchill Livingstone.

*Basmajian JV, Nyberg R: *Rational manual therapies,* Baltimore, Md., 1993, Williams and Wilkins.

Bullock BL, Rosendahl PP: *Pathophysiology adaptations and alteration in function,* ed 3, Philadelphia, 1992, Lippincott.

*Cailliet R: *Foot and ankle pain,* ed 3, Philadelphia, 1997, FA Davis.

*Cailliet R: *Hand pain and impairment,* ed 4, Philadelphia, 1994, FA Davis.

*Cailliet R: *Knee pain and disability,* ed 3, Philadelphia, 1992, FA Davis.

*Cailliet R: *Low back pain syndrome,* ed 5, Philadelphia, 1995, FA Davis.

*Cailliet R: *Neck and arm pain,* ed 3, Philadelphia, 1991, FA Davis.

*Cailliet R: *Shoulder pain,* ed 3, Philadelphia, 1991, FA Davis.

Cailliet R: *Soft tissue pain and disability,* Philadelphia, 1977, FA Davis.

*Cailliet R: *Soft tissue pain and disability,* Philadelphia, 1996, FA Davis.

*Cantu RI, Grodin AJ: *Myofascial manipulation theory and clinical application,* Gaithersburg, Md., 1992, Aspen Publishers.

Chaitow L: *The book of natural pain relief,* New York, 1995, Harper Paperbacks.

*Chaitow L: *Modern neuromuscular techniques,* New York, 1996, Churchill Livingstone.

*Chaitow L: *Muscle energy techniques,* New York, 1996, Churchill Livingstone.

^Chaitow L: *Palpation skills, assessment and diagnosis through touch,* New York, 1997, Churchill Livingstone.

Chaitow L: *Soft-tissue manipulation,* Vermont, 1988, Healing Arts Press.

Chaitow L et al: Breathing dysfunction, *Journal of Bodywork and Movement Therapies* 1(5):252, 1997.

Colby LA, Kisner C: *Therapeutic exercise: foundations and techniques,* ed 3, Philadelphia, 1996, FA Davis.

Dean BZ, Geiringer SR: Physiatric therapeutics. 5. Pain, *Arch Phys Med Rehabil* 71:S271, 1990.

Degenhardt B, Kuchera M: Update of osteopathic medical concepts and the lymphatic system, *Journal American Osteopathic Association* 96(2):97, 1996.

deGroot J, Chusid JG: *Correlative neuroanatomy,* ed 20, San Mateo, Calif., 1985, Appleton & Lange.

DiLima SN, Painter SJ, Johns LT, editors: *Orthopaedic patient education resource manual,* Gaithersburg, Md., 1995, Aspen.

Ernst M, Lee MHM: Sympathetic effects of manual and electrical acupuncture of the Tsusanli knee point: comparison with the Huko hand point sympathetic effects, *Exp Neurol* 1986.

**Fritz S, Paholsky K, Grosenbach M: *Mosby's basic science for soft tissue and movement therapies,* St Louis, 1999, Mosby.

Ganong WF: *Review of medical physiology,* ed 13, Norwalk, Conn., 1987, Appleton & Lange.

Gewirtz D: *Touchpoints* 1(1), 1993.

Greenman PE: *Principles of manual medicine,* Baltimore, 1989, Williams & Wilkins.

*Greenman PE: *Principles of manual medicine,* ed 2, Baltimore, 1996, Williams & Wilkins.

Gunn CC: Clinical research unit, rehabilitation clinic, *J Acupuncture* 6, 1978.

Gunn CC: *Reprints on pain, acupuncture and related subjects,* Seattle, 1992, University of Washington.

Hooper J, Teresi D: *The three pound universe,* New York, 1986, Dell.

Horacek J: *Brainstorms,* Northvale, N.J., 1998, Jason Aronson.

Knaster M: Tiffany Field provides proof positive, scientifically, *Massage Therapy Journal* 37(1):84, 1998.

*Lederman E: *Fundamentals of manual therapy physiology neurology and psychology,* New York, 1997, Churchhill Livingstone.

Leflet DH: *HEMME approach to modalities,* Fla., 1996, Hemme Approach.

Levin SR: *Acute effects of massage on the stress response,* master's thesis, Greensboro, N.C., 1990, University of North Carolina.

Longworth J: Psychophysiological effects of slow stroke back massage in normotensive females, *Adv Nursing Sci* 44, 1982.

*Manheim CJ, Lavett DK: *The myofascial release manual,* Thorofare, N.J., 1989, Slack.

Marieb E: *Human anatomy and physiology,* ed 2, Redwood City, Calif., 1992, Benjamin/Cummings Publishing.

McArdle WD et al: *Exercise physiology energy nutrition and human performance,* ed 3, Philadelphia, 1991, Lea and Febiger.

McCraty R, Tiller WA, Atkinson M: *Head-heart entrainment: a preliminary survey,* 1995, Institute of HeartMath. http://www.heartmath.org/research papers/Head/Hart/Headheart.html

Millenson JR: *Mind matters, psychological medicine in holistic practice,* Seattle, 1995, Eastland Press.

NNIH Funds Massage Studies, *Hands On* 9(4), 1993.

Oschman JL: What is healing energy part 3: silent pulses, *Journal of Bodywork and Movement Therapies* 1(3):179, 1997.

Research at TRI, *Touch Therapy Times* 5(5): 1994.

Selye H: *The healing brain: understanding stress, stress without distress,* Los Altos, Calif., ISHK Paperbacks.

*Selye H: *The stress of life,* ed 2, New York, 1978, McGraw-Hill.

Shealy NC: The neurochemical substrate of behavior, *Psychol Health Immun Dis B* 434, 1992.

*Thibodeau GA, Patton KT: *Anatomy and physiology,* ed 3, St Louis, 1996, Mosby.

Thibodeau GA, Patton KT: *The human body in health and disease,* St Louis, 1992, Mosby.

Thomas CL, editor: *Taber's cyclopedic medical dictionary,* ed 16, Philadelphia, 1985, FA Davis.

Timmons BH, Ley R: *Behavioral and psychological approaches to breathing disorders,* New York, 1994, Plenum Press.

Tortora GJ, Grabowski SR: *Principles of anatomy and physiology,* ed 7, New York, 1992, Harper Collins.

Touch research, *Int J Alternative and Complementary Med* 11:7, 1993.

*Travell JG, Simons DG: *Myofascial pain and dysfunction: the trigger point manual,* Baltimore, 1984, Waverly.

*Travell JG, Simons DG: *Myofascial pain and dysfunction: the trigger point manual: the lower extremities,* vol 2, Baltimore, 1992, Williams and Wilkins.

Trew M, Everett T: *Human movement, an introductory text,* ed 3, New York, 1997, Churchill Livingstone.

van Why R: *History of massage and its relevance to today's practitioner,* 1992 (self-published).

Wale JO: *Tidy's massage and remedial exercises,* Bristol, England, 1987, John Wright & Sons.

Work modification, work hardening, and work rehabilitation (Cassette #22), Physical Medicine Research Foundation, Third International Symposium, 1990, Vancouver, British Columbia.

Yates J: *Physiological effects of therapeutic massage and their application to treatment,* British Columbia, 1989, Massage Therapists Association.

CHAPTER 5

*Anderson KN, Anderson LE, Glanze WD, editors: *Mosby's medical, nursing, and allied health dictionary,* ed 4, St Louis, 1994, Mosby.

Board of Directors of Masseurs—Province of Ontario: *Ontario, Canada therapeutic massage curriculum guidelines,* Toronto, Ontario, Canada, 1992, Authors.

Bulluck BL, Rosendahl PP: *Pathophysiology adaptations and alterations in function,* ed 3, Philadelphia, 1992, Lippincott.

Cailliet R: *Soft tissue pain and disability,* Philadelphia, 1996, FA Davis.

*Cantu RI, Grodin AJ: *Myofascial manipulation theory and clinical application,* Gaithersburg, Md., 1992, Aspen Publishers.

*Chaitow L: *Modern neuromuscular techniques,* New York, 1996, Churchill Livingstone.

*Chaitow L: *Muscle energy techniques,* New York, 1996, Churchill Livingstone.

Chaitow L: *Osteopathic self-treatment,* London, 1990, Thorsons.

*Chaitow L: *Palpation skills, assessment and diagnosis through touch,* New York, 1997, Churchill Livingstone.

Chaitow L: *Palpatory literacy,* London, 1991, Thorsons.

Chaitow L: *Soft-tissue manipulation,* Rochester, Vt., 1988, Healing Arts Press.

Chaitow L: *Soft-tissue manipulation and neuromuscular techniques: improving palpatory literacy and treatment efficiency,* Lapeer, MI, 1991, Soft Tissue Manipulation Seminar.

Chaitow L et al: Breathing dysfunction, *Journal of Bodywork and Movement Therapies* 1(5):252, 1997.

Chopra D: *Restful sleep,* New York, 1994, Crowne Trade Paperbacks.

Colby LA, Kisner C: *Therapeutic exercise: foundations and techniques,* ed 3, Philadelphia, 1996, FA Davis.

Cowan P: *Staying well: advanced pain management for ACPA members,* 1994, American Chronic Pain Association.

Dean BZ, Geiringer SR: Physiatric therapeutics, 5. Pain, *Arch Phys Med Rehabil* 71:S271, 1990.

Degenhardt B, Kuchera M: Update of osteopathic medical concepts and the lymphatic system, *Journal American Osteopathic Association* 96(2):97, 1996.

deGroot J, Chusid JG: *Correlative neuroanatomy,* ed 20, San Mateo, Calif., 1985, Appleton and Lange.

Falvo DR: *Medical and psychosocial aspects of chronic illness & disability,* Gaithersburg, Md., 1991, Aspen.

**Fritz S, Paholsky K, Grosenbach M: *Mosby's basic science for soft tissue and movement therapies,* St Louis, 1999, Mosby.

Ganong WF: *Review of medical physiology,* ed 13, Norwalk, Conn., 1987, Appleton and Lange.

*Greenman PE: *Principles of manual medicine,* ed 2, Baltimore, 1996, Williams & Wilkins.

Hahn DB, Payne WA: *Focus on health,* ed 2, St Louis, 1994, Mosby.

Kruger L, editor: *Pain and touch,* ed 2, San Diego, 1996, Academic Press.

McCraty R, Tiller WA, Atkinson M: *Head-heart entrainment: a preliminary survey,* Boulder Creek, Calif., 1995, Institute of HeartMath. http://www.heartmath.org/research papers/Head/Hart/Headheart.html

Melzack R: TP relationship to mechanisms of pain, *Arch Phys Med Rehabil* 62:114, 1981.

Nimmi ME: *Collagen,* vol 1, Boca Raton, Fla., 1988, CRC Press.

Oregon Board of Massage Technicians: *Sanitation requirements for the state of Oregon,* Portland, Ore., 1991, Oregon Administrative Rules.

Oschman JL: What is healing energy part 3: silent pulses, *Journal of Bodywork and Movement Therapies* 1(3):179, 1997.

*Premkumar K: *Pathology A to Z—a handbook for massage therapists,* Calgary, Ontario, Canada, 1996, VanPub Books.

Scull CW: Massage: physiological basis, *Arch Phys Med* 159, 1945.

*Selye H: *The stress of life,* ed 2, New York, 1978, McGraw-Hill.

Shealy NC: The neurochemical substrate of behavior, *Psychol Health Immun Dis* B434, 1992.

*Sheridan CL, Radmacher SA: *Health psychology: challenging the biomedical model,* New York, 1992, John Wiley and Sons.

Tate P, Seeley RR, Stephens TD: *Understanding the human body,* St Louis, 1994, Mosby.

Thibodeau GA: *Structure and function of the body,* St Louis, 1992, Mosby.

Thibodeau GA, Patton K: *The human body in health and disease,* St Louis, 1992, Mosby.

Thomas CL, editor: *Taber's cyclopedic medical dictionary,* Philadelphia, 1985, FA Davis.

Thompson CW: *Manual of structural kinesiology,* ed 10, St Louis, 1985, Mosby.

Timms R, Connors P: *Embodying healing: integrating bodywork and psychotherapy in recovery from childhood sexual abuse,* Orwell, Vt., 1992, The Safer Society Press.

Waites EA: *Trauma and survival: post-traumatic and dissociative disorders in women,* New York, 1993, Norton.

Walton TH: Contraindications to massage therapy part i: roadblocks on the way to consensus, *Massage Therapy Journal* 37(2):108, 1998.

Yates J: *Physiological effects of therapeutic massage and their application to treatment,* British Columbia, Canada, 1989, Massage Therapist Association.

CHAPTER 6

Board of Directors of Masseurs—Province of Ontario: *Ontario, Canada therapeutic massage curriculum guidelines,* Toronto, Ontario, Canada, 1992, Author.

Bulluck BL, Rosendahl PP: *Pathophysiology adaptations and alterations in function,* ed 3, Philadelphia, 1992, Lippincott.

**Fritz S, Paholsky K, Grosenbach M: *Mosby's basic science for soft tissue and movement therapies,* St Louis, 1999, Mosby.

**Hamann B: *Disease: identification, prevention and control,* St Louis, 1994, Mosby.

Newton D: *Pathology for massage therapists,* ed 2, Portland, Ore., 1995, Simran Publications.

Oregon Board of Massage Technicians: *Sanitation requirements for the state of Oregon,* Portland, Ore., 1991, Author.

*Premkumar K: *Pathology A to Z—a handbook for massage therapists,* Calgary, Canada, Calgary, Ontario, Canada, 1996, VanPub Books.

Sorrentino SA: *Mosby's textbook for nursing assistants,* ed 3, St Louis, 1992, Mosby.

*Thibodeau GA, Patton KT: *Anatomy and physiology,* ed 3, St Louis, 1996, Mosby.

Thibodeau GA, Patton K: *The human body in health and disease,* St Louis, 1992, Mosby.

Vardaxis NJ: *Pathology for the health sciences,* New York, 1995, Churchill Livingstone.

CHAPTER 7

Birnbaum JS: *The musculoskeletal manual,* ed 2, Philadelphia, 1986, WB Saunders.

Colby LA, Kisner C: *Therapeutic exercise: foundations and techniques,* ed 3, Philadelphia, 1996, FA Davis.

Kreighbaum E, Barthels KM: *Biomechanics: a qualitative approach for studying human movement,* ed 2, New York, 1985, Macmillan.

Norkin CC, Levangie PK: *Joint structure and function: a comprehensive analysis,* ed 2, Philadelphia, 1992, FA Davis.

Smith LK, Weiss E, Lehmkuhl L: *Brunnstrom's clinical kinesiology,* ed 5, Philadelphia, 1996, FA Davis.

Sorrentino SA: *Mosby's textbook for nursing assistants,* ed 3, St Louis, 1992, Mosby.

CHAPTER 8

De Domenico G, Wood EC: *Beards massage,* ed 4, Philadelphia 1997, WB Saunders.

Small C: *A handbook for the holistic health practitioner,* Irving, Tex., 1983, self-published.

Sorrentino SA: *Mosby's textbook for nursing assistants,* ed 3, St Louis, 1992, Mosby.

Tappan FM, Benjamin PJ: *Tappan's handbook of healing massage techniques, holistic, classic, and emerging methods,* ed 3, Norwalk, Conn., 1998, Appleton and Lange.

CHAPTER 9

Anderson KE, Anderson LE, Glanze D, editors: *Mosby's medical, nursing, and allied health dictionary,* ed 4, St Louis, 1990, Mosby.

Arvedson J: *Medical gymnastics and massage in general practice,* London, 1930, JA Churchill.

Arvedson J: *The techniques, effects and uses of Swedish medical gymnastics and massage,* London, 1931, JA Churchill.

Basmajian JV, editor: *Manipulation traction and massage,* ed 3, Baltimore, 1985, Williams and Wilkins.

*Basmajian JV, Nyberg R: *Rational manual therapies,* Baltimore, 1993, Williams and Wilkins.

Baumgartner AJ: *Massage in athletics,* Minneapolis, 1947, Brugess.

Beard G: A history of massage technic, *Phys Ther Rev* 32:613, 1952.

Bishop B: Vibratory stimulation, *Phys Ther* 54:1273, 1974.

Breakey BM: An overlooked therapy you can use ad lib, *Registered Nurse* p 50, July 1982.

Butler DS: *Mobilization of the nervous system,* Melbourne, Australia, 1991, Churchill Livingstone.

*Cailliet R: *Soft tissue pain and disability,* Philadelphia, 1996, FA Davis.

*Calais-Germain B: *Anatomy of movement,* Seattle, 1993, Eastland Press.

Carpenter IC: *A practical guide to massage,* Baltimore, 1937, William Wood.

**Chaitow L: *Modern neuromuscular techniques,* New York, 1996, Churchill Livingstone.

**Chaitow L: *Muscle energy techniques,* New York, 1996, Churchill Livingstone.

Chaitow L: *Osteopathic self-treatment,* London, 1990, Thorsons.

**Chaitow L: *Palpation skills, assessment and diagnosis through touch,* New York, 1997, Churchill Livingstone.

Chaitow L: *Palpatory literacy,* London, 1991, Thorsons.

Chaitow L: *Soft-tissue manipulation,* Rochester, Vt., 1988, Healing Arts Press.

Chaitow L: *Soft tissue manipulation and neuromuscular techniques: improving palpatory literacy and treatment efficiency,* Lapeer, Mich., 1991, Soft Tissue Manipulation Seminar.

Cyriax E: Some misconceptions concerning mechano-therapy, *Br J Phys Med* 92, 1938.

Cyriax J: Treatment by movement, *Bri Med J* 1944.

*Danials L, Worthingham C: *Muscle testing techniques of manual examination,* ed 5, Philadelphia, 1986, WB Saunders.

Darian-Smith I: Touch in primates, *Ann Rev* 157, 1982.

DeDomenico G, Wood EC: *Beards massage,* ed 4, Philadelphia, 1997, WB Saunders.

DePuy CE: Remarks on the efficacy of friction in palsy and apoplexy, October 1817.

Despard LL: *Textbook of massage and remedial gymnastics,* ed 3, New York, 1932, Oxford University Press.

Eccles AS: *The practice of massage: its physiological effects and therapeutic uses,* ed 2, London, 1898, Bailliere, Tindall, and Cox.

Frank LK: Tactile communication, *Genet Psychol Monographs* 56:209, 1957.

Gammon GD, Starr I: *Studies on the relief of pain by counterirritation,* Philadelphia, July, 1940, Hospital of the University of Pennsylvania.

Garofano JS: *Therapeutic massage & bodywork,* Stamford, Conn., 1997, Appleton & Lange.

Grafstrom AV: *Medical gymnastics including the Schott movements,* London, 1899, The Scientific Press.

Graham D: The history of massage, *The Medical Record,* approximately 1874.

Graham D: Massage, *Med Surg Rep* XXXL, 1874.

Graham D: *A treatise on massage its history, mode of application and effects,* ed 3, Philadelphia, 1902, JB Lippincott.

*Greenman PE: *Principles of manual medicine,* ed 2, Baltimore, 1996, Williams & Wilkins.

*Hinkle CZ: *Fundamentals of anatomy and movement, a workbook and guide,* St Louis, 1997, Mosby.

*Hislop HJ, Montgomery J: *Daniel and Worthingham's muscle testing,* ed 6, Philadelphia, 1995, WB Saunders.

Hough T: *A review of Swedish gymnastics,* Boston, 1899, George Ellis.

Jensen K: *Fundamentals in massage for students of nursing,* New York, 1936, Macmillan.

Johnson W: *The anatriptic art and medical rubbing,* London, 1866, Simpkin, Marshall and Co.

Kellogg JH: *The art of massage,* Battle Creek, Mich., 1929, Modern Medicine Publishing.

Kisner CD, Taslitz N: Connective tissue massage: influence of the introductory treatment on autonomic functions, *Phys Ther* 48:107, 1967.

Kleen E: *Massage and medical gymnastics,* ed 2, New York, 1921, William Wood Co.

Knapp ME: Massage, physical medicine and rehabilitation, *Postgrad Med* 192, 1968.

Lee D: *Manual therapy for the thorax, a biomechanical approach,* Delta, British Columbia, Canada, 1994, DOPC.

Knott M, Voss D: *Proprioceptive neuromuscular facilitation,* New York, 1956, Harper and Row.

Leflet DH: *HEMME approach to soft-tissue therapy,* Bonifay, Fla., 1992, HEMME Approach Publications.

*Lewit K: *Manipulative therapy in rehabilitation of the locomotor system,* ed 2, Oxford, 1991, Butterworth-Heinemann.

Lindsay DT: *Functional human anatomy,* St Louis, 1996, Mosby.

Lowe WW: *Functional assessment in massage therapy,* ed 2, Bend, Ore., 1995, Omeri.

McMillian M: *Massage and therapeutic exercise,* ed 3, Philadelphia, 1932, WB Saunders.

McNaught AB, Callander R: *Illustrated physiology,* ed 4, New York, 1983, Churchill Livingstone.

Melzack R: Hyperstimulation analgesia, *Clin Anesthesiol* 3:81, 1985.

Mennell JB: *Physical treatment by movement, manipulation, and massage,* London, 1940, JA Churchill.

Mennell JM: *The musculoskeletal system, differential diagnosis from symptoms and physical signs,* Gaithersburg, Md., 1992, Aspen.

Mulliner MR: *Mechano-therapy,* Philadelphia, 1929, Lea and Febiger.

Norkin CC, Levangie PK: *Joint structure & function,* ed 2, Philadelphia, 1992, FA Davis, 1992.

Norstrom G: *Handbook of massage,* New York, 1896, The Faculty of Stockholm.

Post SE: *Massage: a primer for nurses,* New York, 1891, Nightingale Publishing.

Roth M: *Handbook of the movement cure,* London, 1856, Groombridge and Sons.

Scull CW: Massage: physiological basis, *Arch Phys Med* 159, 1945.

Tappan FM: *Massage techniques: a case method approach,* New York, 1961, Macmillan Company.

*Tappan FM, Benjamin PJ: *Tappan's handbook of healing massage techniques, holistic, classic, and emerging methods,* ed 3, Norwalk, Conn., 1998, Appleton and Lange.

Taylor CF: *Theory and practice of the movement cure by the Swedish system,* Philadelphia, 1861, Lindsay and Blakiston.

Taylor GH: *An illustrated sketch of the movement cure: its principle methods and effects,* New York, 1866, self-published.

The elements of Kellgren's manual treatment, New York, 1901, William Wood and Co.

Thibodeau GA: *Structure and function of the body,* St Louis, 1992, Mosby.

Thibodeau GA, Patton K: *The human body in health and disease,* St Louis, 1992, Mosby.

Travell JG, Simons DG: *Myofascial pain and dysfunction: the trigger point manual,* Baltimore, 1984, Williams and Wilkins.

Trew M, Everett T: *Human movement, an introductory text,* ed 3, New York, 1997, Churchill Livingstone.

Wall PD: Pain, itch, and vibration, *Arch Neurol* 2:365, 1960.

*Zahourek J: Myologik an atlas of human musculature. In Clay *Zoologik Systems Kinesthetic Anatomy Maniken,* vol 1-5, 1996, Zahourek Systems.

CHAPTER 10

The Academy of Traditional Chinese Medicine: *An outline of Chinese acupuncture,* Peking, 1975, Foreign Language Press.

Alfaro R: *Applying nursing diagnosis and nursing process: a step-by-step guide,* ed 2, Philadelphia, 1990, Lippincott.

Basmajian JV, editor: *Manipulation traction and massage,* ed 3, Baltimore, 1985, Williams and Wilkins.

Basmajian JV, Nyberg R: *Rational manual therapies,* Baltimore, 1993, Williams and Wilkins.

**Bates B: *A guide to physical examination and history taking,* ed 5, Philadelphia, 1991, Lippincott.

**Biel A: *Trail guide to the body,* Boulder Col., 1997, self-published.

Birnbaum JS: *The musculoskeletal manual,* ed 2, Philadelphia, 1986, WB Saunders.

*Cailleit R: *Foot and ankle pain,* ed 3, Philadelphia, 1997, FA Davis.

*Cailliet R: *Hand pain and impairment,* ed 4, Philadelphia, 1994, FA Davis.

*Cailliet R: *Knee pain and disability,* ed 3, Philadelphia, 1992, FA Davis.

*Cailliet R: *Low back pain syndrome,* ed 5, Philadelphia, 1995, FA Davis.

*Cailliet R: *Neck and arm pain,* ed 3, Philadelphia, 1991, FA Davis.

*Cailliet R: *Shoulder pain,* ed 3, Philadelphia, 1991, FA Davis.

Cailliet R: *Soft tissue pain and disability,* Philadelphia, 1988, FA Davis.

*Cailliet R: *Soft tissue pain and disability,* Philadelphia, 1996, FA Davis.

*Calais-Germain B: *Anatomy of movement,* Seattle, 1993, Eastland Press.

Chaitow L: *Osteopathic self-treatment,* 1990, Thorsons Harper Collins.

*Chaitow L: *Palpation skills, assessment and diagnosis through touch,* New York, 1997, Churchill Livingstone.

Chaitow L: *Palpatory literacy,* Hammersmith, London, 1991, Thorsons Harper Collins.

Chaitow L: *Soft tissue manipulation,* Rochester, Vt., 1988, Healing Arts Press.

Clark J, editor: *The human body,* New York, 1989, Arch Cape Press.

Colby LA, Kisner C: *Therapeutic exercise: foundations and techniques,* ed 3, Philadelphia, 1996, FA Davis.

**Daniels L, Worthingham C: *Muscle testing techniques of manual examination,* ed 6, Philadelphia, 1995, WB Saunders.

Daniels L, Worthingham C: *Therapeutic exercise for body alignment and function,* ed 2, Philadelphia, 1977, WB Saunders.

deGrout J, Chusid JG: *Correlative neuroanatomy,* ed 12, East Norwalk, Conn., 1985, Appleton and Lange.

Greenman PE: *Principles of manual medicine,* Baltimore, 1989, Williams and Wilkins.

**Greenman PE: *Principles of manual medicine,* ed 2, Baltimore, 1996, Williams & Wilkins.

Gunn C: *Bones and joints,* ed 3, New York, 1996, Churchill Livingstone.

Gunn CC: *Treating myofascial pain,* Seattle, 1989, Health Services Center for Educational Resources, University of Washington.

Hall-Craggs ECB: *Anatomy as a basis for clinical medicine,* Baltimore, 1985, Urban and Schwarzenberg.

*Hinkle CZ: *Fundamentals of anatomy and movement, a workbook and guide,* St Louis, 1997, Mosby.

**Hislop HJ, Montgomery J: *Daniel and Worthingham's muscle testing,* ed 6, Philadelphia, 1995, WB Saunders.

Jacobs PH, Anhalt TS: *Handbook of skin clues of systemic diseases,* ed 2, Philadelphia, 1992, Lea & Febiger.

**Kapit W, Elson M: *The anatomy coloring book,* New York, 1977, Harper Collins.

Kreighbaum E, Barthels KM: *Biomechanics: a qualitative approach for studying human movement,* ed 2, New York, 1985, Macmillan.

*Lederman E: *Fundamentals of manual therapy physiology neurology and psychology,* New York, 1997, Churchill Livingstone.

Lee D: *Manual therapy for the thorax, a biomechanical approach,* Delta, British Columbia, Canada, 1994, DOPC.

LeVay D: *Human anatomy and physiology,* Binge Suffolk, England, 1974, Hodder and Stoughton Ltd.

*Lewit K: *Manipulative therapy in rehabilitation of the locomotor system,* ed 2, Oxford, 1991, Butterworth-Heinemann.

**Lowe WW: *Functional assessment in massage therapy,* ed 2, Bend, Ore., 1995, Omeri.

McNaught AB, Callander R: *Illustrated physiology,* ed 4, New York, 1983, Churchill Livingstone.

Memmler RL, Wood DL: *Structure and function of the human body,* ed 3, Philadelphia, 1983, Lippincott.

**Mennell J: *The musculoskeletal system differential diagnosis from symptoms and physical signs,* Gaithersburg, Md., 1992, Aspen.

Norkin CC, Levangie PK: *Joint structure and function: a comprehensive analysis,* ed 2, Philadelphia, 1992, FA Davis.

Smith LK, Lehmkuhl LD: *Brunnstrom's clinical kinesiology,* ed 4, Philadelphia, 1983, FA Davis.

Sorrentino SA: *Mosby's textbook for nursing assistants,* ed 3, St Louis, 1992, Mosby.

Sparks SM, Taylor CM: *Nursing diagnosis reference manual,* ed 2, Springhouse, Penn., 1993, Springhouse.

Tate P, Seeley RR, Stephens TD: *Understanding the human body,* St Louis, 1994, Mosby.

Thibodeau GA: *Structure and function of the body,* ed 9, St Louis, 1992, Mosby.

Thibodeau GA, Patton KT: *Anatomy and physiology,* ed 3, St Louis, 1996, Mosby.

Thibodeau GA, Patton KT: *The human body in health and disease,* St Louis, 1992, Mosby.

*Timmons BH, Ronald Ley: *Behavioral and psychological approaches to breathing disorders,* New York, 1994, Plenum Press.

*Travell JG, Simons DG: *Myofascial pain and dysfunction the trigger point manual,* Baltimore, 1983, Williams and Wilkins.

Wale JO, editor: *Tidy's massage and remedial exercises,* ed 11, Bristol, England, 1987, John Wright & Sons.

Walther DS: *Applied kinesiology synopsis,* Pueblo, Col., 1988, SDC Systems.

CHAPTER 11

*Baldry PE: *Acupuncture, triggers points and musculoskeletal pain,* New York, 1989, Churchill Livingstone.

Basmajian JV, editor: *Manipulation traction and massage,* ed 3, Baltimore, 1985, Williams and Wilkins.

Berube R: *Evolutionary traditions: unique approaches to lymphatic drainage and circulatory massage techniques,* Hudson, N.H., 1988, self-published.

Buchman DD: *The complete book of water therapy: 500 ways to use our oldest natural medicine,* New York, 1979, EP Dutton.

Bugaj R: The cooling analgesic, and rewarming effects of ice massage on localized skin, *Phys Ther* 55:11, 1975.

Cailliet R: *Soft tissue pain and disability,* Philadelphia, 1977, FA Davis.

*Cailliet R: *Soft tissue pain and disability,* Philadelphia, 1996, FA Davis.

*Cantu RI, Grodin AJ: *Myofascial manipulation: theory and clinical application,* Gaithersburg, Md., 1992, Aspen Publishers.

Chaitow L: Extremely light manipulative methods: time for research, *Int J Alternative Complementary Med* 10:12, 1992.

Chaitow L: *Soft-tissue manipulation,* Rochester, Vt., 1988, Healing Arts Press.

Chaitow L: *Workshop notes,* Lapeer, Mich., 1988, 1991, 1992, 1993.

*Chengnan S: *Chinese bodywork, a complete manual of Chinese therapeutic massage,* Berkley Calif., 1993, Pacific View Press.

Ciolek J: Cryotherapy: review of physiological effects on clinical application, *Cleveland Clinic Quarterly* 52:193, 1985.

Cohen MR: *The Chinese way to healing: many paths to wholeness,* New York, 1996, Berkley Publishing Group.

*Connelly DM: *Traditional acupuncture the law of five elements,* ed 2, Columbia, Md., 1994, Traditional Acupuncture Institute.

Coulter J: Interview with Hildegard Wittlinger, *J Soft Tissue Manipulation* 1:12, 1993.

Cyriax J, Coldham M: *The textbook of orthopaedic medicine treatment by manipulation massage and injection,* vol 2, ed 11, East Sussex, England, 1984, Bailliere Tindall.

Daulby M, Mathison C: *Guide to spiritual healing,* London, 1996, Brockhampton Press.

Degenhardt B, Kuchera M: Update of osteopathic medical concepts and the lymphatic System, *Journal American Osteopathic Association* 96 (2):97, 1996.

Ding Li: *Acupuncture meridian theory, and acupuncture points,* San Francisco, 1990, China Books and Periodicals.

Ewig J, Provost STP: *An inaugural essay on the effects of cold upon the human body,* Philadelphia, 1797, Joseph Gales.

Gunn CC: *Reprints on pain, acupuncture and related subjects,* Seattle, 1992, University of Washington.

Gunn CC: *Treating myofascial pain: intramuscular stimulation (IMS) for myofascial pain syndromes of neuropathic origin,* Seattle, 1989, University of Washington Medical School.

Harris R: Edema and its treatment in massage therapy, *J Soft Tissue Manipulation* 1:4, 1993.

Hayden CA: Cyrokinetics in an early treatment program, *J Am Phys Ther Assoc* 44, 1964.

Holmes G: Hydrotherapy and spa treatment, *The Practitioner* CXLI, 1938.

Ingham ED: *Stories the feet have told,* St Petersburg, Fla., 1982, Ingham Publishing.

Johari H: *Ayurvedic massage traditional Indian techniques for balancing body and mind,* Rochester, Vt., 1996, Healing Arts Press.

Kreighbaum E, Barthels KM: *Biomechanics: a qualitative approach for studying human movement,* ed 2, New York, 1985, Macmillan.

Leadbeater CW: *The Chakras,* Wheaton, Ill., 1927, The Theosophical Publishing House.

Lederman E: *Fundamentals of manual therapy physiology neurology and psychology,* New York, 1997, Churchill Livingstone.

Maciocia G: *The foundations of Chinese medicine,* New York, 1994, Churchill Livingstone.

*Manheim CJ, Lavett DK: *The myofascial release manual,* Thorofare, N.J., 1989, Slack.

*Masunaga S, Ohashi W: *Zen Shiatsu: how to harmonize yin and yang for better health,* New York, 1997, Japan Publications.

*Nikola RJ: *Creatures of water-hydrotherapy textbook,* Salt Lake City, 1995, Europa Therapeutic.

*Ohashi W: *Do-it-yourself shiatsu: how to perform the ancient Japanese art of acupuncture without needles,* New York, 1976, Penguin Books.

Philips P: Polarity therapy: bodywork to address our energetic nature, *Massage Magazine* p 28, May/June 1998.

Segal M: *Reflexology,* North Hollywood, Calif., 1976, Hal Leighton.

Singer E: *Fasciae of the human body and their relations to the organs the envelop,* Baltimore, 1935, Williams and Wilkins.

Tappan FM, Benjamin PJ: *Tappan's handbook of healing massage techniques, holistic, classic, and emerging methods,* ed 3, Norwalk, Conn., 1998, Appleton and Lange.

*Travell JG, Simons DG: *Myofascial pain and dysfunction: the trigger point manual,* Baltimore, 1984, Waverly Press.

*Travell JG, Simons DG: *Myofascial pain and dysfunction the trigger point manual: the lower extremities,* vol 2, Baltimore, 1992, Williams and Wilkins.

Walther DS: *Applied kinesiology synopsis,* Pueblo, Col., 1988, SDC Systems.

Yao JH: *Acutherapy,* Libertyville, Ill., 1984, Acutherapy Postgraduate Seminars.

CHAPTER 12

Allison TG: How to counsel patients with chronic fatigue syndrome, *Psychol Health Immun Dis* A:5, 1992.

Bandler R, Grinder J: *Patterns of the hypnotic techniques of Milton H. Erickson, M.D.,* vol 1, Cupertino, Calif., 1975, Meta Publications.

Bass E, Davis L: *The courage to heal: a guide for women survivors of child sexual abuse,* New York, 1988, Harper and Row.

*Benjamin PJ, Lamp CP: *Understanding sports massage,* Champaign, Ill., 1996, Human Kinetics.

Calvert R: Dolores Krieger, PhD and her therapeutic touch, *Massage* Jan/Feb 47:56, 1994.

Cunningham AJ: The healing journey: how to organize healing efforts at the psychological, social, and spiritual levels, *Psych Health Immun Dis* A:63, 1992.

Denny NW, Quadagno D: *Human sexuality,* ed 2, St Louis, 1992, Mosby.

Doore G, editor: *Shaman's path: healing, personal growth and empowerment,* Boston, 1988, Shambhala Publications.

Hahn DB, Payne WA: *Focus on health,* ed 2, St Louis, 1994, Mosby.

Hammerschlag CA: *The dancing healers: a doctor's journey of healing with Native Americans,* San Francisco, 1988, Harper.

Jevne R: Enhancing hope in the chronically ill, *Phychol Health Immun Dis* A:127, 1992.

Kohn A: Shattered innocence, *Psychol Today,* p 54, Feb 1987.

*Kubler-Ross E: *To live until we say goodbye,* Englewood Cliffs, N.J., 1978, Prentice-Hall.

Lee D: Amplifying the power of visualization techniques with neuro-linguistic programming, *Psychol Health Immun Dis* A:215, 1992.

Ludhman R: *The sociological outlook,* ed 3, San Diego, 1992, Collegiate Press.

*Meagher J, Boughton P: *Sportsmassage,* Barrytown, N.Y., 1990, Station Hill Press.

McArdle WD et al: *Exercise physiology: energy nutrition and human performance,* ed 3, Philadelphia, 1991, Lea and Febiger.

McGladrey, Pullen: *The Americans With Disabilities Act* (Rev), New York, 1994, Panel Publishers.

Mower MB: An interview with Clyde Ford, *Massage* p 77, Jan/Feb 1994.

Mower MB: An interview with Tiffany Field, Ph.D. Director of the Touch Therapy Research Institute, *Massage* p 74, Jan/Feb 1994.

Northrup C: *Heal your symptoms naturally,* Potomac, Md., 1996, Phillips.

*Northrup C: *Women's bodies, women's wisdom,* New York, 1994, Bantam Books.

Pearson JC, Spitzberg BH: *Interpersonal communication: concept, components, and contexts,* ed 2, Dubuque, Iowa, 1987, Wm. C Brown

Perry HM, Morley JE, Coe RM: *Aging and musculoskeletal disorders,* New York, 1993, Springer Publishing.

*Selye H: *The stress of life,* ed 2, New York, 1978, McGraw-Hill.

Shaughnessy J, editor: *The roots of ritual,* Grand Rapids, Mich., 1973, William B Eerdmans Publishing.

Shealy NC: The neurochemical substrate of behavior, *Psych Health Immun Dis* B:434, 1992.

*Sheridan CL, Radmacher SA: *Health psychology: challenging the biomedical model,* New York, 1992, John Wiley and Sons.

Siegal BS: *Peace, love and healing,* New York, 1989, Harper and Row.

Sorrentino SA: *Mosby's textbook for nursing assistants,* ed 3, St Louis, 1992, Mosby.

Steefel L: Treating depression: helping the body heal the mind, *Alternative & Complementary Therapies* Jan/Feb 1996.

Tate DA: Health, hope, and healing: a survivor's perspective, *Psychol Health Immun Dis* A:304, 1992.

Tate P, Seeley RR, Stephens TD: *Understanding the human body,* St Louis, 1994, Mosby.

Thibodeau GA, Patton K: *The human body in health and disease,* St Louis, 1992, Mosby.

Timms R, Connors P: *Embodying healing: integrating bodywork and psychotherapy in recovery from childhood sexual abuse,* Orwell, Vt, 1992, The Safer Society Press.

Upledger JE: Tissue memory, energy cysts and somatoemotional release, *Psychol Health Immun Dis* A:323, 1992.

Wade C, Tavris C: *Psychology,* ed 2, New York, 1990, Harper.

Waites E: *Trauma and survival: post-traumatic and dissociative disorder in women,* New York, 1993, WW Norton.

Work modification, work hardening and work rehabilitation, Physical Medicine Research Foundation 3rd International Symposium, Vancouver, British Columbia, Canada, 1990.

CHAPTER 13

Allard N, Barnett G: The power of the breath part II, *Massage and Bodywork Quarterly* Summer 1993, p 47.

*Benson H: *Timeless healing the power and biology of belief,* New York, 1996, Scribner.

Castleman M: *Nature's cures,* Emmaus, N.J., 1996, Rodale Press.

*Chaitow L: *The body/mind purification program,* New York, 1991, Fireside.

Chaitow L et al: Breathing dysfunction, *Journal of Bodywork and Movement Therapies* 1(5):252, 1997.

Chopra D: *Restful sleep,* New York, 1994, Crowne Trade Paperbacks.

Commings DE: *Tourette Syndrome and human behavior,* Duarte, Calif., 1997, Hope Press.

Doctor's little black bag of remedies and cures, vol 1, 1997, Boardroom.

**Fritz S, Paholsky K, Grosenbach M: *Mosby's basic science for soft tissue and movement therapies,* St Louis, 1999, Mosby.

*Golan R: *Optimal wellness,* New York, 1995, Ballantine Books.

Hahn DB, Wayne PA: *Focus on health,* ed 2, St Louis, 1994, Mosby.

Hoffman CJ: *HEV 370 Nutrition,* ed 2, Mount Pleasant, Mich., 1996, Central Michigan University.

Lippert L: *Clinical kinesiology for physical therapist assistants,* Portland, Ore., 1991, Author.

Millenson JR: *Mind matters, psychological medicine in holistic practice,* Seattle, 1995, Eastland Press.

Northrup C: *Heal your symptoms naturally,* Potomac, Md., 1996, Phillips.

Ornstein R, Sobel D: *The healing brain,* New York, 1987, Simon and Schuster.

Sacks O: An anthropologist on Mars, *The New Yorker,* p 106, December 1993.

*Sapolsky RM: *Why zebras don't get ulcers: a guide to stress, stress-related disease and coping,* New York, 1994, WH Freeman.

*Selye H: *The stress of life,* ed 2, New York, 1978, McGraw-Hill.

Shealy NC: The neurochemical substrate of behavior, *The Psychology of Health Immunity and Disease,* vol B, Conn., 1992.

Sheridan CL, Radmacher SA: *Health psychology: challenging the biomedical model,* New York, 1992, John Wiley and Sons.

Tate P, Seeley RR, Stephens TD: *Understanding the human body,* St Louis, 1994, Mosby.

**Timmons BH, Ley R: *Behavioral and psychological approaches to breathing disorders,* New York, 1994, Plenum Press.

**Travis JW, Ryan RS: *Wellness workbook,* ed 2, Berkeley, Calif., 1998, Ten Speed Press.

Whitney EN, Rolfes SR: *Understanding nutrition,* ed 7, Minneapolis-St. Paul, 1996, West.

Zi N: *The art of breathing,* Glendale, 1997, Vivi Company.

CHAPTER 14

Bliss E: *Getting things done,* Boulder, Col., 1986 (cassette series).

Calano J, Salzman J: *Success shortcuts, 25 career skills you were never taught, but must know,* Chicago, Career Track Publications.

*Capo M: *The business of massage: a manual for students and professionals,* New York, 1992, Ten Plus Ten.

Jordan DM: An analysis of existing law governing licensed and unlicensed health practices, *Am Holistic Med* 1, 1979.

Ornstein R, Ehrlich P: *New world new mind: moving toward conscious evolution,* New York, 1989, Doubleday.

**Sohnen-Moe C: *Business mastery,* ed 2, Tucson, Ariz., 1991, Sohnen-Moe Associates.

Successful business handbook, Evergreen, Col., 1997, Associated Bodywork and Massage Professionals.

Touch training directory, Evergreen, Col., 1993, Associated Bodywork and Massage Professionals.

Tracy B: *The psychology of achievement,* Chicago, Brian Tracy Learning Symposium, Solana Beach, Calif. (cassette series).

Verbury K: *Managing the modern Michigan township,* Lansing, Mich., 1990, Community Development Publishers, Michigan State University.

GLOSSARY

abbreviation Shortened forms of words or phrases.

abuse Exploitation, misuse, mistreatment, molestation, neglect.

acquired immunodeficiency syndrome (AIDS) A dysfunction in the body's immune system, which defends the body against disease.

active assisted movement Movement of a joint in which both the client and the therapist produce the motion.

active joint movement Movement of a joint through its range of movement by the client.

active range of motion Movement of a joint by the client without any type of assistance from the massage practitioner.

active resistive movement Movement of a joint by the client against resistance provided by the therapist.

acupressure Methods used to tone or sedate acupuncture points without the use of needles.

acupuncture point Oriental term for a specific point that correlates with a neurologic motor point.

acute A term that describes a condition in which the signs and symptoms develop quickly, last a short time, and then disappear.

acute illness A short-term illness that resolves by means of the normal healing process and, if necessary, supportive medical care.

acute pain A symptom of a disease condition or a temporary aspect of medical treatment. Acute pain acts as a warning signal because it can activate the sympathetic nervous system. It usually is temporary, of sudden onset, and easily localized. The client frequently can describe the pain, which often subsides without treatment.

adaptation A response to a sensory stimulation in which nerve signaling is reduced or ceases.

allied health A division of medicine in which the professional receives training in a specific area of medicine to serve as support for the physician.

anatomic barriers Anatomic structures determined by the shape and fit of the bones at the joint.

antagonism Occurs when massage produces the opposite effect, such as with medications.

antagonists The muscles that oppose the movement of the prime movers.

anxiety A feeling of uneasiness, usually connected with an increase in sympathetic arousal responses.

applied kinesiology Methods of evaluation and bodywork that use a specialized type of muscle testing and various forms of massage and bodywork for corrective procedures.

approximation The technique of pushing muscle fibers together in the belly of the muscle.

arterial circulation Movement of oxygenated blood under pressure from the heart to the body through the arteries.

arthrokinematic movement Accessory movements that occur as a result of inherent laxity or joint play that exists in each joint. The joint play allows the ends of the bones to slide, roll, or spin smoothly on one another. These essential movements occur passively with movement of the joint and are not under voluntary control.

aseptic technique Procedures that kill or disable pathogens on surfaces to prevent transmission.

assessment The collection and interpretation of information provided by the client, the client's family and friends, the massage practitioner, and referring medical professionals.

asymmetric stance The position in which the body weight is shifted from one foot to the other while standing.

athlete A person who participates in sports as an amateur or a professional. Athletes require precise use of their bodies.

autonomic nervous system The body system that regulates involuntary body functions using the sympathetic "fight/flight/fear response" and the restorative parasympathetic "relaxation response." The sympathetic and parasympathetic systems work together to maintain homeostasis through a feedback loop system.

autoregulation Control of homeostasis through alteration of tissue or function.

Ayurveda A system of health and medicine that grew from East Indian roots.

bacteria Primitive cells that have no nuclei. Bacteria cause disease by secreting toxic substances that damage human tissues, by becoming parasites inside human cells, or by forming colonies in the body that disrupt normal function.

beating A form of heavy *tapotement* involving use of the fist.

benign A term that describes the type of tumor that remains localized within the tissue from which it arose and does not undergo malignant changes. Benign tumors usually grow very slowly.

body mechanics Use of the body in an efficient and biomechanically correct way.

body segment The area of the body between joints that provides movement during walking and balance.

body supports Pillows, folded blankets, foam forms, or commercial products that help contour the flat surface of a massage table or mat.

body/mind The interaction between thought and physiology that is connected to the limbic system, hypothalamic influence on the autonomic nervous system, and the endocrine system.

bodywork A term that encompasses all the various forms of massage, movement, and other touch therapies.

boundary Personal space that exists within an arm's length perimeter. Personal emotional space is designated by morals, values, and experience.

burnout A condition that occurs when a person uses up energy faster than it can be restored.

care or treatment plan The plan used to achieve therapeutic goals. It outlines the agreed objectives; the frequency, duration, and number of visits; progress measurements; the date of reassessment; and massage methods to be used.

career A chosen pursuit; a life's work.

centering The ability to focus the mind by screening out sensation.

certification A voluntary credentialing process that usually requires education and testing; tests are administered either privately or by government regulatory bodies.

challenge Living each day knowing that it is filled with things to learn, skills to practice, tasks to accomplish, and obstacles to overcome.

chemical effects The effects of massage produced by the release of chemical substances in the body. These substances may be released locally from the massaged tissue, or they may be hormones released into the general circulation.

chronic A term that describes the type of disease that develops slowly and lasts for a long time, sometimes for life.

chronic illness A disease, injury, or syndrome that shows little change or slow progression.

chronic pain Pain that persists or recurs for indefinite periods, usually for longer than 6 months. It frequently has an insidious onset, and the character and quality of the pain change over time. It frequently involves deep somatic and visceral structures. Chronic pain usually is diffuse and poorly localized.

circulatory Systems that depend on the pumping action of the skeletal muscle (i.e., the arterial, venous, lymphatic, respiratory, cerebrospinal fluid circulatory systems).

client information form A document used to obtain information from the client about health, preexisting conditions, and expectations for the massage.

client outcome The results desired from the massage and the massage therapist.

client/practitioner agreement and policy statement A detailed written explanation of all rules, expectations, and procedures for the massage.

coalition A group formed for a particular purpose.

cognition Conscious awareness and perception, reasoning, judgment, intuition, and memory.

comfort barrier The first point of resistance short of the client's perceiving any discomfort at the physiologic or pathologic barrier.

commitment The ability and willingness to be involved in what is happening around us so as to have a purpose for being.

communicable disease A disease caused by pathogens that are easily spread; a contagious disease.

compensation The process of counterbalancing a defect in body structure or function.

compression Pressure into the body to spread tissue against underlying structures. (This massage manipulation sometimes is classified with *pétrissage*.) Also, the exertion of inappropriate pressure on nerves by hard tissue (e.g., bone).

compressive force The amount of pressure exerted against the surface of the body in order to apply pressure to the deeper body structures; pressure directed in a particular direction.

concentric isotonic contraction Application of a counterforce by the massage therapist while allowing the client to move, which brings the origin and insertion of the target muscle together against the pressure.

condition management The use of massage methods to support clients who are unable to undergo a therapeutic change but who wish to function as effectively as possible under a set of circumstances.

confidentiality Respect for the privacy of information.

connective tissue The most abundant tissue type in the body; it provides support, structure, space, stabilization, and scar formation.

conservation withdrawal A parasympathetic survival pattern that is similar to "playing 'possum" or hibernation.

contamination The process by which an object or area becomes unclean.

contraindication Any condition that renders a particular treatment improper or undesirable.

control The belief that we can influence events by the way we feel, think, and act.

cortisol A stress hormone produced by the adrenal glands that is released during long-term stress. An elevated level indicates increased sympathetic arousal.

counterirritation Superficial stimulation that relieves a deeper sensation by stimulating different sensory signals.

counterpressure Force applied to an area that is designed to match exactly (isometric contraction) or partly (isotonic contraction) the effort or force produced by the muscles of that area.

countertransference The personalization of the professional relationship by the therapist in which the practitioner is unable to separate the therapeutic relationship from personal feelings and expectations for the client.

craniosacral and myofascial approaches Methods of bodywork that work both reflexively and mechanically with the fascial network of the body.

cream A type of lubricant that is in a semisolid or solid state.

credential A designation earned by completing a process that verifies a certain level of expertise in a given skill.

cross-directional stretching Tissue stretching that pulls and twists connective tissue against its fiber direction.

cryotherapy Therapeutic use of ice.

culture The arts, beliefs, customs, institutions, and all other products of human work and thought created by a specific group of people at a particular time.

cupping The type of *tapotement* that involves the use of a cupped hand; it is often used over the thorax.

cutaneous sensory receptors Sensory nerves in the skin.

database All the information available that contributes to therapeutic interaction.

deep inspiration Movement of air into the body by hard breathing to meet an increased demand for oxygen. Any muscles that can pull the ribs up are called into action.

deep transverse friction A specific rehabilitation technique that creates therapeutic inflammation by creating a specific, controlled reinjury of tissues by applying concentrated therapeutic movement that moves the tissue against its grain over only a very small area.

defensive measures The means by which our bodies defend against stressors (e.g., production of antibodies and white blood cells or through behavioral or emotional means).

denial The ability to retreat and to ignore stressors.

depression A condition characterized by a decrease in vital functional activity and by mood disturbances of exaggerated emptiness, hopelessness, and melancholy or of unbridled high energy with no purpose or outcome.

depth of pressure Compressive stress that can be light, moderate, deep, or varied.

dermatome Cutaneous (skin) distribution of spinal nerve sensation.

direction Flow of massage strokes from the center of the body outward (centrifugal), or from the extremities inward toward the center of the body (centripetal). Direction can be circular motions; it can flow from origin to insertion of the muscle following the muscle fibers or can flow transverse to the tissue fibers.

direction of ease The position the body assumes with postural changes and muscle shortening or weakening, depending on how it has balanced against gravity.

disclosure Acknowledging and informing the client of any situation that interferes with or affects the professional relationship.

disinfection The process by which pathogens are destroyed.

dissociation Detachment, discontentedness, separation, isolation.

dopamine A neurochemical that influences motor activity involving movement (especially learned fine movement, such as hand writing), conscious selective selection (what to pay attention to), mood (in terms of inspiration), possibility, intuition, joy, and enthusiasm. If the dopamine level is low, the opposite effects are seen, such as lack of motor control, clumsiness, inability to decide what to attend to, and boredom.

drag The amount of pull (stretch) on the tissue (tensile stress).

drape Fabric used to cover the client and keep the individual warm while the massage is given.

draping The procedures of covering and uncovering areas of the body and turning the client during the massage.

draping material Coverings that provide the client with privacy and warmth. The most commonly used coverings are standard bed linens because they are large enough to cover the entire body and are easy to use for most draping procedures.

dual role Overlap in the scope of practice, with one professional providing support in more than one area of expertise.

duration The length of time a method lasts or stays in the same location.

dysfunction An in-between state in which one is "not healthy" but also "not sick" (i.e., experiencing disease).

eccentric isotonic contraction Application of a counterforce while the client moves the jointed area, which allows the origin and insertion to separate. The muscle lengthens against the pressure.

effleurage (Gliding stroke); horizontal strokes applied with the fingers, hand, or forearm that usually follow the fiber direction of the underlying muscle, fascial planes, or dermatome pattern.

electrical-chemical functions Physiologic functions of the body that rely on or produce body energy; often called *chi, prana,* and *meridian energy.*

employee A person who works for another for a wage.

end-feel The perception of the joint at the limit of its range of motion. The end-feel is either soft or hard. (See *joint end-feel.*)

endangerment site Any area of the body where nerves and blood vessels surface close to the skin and are not well protected by muscle or connective tissue; therefore deep, sustained pressure into these areas could damage these vessels and nerves. The kidney area is included because the kidneys are loosely suspended in fat and connective tissue, and heavy pounding is contraindicated in that area.

endogenous Made in the body.

energetic approaches Methods of bodywork that work with subtle body responses.

enkephalins and endorphins Neurochemicals that elevate mood, support satiety (reduce hunger and cravings), and modulate pain.

entrainment The coordination of movements or their synchronization to a rhythm.

entrapment Pathologic pressure placed on a nerve or vessel by soft tissue.

environmental contact Contact with pathogens found in the environment in food, water, and soil and on various surfaces.

epinephrine/adrenaline A neurochemical that activates arousal mechanisms in the body; the activation, arousal, alertness, and alarm chemical of the "fight or flight" response and all sympathetic arousal functions and behaviors.

essential touch Vital, fundamental, and primary touch that is crucial to well-being.

ethical behavior Right and good conduct that is based on moral and cultural standards as defined by the society in which we live.

ethical decision making The application of ethical principles and professional skills to determine appropriate behavior and resolve ethical dilemmas.

ethics The science or study of morals, values, or principles, including ideals of autonomy, beneficence, and justice; principles of right and good conduct.

exemption A situation in which a professional is not required to comply with an existing law because of educational or professional standing.

experiment A method of testing a hypothesis.

expressive touch Touch applied to support and convey awareness and empathy for the client as a whole.

external sensory information Stimulation from an origin exterior to the surface of the skin that is detected by the body.

facilitation The state of a nerve in which it is stimulated but not to the point of threshold, the point at which it transmits a nerve signal.

fascial sheath A flat sheet of connective tissue used for separation, stability, and muscular attachment points.

feedback A method of autoregulation to maintain internal homeostasis that interlinks body functions; a noninvasive, continual exchange of information between the client and the professional.

forced expiration Movement of air out of the body, produced by activating muscles that can pull down the ribs and muscles that can compress the abdomen, forcing the diaphragm upward.

forced inspiration Movement of air into the body that occurs when an individual is working very hard and needs a great deal of oxygen. This involves not only the muscles of quiet and deep inspiration but also the muscles that stabilize and/or elevate the shoulder girdle in order to directly or indirectly elevate the ribs.

frequency The number of times a method repeats itself in a time period.

friction Specific circular or transverse movements that do not glide on the skin and that are focused on the underlying tissue.

fungi A group of simple parasitic organisms that are similar to plants but that have no chlorophyll (green pigment). Most pathogenic fungi live on tissue on or near the skin or mucous membranes.

gait Walking pattern.

gate control theory A hypothetical gating mechanism that functions at the level of the spinal cord; a "gate" through which pain impulses reach the lateral spinothalamic system. Painful impulses are transmitted by large-diameter and small-diameter nerve fibers. Stimulation of large-diameter fibers prevents the small-diameter fibers from transmitting signals. Stimulating (rubbing, massaging) large-diameter fibers helps to suppress the sensation of pain, especially sharp pain.

general adaptation syndrome The process that calls into play the three stages of the body's response to stress (i.e., the alarm reaction, the resistance reaction, and the exhaustion reaction).

general contraindications Factors that require a physician's evaluation to rule out serious underlying conditions before any massage is indicated. If the physician recommends massage, the physician must help develop a comprehensive treatment plan.

gestures The way a client touches the body while explaining a problem. These movements may indicate whether the problem is a muscle problem, a joint problem, or a visceral problem.

goals Desired outcomes.

Golgi tendon receptors Receptors in the tendons that sense tension.

growth hormone A hormone that promotes cell division; in adults it is implicated in the repair and regeneration of tissue.

hacking A type of *tapotement* that alternately strikes the surface of the body with quick, snapping movements.

hardening A method of teaching the body to deal more effectively with stress; sometimes called *toughening*.

hardiness The physical and mental ability to withstand external stressors.

healing The restoration of well-being.

health Optimal functioning with freedom from disease or abnormal processes.

heavy pressure Compressive force that extends to the bone under the tissue.

hepatitis A viral inflammatory process and infection of the liver.

histamine A chemical produced by the body that dilates the blood vessels.

history Information from the client about past and present medical conditions and patterns of symptoms.

homeostasis Dynamic equilibrium of the internal environment of the body through processes of feedback and regulation.

hormone A messenger chemical in the bloodstream.

human immunodeficiency virus (HIV) The virus that appears to be responsible for AIDS.

hydrotherapy The use of various types of water applications and temperatures for therapy.

hygiene Practices and conditions that promote health and prevent disease.

hyperstimulation analgesia Diminishing the perception of a sensation by stimulating large-diameter nerve fibers. Some methods used are application of ice or heat, counterirritation, acupressure, acupuncture, rocking, music, and repetitive massage strokes.

hyperventilation Deep or rapid breathing in excess of physical demands.

hyperventilation syndrome A complex set of behaviors that leads to overbreathing in the absence of a pathologic condition. Hyperventilation syndrome is considered a functional syndrome because all the parts are working effectively, therefore a specific pathologic condition does not exist.

hypothesis The starting point of research; it is based on the statement, "If this happens, then that will happen."

impingement syndromes Conditions that involve pathologic pressure on nerves and vessels; the two types of impingement are compression and entrapment.

indication A therapeutic application that promotes health or assists in a healing process.

inflammatory response A normal mechanism, characterized by pain, heat, redness, and swelling, that usually speeds recovery from an infection or injury.

informed consent Client authorization for any service from a professional based on adequate information provided by the professional. Obtaining informed consent is a consumer protection process that requires that clients have knowledge of what will occur, that their participation is voluntary, and that they are competent to give consent. Informed consent is an educational procedure that allows clients to make knowledgeable decisions about whether they want to receive a massage.

inhibition A decrease in or the cessation of a response or function.

initial treatment plan A plan that states therapeutic goals, the duration of the sessions, the number of appointments necessary to meet the agreed goals, costs, the general classification of intervention to be used, and the objective progress measurement to be used to identify attainment of goals.

insertion The muscle attachment point that is closest to the moving joint.

integrated approaches Combined methods of various forms of massage and bodywork styles.

integration The process of remembering an event while being able to remain in the present moment, with an awareness of the difference between then and now, to bring some sort of resolution to the event.

intercompetition massage Massage provided during an athletic event.

intimacy A tender, familiar, and understanding experience between beings.

intuition Knowing something by using subconscious information.

isometric contraction A contraction in which the effort of the muscle or group of muscles is exactly matched by a counterpressure, so that no movement occurs, only effort.

isotonic contraction A contraction in which the effort of the target muscle or group of muscles is partly matched by counterpressure, allowing a degree of resisted movement.

job A regular activity performed for payment.

joint end-feel The sensation felt when a normal joint is taken to its physiologic limit. (See *end-feel.*)

joint kinesthetic receptors Receptors in the capsules of joints that respond to pressure and to acceleration and deceleration of joint movement. The two main types of joint kinesthetic receptors are type II cutaneous mechanoreceptors and pacinian (lamellated) corpuscles.

joint movement The movement of the joint through its normal range of motion.

joint play The inherent laxity present in a joint.

law A scientific statement that is true uniformly for a whole class of natural occurrences.

lengthening The process in which the muscle assumes a normal resting length by means of the neuromuscular mechanism.

license A type of credential required by law; licenses are used to regulate the practice of a profession to protect the public health, safety, and welfare.

longitudinal stretching A stretch applied along the fiber direction of the connective tissues and muscles.

lubricant A substance that reduces friction on the skin during massage movements.

lymphatic drainage A specific type of massage that enhances lymphatic flow.

malignant The type of tumor (cancer) that tends to spread to other regions of the body.

manipulation Skillful use of the hands in a therapeutic manner. Massage manipulations focus on the soft tissues of the body and are not to be confused with joint manipulation using a high-velocity thrust.

manual lymph drainage Methods of bodywork that influence lymphatic movement.

marketing The advertising and other promotional activities required to sell a product or service.

massage The scientific art and system of assessment of and manual application of certain techniques to the superficial soft tissue of skin, muscles, tendons, ligaments, and fascia and the structures that lie within the superficial tissue. The hand, foot, knee, arm, elbow, and forearm are used for the systematic external application of touch, stroking *(effleurage)*, friction, vibration, percussion, kneading *(pétrissage)*, stretching, compression, or passive and active joint movements within the normal physiologic range of motion. Massage includes adjunctive external applications of water, heat, and cold for the purposes of establishing and maintaining good physical condition and health by normalizing and improving muscle tone, promoting relaxation, stimulating circulation, and producing therapeutic effects on the respiratory and nervous systems and the subtle interactions among all body systems. These intended effects are accomplished through the physiologic energetic and mind/body connections in a safe, nonsexual environment that respects the client's self-determined outcome for the session.

massage chair A specially designed chair that allows the client to sit comfortably during the massage.

massage environment An area or location where a massage is given.

massage equipment Tables, mats, chairs, and other incidental supplies and implements used during the massage.

massage mat A cushioned surface that is placed on the floor.

massage routine The step-by-step protocol and sequence used to give a massage.

massage table A specially designed table that allows massage to be done with the client lying down.

mechanical methods Techniques that directly affect the soft tissue by normalizing the connective tissue or moving body fluids and intestinal contents.

mechanical response A response that is based on a structure change in the tissue. The tissue change is caused directly by application of the technique.

mechanical touch Touch applied with the intent of achieving a specific anatomic or physiologic outcome.

medications Substances prescribed to stimulate or inhibit a body process or replace a chemical in the body.

mental impairment Any mental or psychologic disorder such as mental retardation, developmental disabilities, organic brain syndrome, emotional or mental illness, and specific learning disabilities.

metastasis Migration of cancer cells.

moderate pressure Compressive pressure that extends to the muscle layer but does not press the tissue against the underlying bone.

motivation The internal drive that provides the energy to do what is necessary to accomplish a goal.

motor point The point where a motor nerve enters the muscle it innervates and causes a muscle to twitch if stimulated.

movement cure Term used in the nineteenth and early twentieth centuries for a system of exercise and massage manipulations focused on treating a variety of ailments.

multiple isotonic contractions Movement of the joint and associated muscles by the client through a full range of motion against partial resistance applied by the massage therapist.

muscle energy techniques Neuromuscular facilitation; specific use of active contraction in individual muscles or groups of muscles to initiate a relaxation response; activation of the proprioceptors to facilitate muscle tone, relaxation, and stretching.

muscle spindles Structures located primarily in the belly of the muscle that respond to both sudden and prolonged stretches.

muscle testing procedures An assessment process that uses muscle contraction. Strength testing is done to determine whether a muscle responds with sufficient strength to perform the required body functions. Neurologic muscle testing is designed to determine whether the neurologic interaction of the muscles is working smoothly. The third type, applied kinesiology, uses muscle strength or weakness as an indicator of body function.

musculotendinous junction The point where muscle fibers end and the connective tissue continues to form the tendon; a major site of injury.

myofascial approaches Styles of bodywork that affect the connective tissues; often called *deep tissue massage, soft tissue manipulation,* or *myofascial release.*

myofascial release A system of bodywork that affects the connective tissue of the body through various methods that elongate and alter the plastic component and ground matrix of the connective tissue.

needs assessment History taking using a client information form and physical assessment using an assessment form. The information is evaluated to develop a care plan.

nerve impingement Pressure against a nerve by skin, fascia, muscles, ligaments, or joints.

neurologic muscle testing Testing designed to determine whether the neurologic interaction of the muscles is proceeding smoothly.

neuromuscular A term describing the interaction between nervous system control of the muscles and the response of the muscles to the nerve signals.

neuromuscular approaches Methods of bodywork that influence the reflexive responses of the nervous system and its connection to muscular function.

neuromuscular mechanism The interplay and reflex connection between sensory and motor neurons and muscle function.

neurotransmitter A messenger chemical in the synapse of the nerve.

norepinephrine/noradrenaline A neurochemical that functions in a manner similar to epinephrine but that is more concentrated in the brain.

occupation A productive or creative activity that serves as a regular source of livelihood.

oil A type of liquid lubricant.

open-ended question A question that cannot be answered with a simple, one-word response.

opportunistic invasion Potentially pathogenic organisms are found on the skin and mucous membranes of nearly everyone that do not cause disease until they have the opportunity, such as in depressed immunity.

Oriental approaches Methods of bodywork that have developed from ancient Chinese methods.

origin The attachment point of a muscle at the fixed point during movement.

osteokinematic movements The movements of flexion, extension, abduction, adduction, and rotation; also known as *physiologic movements.*

oxytocin A hormone that is implicated in pair or couple bonding, parental bonding, feelings of attachment, and care taking, along with its more commonly known functions in pregnancy, delivery, and lactation.

pain and fatigue syndromes Multicausal and often chronic nonproductive patterns that interfere with well-being, activities of living, and productivity.

pain-spasm-pain cycle Steady contraction of muscles, which causes ischemia and stimulates pain receptors in muscles. The pain, in turn, initiates more spasms.

palliative care Care intended to relieve or reduce the intensity of uncomfortable symptoms but that cannot effect a cure.

palpation Assessment through touch.

panic An intense, sudden, and overwhelming fear or feeling of anxiety that produces terror and immediate physiologic change resulting in immobility or senseless, hysteric behavior.

parasympathetic autonomic nervous system The restorative part of the autonomic nervous system. The parasympathetic response often is called the *relaxation response.*

passive joint movement Movement of a joint by the massage practitioner without the assistance of the client.

passive range of motion Movement of a joint in which the therapist, not the client, effects the motion.

pathogenic animals Large, multicellular organisms sometimes called *metazoa.* Most metazoa are worms that feed off human tissue or cause other disease processes.

pathologic barrier An adaptation of the physiologic barrier that allows the protective function to limit rather than support optimal functioning.

pathology The study of disease.

peer support Interaction among those involved in the same pursuit. Regular interaction with other massage practitioners creates an environment in which both technical information and dilemmas and interpersonal dilemmas can be sorted out.

person-to-person contact Pathogens can often be carried in the air from one person to another.

pétrissage Kneading; rhythmic rolling, lifting, squeezing, and wringing of soft tissue.

phasic muscles The muscles that move the body.

physical assessment Evaluation of body balance, efficient function, basic symmetry, range of motion, and ability to function.

physical disability Any physiologic disorder, condition, cosmetic disfigurement, or anatomic loss that affects one or more of the following body systems: neurologic, musculoskeletal, special sense organ, respiratory (including speech organs), cardiovascular, reproductive, digestive, genitourinary, hemic and lymphatic, skin, and endocrine. Extremes in size and extensive burns also may be considered physical impairments.

physiologic barriers The result of the limits in range of motion imposed by protective nerve and sensory functions to support optimal performance.

piezoelectricity The production of an electrical current by application of pressure to certain crystals such as mica, quartz, Rochelle salt, and connective tissue.

placebo A treatment for an illness that influences the course of the disease even if the treatment is not specifically validated.

polarity A holistic health practice that encompasses some of the theory base of Oriental medicine and Ayurveda. Polarity is an eclectic, multifaceted system.

positional release A method of moving the body into the direction of ease (the way the body wants to move out of the position that causes the pain); the proprioception is taken into a state of safety and may stop signally for protective spasm.

positioning Placing the body in such a way that specific joints of muscles are isolated.

postevent massage Massage provided after an athletic event.

postisometric relaxation (PIR) The state that occurs after isometric contraction of a muscle; it results from the activity of minute neural reporting stations called the *Golgi tendon bodies.*

posttraumatic stress disorder A disorder characterized by episodes of flashback memory, state-dependent memory, somatization, anxiety, irritability, sleep disturbance, concentration difficulties, times of melancholy or depression, grief, fear, worry, anger, and avoidance behavior.

postural muscles Muscles that support the body against gravity.

powder A type of lubricant that consists of a finely ground substance.

prefix A word element placed at the beginning of a root word to change the meaning of the word.

premassage activities Any activity that is involved in preparation for a massage, including setting up the massage room, obtaining supplies, and determining the temperature of the room.

pressure Compressive force.

prime movers The muscles responsible for movement.

principle A basic truth or rule of conduct

profession An occupation that requires training and specialized study.

professional A person who practices a profession.

professional touch Skilled touch delivered to achieve a specific outcome; the recipient in some way reimburses the professional for services rendered.

professionalism The adherence to professional status, methods, standards, and character.

prone Lying face down.

proprioceptive neuromuscular facilitation (PNF) Specific application of muscle energy techniques that uses strong contraction combined with stretching and muscular pattern retraining.

proprioceptors Sensory receptors that detect joint and muscle activity.

protozoa One-celled organisms that are larger than bacteria and can infest human fluids and cause disease by parasitizing (living off) or directly destroying cells.

pulsed muscle energy Procedures that involve engaging the barrier and using minute, resisted contractions (usually 20 in 10 seconds), which introduces mechanical pumping as well as PIR or RI.

qualified Criteria that indicated when the goal is achieved.

quantified Goals measured in terms of objective criteria, such as time, frequency, 1 to 10 scale, measurable increase or decrease in the ability to perform an activity, or measurable increase or decrease in a sensation, such as relaxation or pain.

quiet expiration Movement of air out of the body through passive action. This occurs through relaxation of the external intercostals and the elastic recoil of the thoracic wall and tissue of the lungs and bronchi, with gravity pulling the rib cage down from its elevated position.

quiet inspiration Movement of air into the body while resting or sitting quietly. The diaphragm and external intercostals are the prime movers.

range of motion Movement of joints.

rapport The development of a relationship based on mutual trust and harmony.

reciprocal inhibition (RI) The effect that occurs when a muscle contracts, obliging its antagonist to relax in order to allow normal movement to take place.

reciprocity The exchange of privileges between governing bodies.

recovery massage Massage structured primarily for the uninjured athlete who wants to recover from a strenuous workout or competition.

reenactment Reliving an event as though it were happening at the moment.

referral Sending a client to a health care professional for specific diagnosis and treatment of a disease.

referred pain Pain felt in an area other than the source of the pain.

reflex An involuntary response to a stimulus. Reflexes are specific, predictable, adaptive, and purposeful. Reflexive methods work by stimulating the nervous system (sensory neurons), and tissue changes occur in response to the body's adaptation to the neural stimulation.

reflexive methods Massage techniques that stimulate the nervous system, the endocrine system, and the chemicals of the body.

reflexology A massage system directed primarily toward the feet and hands.

refractory period The period after a muscle contraction during which the muscle is unable to contract again.

regional contraindications Contraindications that relate to a specific area of the body.

rehabilitation massage Massage used for severe injury or as part of intervention after surgery.

remedial massage Massage used for minor to moderate injuries.

resourceful compensation Adjustments made by the body to manage a permanent or chronic dysfunction.

resting position The first stroke of the massage; the simple laying on of hands.

rhythm The regularity of application of a technique. If the method is applied at regular intervals, it is considered even or rhythmic. If it is choppy or irregular, it is considered uneven or not rhythmic.

right of refusal The entitlement of both the client and the professional to stop the session.

rocking Rhythmic movement of the body.

root word The part of a word that provides the fundamental meaning.

safe touch Secure, respectful, considerate, sensitive, responsive, sympathetic, understanding, supportive, and empathetic contact.

sanitation The formulation and application of measures to promote and establish conditions favorable to health, specifically public health.

science The intellectual process of understanding through observation, measurement, accumulation of data, and analysis of findings.

scope of practice The knowledge base and practice parameters of a profession.

self-employment To work for oneself rather than another.

serotonin The neurochemical that regulates mood in terms of appropriate emotions, attention to thoughts, calming, quieting, and comforting effects; it also subdues irritability and regulates drive states.

service An action performed for another person that results in a specific outcome.

sexual misconduct Any behavior that is sexually oriented in the professional setting.

shaking A technique in which the body area is grasped and shaken in a quick, loose movement; sometimes classified as rhythmic mobilization.

shiatsu An acupressure and meridian-focused bodywork system from Japan.

side-lying The position in which the client is lying on his or her side.

skin rolling A form of *pétrissage* that lifts skin.

slapping A form of tapotement that uses a flat hand.

SOAP charting A problem-oriented method of medical record keeping; the acronym SOAP stands for *s*ubjective, *o*bjective, *a*ssessment (*a*nalysis), and *p*lan.

soft tissue The skin, fascia, muscles, tendons, joint capsules, and ligaments of the body.

somatic Pertaining to the body.

somatic pain Pain that arises from stimulation of receptors in the skin (superficial somatic pain) or in skeletal muscles, joints, tendons, and fascia (deep somatic pain).

speed Rate of application (i.e., fast, slow, varied).

spindle cells Sensory receptors in the belly of the muscle that detect stretch.

stabilization Holding the body in a fixed position during joint movement, lengthening, and stretching.

standards of practice The principles that form specific guidelines to direct professional ethical practice and quality care, including a structure for evaluating the quality of care. Standards of practice represent an attempt to define the parameters of quality care.

start-up costs The initial expenses involved in starting a business.

state-dependent memory The encoding and storing of a memory based on the effects of the autonomic nervous system and the resulting chemical levels of the body. The memory is retrievable only during a similar physiologic experience in the body.

sterilization The process by which all microorganisms are destroyed.

stimulation Excitation that activates the sensory nerves.

strength testing Testing intended to determine whether a muscle is responding with sufficient strength to perform the required body functions. Strength testing determines a muscle's force of contraction.

stress Any substantial change in routine or any activity that forces the body to adapt.

stressors Any internal perceptions or external stimuli that demand a change in the body.

stretching Mechanical tension applied to lengthen the myofascial unit (muscles and fascia); two types are longitudinal and cross-directional stretching.

stroke A technique of therapeutic massage that is applied with a movement on the surface of the body, whether superficial or deep.

structural and postural integration approaches Methods of bodywork derived from biomechanics, postural alignment, and the importance of the connective tissue structures.

subtle energies Weak electrical fields that surround and run through the body.

suffering An overall impairment of a person's quality of life.

suffix A word element placed at the end of a root word to change the meaning of the word.

superficial fascia The connective tissue layer just under the skin.

superficial pressure Pressure that remains on the skin.

supervision Support from more experienced professionals.

supine The position in which the client is lying face up.

symmetric stance The position in which body weight is distributed equally between the feet.

sympathetic autonomic nervous system The energy-using part of the autonomic nervous system, the division in which the fight-or-flight response is activated.

symptoms The subjective abnormalities felt only by the patient.

syndrome A group of different signs and symptoms that usually arise from a common cause.

synergistic The interaction of medication and massage to stimulate the same process or effects.

system A group of interacting elements that function as a complex whole.

systemic massage Massage structured to affect one body system primarily. This approach usually is used for lymphatic and circulation enhancement massage.

tapotement Springy blows to the body at a fast rate to create rhythmic compression of the tissue; also called *percussion*.

tapping A type of tapotement that uses the fingertips.

target muscle The muscle or groups of muscles on which the response of the methods is specifically focused.

techniques Methods of therapeutic massage that provide sensory stimulation or mechanical change of the soft tissue of the body.

tendon organs Structures found in the tendon and musculotendinous junction that respond to tension at the tendon. Articular (joint) ligaments contain receptors that are similar to tendon organs and adjust reflex inhibition of the adjacent muscle when excessive strain is placed on the joints.

therapeutic applications Healing or curative powers.

therapeutic change Beneficial change produced by a bodywork process that results in a modification of physical form or function that can affect a client's physical, mental, and/or spiritual state.

therapeutic relationship The interpersonal structure and professional boundaries between professionals and the clients they serve.

tonic vibration reflex Reflex that tones a muscle with stimulation through vibration methods at the tendon.

touch Contact with no movement.

touch technique The basis of soft tissue forms of bodywork methods.

toughening/hardening The reaction to repeated exposure to stimuli that elicit arousal responses.

traction Gentle pull on the joint capsule to increase the joint space.

transference The personalization of the professional relationship by the client.

trauma Physical injury caused by violent or disruptive action, toxic substances, or psychic injury resulting from a severe long- or short-term emotional shock.

trigger point An area of local nerve facilitation; pressure on the trigger point results in hypertonicity of a muscle bundle and referred pain patterns.

universal precautions Procedures developed by the Centers for Disease Control and Prevention (CDC) to prevent the spread of contagious diseases.

vibration Fine or coarse tremulous movement that creates reflexive responses.

viruses Microorganisms that invade cells and insert their genetic code into the host cell's genetic code. Viruses use the host cell's nutrients and organelles to produce more virus particles.

wellness The efficient balance of body, mind, and spirit, all working in a harmonious way to provide quality of life.

yang The portion of the whole realm of function of the body, mind, and spirit in Eastern thought that corresponds with sympathetic autonomic nervous system functions.

yin The portion of the whole realm of function of the body, mind, and spirit in Eastern thought that corresponds with parasympathetic autonomic nervous system functions.

INDICATIONS AND CONTRAINDICATIONS TO MASSAGE

BECAUSE each situation is different, it is difficult to make recommendations on when to give a massage and when not to give one. Each situation needs to be evaluated to determine whether massage is indicated or contraindicated. The existence of contraindications does not always mean that therapeutic massage is inappropriate. What most contraindications require is *caution*, which may call for modification of the massage treatment and, in some cases, supervision by and cooperation with the health care team. The clinical reasoning model is a valuable tool for making decisions about contraindications. This appendix presents two models of a guideline system for determining the indications and contraindications for massage. Specific conditions, symptoms, indications, and contraindications for massage follow. Use a medical dictionary to look up unfamiliar terms.

THE ONTARIO MODEL

The following are absolute contraindications (CI) to massage (i.e., massage treatment should not be given).

General

1. Acute-stage pneumonia
2. Advanced kidney failure (modified treatment may be possible with medical consent)
3. Advanced respiratory failure (modified treatment may be possible with medical consent)
4. Diabetes with complications (e.g., gangrene, advanced heart or kidney disease, very high or unstable blood pressure)
5. Eclampsia-toxemia in pregnancy
6. Hemophilia
7. Hemorrhage
8. Liver failure (modified treatment may be possible with medical consent)
9. Postcerebrovascular accident (CVA, stroke), condition not yet stabilized
10. Postmyocardial infarction (MI, heart attack), condition not yet stabilized
11. Severe atherosclerosis
12. Severe hypertension (if unstable)
13. Shock (all types)
14. Significant fever (higher than 101° F [38.3° C])
15. Some acute conditions that require first aid or medical attention
    - Anaphylaxis
    - Appendicitis
    - CVA
    - Diabetic coma, insulin shock
    - Epileptic seizure
    - MI
    - Pneumothorax, atelectasis
    - Severe asthma attack, status asthmaticus
    - Syncope (fainting)
16. Some highly metastatic cancers not judged to be terminal
17. Systemic contagious/infectious condition

Local (Regional)

1. Acute flare-up of inflammatory arthritis (e.g., rheumatoid arthritis, systemic lupus erythematosus, ankylosing spondylitis, Reiter's syndrome); may be general CI, depending on case
2. Acute neuritis
3. Aneurysms deemed life-threatening (e.g., of the abdominal aorta); may be general CI, depending on location
4. Ectopic pregnancy

5. Esophageal varicosities (varices)
6. Frostbite
7. Local contagious condition
8. Local irritable skin condition
9. Malignancy (especially if judged unstable)
10. Open wound or sore
11. Phlebitis, phlebothrombosis, arteritis; may be general CI if located in a major circulatory channel
12. Recent burn
13. Sepsis
14. Temporal arteritis
15. Twenty-four to 48 hours after antiinflammatory treatment (target tissue and immediate vicinity)
16. Undiagnosed lump

General

The following conditions require an awareness of the possibility of adverse effects from massage therapy. Substantial treatment adaptation may be appropriate. Medical consultation often is needed.

1. Any condition of spasticity or rigidity
2. Asthma
3. Cancer (including finding appropriate relationships to other current treatments)
4. Chronic congestive heart failure
5. Chronic kidney disease
6. Client taking antiinflammatory drugs, muscle relaxants, anticoagulants, analgesics, or any other medications that alter sensation, muscle tone, standard reflex reactions, cardiovascular function, kidney or liver function, or personality
7. Coma (may be absolute CI, depending on cause)
8. Diagnosed atherosclerosis
9. Drug withdrawal
10. Emphysema
11. Epilepsy
12. Hypertension
13. Immunosuppressed client
14. Inflammatory arthritides
15. Major or abdominal surgery
16. Moderately severe or juvenile-onset diabetes
17. Multiple sclerosis
18. Osteoporosis, osteomalacia
19. Pregnancy and labor
20. Post-MI
21. Post-CVA
22. Recent head injury

Local (Regional)

1. Acute disk herniation
2. Aneurysm (may be general CI, depending on location)
3. Any acute inflammatory condition
4. Any antiinflammatory treatment site
5. Any chronic or long-standing superficial thrombosis

6. Buerger's disease (may be general CI if unstable)
7. Chronic arthritic conditions
8. Chronic abdominal or digestive disease
9. Chronic diarrhea
10. Contusion
11. Endometriosis
12. Flaccid paralysis or paresis
13. Fracture (while casted and immediately after cast removal)
14. Hernia
15. Joint instability or hypermobility
16. Kidney infection, stones
17. Mastitis
18. Minor surgery
19. Pelvic inflammatory disease
20. Pitting edema
21. Portal hypertension
22. Prolonged constipation
23. Recent abortion/vaginal birth
24. Trigeminal neuralgia

Other Important Considerations

1. Massage therapists are expected to know how and when to consult with physicians and other health professionals.
2. Most emotional or psychiatric conditions affect massage treatment. Individual decisions must be made according to case circumstances and, in many instances, medical advice. Medications may be a factor.
3. The client may be allergic to certain massage oils and creams, or cleansers or disinfectants used on sheets and tables.
4. The presence of pins, staples, or artificial joints may alter treatment indications.

The massage therapist should be aware of the role of common chronic conditions that affect public health (e.g., cardiovascular disease, cancer, substance abuse, chronic mental diseases).

The local Health Department can provide additional information on public mental health services, environmental hazards, occupational health, or various health care organizations available in the community.

THE OREGON MODEL: INDICATIONS AND CONTRAINDICATIONS BY BODY SYSTEM

This extensive list was developed by the Oregon Board of Massage. However, no specific recommendations regarding indications or contraindications for massage were made. The descriptions of the disease processes and the massage recommendations were added by this author, using a very conservative approach. If an indication for massage is not listed for a disease process, massage has no direct benefit; such cases are designated *N/A*. This textbook covers basic massage. Advanced training in the medical application of massage, as well as direct supervision by a physician, chiropractor, physical therapist, psychologist, dentist, podiatrist, or other health care professional, will greatly expand the application of massage in rehabilitative situations.

The Integumentary System

Assessment parameters include color (e.g., pallor, jaundice, cyanosis, erythema, mottling), texture (e.g., dry, moist, scaly), scars (normal and keloid), vascularity (e.g., dilated veins, angiomas, varicosities, ecchymoses, petechiae, purpura), temperature, rashes, lesions, nail condition, hair condition, contour, hydration, and edema.

Deviations that suggest the need for evaluation and referral include lumps or masses, rashes of unknown origin, lesions, burns, urticaria, itching of unknown origin, cyanosis, jaundice, ulcerations, multiple bruises, and petechiae.

Specific Disease Processes and Bacterial Conditions

Acne
Definition/symptoms: Inflammation of the skin affecting the sebaceous gland ducts
Indications: Massage increases systemic circulation; may assist healing
Contraindications: Regional; avoid affected area; do not use ointments that clog pores

Carbuncle
Definition/symptoms: Mass of connected boils
Indications: Massage may increase systemic circulation and may assist healing
Contraindications: Refer client to physician; regional; avoid affected area

Cellulitis
Definition/symptoms: Inflammation of subcutaneous tissue with redness and swelling
Indications: Avoid
Contraindications: Regional; may be associated with erysipelas, a contagious condition; refer client to physician

Folliculitis
Definition/symptoms: Inflammation of hair follicle
Indications: Massage may increase systemic circulation and assist healing
Contraindications: Regional; refer client to physician; avoid affected area

Furuncle (boil)
Definition/symptoms: Pus-filled cavity formed by infection of hair follicle
Indications: Massage may increase systemic circulation and assist healing

Contraindications: Regional; refer client to physician; avoid affected area

Impetigo
Definition/symptoms: Highly contagious bacterial skin infection that occurs most often in children; begins as a reddish discoloration and develops into vesicles with a yellow crust
Indications: Massage may increase systemic circulation and assist healing
Contraindications: Regional; refer client to physician; avoid affected area

Syphilis
Definition/symptoms: Primary stage: a usually painless lesion (chancre) present on exposed skin; secondary stage: begins about 2 months after chancre disappears and produces a variety of symptoms, including skin rash
Indications: N/A
Contraindications: General; rash is contagious; refer client to physician

Viral Conditions

Bell's palsy
Definition/symptoms: Infection of seventh cranial nerve; primary symptom is paralysis of facial features, including the eyelids and mouth
Indications: Relaxation massage may facilitate healing
Contraindications: Regional; refer client to physician for diagnosis

Herpes simplex
Definition/symptoms: Acute viral disease marked by groups of watery blisters on or near mucous membranes
Indications: Recurrence is stress induced; massage may reduce stress levels
Contraindications: Regional; contagious; avoid affected area

Herpes zoster (shingles)
Definition/symptoms: Viral infection that usually affects the skin of a single dermatome; produces a red, swollen plaque that ruptures and crusts
Indications: Condition is painful; general massage may ease pain
Contraindications: Regional; avoid affected area; may need to refer client to physician

Warts
Definition/symptoms: Usually benign, excess cell growth of the skin
Indications: N/A
Contraindications: Regional; avoid affected area; contagious; may become malignant; if any changes in wart occur, refer client to physician

Fungal Conditions

Ringworm, athlete's foot, fungal infection of the nails
Definition/symptoms: Scaly and crusty cracking of the skin
Indications: Keep area dry; do not use lubricants
Contraindications: Regional; do not use lubricants near the area because fungi thrive in a moist environment

Allergic Reactions

Atopic dermatitis (eczema)

Definition/symptoms: Common inflammation of the skin marked by papules, vesicles, and crusts

Indications: Symptom of an underlying condition; refer client to physician for diagnosis

Contraindications: Regional; avoid affected area

Contact dermatitis

Definition/symptoms: Inflammation that occurs in response to contact with an external agent

Indications: Use unscented lubricants (scents often cause allergic reactions)

Contraindications: Regional; avoid affected area

Urticaria (hives)

Definition/symptoms: Red, raised lesions caused by leakage of fluid from skin and blood vessels; primary symptom is severe itching

Indications: Do not use scented products; hives may have an emotional component

Contraindications: Regional; avoid affected area

Benign Conditions

Mole

Definition/symptoms: Pigmented, fleshy growth of skin

Indications: Watch for any change in a mole; refer client to physician if a change is noted

Contraindications: Regional; avoid mole

Psoriasis

Definition/symptoms: Chronic inflammation of the skin; probably genetic; symptoms include scaly plaque and excessive growth rate of epithelial cells

Indications: May be stress induced; massage reduces stress

Contraindications: Regional; avoid affected area

Scleroderma

Definition/symptoms: Autoimmune disease that affects blood vessels and connective tissue of the skin; primary symptom is hard, yellowish skin

Indications: N/A

Contraindications: Regional (except in systemic cases); refer client to physician

Malignant Conditions

Skin cancer

Definition/symptoms: Squamous cell carcinoma, basal cell carcinoma, melanoma, Kaposi's sarcoma

Indications: N/A

Contraindications: Watch for any change in a mole or existing skin condition; if this occurs, refer client to physician immediately

The Skeletal System, Muscular System, and Articulations

Assessment parameters include range of motion, swelling, masses, deformity, pain or tenderness, temperature, crepitus, spasm, paresthesia, pulses, skin color, paralysis, atrophy, and contracture.

Deviations that suggest the need for evaluation and referral include malalignment of an extremity, asymmetry of musculoskeletal contour, progressive or persistent pain, masses or progressive swelling, numbness and/or tingling with loss of function, diminished or absent peripheral pulses, pallor and/or coolness of one extremity, redness and/or increased temperature of one extremity, and difference in size of extremities.

Specific Disease Processes

Atonicity (flaccidity)

Definition/symptoms: Reduced ability or inability of the muscle to contract (hypotonicity)

Indications: Massage to tone; relaxation of opposing muscle groups

Contraindications: Regional; refer client to physician for diagnosis before proceeding

Contracture

Definition/symptoms: Fixed resistance to passive stretching of muscles; usually the result of fibrosis or tissue ischemia

Indications: Massage and stretch

Contraindications: Do not stretch past fixed barrier

Convulsion

Definition/symptoms: Sudden, involuntary series of muscle contractions, sometimes called a *seizure*

Indications: N/A

Contraindications: Refer client to physician immediately

Fibrillation

Definition/symptoms: A small local contraction of muscle that is invisible under the skin; results from spontaneous, synchronous activation of single muscle cells

Indications: Massage, direct pressure

Contraindications: If continuous, refer client to physician for diagnosis

Hypertonicity

Definition/symptoms: Increased muscle tone

Indications: Massage and stretch

Contraindications: Recurrence without explanation; refer client to physician for diagnosis

Spasms (cramp)

Definition/symptoms: Sudden, painful onset of muscle contraction

Indications: Use reciprocal inhibition; push muscle belly together and slowly stretch

Contraindications: If recurring and transient, refer client to physician

Tic

Definition/symptoms: Spasmodic twitching; often occurs in the face

Indications: May be stress induced; massage is beneficial in reducing stress

Contraindications: Refer client to physician for diagnosis to rule out underlying pathologic condition

Soft Tissue Injuries

Dislocation

Definition/symptoms: Displacement of a bone within a joint

Indications: N/A

Contraindications: Immediately refer client to physician

Sprains

Definition/symptoms: Traumatic injury of ligaments that form a skeletal joint; may involve injury (strain) of muscles or tendon

Indications: RICE (*r*est, *i*ce, *c*ompression, *e*levation), first aid, gentle massage, and range of motion facilitate healing

Contraindications: Regional; all traumatic injuries should be evaluated by a physician

Strains

Definition/symptoms: Traumatic injury caused by overstretching or overexertion of muscle or tendon tissue

Indications: RICE, first aid, gentle massage, and range of motion may facilitate healing

Contraindications: Regional; all traumatic injuries should be evaluated by a physician

Subluxation

Definition/symptoms: Any deviation from the normal relationship in which the articular cartilage is touching any portion of its mating cartilage

Indications: Massage may help relieve muscle spasm

Contraindications: Refer client to physician

Infectious Processes

Osteomyelitis

Definition/symptoms: Bacterial infection of the bone; symptoms include deep pain and fever

Indications: N/A

Contraindications: General; immediately refer client to physician; difficult to diagnose and treat

Inflammatory Processes

Ankylosing spondylitis

Definition/symptoms: Chronic inflammatory disease; can be progressive; usually involves the sacroiliac joint and spinal articulations; cause is unknown, appears to be genetic; if progressive, calcification of the joints and articular surfaces occurs; begins with feelings of fatigue and intermittent low back pain; synovial tissue around the involved joints becomes inflamed; heart disease also may occur

Indications: Massage may be helpful under direct supervision of a physician

Contraindications: General; refer client to physician; avoid any area of inflammation

Bursitis

Definition/symptoms: Inflammation of bursa

Indications: Massage may take pressure off joint by relaxing and normalizing surrounding musculature; ice

Contraindications: Regional; avoid affected area; work above and below jointed area

Fibromyalgia

Definition/symptoms: General disruption in connective tissue muscle component; symptoms include tender point activity; vague symptoms of pain and fatigue

Indications: Massage may be beneficial; work with physician

Contraindications: General; refer client to physician for diagnosis. Do not use therapeutic inflammation methods.

Gouty arthritis

Definition/symptoms: Metabolic condition in which sodium urate crystals trigger a chronic inflammatory process

Indications: Dietary adjustment necessary

Contraindications: Regional; avoid area of inflammation

Lupus erythematosus

Definition/symptoms: Chronic inflammatory disease that affects many body tissues; common symptom is a red rash on the face

Indications: Massage may be beneficial under physician's close supervision

Contraindications: General; systemic disease

Osgood-Schlatter disease

Definition/symptoms: Osteochondrosis (inflammation of bone and cartilage) of the tibial tuberosity

Indications: N/A

Contraindications: Regional; avoid affected area

Rheumatoid arthritis

Definition/symptoms: Autoimmune inflammatory joint disease characterized by synovial inflammation that spreads to other tissues

Indications: Stress responsive; massage can be helpful under medical supervision

Contraindications: General; work closely with physician

Tendinitis

Definition/symptoms: Inflammation of tendon and tendon-muscle junction

Indications: Massage may assist healing; ice

Contraindications: Regional; avoid affected area; work above and below the area

Tenosynovitis

Definition/symptoms: Inflammation of tendon sheath, usually from repetitive movement

Indications: Massage may relieve muscle hypertension and assist healing of area; ice

Contraindications: Regional; avoid affected area; work above and below the area

Compression Processes

Carpal tunnel syndrome

Definition/symptoms: Inflammation in tendon sheaths in the carpal tunnel that creates pressure on the median nerve; symptoms include weakness and tingling in the hand

Indications: Symptoms often are confused with thoracic outlet syndrome; massage is proving to be beneficial

Contraindications: Regional; refer client to physician for diagnosis

Degenerative Processes

Muscular dystrophy

Definition/symptoms: A group of muscle disorders characterized by atrophy of skeletal muscle without nerve involvement

Indications: Massage is beneficial; work closely with supervising physician

Contraindications: General

Osteoarthritis

Definition/symptoms: Degenerative joint disease of the articular cartilage; age and joint damage are risk factors

Indications: Massage is beneficial

Contraindications: Regional; avoid area of inflammation

Osteoporosis

Definition/symptoms: Loss of minerals and collagen from bone matrix, resulting in reduced volume and strength of skeletal bone

Indications: Gentle massage is beneficial; use care and caution

Contraindications: General

Abnormal Spinal Curve

Kyphosis

Definition/symptoms: Abnormal increased convexity of the thoracic spine

Indications: Massage is beneficial as part of the treatment plan

Contraindications: Regional; in severe cases proceed after obtaining physician's recommendation

Lordosis

Definition/symptoms: Abnormal increased concavity in the curvature of the lumbar spine

Indications: Massage is beneficial as part of the treatment plan

Contraindications: Regional; in severe cases proceed after obtaining physician's recommendation

Scoliosis

Definition/symptoms: Lateral curve of vertebral column

Indications: Massage is beneficial as part of the treatment plan

Contraindications: Regional; in severe cases proceed after obtaining physician's recommendation

Disordered Muscular Processes

Low back pain

Definition/symptoms: May be of many varieties: muscular, nerve entrapment, or disk problem

Indications: Massage can be beneficial as part of the treatment plan

Contraindications: Regional; important to refer client to physician to rule out serious condition of the spine or viscera

Spasmodic torticollis

Definition/symptoms: A contracted state of the cervical muscles that causes pain and rotation of the head

Indications: Massage is beneficial

Contraindications: Regional; refer client to physician for diagnosis to rule out serious disease

Temporomandibular joint (TMJ) dysfunction

Definition/symptoms: Dysfunction in the TMJ; pain and muscle contraction

Indications: Massage is beneficial; work closely with dentist and physician

Contraindications: Regional if painful

Neurologic Conditions

Assessment parameters include mental status, the presence of involuntary movements, coordination and balance, muscle tone and strength, changes in sensory perception (i.e., touch, pain, temperature, vibration, position sense, hearing, vision).

Deviations that suggest the need for evaluation and referral include inequality of pupil size; diplopia; abnormal Babinski's sign (extensor plantar response); seizures (partial or generalized); significant personality changes; changes in sensorium; progressively worsening or persistent headache; temporary loss of speech, vision, or motion; triad of fever, headache, and nuchal rigidity; vomiting; and change in pupil size with head injury.

Specific Disease Processes

Dyskinesia

Definition/symptoms: Impairment of the power of voluntary movement, resulting in fragmentary or incomplete movement and possibly pain

Indications: Massage is beneficial as part of a physician-directed treatment plan

Contraindications: General; refer client to physician for diagnosis and treatment plan

Dystonia

Definition/symptoms: Disordered, random tonicity of muscles

Indications: Massage is beneficial as part of a physician-directed treatment plan

Contraindications: General; refer client to physician for diagnosis and treatment plan

Insomnia

Definition/symptoms: Inability to sleep or interrupted sleep

Indications: Massage is beneficial

Contraindications: Regional; refer client to physician for specific diagnosis to rule out serious underlying condition

Peripheral neuropathy

Definition/symptoms: General functional disturbances and/or pathologic changes in the peripheral nervous system caused by diabetic neuropathy, ischemic neuropathy, or traumatic neuropathy; symptoms include numbness, burning, and pain

Indications: Massage is beneficial as part of the treatment plan

Contraindications: General; refer client to physician for diagnosis to determine underlying condition

Tinnitus

Definition/symptoms: Noise in the ear; symptoms include ringing, buzzing, roaring, or clicking

Indications: N/A

Contraindications: Regional; refer client to physician for specific diagnosis

Vertigo

Definition/symptoms: Sensation of movement, not to be

confused with dizziness

Indications: N/A

Contraindications: General; usually symptomatic of underlying condition; physician's diagnosis required

Vascular Processes

CVA

Definition/symptoms: Stroke; a disturbance in cerebral circulation; major causes include atherosclerosis (thrombosis), embolism, hypertensive intracerebral hemorrhage or ruptured saccular aneurysm; symptoms differ depending on where the disturbance in circulation occurs; general symptoms include weakness or paralysis of the arm or leg, headache, numbness, blurred or double vision, and confusion or dizziness; often only one side is affected; symptoms persist for at least 24 hours, usually much longer.

Indications: Massage may be beneficial during recovery under physician's supervision and during long-term care for continued support

Contraindications: Refer client to physician for diagnosis

Headache

Definition/symptoms: Pain or dull ache in the head and upper neck; can have a variety of causes such as muscle tension, sinus pressure, pinched nerve, vascular disruption (e.g., migraine headache, cluster headaches), and toxins

Indications: Massage may be beneficial

Contraindications: Refer all clients with a persistent, severe headache to physician for specific diagnosis

Head injury

Definition/symptoms: Contusion (bump on the head); laceration (cut or break in the skin); subdural and epidural injury may produce disorientation, nausea, and uneven pupil dilation

Indications: Immediately refer client to physician if any of the signs listed above are noted

Contraindications: General; all traumatic injuries must be evaluated by a physician

Transient ischemic attack (TIA)

Definition/symptoms: Episodes of neurologic dysfunction that usually are of short duration (a few minutes) but may persist for 24 hours; reversible; symptom pattern is the same with each attack because the same vessel is involved; small strokes, seizures, migraine symptoms, postural hypotension, and Stokes-Allen syndrome may be misdiagnosed as TIAs

Indications: Massage may be beneficial under physician's supervision

Contraindications: Refer client to physician for diagnosis

Infectious Processes

Conjunctivitis

Definition/symptoms: Inflammation and/or infection of mucous membranes of the eye

Indications: N/A

Contraindications: Regional; refer client to physician; may be contagious; avoid affected area

Parkinson's disease

Definition/symptoms: Nervous disorder characterized by abnormally low levels of the neurotransmitter dopamine, resulting in involuntary trembling and muscle rigidity

Indications: Massage is beneficial as part of a physician-directed treatment plan

Contraindications: General

Poliomyelitis

Definition/symptoms: Viral infection of nerves that control skeletal muscles

Indications: Massage is beneficial as part of a physician-directed treatment plan

Contraindications: General

Postpolio syndrome

Definition/symptoms: Symptoms of fatigue and general muscle weakness appear years after resolution of poliomyelitis

Indications: Massage is beneficial as part of a physician-directed treatment plan

Contraindications: Regional; refer client to physician for specific diagnosis

Neuromuscular Processes

Multiple sclerosis

Definition/symptoms: Primary disease of the central nervous system marked by degeneration of myelin

Indications: Massage is beneficial as part of a physician-directed treatment plan

Contraindications: General

Spinal cord injury

Definition/symptoms: Traumatic injury or degenerative process of the spinal cord; may result from compression, cut, or tissue replacement in scarring

Indications: Massage is beneficial as part of a physician-directed treatment plan

Contraindications: Regional

Trigeminal neuralgia (tic douloureux)

Definition/symptoms: Compression or degeneration of fifth cranial nerve; primary symptom is recurring episodes of stabbing pain in the face

Indications: Avoid entire area of trigeminal nerve innervation; massage may trigger pain response

Contraindications: Regional

Miscellaneous Disorders

Seizure disorders

Definition/symptoms: Sudden bursts of abnormal neuronal activity that cause temporary changes in brain activity; may vary from mild, affecting conscious motor control or sensory perception, to severe, resulting in convulsion

Indications: Massage may be beneficial

Contraindications: General; follow physician's recommendation for massage

Sleep apnea

Definition/symptoms: Cessation of breathing during sleep

Indications: Stress may be a factor; massage is beneficial in reducing stress

Contraindications: Regional

Thoracic outlet syndrome

Definition/symptoms: Compression of brachial nerve plexus; primary symptom is pain that radiates to the shoulder and arm

Indications: Massage is beneficial as part of the treatment plan

Contraindications: Regional; refer client to physician for specific diagnosis

Endocrine System

Assessment parameters include fatigue, depression, changes in energy level, hyperalertness, sleep patterns, and mood. These can affect the skin, hair, and personal appearance.

Deviations that suggest the need for evaluation and referral include cold, clammy skin; numbness of fingers, toes, or mouth; rapid heartbeat, a feeling of faintness; vertigo; tremors, dyspnea (difficulty breathing); thyroid nodule; unusually warm hands and feet; and lethargy.

Specific Disease Processes

Diabetes mellitus

Definition/symptoms: Metabolic disorder; body loses the ability to oxidize carbohydrates because of faulty pancreatic activity, especially of the islets of Langerhans, which affects insulin production; symptoms include thirst, hunger, and acidosis; severe symptoms include difficulty breathing and changes in blood chemistry that lead to coma

Indications: Massage is given under supervision of the primary care physician; it is beneficial for circulation enhancement and stress reduction; exercise also is beneficial

Contraindications: General; work only under physician's supervision

Hyperglycemia

Definition/symptoms: High blood sugar, resulting from inadequate insulin in the blood; symptoms are the same as those for diabetes mellitus

Indications: See *Diabetes mellitus*

Contraindications: See *Diabetes mellitus*

Hypoglycemia

Definition/symptoms: Low blood glucose, resulting from an excess of insulin in the blood; symptoms include lightheadedness, anxiety, and forgetfulness

Indications: Dietary changes; massage is helpful and may relieve stress

Contraindications: Refer client to physician to determine the cause of low blood sugar

Hyperthyroidism

Definition/symptoms: Overproduction of thyroid hormone; can be caused by a tumor or by problems with the self-regulatory mechanism in the pituitary gland; symptoms include anxiety, bulging eyes, high metabolic rate, and nervousness

Indications: Massage is beneficial for relaxing the client

Contraindications: General; work within physician's recommendations

Hypothyroidism

Definition/symptoms: Underproduction of thyroid hormone; symptoms include sensitivity to cold, weight gain, fatigue, and dullness

Indications: Massage is beneficial for stimulating metabolic function

Contraindications: General; work within physician's recommendations

Neuropathy

Definition/symptoms: Functional disturbance or pathologic change in peripheral nervous system; symptoms include numbness, burning, and tingling pain

Indications: Massage is beneficial under medical supervision; may calm hypersensitive nerves

Contraindications: General; work under physician's direction

Cardiovascular System

Assessment parameters include skin color and appearance, respiratory rate and effort, condition of nails and nail beds (e.g., clubbing, cyanosis), pain or tenderness and points of radiation, swelling, and symmetry of chest cavity.

Deviations that suggest the need for evaluation and referral include pulse over 90 or under 60 beats per minute; dyspnea; pitting edema; distended neck veins; glossy appearance of the skin; positive Homans' sign (calf tenderness with dorsiflexion of the foot); asymmetry of limb circumference; red, warm, tender, and hard veins; edema, pain and tenderness of extremity; clubbing of nail beds; chest pain (especially if radiating to left arm); central or peripheral cyanosis; pallor; mottling or cyanosis of a limb; stasis ulcers; and splinter hemorrhages (small red to black streaks under fingernails).

Physiologic Processes

Anemia

Definition/symptoms: Reduced red blood cell count or hemoglobin; symptoms include fatigue and pallor

Indications: Massage can be beneficial as part of the treatment plan

Contraindications: General; refer client to physician for diagnosis and proceed under physician's direction

Aneurysm

Definition/symptoms: Abnormal widening of the arterial wall; tends to form thrombi and also to burst; a pulsating bulge and pressure is felt with accompanying symptoms of pain

Indications: N/A

Contraindications: Regional; immediately refer client to physician; avoid direct heavy pressure into arterial vessels

Angina pectoris

Definition/symptoms: Chest pain caused by inadequate oxygen to heart (usually from blocked coronary arteries)

Indications: Massage is beneficial as part of a lifestyle change

Contraindications: General; massage is performed under physician's supervision

Arteriosclerosis and atherosclerosis

Definition/symptoms: Hardening of the arteries; a type of coronary heart disease; symptoms may be mild to severe; may be mistaken for other problems

Indications: Massage is beneficial as part of a lifestyle change

Contraindications: General; perform massage under physician's supervision

Congestive heart failure

Definition/symptoms: Left heart failure; inability of the left ventricle to pump effectively; one symptom is increased fluid retention

Indications: Massage is beneficial in helping diuretics remove excess fluid

Contraindications: General; must work under physician's supervision; client may have difficulty breathing in a supine position

Deep vein thrombosis

Definition/symptoms: Blood clot in deep veins; risk factor for pulmonary embolism (blood clot in the heart); often asymptomatic; symptoms may include swelling, edema, and pain described as aching and throbbing

Indications: N/A

Contraindications: Regional to general, depending on the severity of symptoms; always refer client to physician for unexplained pain; never massage over such areas

Hemophilia

Definition/symptoms: Blood clotting disorder; primary symptom is spontaneous bleeding due to inability to form clots

Indications: Extremely light energy type of massage given only under physician's direction

Contraindications: General; work only under physician's supervision

MI (myocardial infarction)

Definition/symptoms: Death of cardiac muscle cells, usually from inadequate blood supply, often from coronary thrombosis or coronary artery disease; symptoms include severe pain in the chest or left arm, difficulty breathing, and weakness

Indications: During rehabilitation massage can be beneficial when supervised by a physician

Contraindications: General; refer client to physician immediately

Mononucleosis

Definition/symptoms: Induced by Epstein-Barr virus; symptoms include fever, fatigue, and swollen glands

Indications: Massage is beneficial as part of the treatment plan; care must be taken with contagious conditions

Contraindications: General; refer client to physician for specific diagnosis

Phlebitis

Definition/symptoms: Inflammation of a vein; may be caused by a blood clot; symptoms include edema, stiffness, and pain; veins may streak red

Indications: N/A

Contraindications: Regional to general; see *Deep vein thrombosis*

Raynaud's syndrome

Definition/symptoms: Arteriospastic condition caused by vasospasms of the small cutaneous and subcutaneous arteries and arterioles; usually activated by cold but can be emotionally triggered; symptoms include skin pallor and pain

Indications: Care must be taken to avoid triggering the symptoms; interview client carefully; massage may be beneficial for stress reduction

Contraindications: Refer client to physician for specific underlying diagnosis; condition may be symptomatic of serious disorder

Syncope

Definition/symptoms: Sudden loss of strength; fainting; may be caused by a cardiac spasm resulting from closure of coronary arteries

Indications: N/A

Contraindications: General; immediately refer client to physician

Varicose veins

Definition/symptoms: Enlarged veins in which blood pools; caused by collapse of valve system; tend to form thrombi

Indications: N/A

Contraindications: Regional; avoid affected area

Lymphatic and Immune Systems

Assessment parameters include skin color and condition, evidence of eye irritation, lymph nodes, and nasal discharge/irritation.

Deviations that suggest the need for evaluation and referral include client history of chronic fatigue or recurrent physical ailments (e.g., skin, respiratory, gastrointestinal) in the absence of general illness; history of food intolerance; failure to gain weight; unexplained weight loss; rashes of unknown origin; urticaria; enlarged, tender nodes; and excessive or persistent dryness and scaliness of skin.

Specific Disease Processes

Allergy

Definition/symptoms: Hypersensitivity of immune system to relatively harmless environmental antigens; symptoms include increased mucous membrane inflammation, occasionally spastic bladder

Indications: Massage is beneficial

Contraindications: Refer client to physician for specific diagnosis

Autoimmune disease

Definition/symptoms: Disease in which the immune system attacks the body's own tissues; symptoms include inflammation, fatigue, and allergy

Indications: Massage is beneficial with physician's recommendation

Contraindications: General; refer client to physician for specific diagnosis

Chronic fatigue syndrome

Definition/symptoms: May be induced by a virus; symptoms include swollen glands, low-grade fever, muscle and joint aches, headache, and fatigue

Indications: Massage is beneficial

Contraindications: General; refer client to physician for specific diagnosis

Human immunodeficiency virus (HIV) infection

Definition/symptoms: Viral infection transmitted by means of body fluids; causes immunosuppression

Indications: Massage is beneficial with physician's recommendation; follow antiviral precautions for control of virus; 10% bleach solution; avoid body fluid contact

Contraindications: General; work with physician

Lymphedema

Definition/symptoms: Swelling of tissue caused by partial or complete blockage of lymph vessels

Indications: Massage is beneficial as part of the treatment plan and is given under the supervision of the primary care physician

Contraindications: Refer client to physician for diagnosis

The Respiratory System

Assessment parameters include the rate and pattern of respiration, chest movement, color, nodes, chest configuration, ease of chest excursions, fremitus, and pain.

Deviations that suggest the need for evaluation and referral include inspiratory flaring of the nostrils; use of accessory muscles; intercostal retractions or bulging; pursed lips on exhalation; splinting; uneven chest movement; altered tactile fremitus/crepitus (increased or decreased); cyanosis or pallor; enlarged, tender nodes; pain with breathing; and a respiratory rate over 20 respirations per minute in the absence of exertion or strong emotion.

Specific Infectious Disease Processes

Asthma

Definition/symptoms: Recurring muscle spasms in the bronchial wall accompanied by fluid retention and production of mucus; stress-specific condition

Indications: Massage is beneficial; monitor breathing closely

Contraindications: Work under direction of primary care physician

Tuberculosis

Definition/symptoms: Infectious disease caused by *Mycobacterium tuberculosis;* early stage requires testing to reveal infection; advanced cases are marked by lung destruction, coughing, fatigue, weakness, and weight loss; may be confused with bronchitis and pneumonia

Indications: Droplet transmission; contagious; be aware of sanitation

Contraindications: General; work only if physician recommends and clears for contagious condition

Upper respiratory infection (bronchitis, common cold, sinusitis, pneumonia)

Definition/symptoms: Viral or bacterial in origin; symptoms include increased production of mucus, fever, body aches, and headaches

Indications: Light massage may be beneficial to ease body ache; avoid heavy pressure; watch for contamination

Contraindications: Refer client to physician if symptoms are severe or persist longer than 2 weeks

The Gastrointestinal System

Assessment parameters include skin (see The Integumentary System, p. 619); contour of abdomen (flat, rounded, concave, protuberant, distended); symmetry; observable masses; palpable masses; movement; tenderness or pain; and location and contour of umbilicus.

Deviations that suggest the need for evaluation and referral include a history of persistent or recurring nausea or vomiting; abdominal pain of unknown origin; rebound tenderness; epigastric pain that occurs 1 to 3 hours after meals; rigid or boardlike abdomen (unrelated to calisthenic exercise); persistent or increasing abdominal or epigastric pain; history of blood in stools or vomitus; difficulty swallowing; masses or nodules; enlarged, tender nodes; bulge or swelling in abdomen; change in location or inversion/eversion of umbilicus; and lesions in oral cavity or on lips or tongue.

Specific Disease Processes

Constipation

Definition/symptoms: Slow movement of bowels; hard, compacted, dry stool

Indications: Massage is beneficial; increase fiber and water consumption and moderate exercise; may be drug related

Contraindications: Refer client to physician if severe or persistent or if a mass is felt in the large intestine

Diarrhea

Definition/symptoms: Loose bowels; excessive loss of water in stool; can be caused by a virus or bacterium or can be a symptom of other disease processes

Indications: Loose stool is not uncommon 24 hours after vigorous massage

Contraindications: Refer client to physician if symptoms persist or dehydration is present

Flatulence

Definition/symptoms: Intestinal gas

Indications: May be diet or stress related; massage may reduce stress

Contraindications: Refer client to physician if intestinal tract is painfully distended or to rule out severe underlying condition

Halitosis

Definition/symptoms: Bad breath; may indicate digestive problems or sinus infection

Indications: N/A

Contraindications: Refer client to physician for specific diagnosis

Inflammatory Processes

Appendicitis

Definition/symptoms: Inflammation of the mucosal lining of the appendix, caused by trapped food or fecal matter; more common in individuals under age 25; symptoms include mild periumbilical pain, nausea, vomiting, increasing pain in the lower right quadrant, muscle spasm, and rebound tenderness

Indications: N/A

Contraindications: Immediately refer client to physician

Cholelithiasis and cholecystitis

Definition/symptoms: Gall stones formed as a result of inflammation; primary symptom is severe pain in upper abdomen radiating to back and right shoulder

Indications: N/A

Contraindications: Immediately refer client to physician

Cirrhosis of the liver

Definition/symptoms: Chronic disease that replaces liver tissue with connective tissue; major cause is alcohol consumption; early symptoms include gas, change in bowel habits, slight weight loss, nausea in the morning, and a dull, heavy ache in the right upper quadrant of the abdomen; advanced symptoms include jaundice, peripheral edema, bleeding, and red palms

Indications: Massage is beneficial in stress reduction and drug withdrawal

Contraindications: Refer client to physician for diagnosis; work under physician's supervision

Colitis

Definition/symptoms: Inflammatory condition of the large intestine; one type (irritable bowel syndrome) is brought on by stress

Indications: Painful condition; massage may be helpful in general stress and pain reduction

Contraindications: Immediately refer client to physician; work with chronic conditions under direct supervision of physician

Crohn's disease (regional enteritis)

Definition/symptoms: Chronic relapsing inflammatory disease of the intestinal tract; symptoms include intermittent diarrhea, colicky pain in lower abdomen, fatigue, low-grade fever

Indications: Painful condition; massage may be helpful in general stress and pain reduction

Contraindications: Refer client to physician immediately; with chronic conditions, work under physician's direct supervision

Diverticulosis

Definition/symptoms: Formation of small pockets in the large intestine, caused by herniation of the mucosa; if pockets become inflamed, condition is called *diverticulitis;* symptoms include gas, diarrhea, and pain

Indications: Diet may need adjustment to include more fiber

Contraindications: Refer client to physician if pain or symptoms persist

Duodenal ulcer

Definition/symptoms: Ulcer caused by hyperacidity in duodenal bulb; stress related; symptoms include burning pain that feels better after eating

Indications: Massage is beneficial for reducing stress; lifestyle and diet changes may be necessary

Contraindications: Refer client to physician for specific diagnosis; support physician's treatment plan

Hepatitis

Definition/symptoms: Infectious disease that has generalized effects in the body but that predominantly affects the liver; type A is common in children and in people living in institutions; it is transmitted by fecal matter, orally through contaminated food and water; usual symptoms are mild and flulike; types B and C affect all age groups and are transmitted through blood, needles, the fecal/oral route, and sexual contact

Indications: Careful use of aseptic procedures

Contraindications: General; refer client to physician and work only with physician's recommendation and guidelines concerning contagious condition

Gastritis

Definition/symptoms: Acute inflammation of the stomach; a common condition usually caused by irritant such as alcohol or aspirin; symptoms include pain, nausea, and belching

Indications: Massage is beneficial because gastritis sometimes is stress related and massage may reduce stress

Contraindications: Refer client to physician for specific diagnosis

Hernia

Definition/symptoms: Protrusion of a loop or piece of an organ or tissue through an abnormal opening; hiatal—protrusion of any structure (usually the esophagus or end of the stomach) through the hiatus of the diaphragm; inguinal—protrusion through the inguinal ring, causing swelling of the scrotum and possibly a medical emergency; umbilical—protrusion at the umbilicus; in inguinal and umbilical hernias, weakness may be felt in the abdominal wall

Indications: N/A

Contraindications: Refer client to physician; avoid area

Pancreatitis

Definition/symptoms: Inflammation of the pancreas; may

be present with diabetes and is aggravated by consumption of alcohol; one symptom is severe abdominal pain

Indications: Painful condition; massage may be helpful in general stress and pain reduction

Contraindications: Refer client to physician immediately; with chronic conditions, work under physician's direct supervision

Stress ulcer

Definition/symptoms: Ulcer related to severe stress (e.g., trauma, burns, long-term illness); symptoms similar to those seen in gastritis

Indications: Massage is beneficial for reducing stress; lifestyle and dietary changes may be necessary

Contraindications: Refer client to physician for specific diagnosis; support physician's treatment plan

Ulcer

Definition/symptoms: Peptic ulcer—break or open sore not covered by protective mucus in the gastrointestinal wall that is exposed to pepsin and gastric juice; often caused by alcohol, pepsin, bile salts, and stress

Indications: Massage is beneficial to reduce stress levels; lifestyle and dietary changes may be necessary

Contraindications: Refer client to physician for specific diagnosis; support physician's treatment plan

The Metabolic System

Assessment parameters include eating patterns, skin, hair, nails, weight and height data, and general health status.

Deviations that suggest the need for evaluation and referral include significant underweight or overweight, evidence of nutritional deficiencies (e.g., dry hair or skin, fatigue), and respiratory problems.

Specific Disease Processes

Cystic fibrosis

Definition/symptoms: Inherited disorder that disrupts cell transport and causes exocrine glands to produce thick secretions; thick pancreatic secretions may block the pancreatic duct

Indications: Massage is beneficial with specific training to loosen mucus with percussive techniques

Contraindications: General; work under direct care of physician

Malnutrition

Definition/symptoms: Deficiency of calories in general and often in protein; malnutrition may be caused by increased nutrient demand on the body without sufficient food intake, (e.g., severe burns, illness, or lack of food, especially protein); symptoms include flaking skin, brittle hair, hair loss, slow-healing sores, bruising, susceptibility to infection, and fatigue; more common in children and the elderly and with drug and alcohol abuse; be aware of eating disorders. (NOTE: Malnutrition also can be caused by insufficient or improper digestion and absorption of food.)

Indications: With anorexia or bulimia, massage may be beneficial for stress reduction

Contraindications: Refer client to physician for diagnosis and treatment plan

Obesity

Definition/symptoms: Excess body fat (over 30% of normal body weight); risks of obesity include diabetes, stroke, heart attack, gallstones, and high blood pressure

Indications: Morbid obesity (over 60% of normal body fat) may cause difficulty positioning client; fluid retention, risk of blood pressure fluctuation, and interference with breathing are other possible problems; may need to alter massage position

Contraindications: Refer client for nutritional and dietary consultation

The Genitourinary System

Assessment parameters include pain (groin, periumbilical, flank, abdominal, dysuria), patterns of urination and output, urine consistency (color, concentration, or hematuria), edema (facial, ankle), weight changes, skin changes, discharge, and masses.

Deviations that suggest the need for evaluation and referral include a history of unusual vaginal, urethral, or nipple discharge; breast, penile, scrotal, or inguinal masses or lumps; genital blisters, lesions, or growths; changes in urinary frequency, output, or control or in urine characteristics; sudden weight gain, abnormal periods, edema, skin abnormalities, pain or tenderness (costovertebral angle, abdominal area, or low back), masses or lumps, and tender or enlarged nodes.

Specific Disease Processes

Breast cancer

Definition/symptoms: Abnormal, malignant tissue growth on or in the breast; most common cause of cancer in women; encourage monthly breast self-examination and regular checkups

Indications: Be aware of changes in tissue around axillary region

Contraindications: If changes are noted, refer client to physician; early diagnosis is important

Dysmenorrhea

Definition/symptoms: Painful menstruation; may be caused by endometriosis (abnormal growth and distribution of uterine lining); symptoms include heavy periods and clotting

Indications: Massage is beneficial for stress reduction and pain

Contraindications: Refer client to physician for diagnosis

Pelvic inflammatory disease

Definition/symptoms: Inflammation of the uterus, fallopian tubes, ovaries, and surrounding tissue; infection often is introduced by intercourse; symptoms include pain and tenderness in the lower abdomen, backache, pain during intercourse, heavy periods, and vaginal discharge

Indications: N/A

Contraindications: Refer client to physician for diagnosis

Premenstrual syndrome (PMS)

Definition/symptoms: Occurs approximately 1 week before onset of period; symptoms include breast tenderness and swelling, fluid retention, headache, irritability, anxiety, depression, and poor concentration

Indications: Massage is beneficial

Contraindications: Refer client to physician if symptoms are severe

Testicular cancer

Definition/symptoms: Malignant growth in testicle; usually a slow-growing lump

Indications: N/A

Contraindications: Refer client to physician immediately if he mentions such a symptom

Toxic shock syndrome

Definition/symptoms: Staphylococcal bacterial infection that can arise from the use of tampons; can be life-threatening; initial flulike symptoms with red rash; can be prevented by changing tampons several times a day. (NOTE: This condition has occurred in women who do not use tampons.)

Indications: N/A

Contraindications: Immediately refer client to physician

Urinary tract infection

Definition/symptoms: Acute pyelonephritis—inflammation of kidney and pelvis; usually occurs in women with abrupt onset of fever, chills, malaise, and back pain, also tenderness on palpation over the costovertebral region; cystitis—affects men and women, usually caused by transmission of bacteria through the urethra due to improper cleansing after bowel movement; may cause pain in lower abdomen above pubic bone and low back ache

Indications: N/A

Contraindications: Refer client to physician for diagnosis and treatment

Sexually Transmitted Diseases

Genital herpes

Definition/symptoms: Viral infection; primary symptom is blisterlike lesions

Indications: N/A

Contraindications: Refer client to physician; follow sanitation requirements

Gonorrhea

Definition/symptoms: Bacterial infection; may be asymptomatic, or symptoms may include painful urination and pus or cloudy discharge

Indications: N/A

Contraindications: Refer client to physician; contagious; follow sanitation requirements

HIV infection

Definition/symptoms: Viral infection transmitted by blood and body fluids

Indications: Massage is beneficial with physician's recommendation; follow antiviral precautions for control of virus with 10% bleach solution; avoid body fluid contact; immediately wash area thoroughly with antiviral agent should body fluid contact occur

Contraindications: Refer client to physician for treatment; follow sanitation requirements.

Syphilis

Definition/symptoms: Bacterial infection; in stage one, red sore (chancre) appears; in stage two, flulike symptoms develop; in stage three, the disease attacks the brain and nervous tissue

Indications: N/A

Contraindications: Refer client to physician; contagious; follow sanitation requirements

Psychiatric Disorders

Assessment parameters include general appearance and behavior, sensorium, mood and affect, thought content, and intellectual capacity.

Deviations that suggest the need for evaluation and referral include marked changes in posture; dress and hygiene; motor activity; speech and facial expression; lack of orientation to time, place, or person; inappropriate manifestation of anxiety, agitation, anger, euphoria, or depression; presence of hallucinations, delusions, paranoia, and illusions; changes in usual intellectual capacity; or suicidal or homicidal ideation.

Specific Disease Processes

Anxiety, depression (bipolar or manic/depressive disorders)

Definition/symptoms: All types of emotionally erratic or unusual behavior may be symptomatic; listen to conversation carefully; often symptoms are subtle and client may try to hide discomfort; symptoms may include anorexia (self-starvation); bulimia (eating and vomiting and/or laxative abuse); addictive disorders; chemical and compulsive behavior; somatization disorder; manifestation of physical pain or symptoms from emotional causes; and posttraumatic stress disorders, often associated with sexual and physical childhood abuse

Indications: Massage is beneficial under the direction of a psychiatrist or psychologist; always work within physician's or counselor's treatment parameters

Contraindications: Refer client to physician for counseling care; client often will dissociate from the body or will be hypersensitive to stimulation; the therapist must be sensitive to psychiatric issues because often the massage therapist is the first person with whom the client shares these issues; it is important to refer the client for competent counseling and psychiatric care

SKIN PATHOLOGY

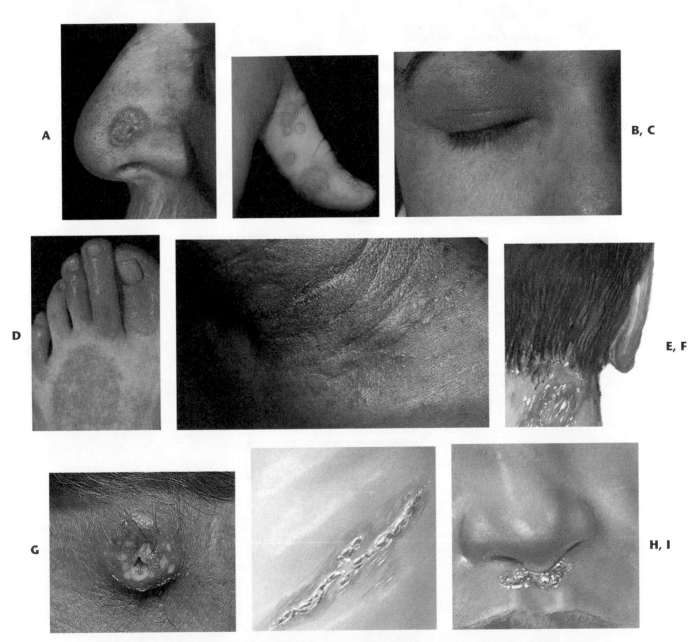

Common skin disorders. NOTE: Skin problems may result from various causes, such as parasitic infestations; fungal, bacterial, or viral infections; reactions to substances encountered externally or taken internally; or new growths. Many of the skin manifestations have no known cause; others are hereditary. **A,** Basal cell carcinoma. **B,** Common warts. **C,** Contact dermatitis from shampoo. **D,** Contact dermatitis from shoes. **E,** Contact dermatitis from application of Lanacane. **F,** Dermatitis. **G,** Furuncle (boil). **H,** Herpes zoster (shingles). **I,** Impetigo contagiosa.

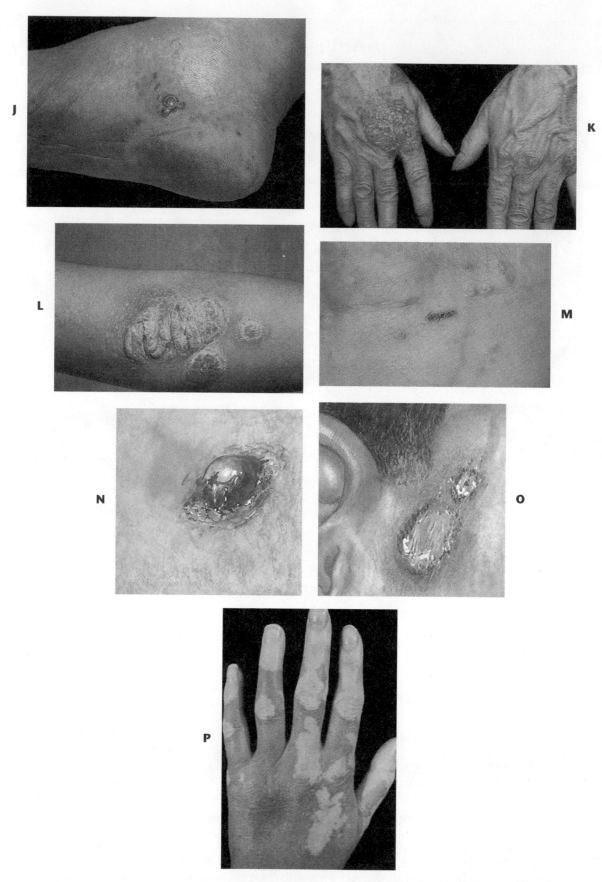

J, Kaposi's sarcoma. **K,** Nummular eczema. **L,** Psoriasis. **M,** Scabies. **N,** Squamous cell carcinoma. **O,** Tinea corporis (ringworm). **P,** Vitiligo. (From Fritz S, Paholsky KM, Grosenbach MJ: *Mosby's basic science for soft tissue and movement therapies,* St Louis, 1999, Mosby.)

COMMON MEDICATIONS AND POSSIBLE IMPLICATIONS FOR MASSAGE

THE following information will help massage practitioners decide what interaction (if any) massage may have with a pharmaceutical. General categories and examples are given in each classification. This is not meant to be an exhaustive list but a general guide. It is important to research any medication, vitamin, or herb a client is taking for the action in the body and possible interaction with massage. This section provides assistance in that process.

Prescription medications fall into a number of groups according to the conditions for which they are prescribed.

CARDIOVASCULAR MEDICATIONS

Vasodilators

Examples: nitroglycerin, isosorbide dinitrate

Vasodilating medications cause the blood vessels to dilate (widen). Some of the antihypertensive agents lower blood pressure by dilating the arteries or veins. Other vasodilators are used in the treatment of stroke and diseases characterized by poor circulation.

Implications for Massage

Massage has a mild peripheral vasodilation effect. The action of the medications may increase the effect of the massage.

Antianginals

Antianginals are prescribed in cases of an insufficient supply of blood, and consequently oxygen, to the heart. These medications act by increasing the amount of oxygen that reaches the heart muscle.

Implications for Massage

See implications for vasodilators.

Beta Blockers

Examples: acebutolol, atenolol, betaxolol, bisoprolol, labetalol, metoprolol, nadolol, pindolol, propranolol, timolol

Beta-blocking medications block nerve stimulation of the heart and blood vessels, slowing the heart rate and reducing high blood pressure. They are used in the treatment of a wide range of diseases, including angina, hypertension, migraine headaches, and arrhythmias.

Implications for Massage

These drugs may distort the expected effect for the massage. Caution is warranted to watch for any exaggerated effects. The client may be susceptible to cold. Massage may help with constipation. The blood pressure–lowering effect of massage may result in dizziness after the massage. Have the client contract and relax the leg muscles for a minute or two before getting off the massage table.

Calcium Channel Blockers

Examples: diltiazem, nifedipine, verapamil

This group of medications is thought to prevent angina and arrhythmias by blocking or slowing calcium flow into muscle cells, which results in vasodilation (widening of the blood vessels) and greater oxygen delivery to the heart muscle.

Implications for Massage

Expected effect for the massage may be distorted. Care must be taken to watch for any exaggerated effects. Massage may help with constipation. The blood pressure–lowering effect of massage may result in dizziness after the massage. Have the client contract and relax the leg muscles for a minute or two before getting off the massage table.

Antiarrhythmics

Examples: disopyramide, mexiletine, procainamide, propranolol, tocainide, quinidine

Antiarrhythmics are prescribed when the heart does not beat rhythmically or smoothly (a condition called *arrhythmia*).

Implications for Massage

Client may complain of joint and muscle pain and swelling in the extremities that is medication related. If this occurs, refer to prescribing physician. Massage may help with constipation. The client may experience dizziness after the massage. Have the client contract and relax the leg muscles for a minute or two before getting off the massage table.

Antihypertensives and Diuretics

Examples of antihypertensives: beta blockers, calcium channel blockers, angiotensin-converting enzyme (ACE) inhibitors (including captopril, enalapril, lisinopril, benazepril, quinapril), prazosin, terazosin, clonidine, and hydralazine

Examples of diuretics: chlorothiazide, chlorthalidone, furosemide, hydrochlorothiazide, spironolactone chlorothiazide, hydrochlorothiazide furosemide, spironolactone, triamterene, amiloride spironolactone and hydrochlorothiazide combination, triamterene and hydrochlorothiazide combination, and amiloride and hydrochlorothiazide combination

High blood pressure, or hypertension, occurs when the pressure of the blood against the walls of the blood vessels is higher than what is considered normal; it can eventually cause damage to the brain, eyes, heart, and kidneys. Diuretics are used in antihypertensive therapy. Diuretics

may deplete the body of potassium, and a potassium supplement or food source high in potassium may be recommended by the physician.

Implications for Massage

Expected effect for the massage may be distorted. Care must be taken to watch for any exaggerated effects. Massage may help with constipation. The blood pressure–lowering effect of massage may result in dizziness after the massage. Have the client contract and relax the leg muscles for a minute or two before getting off the massage table. The stress-reducing effect of massage may affect the dosage of these medications. Have clients monitor themselves carefully and ask their physicians to watch for possible need to reduce dosage or change medication. Massage has the effect of increasing fluid movement and may enhance the diuretic effect temporarily.

Cardiac Glycosides

Examples: digitalis, digoxin, digitoxin

Cardiac glycosides slow the heart rate but increase contraction force; they act both as heart depressants and stimulants. Their uses include regulating irregular heart rhythm, increasing the volume of blood pumped by the heart, and medicating congestive heart failure.

Implications for Massage

Monitor heart rate. Massage tends to slow the heart rate. If rate falls below 50 beats per minute, stop massage and refer immediately to the client's physician. Regular use of massage may affect the dosage of this medication. Have client monitor dose carefully with physician.

Anticoagulants

Examples: Coumadin, Panwarfin, Sofarin, warfarin sodium heparin

Anticoagulants include medications that prevent blood clotting (blood thinners). They fall into two categories. In one category is heparin. It must be given by injection, so its use is generally restricted to hospitalized patient. The second type includes oral anticoagulants, which are derivatives of the medication warfarin. Warfarin may be used in treatment of conditions such as stroke, heart disease, and abnormal blood clotting. It is also used to prevent the movement of a clot. It acts by preventing the liver from manufacturing the proteins responsible for blood clot formation.

Implications for Massage

Response to stress levels can affect the action of anticoagulants. Massage alters the body's response to stress and may interact with dosage of this medication. Avoid any massage methods that may cause bruising, including compression, friction, tapotement, and skin rolling. Watch for bruising and report any bruising to the client. Joint swelling and aching may result from use of these medications. Refer any joint symptoms to physician.

Antihyperlipidemics

Examples: cholestyramine, colestipol, lovastatin, pravastatin, clofibrate

Medications used to treat atherosclerosis act to reduce the serum levels of cholesterol and triglycerides, which form plaque on the walls of arteries. Some antihyperlipidemics bind to bile acids in the gastrointestinal tract, decreasing the body's production of cholesterol.

Implications for Massage

Occasional muscle pain and joint pain can occur when using these medications. Refer clients who complain of these conditions to a physician. Massage may help constipation. Some people experience occasional dizziness. Watch client carefully as he or she gets up from the massage table.

GASTROINTESTINAL MEDICATIONS
Anticholinergics and Narcotics

Examples of anticholinergics: dicyclomine (Antispas, Bentylol, Cyclobec, Dibent, Lomine)
Examples of narcotics and anticholinergics: diphenoxylate and atropine

Anticholinergic medications slow or block nerve impulses at parasympathetic nerve endings, preventing muscle contraction and gland secretion of organs involved. Because these medications slow the action of the bowel by relaxing the muscles and relieving spasms, they are said to have an antispasmodic action. Narcotics and anticholinergics slow the action of the bowel and can thereby help alleviate diarrhea.

Implication for Massage

Client response to relaxation effects because of alteration of parasympathetic action may be altered.

Antiulcer Medications

Examples: cimetidine (Tagamet), peptol, tagan, famotidine, omeprazole, ranitidine, sucralfate

These medications relieve symptoms and promote healing of gastrointestinal ulcers. The antisecretory ulcer medications work by suppressing the production of excess stomach acid. Sucralfate works by forming a chemical barrier over an exposed ulcer, protecting the ulcer from stomach acid.

Implications for Massage

The stress-reduction capacity of massage may enhance the effectiveness of these medications.

HORMONES

A hormone is a substance produced and secreted by a gland. Hormones stimulate and regulate body functions. Most often hormone medications are used to replace naturally occurring hormones that are not being produced in amounts sufficient to regulate specific body functions. This category of medication also includes oral contraceptives and certain types of medications that are used to combat inflammatory reactions.

Antidiabetic Medications

Treatment of diabetes mellitus may involve the administration of insulin or oral antidiabetic medications. Glucagon is given only in emergencies (for example, insulin shock, when blood-sugar levels must be raised quickly).

Oral antidiabetic medications induce the pancreas to secrete more insulin by acting on small groups of cells within the pancreas that make and store insulin. Insulin-dependent (juvenile-onset, or Type I) diabetics must have their blood-sugar levels controlled with injections of insulin.

Implications for Massage

Changes in stress levels may affect the dose. Client's physicians should monitor dosage if massage is used on a regular basis. Do not provide vigorous massage because it may put undue stress on the system, requiring blood sugar level to adjust.

Sex Hormones

Examples: estrogens (Estradiol, Premarin, Feminone), oral contraceptives; progesterones—medroxyprogesterone (Provera); androgens—testosterone

Estrogens are used as replacement therapy to treat symptoms of menopause in women whose bodies are no longer producing sufficient amounts of estrogen. Medroxyprogesterone is used to treat uterine bleeding and menstrual problems.

Most oral contraceptives (birth control pills) combine estrogen and progesterone, but some contain only progesterone.

Testosterone stimulates cells that produce male sex characteristics, replace hormone deficiencies, stimulate red bloods cells, and suppress estrogen production. Athletes sometimes take medications called *anabolic steroids* (chemicals similar to testosterone) to reduce elimination of protein from the body, producing an increase in muscle size. This use of these medications is dangerous. Anabolic steroids can adversely affect the heart, nervous system, and kidneys.

Implications for Massage

Estrogens can change blood clotting abilities. Watch for bruising and adjust pressures as needed. Be aware of any symptoms of blood clots and refer immediately. Estrogen and progesterone can cause increased fluid retention. Massage may temporarily increase fluid movement, reducing swelling. Unusual fluid retention should be referred to the prescribing physician immediately. Hormones have a widespread effect on the body and mood. Emotional states may fluctuate and the ability to handle stress changes with the fluctuations of hormones. Massage can reduce stress levels and help to even out the mood and provide for a sense of well-being.

Steroids

Examples: cortisone, prednisolone, prednisone
Examples of steroid hormone creams or ointments: triamcinolone, hydrocortisone

Oral steroid preparations may be used to treat inflammatory diseases such as arthritis or conditions such as poison ivy, hay fever, or insect bites. Steroids may also be applied to the skin to treat certain inflammatory skin conditions.

Implications for Massage

Changes in stress levels may affect the dose. Client's physician should monitor dosage if massage is used on a regular basis. Avoid any massage methods that may create inflammation such as friction, skin rolling, or stretching methods that pull excessively on the tissue.

Thyroid Medications

Examples: levothyroxine (Synthroid, Levoxine)

Implications for Massage

Changes in stress levels may affect the dose. Client should monitor dosage if massage is used on a regular basis.

ANTIINFECTIVES

Examples of antibiotics: aminoglycoside, cephalosporin, erythromycin, penicillin (including ampicillin and amoxicillin), quinolone, tetracycline

Antibiotics are used to treat a wide variety of bacterial infections. Antibiotics do not counteract viruses such as those causing the common cold.

Antivirals

Examples: acyclovir (Zovirax)

Antiviral medications are used to combat viral infections. They do not eliminate or cure viral infections.

Antifungals

Example: nystatin

Fungal infections are treated to prevent the growth of fungi.

Anthelmintics

Anthelmintics are used to treat worm infestations.

Scabicides

Examples: lindane, crotamiton

Scabicides are used to treat scabies.

Pediculicides

Example: lindane

Pediculicides are used to treat lice.

Implications for Massage for Antiinfective Medications

Anyone taking antiinfective medications is immune compromised. It is important to avoid overstressing the system when providing massage or exposing clients to contagious disease such as colds. Postpone appointments if necessary. Gastrointestinal side effects are common. Massage may calm symptoms temporarily.

Universal precautions are required when dealing with any bacterial, viral, or other pathogenic pathology.

ANTINEOPLASTICS

Antineoplastic medications are used in the treatment of cancer. Most of the medications in this category prevent the growth of rapidly dividing cells such as cancer cells. Antineoplastics are without exception extremely toxic and can cause serious side effects.

Implications for Massage

Individuals undergoing chemotherapy are physiologically stressed because of the toxicity of the medications. Work gently and under the direct supervision of the client's physician.

CENTRAL NERVOUS SYSTEM MEDICATIONS

Antianxiety/Sedatives

Examples: benzodiazepines, diazepam (Valium), clonazepam (Klonopin), alprazolam (Xanax), barbiturates, buspirone diphenhydramine, doxepin, hydroxyzine, triazolam (Halcion)

Medications used in the treatment of anxiety, panic disorder, and insomnia selectively reduce the activity of certain chemicals in the brain.

Implications for Massage

These medications generally act as central nervous system depressants. Massage can increase or decrease the effect of these medications, depending on whether the massage is structured to have a more stimulating or relaxing effect. Careful monitoring of the dosage needs to be maintained when used in conjunction with massage. Dose may be able to be lowered if massage is used on a regular basis. Work in conjunction with the prescribing physician.

Antipsychotics

Examples: phenothiazines (such as chlorpromazine and thioridazine), haloperidol

Major tranquilizers or antipsychotic agents are usually prescribed for patients with psychoses (certain types of mental disorders). These medications calm certain areas of the brain but permit the rest of the brain to function normally. They act as a screen that allows transmission of some nerve impulses but restricts others.

Implications for Massage

These medications generally act as central nervous system depressants. Massage can increase or decrease the effect of these medications depending on whether the massage is structured to have a more stimulating or relaxing effect. Careful monitoring of the dosage needs to be maintained when used in conjunction with massage. These medications are used to treat severe mental disorders. Work only with direct supervision from the prescribing physician. Dosage may be able to be lowered if massage used on a regular basis. Massage can help with constipation.

Antidepressants

Examples: tricyclic antidepressants (amitriptyline [Amitril, Endep]), selective serotonin reuptake inhibitors (fluoxetine [Prozac], sertraline [Zoloft], paroxetine) tetracyclic antidepressants (maprotiline), and monoamine oxidase inhibitors (MAOIs)(phenelzine)

Antidepressants are used to combat depression. Antidepressants are also used in the preventative treatment of migraine headaches and other types of pain, although the manner in which they help to provide pain relief is not clearly understood. Tricyclic antidepressants are thought to work by increasing the concentration of certain chemicals necessary for nerve transmission in the brain.

Implications for Massage

Massage nonspecifically causes a shift in neurotransmitters and other brain chemicals. Massage has a stimulating effect on the central nervous system even when used for relaxation. The relaxation effect is a secondary result of the nervous system stimulation. Massage can increase serotonin levels. Watch carefully for any increase or decrease in effect of the medications. Work with supervision of the prescribing physician to adjust the dosage when massage is used as part of therapy. Massage can help with constipation.

Amphetamines

Examples: methylphenidate (Ritalin, Benzedrine)

Amphetamines or adrenergic medications are nervous system stimulants commonly used as anorectics (medications used to reduce the appetite). These medications temporarily quiet the part of the brain that causes hunger, but they also keep a person awake, speed up the heart, and raise blood pressure. After 2 to 3 weeks, these medications begin to lose their effectiveness as appetite suppressants. They are also used to treat narcolepsy.

Amphetamines stimulate most people, but they have the opposite effect on hyperkinetic children and adults. When hyperkinetic children and adults take amphetamines or adrenergic medications, their level of activity is reduced. Most likely, amphetamines selectively stimulate parts of the brain that control activity.

Implications for Massage

Massage nonspecifically causes a shift in neurotransmitters and other brain chemicals. Massage has a stimulating effect on the central nervous system even when used for relaxation. The relaxation effect is a secondary result of the nervous system stimulation. Watch carefully for any increase or decrease in effect of the medications. Work with supervision from the prescribing physician to adjust the dosage when massage is used as part of therapy. Massage can help with constipation.

Anticonvulsants

Examples: phenobarbital (Barbita, Solfoton)

Anticonvulsants are used to control seizures and other symptoms of epilepsy. They selectively reduce excessive stimulation in the brain.

Implications for Massage

Massage has a stimulating effect on the central nervous system even when used for relaxation. The relaxation effect is a secondary result of the nervous system stimulation. Watch carefully for any increase or decrease in effect of the medications. Work with supervision from the prescribing physician to adjust the dosage when massage is used as part of therapy.

Antiparkinsonism Agents

Examples: benztropine, trihexyphenidyl, levodopa, bromocriptine

Parkinson's disease is a progressive disorder that is caused by a chemical imbalance of dopamine in the brain. These medications are used to correct the chemical imbalance, thereby relieving the symptoms of the disease. Benztropine and trihexyphenidyl are also used to relieve tremors caused by other medications.

Implications for Massage

Massage nonspecifically causes a shift in neurotransmitters and other brain chemicals, including dopamine. Massage has a stimulating effect on the central nervous system even when used for relaxation. The relaxation effect is a secondary result of the nervous system stimulation. Watch carefully for any increase or decrease in effect of the medications. Work with supervision from the prescribing physician, who may adjust the dosage when massage is used as part of therapy. Massage can help with constipation.

Analgesics

Analgesics are used to relieve pain. They may be either narcotic or nonnarcotic. Narcotics act on the brain to cause deep analgesia and often drowsiness. Narcotics relieve pain and give the patient a feeling of well-being. They are also addictive.

A number of analgesics contain codeine or other narcotics combined with nonnarcotic analgesics (such as aspirin or acetaminophen). Darvon is one example. These analgesics are not as potent as pure narcotics but are frequently as effective.

Nonnarcotic pain relievers include the following:
- Salicylate—aspirin
- Acetaminophen (relieves pain but does not reduce inflammation)
- Naproxen, piroxicam (Feldene), ketoprofen (Orudis) (inhibits prostaglandin)

Implications for Massage

Massage reduces pain perception in several ways; through gate control hyperstimulation analgesia and counterirritation and by stimulating the release of pain-inhibiting or pain-modifying chemicals in the body. Massage supports analgesics and has the potential to reduce the dosage and duration of treatment. Aspirin thins the blood. Watch for bruising.

Pain perception is inhibited when taking analgesics. Feedback mechanisms for pressure and massage intensity are not accurate. Reduce the intensity of massage and avoid methods that cause inflammation. Narcotics are constipating. Massage can help with constipation. Dizziness may result with the use of these medications. Have the client relax and contract the muscles of the legs for a few minutes before getting off the table.

Antiinflammatory Medications

Antiinflammatory medications reduce the body's inflammatory response. Inflammation is the body's response to injury. It causes swelling, pain, fever, redness, and itching.

Examples include the following:
- Nonsteroidal antiinflammatory medications (NSAIDs) such as aspirin, fenoprofen, ibuprofen, indomethacin, naproxen, and tolmetin
- Steroids: adrenocorticosteroids (cortisone is also used to treat inflammatory diseases)

NOTE: Skeletal muscle relaxants are often given in combination with an antiinflammatory medication such as aspirin. However, some doctors believe that aspirin and rest are better for alleviating the pain and the inflammation of muscle strain than are skeletal muscle relaxants. When sore muscles tense, increasing muscle tone, they cause pain, inflammation, and spasm. Skeletal muscle relaxants (e.g., orphenadrine, aspirin, and caffeine combination; meprobamate and aspirin combination; and chlorzoxazone and acetaminophen combinations) can relieve pain and these symptoms.

Implications for Massage

Massage therapists should not perform any techniques that create inflammation or damage tissue. Mood may be altered as well as pain perception. Feedback mechanisms for pressure and massage intensity are not accurate. Reduce the intensity of massage. Massage can reduce muscle spasm, reducing the need for muscle relaxants. Muscle spasm is often a protective response acting to immobilize an injured area. Use massage to reduce but not remove these protective spasms. Many of these medications are available over the counter, and the client may neglect to report them. Question clients about any over-the-counter medications.

RESPIRATORY MEDICATIONS

Antitussives

Examples of antitussives: dextromethorphan, codeine

Antitussives control coughs.

Expectorants

Examples: ammonium chloride, guaifenesin, potassium guaiacolsulfonate, and terpin hydrate

Expectorants are used to change a nonproductive cough to a productive one (one that brings up phlegm). Expectorants are supposed to increase the amount of mucus produced. However, drinking water or using a vaporizer or humidifier is probably as effective for increasing mucus production.

Decongestants

Examples: ephedrine, pseudoephedrine, phenylephrine, phenylpropanolamine hydrochloride

Decongestants constrict blood vessels in the nose and sinuses to open air passages. Adrenergists (decongestants) are available as oral preparations, nose drops, and nose sprays. Oral decongestants are slow acting but do not interfere with production of mucus or movement of the cilia (special hairlike structures) of the respiratory tract. They can increase blood pressure, so they should be used cautiously by patients with high blood pressure. Topical decongestants (nose drops or spray) provide fast relief. They do not increase blood pressure as much as oral decongestants, but they do slow cilia movement.

Topical decongestants should not be used for more than a few days at a time.

Bronchodilators

Examples: theophylline, aminophylline, albuterol, metaproterenol

Bronchodilators (agents that open airways in the lungs) and agents that relax smooth-muscle tissue (such as that found in the lungs) are used to improve breathing. Oral bronchodilators are commonly used to relieve the symptoms of asthma and pulmonary emphysema. Inhalant bronchodilators act directly on the muscles of the breathing tubes.

Antihistamines

Examples: diphenhydramine, brompheniramine, chlorpheniramine, meclizine

Histamine is a body chemical that, when released in the body, typically causes swelling and itching. Antihistamines counteract these symptoms of allergy by blocking the effects of histamine. For mild respiratory allergies such as hay fever antihistamines can be used. Some types of antihistamines are also used to prevent or treat the symptoms of motion sickness.

Implications for Massage for All Respiratory Medications

Respiratory medications can reduce sweating, so it is wise to avoid heat hydrotherapy. Bronchodilators are sympathomimetic and act on sympathetic nerve stimulation. Antihistamines can excite or depress the central nervous system. Most of these medications can cause drowsiness and anxiety. Because they act on the central nervous system, expected results of the massage can be distorted. Client may be unable to relax or may be excessively drowsy and dizzy after the massage. Many massage methods produce a skin reddening caused by the release of histamine. Reaction may be altered and feedback may be inaccurate in clients taking antihistamines. Avoid this type of work with such clients. Codeine can cause constipation. Massage may prove beneficial.

Many of these medications are available over the counter, and clients may neglect to report their use to the therapist. Make sure clients are questioned about any over-the-counter medications.

VITAMINS AND MINERALS

Vitamins and minerals are chemical substances that are vital to the maintenance of normal body function. Many people take supplemental vitamins and minerals. High intake of supplements, especially individual vitamins, can cause adverse reactions or may have implications for massage. The practitioner will need to investigate further to determine any suspected interaction. At this point, specific research has not been done to determine what the specific interactions might be. It is necessary to compare the effects of the vitamin and/or mineral with the type of massage application to determine whether the two together are inhibitory or synergistic. This is too comprehensive of an information base to detail in this format.

HERBS

Herbs are medicinal plants. They act in similar ways as pharmaceutical medications. Many medications are derivatives of herbs. Question clients in the use of herbs and their reasons for taking them. The practitioner will need to investigate further to determine any suspected interac-

tions. At this point, specific research has not been done to determine what the specific interactions might be. It is necessary to compare the effects of the herb with the type of massage application to determine whether the two together are inhibitory or synergistic. This is too comprehensive of an information base to detail in this format.

REFERENCES

Consumers Guide Editors: *Prescription medications*, Lincolnwood, Ill., 1995, Signet.

Corey, Corey, Callanan: *Issues and ethics in the helping professions*, ed 4, Belmont, Calif., 1993, Brooks/Cole.

Griffith H: *Complete guide to prescription and non-prescription medications*, Los Angeles, 1990, The Body Press Division of Price Stern Sloan.

Keen J et al: *Mosby's critical care and emergency medication reference*, St Louis, 1994, Mosby.

RESOURCE LIST

T HE following resource list is offered for informational purposes only. It is not meant to be an exhaustive list and is not intended as an endorsement of any publication, organization, or business service.

PUBLICATIONS

Journal of Bodywork and Movement Therapies
Churchill Livingstone
P.O. Box 77
Harlow, Essex CM195BQ UK
44-127-962-3924

Massage & Bodywork Quarterly
28677 Buffalo Park Rd.
Evergreen, CO 80439-7347
800-458-2267

Massage Magazine
1315 W. Mallon
Spokane, WA 99201
800-872-1282
http://www.massagemag.com

Massage Therapy Journal
820 Davis St.
Suite 100 Subscriptions
Evanston, IL 60201-4444
847-864-0123

The Journal of Soft Tissue Manipulation
(An International Journal Sponsored by the Ontario Massage Therapist Association—OMTA)
950 Yonge St.
Suite 1007
Toronto, ON M4W 2J4
416-968-6818

BOOKS

Planning Your Career in Alternative Medicine
Dianne J. B. Lyons
Avery Publishing Group, Garden City Park, New York
ISBN 0-89529-802

Massage: A Career at Your Fingertips
Martin Ashley, J.D., L.M.T.
Stanton Hill Press, Inc., Barrytown, New York 12507
Distributed by The Talman Company
ISBN 0-88268-135-4

Business Mastery
Cherie Sohnen-Moe
Sohnen-Moe Associates
3906 W. Ina Rd. #200-348
Tucson, AZ 85741

The Insurance Reimbursement Manual
Christine Rosche
1-800-888-1516
10441 Pharlap Dr.
Cupertino, CA 95014

PROFESSIONAL ORGANIZATIONS IN EXISTENCE 5 YEARS OR LONGER

ABMP (Associated Bodywork and Massage Professionals)
28677 Buffalo Park Rd.
Evergreen, CO 80439-7347
800-458-ABMP or 303-674-8478
e-mail: expectmore@abmp.com
Web site: http://www.abmp.com

AMTA (American Massage Therapy Association)
820 Davis St.
Suite 100
Evanston, IL 60201-4444
708-864-0123
Web site: http://www.amtamassage.org

IMF (International Myomassetics Federation)
1720 Willow Creek Circle, Suite 517
Eugene, OR 97402
800-433-4IMF (4463)

International Massage Association
3000 Connecticut Ave. N.W., Suite 308
Washington, DC 20008
202-332-6555

OTHER ORGANIZATIONS THAT SUPPORT BODYWORK PROFESSIONALS OR CONDUCT RESEARCH

American Oriental Bodywork Therapy Association
Laurel Oak Corp. Ctr.
1010 Haddonfield-Berlin Rd. Ste #408
Voorhees, NJ 08043
609-782-1616

American Polarity Therapy Association
2888 Bluff Street #149
Boulder CO 80301
303-545-2161

Bastyr University
14500 Juanita Drive Northeast
Bothell, Washington 98011
425-823-1300
Website: http://www.bastry.edu

International Association of Infant Massage Instructors
P.O. Box 10103
Portland, OR 97216

International Institute of Reflexology
P.O. Box 12642
St. Petersburg, FL 35733

International Society for the Study of Subtle Energies and Energy Medicine
356 Goldco Circle
Golden, CO 80403
303-425-4625
Website: http://vitalenergy.com/issseem

National Certification Examination Board for Therapeutic Massage and Bodywork
8201 Greensboro Drive, Suite 300
Mclean, VA 22102
1-800-296 0664 or 703-610-9015
Web site: http://www.NCBTMB.com

Physical Medicine Research Foundation
#510-207 West Hastings St.
Vancouver, BC, Canada V6B 1H7
604-684-6247

Therapeutic Touch (Delores Krieger)
c/o Nurse Healers and Professional Associates Cooperative, Inc.
175 Fifth Avenue, Suite 3399
New York, NY 10010

Touch for Health Foundation
1174 North Lake Avenue
Pasadena, CA 91104

Touch Research Institute
University of Miami School of Medicine
Department of Pediatrics
P.O. Box 016820
Miami FL 33101
Web site: http://www.miami.edu/touch_research
305-243-6781

Van Why, Richard (bodywork knowledge base and research)
123 East Eighth Street
Suite 121
Frederick, MD 21701

RESOURCES FOR ADDITIONAL INFORMATION

American Holistic Health Association 714-779-6152

American Preventive Medical Association 703-759-0622

Association of Massage Therapists New South Wales Ltd. (Australia) 352-795-7336

Canadian Massage Therapist Alliance 416-968-2149

Massage Therapist Association of British Columbia (Canada) 604-873-4467

Massage Therapy Association of Manitoba (Canada) 204-254-0406

The Office of Alternative Medicine at the National Institutes of Health
Web site: http://altmed.od.nih.gov/

Saskatchewan Massage Therapist Association (Canada)
306-653-5650

BUSINESS SERVICES

Service Corps of Retired Executives (SCORE)
1825 Connecticut Avenue NW
Suite 503
Washington, DC 20009
800-634-0245
202-653-6279

U.S. Chamber of Commerce
1615 H Street NW
Washington, DC 20062
800-638-6582
202-659-6000

U.S. Small Business Administration (SBA)
Federal Office 409 Third St. S.W.
Washington, DC 20416
800-827-5722
202-653-6822

SELF-MASSAGE*

THIS appendix is intended to help you, the massage therapist or student, teach clients how to perform self-massage. The pages that follow are for the client. Please feel free to photocopy them and provide them to clients for use at home.

---

*Photos and text modified from Fritz S: *Mosby's visual guide to massage essentials,* St Louis, 1996, Mosby.

SELF-MASSAGE

Massaging oneself can be very effective for stress management and pain control. Because of the way the brain processes sensory input, some forms of self-massage are more effective than others.

The brain contains areas called the *somatic sensory cortex* and the *motor cortex*. The *somatic sensory cortex* determines the source and quality of various sensory stimuli. The motor cortex activates voluntary muscular movement. The body is represented in both of the areas. Because of the number and sensitivity of nerve receptors, the brain does not see the body as we do. The hands, fingers, face, lips, and feet are the most sensitive body areas, and therefore larger in the brain's view of the body than the legs, arms, back, and chest.

This is important when we consider what areas will respond best to self-massage. Because the hand has such a large sensory and motor distribution, during self-massage the brain neurologically pays the most attention to the sensations coming from the hand. When an individual massages his or her own neck, which has little sensory distribution, the brain tends to interpret the stronger sensation from the hand. That is why it feels better when someone else massages your neck. When someone gives us a massage, the brain is not splitting sensory signals and can pay full attention to the feeling coming from the area being massaged.

If we massage our own hands, face, and feet, the sensory information from the hands and the area being massaged is more balanced. This allows the brain to pay attention to both the area being massaged and the hand doing the massage work. Using massage tools helps because it eliminates the hand sensations and allows the brain to concentrate on the area being massaged.

Self-Massage Tools

Everyday household items make excellent and inexpensive massage tools (Fig. E-1):

- Various sizes and densities of balls (e.g., tennis balls, golf balls, softballs)
- Marbles
- Tube socks
- Wooden knobs
- Rubber mats, foam, or towels rolled up to 3- and 6-inch diameters around a 1-inch wooden dowel
- Rolling pin
- Bicycle tire inner tubes
- 1-, 2-, and 5-pound rice or sand bags
- Frozen vegetables in plastic bags for ice packs

Self-Massage for the Head and Face

The face is easy to massage yourself. The high neurologic activity of the hands and face make self-massage effective. A 1- or 2-pound bag of rice wrapped in a towel and placed over the face, just above the nose, provides an effective compression that many find relaxing (Figs. E-2 and E-3).

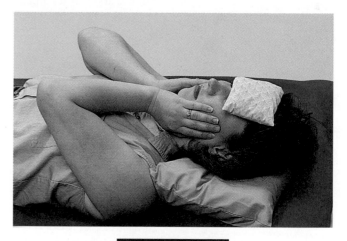

fig. E-2

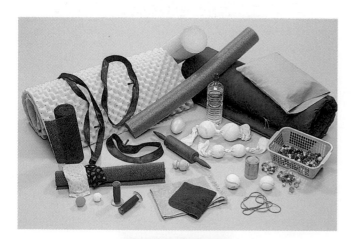

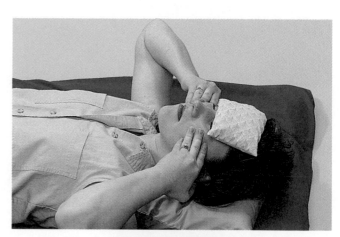

fig. E-1

fig. E-3

Self-Massage for the Neck

A massage tool for the neck can be made by placing two tennis balls in a long sock and securing them (with knots) in the position that best fits the neck. A section of the sock should be left at the end to use as a handle. You can either lie on the floor with the balls under your neck and use the handle to move the position of the balls or roll back and forth on the tennis balls (Fig. E-4). In an upright position you can use the balls to massage the neck by placing them against the neck and pulling on the handles. The effect can be increased by rolling the neck back on the balls in a semicircular pattern from left to right against the pressure of the balls (Figs. E-5 and E-6).

Tilt the head straight back to slacken the tissue at the back of the neck. Using one hand, firmly squeeze the tissue at the back of the neck and lift it as a cat would lift a kitten (Fig. E-7). Still holding the tissue tightly, roll the neck forward and move the head left and right. Attempt

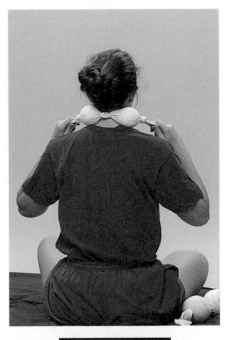

fig. E-6

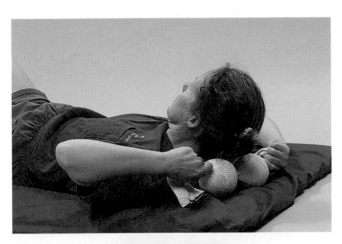

fig. E-4

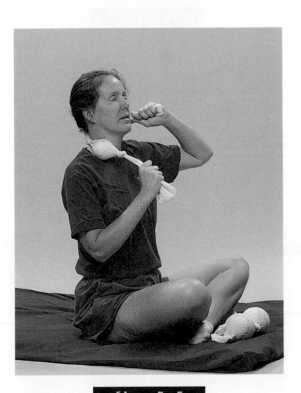

fig. E-5

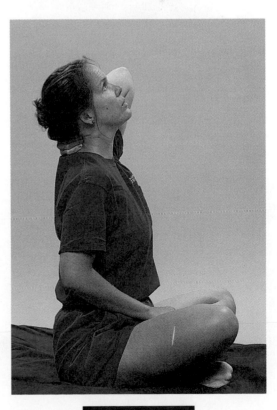

fig. E-7

to hold the stretch for 30 seconds (Fig. E-8). Because this is a connective tissue stretch, the feeling may be intense and slightly uncomfortable while performed, but will result in freer neck motion.

Self-Massage for the Shoulders

Range of motion is the most effective method for self-massage of the shoulders. Moving against resistance in-creases the effectiveness of massage. A bicycle tire inner tube can be used to provide the resistance, and its circular shape lends itself to many different movement positions.

Because the shoulder is stabilized at the hip and low back area, self-stretching by bringing the elbow above the head and bending to one side is effective. Changing the angle of the elbow and the direction of the bend addresses the multidirectional aspects of the tissue in this area (Figs. E-9, E-10, and E-11).

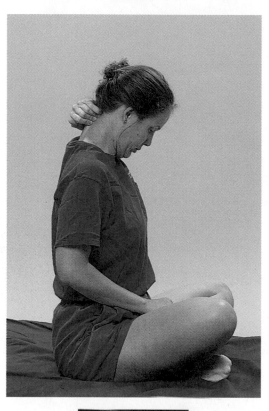

fig. E-8

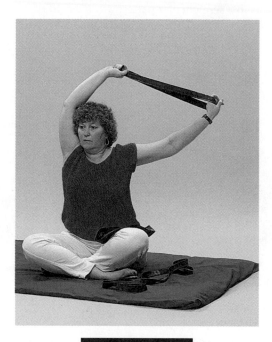

fig. E-10

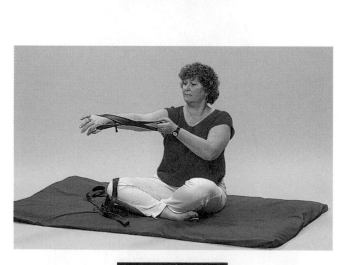

fig. E-9

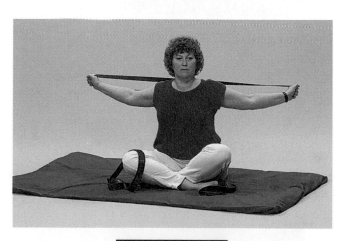

fig. E-11

A wood knob mounted on the wall at shoulder height can provide a stable force to push against (Figs. E-12 and E-13). Using a ball of some type on the floor and lying or rolling on the ball can also be effective (not pictured).

Self-Massage for the Arm

Place the arm to be massaged on a firm surface. Use the opposite hand or forearm to apply compression to the arm being massaged (Fig. E-14). While applying the compression, turn the arm palm upward and palm downward to massage the tissue. Another method is to grasp the arm to be massaged firmly with the opposite hand and while grasping, turn the palm upward and downward, which will provide massage to the arm. Move up the arm with the grasping hand until you reach the elbow (Figs. E-15 and E-16).

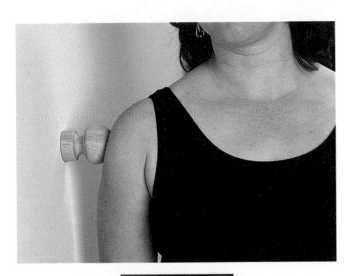

fig. E-12

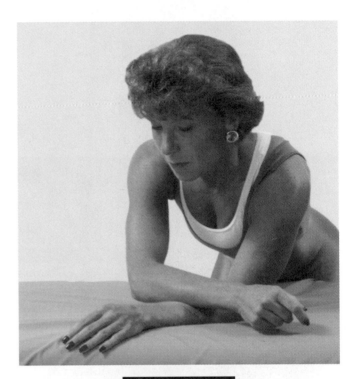

fig. E-14

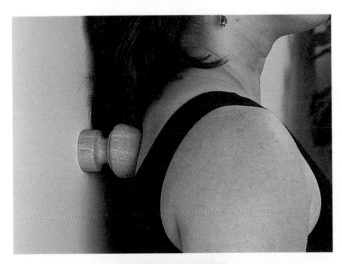

fig. E-13

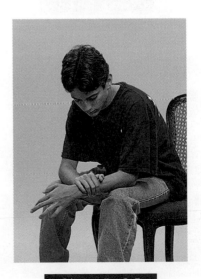

fig. E-15

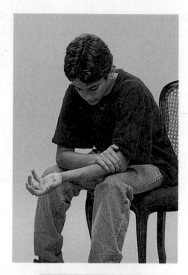

fig. E-16

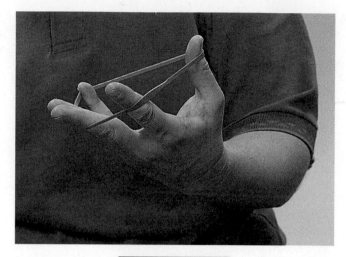

fig. E-19

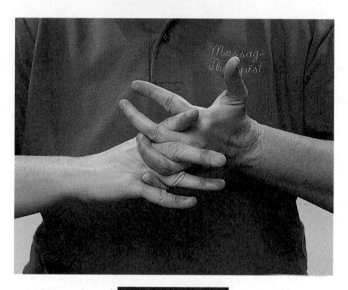

fig. E-17

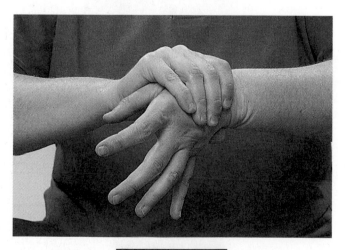

fig. E-18

Self-Massage for the Hand and Wrist

It is easy to massage your own hands and it is very calming. People tend to wring their hands when anxious, subconsciously attempting to calm themselves. It is important to be deliberate and slow as you perform the wringing action (Figs. E-17 and E-18). Squeezing a ball or playing with clay is effective, especially for the flexor muscles. The extensor muscles need stimulation as well. Place a thick rubber band around the fingertips and thumb. Open your hand against the resistance of the rubber band (Fig. E-19).

Self-Massage for the Chest

While lying on your back, use your fingertips to massage between the ribs, especially next to the sternum (Fig. E-20). With one hand, grasp and pull as much tissue in the armpit as possible. Hold the tissue firmly while moving the arm and shoulder slowly through a full range of motion (Fig. E-21).

Lie prone or on your side with a foam cylinder between your chest and the floor, and roll back and forth on the floor (Fig. E-22). By changing the angle and position, you can massage the chest. When you find an area that is tender, stop and let the pressure of the weight of your body provide compression and direct pressure. It is beneficial to lengthen and stretch the area after direct pressure.

Place weighted sand or rice bags (2 to 5 pounds) on the upper shoulders while seated and breathe slowly for 15 minutes (not pictured). The weight on the shoulders helps reduce chest and shoulder breathing, which can lead to muscle tension.

Self-Massage for the Abdomen

Rolling a large softball on the abdomen is an effective method (Fig. E-23). Begin with the ball placed in the lower

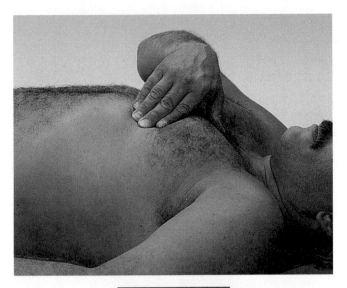

fig. E-20

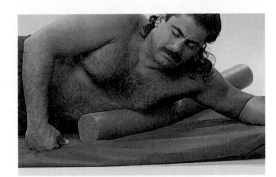

fig. E-22

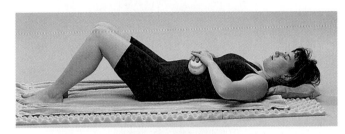

fig. E-23

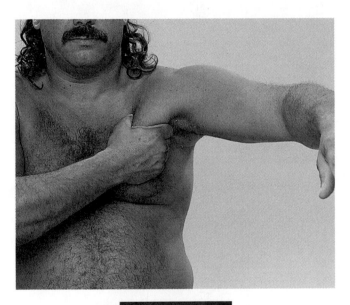

fig. E-21

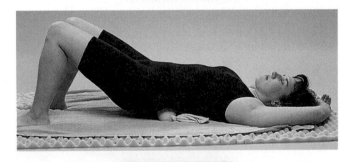

fig. E-24

right of the abdominal area. Roll the ball up, around, and under the rib cage to the left, coming back to the starting point. Continue to make circles in this pattern.

Self-Massage for the Back

Tie two tennis balls in a long sock so that the spine fits safely between the balls. Lie down on the balls and roll back and forth. When a tender area is located, let your body weight slowly increase direct pressure against the area (Fig. E-24). Lengthen and stretch the area after direct pressure has been applied. Using a rolled foam or rubber mat to massage the back by rolling on it is especially effective (Figs. E-25 and E-26).

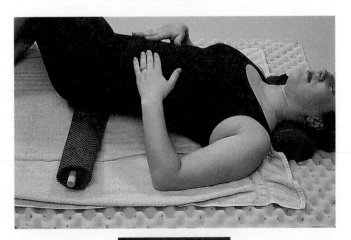

fig. E-25

Self-Massage for the Gluteals and Hips

Rolling on softballs works well. When an area of tenderness is located, let your body weight slowly increase the pressure, providing a compressive force against the area (Fig. E-27). Do not maintain the pressure for longer than 30 seconds at a time to protect any nerves in the area. Reduce the pressure for 60 seconds and then repeat. The area should be lengthened and stretched after compression.

Rolling on rolled foam or rubber mats to massage gluteals and hips is also effective (Fig. E-28).

Self-Massage for the Leg

In a seated position, cross one leg over the other so that the lower leg and ankle are in contact with the thigh (Fig. E-29). Use the crossed leg to massage the other leg (Fig. E-30). Drop the crossed leg down so that the calf is in contact with the knee of the opposite leg. Use pressure

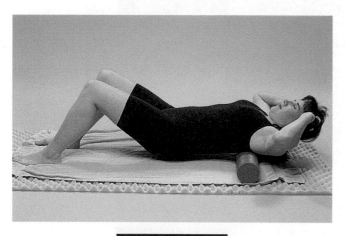

fig. E-26

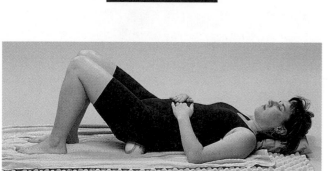

fig. E-27

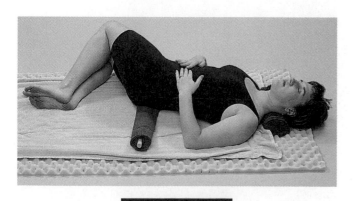

fig. E-28

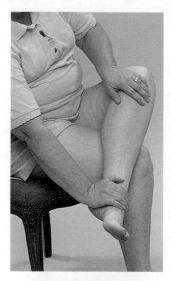

fig. E-29

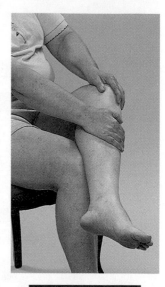

fig. E-30

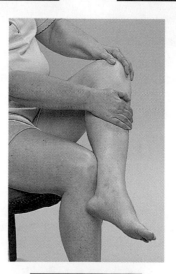

fig. E-31

against the knee to massage the calf (Fig. E-31). In the seated position you can use the forearm for self-massage of the leg. A rolling pin works well for self-massage of the legs. It is especially effective for massaging the iliotibial band as well as the lateral side of the thigh (Figs. E-32 and E-33).

Self-Massage for the Foot and Ankle

Rolling the feet on marbles is an effective massage approach. Standing on marbles placed in a box or basket provides intense stimulation to the bottoms of the feet

(Fig. E-34). Rolling the feet on a large wood dowel or a golf ball is also a good self-massage technique (Fig. E-35).

Massaging your feet with your hands is an effective combination. The sensory distribution is similar, so the body can pay attention to both sensations without the hands overriding the sensory input. Because both the hands and feet are prime sources of sensory information, massaging one's own feet floods the nervous system with impulses and often blocks sensory input from other areas. This stimulation is excellent for temporary pain control and tension relief. The heel of one foot can also be used to massage the other foot (Fig. E-36).

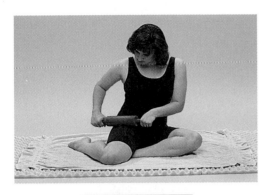

fig. E-32

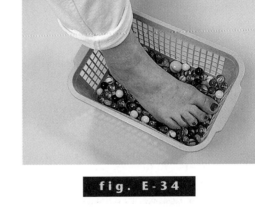

fig. E-34

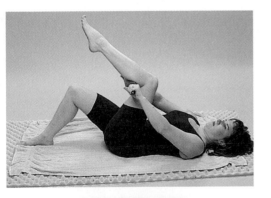

fig. E-33

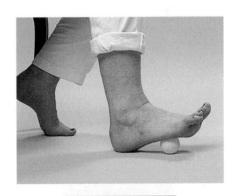

fig. E-35

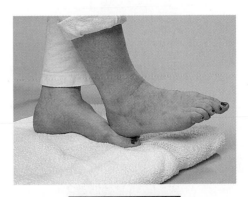

fig. E-36

INDEX*

---

*Page numbers in italics indicate illustrations; *t* indicates tables.